CONCEPTUAL NURSING CARE PLANNING

CONCEPTUAL NURSING CARE PLANNING

SECOND EDITION

MARIANN HARDING, PhD, RN, CNE, FAADN
Nursing Program Director and Professor of Nursing
Kent State University Tuscarawas
United States

DEBRA HAGLER, PhD, RN, ACNS-BC, CNE, CHSE, ANEF, FAAN
Clinical Professor
Edson College of Nursing and Health Innovation
Arizona State University
United States

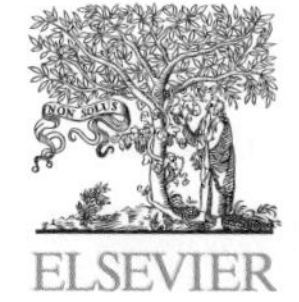

ELSEVIER

Elsevier
3251 Riverport Lane
St. Louis, Missouri 63043

CONCEPTUAL NURSING CARE PLANNING, SECOND EDITION ISBN: 978-0-443-10528-9

Senior Content Strategist: Sandra Clark
Content Development Specialist: Meredith Madeira
Publishing Services Manager: Deepthi Unni
Project Manager: Haritha Dharmarajan
Design Direction: Renee Duenow

Printed in India

Last digit is the print number: 9 8 7 6 5 4 3 2 1

Preface

THE CONCEPTUAL APPROACH TO PLANNING NURSING CARE

The knowledge you need to provide effective nursing care is growing by the minute. It is not possible for any nurse to know about every health condition, every intervention, or every medication. To help you be prepared with a strong foundation for clinical practice, this book uses a concept-based approach to organize and classify information. The general idea is that organizing information around concepts, or key ideas, will help you understand those ideas and transfer knowledge to related situations.

For example, nutrition is a concept of focus. Interventions that support optimal nutrition are needed for the care of persons across the lifespan with diverse health conditions. Learning a general set of assessments and interventions for promoting optimal nutrition along with specific interventions for specific populations prepares the nurse to care for many more patients who have nutrition problems.

CONCEPTS AND CLINICAL PROBLEMS

A **concept** is a general classification for related information. Each chapter in this book is framed around one concept that nurses use when directly planning patient care. There are 43 concepts, organized by common themes. In school, you also may learn about other important concepts related to nurse attributes or health systems, such health care law. Those concepts are not included in this book.

A **clinical problem** is an issue for which nurses commonly assess, analyze, plan, implement, and/or evaluate care. Clinical problems may also reflect concerns expressed by the patient or caregiver or identified by another health care team member. There are one to four clinical problems described for each concept. The clinical problems are those considered most commonly used within that particular concept. They are defined for you in Table 1. Use this book as a reference to study each concept and its clinical problems as you progress through your course work. Refer back to pertinent clinical problems as you encounter patients and plan their nursing care.

Table 1 Clinical Problems With Definitions

1. Acid–Base Imbalance: Imbalance in the state of equilibrium between the acidity and alkalinity of body fluids
2. Activity Intolerance: Inadequate energy to complete daily activities or desired activities
3. Allergy: Hypersensitivity induced by exposure to an allergen, resulting in harmful immune responses on subsequent exposures
4. Altered Blood Pressure: Force propelling blood through the body at a level inadequate for perfusion
5. Altered Glucose Level: Impaired ability to maintain optimal glucose levels
6. Altered Temperature: Not having a core body temperature between 36.2°C and 37.6°C (97.0°F to 100°F)
7. Anxiety: Subjectively distressful experience based on perception of threat, which has both a potential psychologic and physiologic cause and expression
8. Body Weight Problem: Being overweight or underweight
9. Caregiver Role Strain: Distress of performing responsibilities of providing health-related care for a family member or significant other
10. Continuity of Care Problem: Inadequate coordination across aspects of health care, including a lack of consistency in being able to see the same provider, poor communication and transfer of information across providers and settings, and a lack of follow-up/ongoing monitoring
11. Cultural Belief Conflict: Differences in values and beliefs that place a person at odds with health care providers or health recommendations
12. Deficient Knowledge: Lacking information on a specific topic
13. Depressed Mood: Depressed mood lasting 2 weeks or longer and accompanied by lack of pleasure or interest in most other activities
14. Difficulty Coping: Inadequate personal ability to manage problems, stress, or responsibilities
15. Dying Process: Progress toward the end of life
16. Electrolyte Imbalance: Higher or lower than normal concentrations of an electrolyte
17. Emotional Problem: Emotional problem that interferes with or results in functional impairment
18. Fatigue: Lack of physical and/or mental energy that interferes with usual and desired activities
19. Fluid Imbalance: Any change in or modification of body fluid balance
20. Grief: Pattern of physical and emotional responses to bereavement, separation, or loss
21. Health Care–Associated Complication: Detrimental patient condition that occurs during the process of receiving health care
22. Health Maintenance Alteration: Impaired ability to manage health or and access help to maintain health
23. Impaired Bowel Elimination: Difficulty with formation and evacuation of stool

Continued

Table 1 Clinical Problems With Definitions—cont'd

24. Impaired Cardiac Function: Inadequate blood pumped from the heart to meet the body's needs
25. Impaired Cognition: Observable or measurable disturbance in one or more of the thinking processes
26. Impaired Communication: Impediment or blockage to exchanging thoughts, messages, or information
27. Impaired Endocrine Function: Problem involving the mechanisms that regulate the secretion and action of hormones of the endocrine system
28. Impaired Family Function: Inability of the family to meet family members' needs
29. Impaired Fertility: Impaired capacity to reproduce or conceive
30. Impaired Gastrointestinal Function: Impaired ability of the gastrointestinal system to ingest, absorb, and/or digest food
31. Impaired Growth and Development: Delay or decline in growth or one or more areas of development
32. Impaired Immunity: Impaired ability of the body to resist disease
33. Impaired Respiratory Function: Inability to ventilate, clear the airway, and/or diffuse oxygen and carbon dioxide
34. Impaired Role Performance: Impaired ability to perform normal daily activities required to fulfill usual roles in the family, workplace, and community
35. Impaired Socialization: Insufficient or ineffective quality of human interaction
36. Impaired Psychologic Status: State in which there is a loss of contact with reality
37. Impaired Sexual Function: Presence of a problem with sexual function that prevents the person from experiencing satisfaction from sexual activity
38. Impaired Sleep: Not obtaining adequate sleep
39. Impaired Tissue Integrity: Damage, inflammation, or lesion to the skin or underlying structures
40. Impaired Tissue Perfusion: Inadequate blood circulation to a particular area of the body
41. Impaired Urinary Elimination: Difficulty with the collection and discharge of urine
42. Inadequate Community Resources: Deficiency in environmental support for health
43. Increased Intracranial Pressure: Potentially life-threatening situation that results from an increase in brain tissue, blood, and/or cerebrospinal fluid within the skull
44. Infant Feeding Problem: Difficulty with the effective feeding of an infant
45. Infection: Disease caused by the invasion of the body by pathogenic microorganisms
46. Inflammation: Immunologic response to tissue injury, infection, or allergy
47. Health Literacy Problem: Limited ability to obtain and understand basic health information needed to make appropriate health decisions
48. Musculoskeletal Problem: Impaired ability to move one or more extremities
49. Negative Self-Image: Negative evaluation of oneself
50. Neurologic Problem: Impaired cognition, motor, sensory, and/or regulatory functions of the central or peripheral nervous system
51. Nutritionally Compromised: Poor nutrition due to intake of unbalanced or insufficient quality of nutrients
52. Pain: Unpleasant sensory and emotional experience associated with actual or potential tissue damage
53. Parenting Problem: Inability or change of the parent to provide care that promotes optimal growth and development of the child
54. Personal Care Problem: Impaired ability to adequately perform personal care
55. Risk for Clotting: Risk of blood clots forming where they are not needed
56. Risk for Disease: Characteristic, condition, or behavior that increases the likelihood of developing a disease or health problem
57. Risk for Environmental Injury: Risk for adverse health outcomes associated with exposure to environmental contaminants
58. Risk for Impaired Skin Integrity: At risk for loss of intact skin/tissue barrier
59. Risk for Infection: Increased risk for a disease caused by the invasion of the body by pathogenic microorganisms
60. Risk for Injury: State in which a person is at an increased risk for harm
61. Risk for Perinatal Problems: Increased risk for problems during the perinatal period
62. Sensory Deficit: Impaired ability to hear, see, taste, smell, or correctly perceive touch
63. Socioeconomic Difficulty: Challenges to health based on income, education, financial security, and subjective perceptions of social status and social class
64. Spiritual Problem: Distress associated with conflicts about meaning and purpose in life
65. Substance Use: Dependence on a substance that leads to detrimental effects to the person's physical or mental health, or the welfare of others
66. Victim of Violence: Having been harmed or under threat of harm by another person
67. Violent Behavior: Force, physical or emotional, exerted to cause injury to others or destruction of property

How to Use This Book

Each clinical problem chapter begins with a definition of the clinical problem followed by a description of the clinical problem, why that clinical problem occurs, the clinical problem's relationship to other problems, and key nursing responsibilities. This introduction is followed by a list of associated clinical problems with their definitions. Associated clinical problems describe specific conditions linked back to the clinical problem (Fig. 1). You may choose to use an associated clinical problem instead of the clinical problem in specific patient situations or if that term is an option when you are documenting in an electronic health record.

Associated Clinical Problems

- Abnormal Breath Sounds: unusual sounds heard over the airways and lung fields, such as fine and coarse crackles, wheezes, pleural rubs, and stridor
- Abnormal Sputum: material of an unusual amount, color, or components that is coughed up from the lungs
- Apnea: absence of spontaneous respirations

These associated clinical problems are related to Impaired Respiratory Function. You can use Impaired Respiratory Function in planning care or choose a more specific associated clinical problem.

FIG. 1 Associated clinical problems example.

The last part of the introductory section lists common health conditions or situations that may be common causes, contributing factors, or risk factors for the clinical problem (Fig. 2) and common manifestations of the clinical problem (Fig. 3). The manifestation section concludes with diagnostic testing results. Evaluating these lists will help you determine whether the clinical problem is applicable to your patient's situation. On many care planning forms and in electronic health records, this information is documented as the supporting data, defining characteristics, or related factors.

Common Causes and Risk Factors

- Acute respiratory distress syndrome
- Acute respiratory failure
- Age-related changes, such as stiff chest wall, weak muscles, and decreased alveolar surface area

These are common factors that contribute to a patient's having Impaired Respiratory Function.

FIG. 2 Sample listing of common factors contributing to a clinical problem.

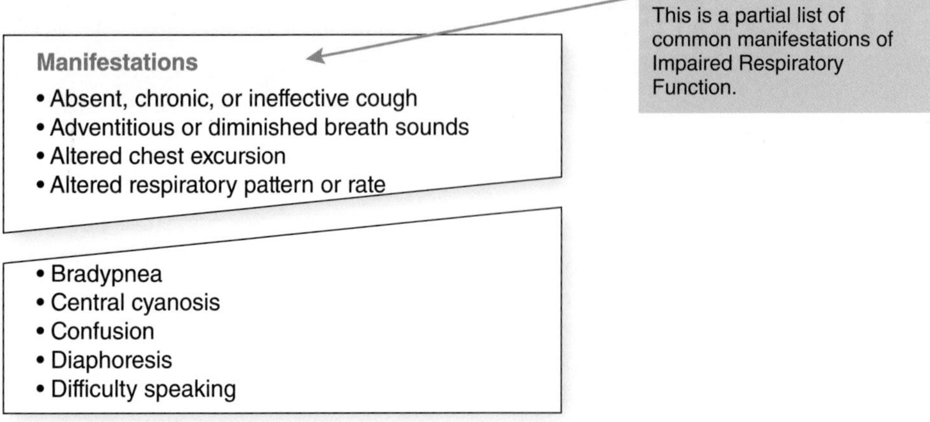

FIG. 3 Sample listing of manifestations of a clinical problem.

The sequence of information for developing a plan of care for each clinical problem follows the steps of assessment (Fig. 4); planning, with expected outcomes; interventions, with attention to patient teaching and referrals; and evaluation, which includes key information to document in the health record. The items listed in each section are suggestions for you to consider as a starting point. Based on the data you collect (assessment), you decide which interventions are a good fit for the patient and specific situation. Individualizing the interventions based on your knowledge of the specific patient and situation is a critical step of planning nursing care.

Some clinical problem chapters include specific labels designating common causes and risk factors, manifestations, assessment, and interventions that apply to the care of pediatric, women's health, and older adult patients. These are provided when additional consideration for a special population is needed. For example, in Fig. 4, knowing about the presence of respiratory assessment manifestations, such as nasal flaring, that are specific to a pediatric patient is important when assessing impaired respiratory function in an infant or young child and planning effective care.

These are common actions nurses perform when assessing respiratory function.

ASSESSMENT OF RESPIRATORY FUNCTION	RATIONALE
Identify patients in need of emergency management of respiratory problems.	Identifying the presence of a respiratory problem allows for the patient to be immediately stabilized.
Assess for risk factors for impaired respiratory function.	Identifying a patient's risk factors for impaired respiratory function allows early intervention.
Determine the potential cause of impaired respiratory function.	It is more effective to treat the cause rather than the imbalance.
Obtain a thorough history of any respiratory symptoms, such as cough or dyspnea, including: • When symptoms started • Onset, sudden or gradual • Frequency • Intensity or severity • Alleviating and aggravating factors • Any pattern to the symptoms	A thorough history aids in evaluating the degree of the patient's respiratory problem and helps direct treatment.

This assessment information is specific to a pediatric patient.

ASSESSMENT OF RESPIRATORY FUNCTION	RATIONALE
Pediatric	
Promptly address the presence of bradypnea, dyspnea, nasal flaring, orthopnea, tachypnea, and the use of accessory muscles to breathe.	These signs indicate ineffective breathing in children who may not communicate verbally.

FIG. 4 Navigating the assessment section.

In the assessment and intervention sections for each clinical problem, you will see that some entries include a concept connection. A concept connection, highlighted in bold print, indicates a relationship between that assessment or intervention and another key concept. If you want to more information about that nursing action, refer to the concept noted (Fig. 5).

If you need further information about nursing interventions actions associated with substance use, nutrition, or anxiety, refer to those concepts for details.

INTERVENTIONS FOR PROMOTING RESPIRATORY FUNCTION	RATIONALE
INFECTION: Administer vaccinations as needed, according to recommended schedules and patient need.	Vaccinations can be effective in preventing common infections, such as Influenza, pertussis, diphtheria, and pneumonia.
SUBSTANCE USE: Implement measures to address substance use, particularly smoking or vaping behaviors, if present.	Vaccinations can be effective in preventing common infections, such as Influenza, pertussis, diphtheria, and pneumonia.
NUTRITION: Ensure adequate nutrition with small, frequent meals and supplements during the acute phase.	Dyspnea may prevent oral intake of adequate calories, and loss of muscle mass may impair respiratory effort.
Assist the patient with developing a regular physical activity plan, considering capabilities, daily routine, and personal preferences.	Regular physical activity is an important part of care for many patients, because it builds endurance and maintains the strength of the respiratory muscles.
ANXIETY: Provide measures to promote comfort and reduce anxiety, as appropriate.	These measures reduce oxygen consumption and minimize hyperventilation.

FIG. 5 Promoting respiratory function concept connection.

Some clinical problems include specific assessment and intervention tables that describe nursing actions specific for a certain associated clinical problem. These are provided when additional consideration for the associated clinical problem is needed. For example, in Fig. 6, knowing about the key interventions common to decreasing the risk for aspiration is important when providing safe, effective care for patients specifically at risk for aspiration.

INTERVENTIONS TO DECREASE RISK FOR ASPIRATION	RATIONALE
Collaborate with speech and occupational therapists to provide an appropriate patient plan, including diet and use of assistive devices.	Speech and occupational therapists provide in-depth clinical assessment and recommend strategies to treat swallowing problems.
Provide food and fluids of the appropriate consistency, based on the swallowing evaluation.	Modifying the consistency of foods and fluids improves the patient's ability to swallow, with a reduced risk of choking.
Provide an environment to promote swallowing: • Remove distractions. • Have the patient in an upright position, with the head flexed forward. • Keep the patient upright for 30 minutes after eating.	These measures assist with reducing the risk of aspiration associated with a swallowing problem.

FIG. 6 Interventions for associated clinical problems.

At the end of each clinical problem section, you will find a graphic showing key related concepts. This will help you expand your thinking about planning patient care.

EXEMPLARS WITH CLINICAL PROBLEMS

An **exemplar** is a specific health condition that serves as a representative example of the concept. A list of exemplar conditions with clinical problems that may be applicable in a particular patient situation are found in the second part of this book. Use the lists to cross reference patient conditions when you are not yet certain which concepts or clinical problems will apply to the patient's care. The exemplars included here were chosen to illustrate each concept in common and important health conditions across the lifespan and patient situations.

Let us apply the use of clinical problems in planning patient care to the following example.

Case Study Example

You are working on the surgical unit. One of your patients, M.M., a 78-year-old man, was admitted yesterday with cellulitis of the right lower leg. He said that his wife accidentally injured his leg with the car door when she was helping him transfer from his wheelchair to the car after church services 6 days ago. He was seen in the emergency department that evening, where the staff cleansed and dressed the wound and administered tetanus prophylaxis. Over the past 5 days, the wound became progressively redder and more edematous, and the primary care provider admitted him for IV antibiotic therapy. M.M. has an extensive history, including diverticulitis with a colon resection, anterior wall myocardial infarction, osteoarthritis, pancreatic cancer with a Whipple procedure, and a benign pituitary tumor with a complete resection of the gland. His current home medications include levothyroxine, testosterone, atenolol, losartan, and cortisol.

Your assessment reveals a 4 × 4 dressing with a small amount of bloody drainage on the medial part of the mid right lower leg. The provider's note describes the wound as being "V-shaped," measuring 6 × 8 × 5 cm with layered sutures. The top layer is open and covered with petroleum-impregnated gauze. You note redness and warmth extending 3 inches out all around the dressing. He reports moderate, burning pain at a level 7/10 that interfered with his being able to sleep the prior night. He has 1+ peripheral pulses with 2+ pitting edema and a capillary refill time of greater than 3 seconds in both lower extremities. The skin of both extremities from the knees down is thin, reddish brown, with numerous purplish areas. His current vital signs are blood pressure 110/60 mm Hg, pulse 108 bpm, respirations 20 breaths/min, temperature 100.8°F (38.2°C), and oxygen saturation 97%. His white blood cell count is elevated at 17,000 cells/mm^3. He says he feels "horrible" and has no appetite, refusing his meal tray. Heart regular S1 S2; telemetry shows sinus rhythm with occasional PVCs. An IV line of normal saline is infusing at 75 mL/hr with 500 mg cefazolin IV every 6 hours. He is ordered to be up to the chair twice daily with the assistance of two persons. A bedside commode with a raised seat and his wheelchair are present. The wound care nurse (WOCN) is scheduled to see M.M. later this morning.

A number of clinical problems appear to exist for M.M.: these include

- Altered Temperature
- Impaired Endocrine Function
- Impaired Sleep
- Impaired Tissue Integrity
- Inadequate Tissue Perfusion
- Infection
- Inflammation
- Musculoskeletal Problem
- Nutritionally Compromised
- Pain
- Personal Care Problem

You determine that the priority clinical problems for M.M. include addressing his infection, which you believe should help to manage the related inflammation, anorexia, sleep problems, and pain present, and instituting measures to promote wound healing.

Clinical Problem 1: Infection

Manifestations
- Temperature 100.8ºF (38.2ºC), pulse 108 bpm
- White blood cell count 17,000 cells/mm^3
- Redness and warmth extending 3 inches out around the dressing
- Anorexia
- Reporting pain at a level of 7/10

Ongoing Assessments Needed
- Vital signs
- Manifestations of wound infection
- White blood cell count with differential
- Effect of the infection on his ability to perform activities of daily living

Expected Outcomes
The patient will:
- Be free from infection
- Be free from complications associated with the infection
- Adhere to the prescribed therapeutic regimen

Interventions With Rationale
- Administer antibiotic therapy as prescribed. *The appropriate antibiotic therapy is necessary to treat an existing infection.*
- ***Pain***: Implement pain management measures, including analgesic administration and the use of nonpharmacologic methods of pain relief. *Analgesics and pain relief measures are instituted to relieve pain caused by inflammation.*
- ***Impaired Sleep***: Provide the patient with opportunities for adequate sleep. *Adequate rest provides the body with energy needed for optimal functioning of the immune system and resolution of infection.*
- Implement strict hand hygiene by the patient and all who have contact with the patient. *Hand hygiene is an important preventative measure that should be done before, during, and after patient contact.*
- ***Altered Temperature***: Implement measures to reduce fever. Antipyretics and other measures can lower fever, which is a common physiological response to inflammation and infection.
- ***Fluid Imbalance***: Provide intravenous fluids as ordered and encourage increased oral fluid intake. *Increased fluid intake will replace fluid loss from fever and help reduce the risk of fluid i mbalance.*
- ***Inflammation***: Administer corticosteroid replacement therapy as ordered. *Corticosteroids are effective in reducing the swelling and pain that accompany inflammation and are required replacement therapy after pituitary removal.*
- Notify the health care provider if manifestations of the infection worsen. *Achieving an effective treatment plan may require adjustments in his therapy.*

Teaching
- Manifestations of infection and signs of improvement
- Diagnostic and laboratory tests being done to monitor infection
- Measures being used to manage the infection
- Hand hygiene techniques
- Safe use of medications, including side effect management and how they fit into the overall management plan

Documentation
Assessment
- Assessments performed
- Laboratory test results
- Manifestations of wound infection

Interventions
- Medications given
- Notification of health care provider about patient status
- Therapeutic interventions and the patient's response
- Teaching provided

Evaluation
- Patient's status: improved, stable, or declined
- Presence of any manifestations of infection
- Response to teaching provided
- Response to therapeutic interventions

Clinical Problem 2: Impaired Tissue Integrity

Manifestations
- Wound present on the medial part of the mid right lower leg: Described as being "V-shaped," measuring 6 × 8 × 5 cm with layered sutures; top layer is open and covered with petroleum-impregnated gauze; redness and warmth extend 3 inches out all around the dressing

Assessments Needed
- Patient's underlying health status, noting factors that may delay wound healing
- Wound assessment, noting signs of infection, with each dressing change
- Perfusion, including pulse, sensation, color, capillary refill, temperature, in the wound area
- Nutrition status, including usual daily caloric intake, dietary choices, and use of nutritional support
- Patient's feelings related to the wound, such as fear of depression, sadness, and their impact on self-image

Expected Outcomes
The patient will:
- Experience progress in wound healing
- Experience resolution of wound infection
- Demonstrate effective wound care

Interventions With Rationale
- Provide appropriate wound care in consultation with the WOCN. *The WOCN will prescribe measures to promote optimal tissue integrity.*
- Position the patient to avoid placing tension on the wound. *Pressure impedes blood flow needed for healing.*
- ***Impaired Tissue Perfusion***: Implement venous thromboembolism prophylaxis. *Enhancing venous return and reducing the incidence of venous thromboembolism promotes fluid mobilization and adequate circulation to promote wound healing.*
- Follow aseptic procedures, including strict handwashing, not allowing the patient to touch the wound except during dressing changes, and keeping the environment as free as possible from

Continued

Clinical Problem 2: Impaired Tissue Integrity—cont'd

contamination. *Aseptic procedures help to keep the wound free from further contamination.*
- ***Nutritionally Compromised***: Provide nutritionally adequate diet, high in protein and vitamins. *Proper nutrition is needed to provide the nutrients necessary to support wound healing.*
- ***Pain***: Administer prescribed analgesics, timed to provide peak action during wound care. *Timing of analgesics can reduce the pain experience of major wound procedures.*
- ***Negative Self-Image***: Assist the patient with managing any feelings of depression or body image concerns. *The patient may be distressed because of the impact of the wound on quality of life.*
- ***Pain***: Encourage nonpharmacologic methods of pain control, such as guided imagery and distraction. *Nonpharmacologic methods may decrease the needed dose or frequency of analgesic medications.*

Referrals
- WOCN. *The WOCN can assess the patient and prescribe measures to promote optimal tissue integrity.*
- Dietician. *The dietitian can prescribe a diet with protein and other nutrients needed for wound healing.*

Teaching
- Process of wound healing and factors that will affect wound healing
- Wound care regimen
- Prescribed topical and systemic medications, including proper administration, side effects
- Importance of proper nutrition, adequate rest
- How to protect the wound
- Follow-up needed with WOCN or health care provider for dressing changes
- When to notify the health care provider, WOCN

Documentation
Assessment
- Wound assessments

Interventions
- Discussions with other members of the interprofessional team
- Medications given
- Notification of health care provider about patient status, assessment findings
- Therapeutic interventions and the patient's response
- Teaching provided
- Referrals initiated

Evaluation
- Patient's status: improved, stable, declined
- Wound assessment
- Response to therapeutic interventions
- Response to teaching provided

Contents

CONCEPTUAL NURSING CARE PLANNING

Cultural Belief Conflict 1

Definition

Differences in values and beliefs that place a person at odds with health care providers or health recommendations

Culture is a pattern of shared attitudes, beliefs, self-definitions, norms, roles, and values expressed by members of a group. The group may be defined by having common experiences, such as speaking a particular language or living in a defined geographic region. These shared dimensions guide such areas as social relationships; expression of thoughts, emotions, and morality; religious beliefs and rituals; and use of technology. Cultural norms affect aspects of life, including interpersonal relationships, family dynamics, childrearing practices, gender roles, dietary preferences, communication patterns, clothing choices, and health practices.

Acculturation is the process of acquiring new attitudes, roles, customs, or behaviors based on contact with another culture. Both the host culture and the culture of origin are changed because of reciprocal influences. Unlike acculturation, *assimilation* is a process by which a person gives up their original identity and develops a new cultural identity by becoming absorbed into the more dominant cultural group. In *biculturalism*, the person has a dual pattern of identification and chooses aspects of both the new culture and the original culture.

All cultures have systems of health beliefs to explain perceptions of health and illness, how illnesses should be treated, and self-care practices. Cultural norms significantly influence how people make decisions about treatment preferences and who is involved in that process. How patients perceive their treatment affects treatment preferences and adherence. In some cultures, admitting to the presence of depression, pain, or stress is unacceptable. Conflicts can arise when the patient's health beliefs, practices, and values are in direct conflict with medical and nursing guidelines.

Nurses strive to provide culturally sensitive and patient-centered care. This involves incorporating respect and understanding of the patient's cultural values and individual values, which may or may not be consistent with others of their cultures, into planning nursing care. Nurses practice cultural humility by (1) identifying their own cultural backgrounds, values, and beliefs, especially as related to health and health care, and (2) examining their own cultural biases about people whose cultures differ from their own. The nurse works to develop a sense of trust and partnership with patients in planning care.

Common Causes and Risk Factors

- Differences in cultural health practices
- Differences in perception of illness and treatment
- Disagreement between the patient and the health care team members
- Cultural ignorance and insensitivity
- Lack of awareness of different societal lifestyle practices
- Longstanding conflict between different nationalities, religious, or ethnic groups

Manifestations

- Decisional conflict
- Discomfort with health care team members or recommendations
- Level of information sharing more or less than expected
- Nonadherence
- Variable health outcomes

Key Conceptual Relationships

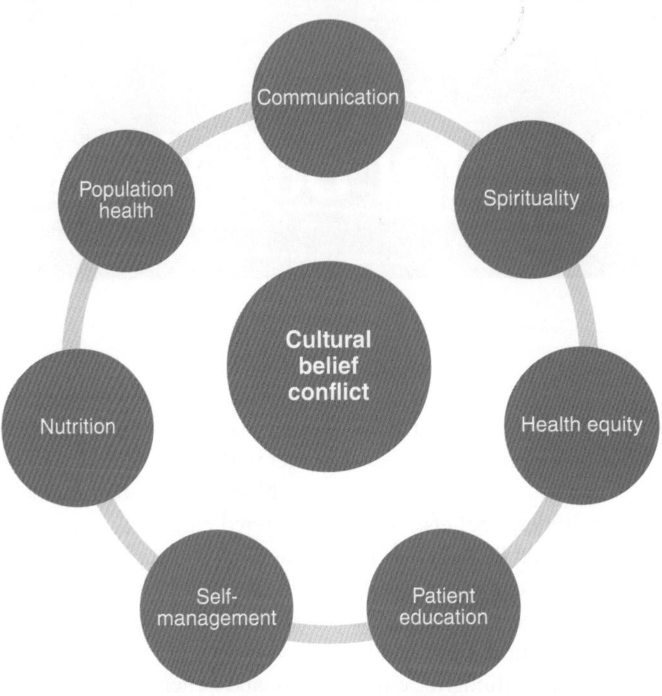

ASSESSMENT OF CULTURAL BELIEFS	RATIONALE
Assess for cultural traits and preferences based on an understanding of generalizations about a cultural group but validate any assumptions with the individual.	Develop cultural knowledge, including key aspects of a culture in relation to health and health care practices. Patients are the best source of information about how they enact their cultures as individuals.
Be alert for unexpected responses with patients, especially as related to cultural issues.	Develop cultural skill in collecting relevant cultural data and performing a cultural assessment.
Complete a cultural assessment in the following areas: *Origins and family* • Where born; if in other country, length of time in United States and circumstances • Decision making within family • Cultural group(s) patient identifies with; social networks • Important cultural practices *Communication* • Languages spoken; skill in speaking, reading, and writing in English • Preferred methods to communicate with patient and/or family member (how to be addressed, to whom questions are directed) • Ways respect is shown to others • Eye contact, interpersonal space *Personal beliefs about health and illness* • Meaning and beliefs about cause of illness • Perception of control over health • Practices or rituals used to improve health • Perception of severity of illness • Expectations for treatment, remedies, and alternative medicine • Practices that violate beliefs • Concerns or fears about illness or process of treatment • Acceptability of direct care by health care providers *Daily practices* • Dietary preferences and practices • Beliefs about food in health and illness • Spiritual beliefs and religious practices or rituals	Knowing information about the person's cultural beliefs provides a basis for collaboratively planning individualized care.

ASSESSMENT OF CULTURAL BELIEFS	RATIONALE
Observe physical and environmental cues during patient and caregiver encounters, such as: • Who is present with the patient • Patient and caregiver interactions • Dress and grooming • Who speaks during encounters	Assessment validates information about the person's cultural beliefs, guides further questioning, and provides a basis for planning individualized care.
Determine whether there is any conflict between the patient's beliefs and wishes and recommendations of the health care team.	A contributing factor to decisional conflict and nonadherence is when the patient or patient's decision maker disagrees with the position of the health care team.

Expected Outcomes

The patient will:

- explore their personal and cultural beliefs about health and health care.
- make choices that promote health.
- adhere to the prescribed therapeutic regimen.

INTERVENTIONS FOR MANAGING CULTURAL BELIEF CONFLICTS	RATIONALE
Establish a therapeutic relationship with the patient: • Build rapport and trust. • Find common ground. • Show genuine interest. • Admit to what you do not know.	This helps to establish a positive relationship and build trust.
Provide the patient the opportunity to share their story.	Listening to the patient's story gives the nurse information about what is influencing the patient's cultural belief conflict.
Use standardized, evidence-based care guidelines for diagnosis and treatment.	Racial or cultural differences in outcomes are reduced when pertinent guidelines are followed.
Provide options for care delivery that incorporate the patient's cultural beliefs.	Incorporating the patient's beliefs shows respect for persons and their cultures.
SPIRITUALITY: Identify preferences related to spiritual and religious practices that can be facilitated in the health care environment.	Maintaining usual practices may provide comfort.
PATIENT EDUCATION: Provide information attuned to the patient's level of health literacy.	The degree to which individuals can obtain, process, and understand basic health information and services needed to make appropriate health decisions affects health outcomes.
COMMUNICATION: For language translation, use a trained medical interpreter who knows how to interpret, has a health care background, understands patients' rights, and can provide advice about the cultural relevance of the health care plan and instructions. When working with an interpreter: • Speak slowly. • Maintain eye contact and talk to the patient, not the interpreter. • Use simple language with as few medical terms as possible. • Speak one or two sentences at a time to allow for easier interpretation. • Avoid raising your voice during the interaction. • Obtain feedback to be certain the patient understands. • Plan for extra time, possibly twice as long, to complete the interaction.	Using a trained medical interpreter ensures professional and effective communication in the patient's preferred language. Communicating via an interpreter requires extra effort for effective messaging.
Implement measures to assist with any decisional conflict that may be present.	A contributing factor to cultural belief conflicts occurs when the patient and the health care team disagree.
Assist the patient in determining the resources needed to be able to follow any prescribed therapeutic regimen.	This will help close any gaps that exist between expected and actual self-care.

Continued

INTERVENTIONS FOR MANAGING CULTURAL BELIEF CONFLICTS	RATIONALE
NUTRITION: Collaborate with the patient and caregivers to identify and provide a culturally acceptable prescribed diet appropriate for nutrition goals.	An appropriate diet is a critical part of achieving balanced nutrition.
Women's Health	
Implement a birth plan that is sensitive to cultural differences and individual preferences.	Including patient preferences in the plan of care demonstrates respect and increases the likelihood of a positive birth experience.

COLLABORATION	RATIONALE
Cultural broker	Cultural brokers act as liaisons, mediating between the health care team and the patient to facilitate a positive health outcome.
HEALTH EQUITY: Social worker or case manager	These professionals can explore resources that may be available to help the patient obtain access to appropriate health care and other resources.
NUTRITION: Dietitian	Collaborating with a dietitian offers the patient further information and support for implementing a culturally appropriate prescribed diet.

PATIENT AND CAREGIVER TEACHING

- How to discuss preferences with health care providers and request cultural accommodations
- Manifestations and management of health problems
- Purpose of medications and treatments
- How to access resources

DOCUMENTATION

Assessment

- Cultural preferences
- Manifestations of cultural belief conflicts

Interventions

- Facilitation of cultural practices
- Teaching provided
- Referrals initiated
- Discussions with other members of the interprofessional team

Evaluation

- Health-related choices and behaviors
- Response to teaching provided

Impaired Growth and Development 2

Definition

A delay or decline in growth or one or more areas of development

Human development is a dynamic, organized process. It follows a similar, predictable sequence, with people evolving at their own rate throughout their lifespan. We track development using development milestones. A development milestone is a behavior or physical skill that most people can accomplish within a certain age range. They are behaviors that emerge over time, forming the basis for growth and continued learning. The person who does not accomplish milestones within a specified age range may be identified as having impaired development.

Typical milestones mark changes that involve motor, emotional, cognitive, and communication skills. Some categories of these behaviors include:

Cognitive: thinking, learning, problem solving

Motor: gross and fine motor skills, coordination

Social Emotional: ability to communicate and form relationships with others, expression and management of emotions, following rules and directions

Language Communication: using words and sentences to express wants, needs, or ideas; understanding spoken information

Like development, growth follows a similar, predictable sequence, with no two people growing at the exact same rate. Growth and development are interdependent and proceed from the simple to the complex. Common influences on growth and development include genetics, prenatal exposures, health, nutrition, culture, family, and environment. Development problems usually affect daily function and often last throughout the person's lifetime. Persons who have reached a development milestone rarely lose that ability unless they have a significant stressor (hospitalization, new health problem).

Most often, we apply the concept of impaired growth and development to children because they undergo rapid changes in growth and development. Nurses need to understand the concept of impaired growth and development so that they can provide nursing care that promotes optimal growth and development based on the patient's specific needs.

Associated Clinical Problems

- Frail Elderly Syndrome: decreased reserves and functions across multiple systems, resulting in a decreased ability to cope with stressors
- Frailty Syndrome: state of decline of a functional, physical, and cognitive nature
- Growth Faltering: children whose attained weight for length or body mass index is below expected on age- and sex-specific growth charts
- Impaired Development: a delay in one or more areas or subcategories of development
- Impaired Newborn Development: delay in a newborn in one or more areas of development
- Impaired Infant Development: delay in an infant in one or more areas of development for their mental age
- Impaired Child Development: delay in a child in one or more areas of development for their mental age
- Impaired Adolescent Development: delay in an adult in one or more areas of development for their mental age
- Impaired Adult Development: delay in an adult in one or more areas of development for their mental age
- Impaired Older Adult Development: delay in an older adult in one or more areas of development for their mental age
- Risk for Delayed Growth: a child younger than age 5 who is at increased risk for poor or abnormally slow height or weight gains
- Risk for Impaired Development: increased risk for a delay in one or more areas of development for a person's mental age

Common Influencing Factors

- Birth trauma
- Chromosomal, congenital, genetic conditions
- Chronic illness, such as cancer, diabetes, cystic fibrosis, heart problems
- Chronic stress
- Depression
- Exposure to environment toxins
- Hospitalizations, prolonged and/or multiple
- Housing, food, and/or energy insecurity

- Inadequate caretaking
- Immunodeficiency
- Impaired cognition
- Impaired family function
- Impaired nutrition, including malnutrition, abnormal weight gain
- Large family size
- Limited access to health care
- Physical disability
- Poor health of family members
- Poverty
- Sensory deficits
- Separation from or loss of caregivers, family, or significant others
- Social, emotional, or development delay disorder, such as autism spectrum disorder
- Social isolation
- Substance use
- Traumatic or severe injuries, such as brain injury
- Victim of interpersonal violence, including abuse, neglect, bullying, domestic violence

Pediatric

- Intrauterine growth retardation
- Maternal education level
- Prematurity, low birth weight
- Prenatal exposure to toxins, alcohol, drugs, smoking

Manifestations

- Apathy
- Behavior problems
- Decline from prior level of functioning
- Exacerbation of chronic health problems
- Growth faltering
- Impaired growth or growth arrest
- Impaired role performance for mental age
- Impaired sleep
- Inability to carry out activities of daily living appropriate for mental age
- Learning disabilities
- Malnutrition
- Mood problems, including depression, anxiety, avoidance, and dull affect
- Problems with any of the following:
  - Cognitive development
  - Communication, including speech and language
  - Emotional control
  - Emotional development
  - Fine motor skills
  - Gross motor skills
  - Physical characteristic development
  - Social skills
- Skeletal muscle loss
- Weight loss greater than 5%

Pediatric

- Feeding problems
- Slower-than-normal rate of growth in a short period of time

Key Conceptual Relationships

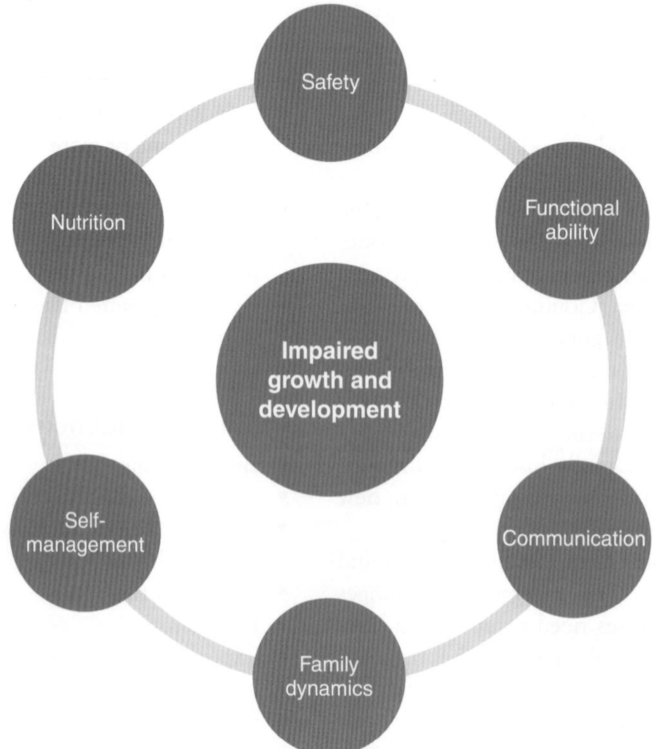

ASSESSMENT OF GROWTH AND DEVELOPMENT	RATIONALE
Assess for factors that influence the patient's growth and development.	A thorough history related to all risk factors that may affect growth and development is essential for early identification of patients at risk for impaired growth and development.
Determine the potential cause of impaired growth and development.	Effective treatment includes addressing the cause of an impairment.
Evaluate the patient's underlying health status.	Underlying health status has a major influence on growth and development.
Perform a physical assessment and monitor indicators at each encounter, including: • Neurologic assessment, including cranial nerves, tone, strength, postural reactions, and reflexes (including primitive reflexes for infants)	A nervous system problem can cause impaired growth and development, so early identification may help find the cause and decrease long-term complications.
• **COMMUNICATION:** Speech and language assessment, including auditory processing, receptive and expressive language, articulation, voice, and fluency	Detecting speech and language problems is important in planning interventions that will assist the patient with interactions and learning.
• **SENSORY PERCEPTION:** Sensory deficits, particularly vision and hearing	Sensory deficits interfere with the ability to interact with people and objects.
• **NUTRITION:** Diet history, including usual daily caloric intake, diet choices, and use of nutrition support	A history can help identify nutrition problems and aid in determining the treatment plan.
Evaluate the results of laboratory studies, such as complete blood count (CBC) with differential, chemistry panel, electrolytes, iron, kidney and thyroid studies, liver function tests, and urinalysis.	Laboratory studies may reveal an underlying health problem that is influencing growth and development.
CULTURE: Assess the role of culture on the patient's growth and development.	The age at which a person is expected to master certain development tasks may be determined by cultural expectations.
INTERPERSONAL VIOLENCE: Screen the patient and parent/caregiver at each encounter for interpersonal violence.	Being a victim of interpersonal violence increases the risk of impaired growth and development and may require action to promote patient safety.
FUNCTIONAL ABILITY: Perform a functional assessment, evaluating for role-performance effects, including the ability to perform work and household duties, perform personal care, and engage in physical and social activities.	Impaired growth and development can result in impaired role performance and impaired ability to carry out activities of daily living.
MOOD AND AFFECT: Screen for coexisting psychological problems.	Identifying depression or other psychologic problems and initiating treatment can improve patient outcomes.
SUBSTANCE USE: Screen the patient and parent/caregiver for substance use.	Identifying substance use is important for initiating care.
Evaluate the effectiveness of measures used to influence growth and development through ongoing assessment.	Monitoring growth and development allows for evaluation of therapy effectiveness.
Pediatric	
Obtain a thorough development history, including: • Age when milestones were achieved • Toileting patterns • Sleep habits • Personal habits • How the patient relates, plays, and talks with others	A diagnosis of impaired growth and development requires a thorough history.
Perform an initial screening for development risks and delays at each encounter, particularly as part of well-child visits, using valid and reliable screening instruments, such as the Ages and Stages Questionnaire, the Parents Evaluation of Developmental Status, or the Child Development Inventory.	Early identification and intervention are among the most important interventions when impaired growth and development are suspected.
When a delay is suspected in an area of growth and development, perform a more in-depth assessment with a tool specific to that particular area.	Screening tools do not provide a diagnosis but indicate if further evaluation is needed.

Continued

ASSESSMENT OF GROWTH AND DEVELOPMENT	RATIONALE
Perform a complete physical assessment and monitor indicators of growth and development at each encounter, including:	
• Measurement and graphing of height, weight, and head circumference	Plotting serial measurements regularly on a standardized growth curve for age and gender is a reliable method of monitoring growth.
• Child's ability to take part in age- and development-appropriate play and activities.	A child's normal role includes play activity.
Elicit information from parent/caregiver regarding concerns they have at each encounter.	Parent/caregiver concern may signal impaired growth and development.
FAMILY DYNAMICS: Evaluate parent/caregiver level of knowledge, support systems, resources, and functioning.	Family functioning and parent/caregiver–child relationships have significant interacting effects on all family members' functioning.
Assess the interactions between the parent/caregiver and child.	The parent/caregiver–child relationship is a powerful influence on a child's growth and development.

Expected Outcomes

The patient will:

- meet expected development milestones.
- display age-appropriate behaviors.
- resume or achieve highest level of functioning possible.
- have resolution of failure to thrive.
- take part in role responsibilities and attend to self-care.
- maintain ongoing contact with the appropriate community resources.

INTERVENTIONS TO ADDRESS IMPAIRED GROWTH AND DEVELOPMENT	RATIONALE
Notify the health care provider (HCP) if manifestations of impaired growth and development are present.	Reporting manifestations of growth and development problems allows for early intervention.
Implement collaborative interventions addressed at treating underlying factors that are contributing to impaired growth and development.	Treatment of underlying causative or risk factors can assist in addressing growth and development problems.
NUTRITION: Encourage the patient and parent/caregiver to provide or follow a healthy, well-balanced diet.	Impaired nutrition status contributes to delayed growth and impaired development.
FUNCTIONAL ABILITY: Encourage the use of adaptive devices for mobility and activities of daily living.	The use of adaptive devices improves function and promotes independence.
Provide sensory stimulation appropriate to the patient's development level.	Stimulation of sensory pathways promotes normal growth and development.
INTERPERSONAL VIOLENCE: Provide the patient and parent/caregiver with adequate referrals or removal from the situation when interpersonal violence is present.	Effective interventions can reduce the negative effects of violence on growth and development.
FAMILY DYNAMICS: Institute measures to promote optimal family functioning.	Family functioning and parent/caregiver–child relationships have significant interacting effects on all family members' functioning.
SAFETY: Help the patient in obtaining necessary adaptive or personal protective equipment and making environment adaptations to promote independence and safety.	Use of adaptive or personal protective equipment and making needed environment modifications can reduce the risk for injury.
Encourage the patient to take part in social relationships and activities that promote feeling useful.	Engagement in productive activities promotes overall well-being.

INTERVENTIONS TO ADDRESS IMPAIRED GROWTH AND DEVELOPMENT	RATIONALE
COMMUNICATION: Institute measures to establish functional communication.	Functional communication can reduce frustration and provide the patient with an alternative means of communicating.
Pediatric Encourage the child to take part in play activities appropriate to age, development level, and abilities.	A child's normal role includes play activity.
FAMILY DYNAMICS: Help the parent/caregiver with establishing discipline and providing positive parenting appropriate to functional age.	All children need appropriate parent–child roles tailored to the child's functional age.
STRESS AND COPING: Offer emotional support and counseling to the parent/caregiver and refer to appropriate community and counseling resources.	Caregivers require ongoing training and support to be able to effectively manage problems related to parent/caregiver–child interaction and impaired development.
Facilitate the patient's enrollment in an early intervention program and continued involvement in school and structured programs.	Structured programs offer child-specific interventions that promote optimal growth and development.
Assist with investigating and evaluating programs and helping parents adjust to the decision for facility placement	Parents/caregivers may not be able to continue care responsibilities, depending on the child's needs.

COLLABORATION	RATIONALE
FAMILY DYNAMICS: Behavior parenting therapy	Behavior parenting therapy teaches parents/caregivers to skills to help manage a child's behavior problems, promoting optimal treatment outcomes.
Parent/caregiver–child interaction therapy	Parent/caregiver–child interaction therapy can improve communication between a child with language problems and the parent/caregiver.
MOBILITY: Physical therapy	Physical therapists assess, plan, and implement interventions that help the patient function at their maximum physical ability.
Speech therapy	Speech therapists assess, plan, and implement interventions that help the patient achieve maximum speech and language development.
NUTRITION: Dietitian	A dietitian can offer the patient a detailed diet plan with appropriate interventions to meet nutrition needs.
FUNCTIONAL ABILITY: Occupational therapy	Occupational therapy can recommend assistive devices and assist with skill development to help the patient function at their maximum ability.
FAMILY DYNAMICS: Family-centered treatment	Family functioning and parent/caregiver–child relationships have significant interacting effects on all family members' development.
Behavior modification therapy	Behavior modification therapy can help those with a development problem with controlling behavior, acting appropriately in social settings, and communicating more effectively.
Support groups	The parents/caregivers of those with impaired growth and development require ongoing support to be able to effectively manage the complex needs of a child with impaired growth and development.
CARE COORDINATION: Social services or case management	Many families bear significant financial and employment burdens because of the numerous needed services of the person with impaired growth and development.
Home safety evaluation	A home safety evaluation assesses the patient's home environment with the goal of increasing the safety for all the people who live there.
MOOD AND AFFECT: Treatment for coexisting psychological problems, including depressed mood and emotional problems	Treatment of underlying depression or other psychological problems can improve patient outcomes.

PATIENT AND CAREGIVER TEACHING

- Cause of impaired growth and development, if known
- Factors that predispose the patient to impaired growth and development
- Manifestations of impaired growth and development
- Management of an underlying condition contributing to impaired growth and development
- Anticipatory guidance about expected physiologic and emotional changes at each stage
- Anticipatory guidance about expected development milestones and expected age-related behaviors
- Measures used to address impaired growth and development
- Recommended health screenings and immunizations
- Importance of proper nutrition
- Modifications in the environment to promote safety
- Sources of information
- Community resources available
- Role of case management
- Importance of regular well-child visits and long-term follow-up
- When to notify the HCP

DOCUMENTATION

Assessment

- Assessments performed
- Diagnostic and laboratory test results
- Growth chart
- Manifestations of impaired growth and development
- Screening test results

Interventions

- Discussions with other interprofessional team members
- Notification of the HCP about patient status
- Therapeutic interventions and the patient's response
- Teaching provided
- Referrals initiated

Evaluation

- Patient's status: improved, stable, declined
- Manifestations of impaired growth and development
- Response to teaching provided
- Response to therapeutic interventions

Negative Self-Image 3

Definition

Negative evaluation of oneself

Self-image is a person's evaluation of their social value. It is made up of the ideas a person has about who they are and their worth to other people. Self-image is important for a person's confidence, motivation, and sense of achievement. Self-image depends mainly on body image and roles but also includes aspects of psychology and spirituality. A person with a healthy self-image has a positive, accurate body image; positive self-concept; high sense of esteem; and clear sense of identity.

Cultural and religious beliefs strongly influence self-image. Societal views of characteristics of people who are attractive are portrayed through the media and internet. Comparing one's body image to models and digitally enhanced persons can make someone feel less than what they are. Many people portray themselves on social media in a very positive light, which may make some people feel inadequate. Culture also plays a role in which experiences are likely to induce shame or stigma. Some persons have a negative self-image associated with a life event. They may have been a victim of interpersonal violence or had an injury or surgery that altered their appearance.

A negative self-concept can affect many aspects of life, including relationships, role performance, and health. It influences how a person perceives their sexual attractiveness and can make it difficult for the person to be intimate. A person with self-image problems may no longer be able to meet role expectations, leading to strained relationships. They may develop anxiety or depression that further interferes with engaging in activities.

Associated Clinical Problems

- Disturbed Body Image: altered personal perception of one's own body
- Lack of Pride: lack of sense of self-worth
- Low Self-Esteem: negative feelings about oneself or capabilities
  - Chronic Low-Self Esteem: long-standing negative feelings about oneself or capabilities
  - Situational Low Self-Esteem: negative feelings about oneself or capabilities in response to a specific situation
- Personal Identity Confusion: lack of direction and definition of self
- Powerlessness: perceived lack of control over the outcome of a specific situation
- Stigma: a specific personal trait that is perceived as or is physically, socially, or psychologically disadvantageous

Common Risk Factors

- Abandonment, including divorce, death
- Burn injury
- Change in body function
- Disfigurement
- Disrupted peer relationships, friendships
- Eating disorder
- Hospitalization
- Identity problems
- LGBTQIA
- Loss of body part
- Loss of job or ability to work
- Marital problems
- Obesity, changes in weight
- Parental rejection
- Radical surgery
- Repeated failures or lack of success at endeavors
- Trauma
- Victim of violence

Pediatric

- Repeated negative feedback from parents or caregivers
- School problems
- Separation from parents or caregivers

Manifestations

- Continually seeks reassurance or approval
- Does not attend to self-care (appearance, hygiene)
- Eating disorders
- Exaggerates negative feedback about self while rejecting positive feedback
- Expresses shame, embarrassment, helplessness, revulsion, guilt
- Expresses feelings about inability to control situation
- Identity problems
- Inability to trust others
- Impaired sexual function
- Intentional hiding or overexposing body part
- Lack of assertiveness
- Lack of culturally appropriate body presentation (posture, eye contact, movements)
- Lack of or poor problem-solving ability

- Refusal to look at or touch a body part(s)
- Passivity
- Poor eye contact
- Rejects attention and positive comments from others
- Resignation
- Self-destructive behaviors, such as mutilation
- Self-negating verbalization about oneself
- Sensitive to criticism
- Social isolation
- Suicidal ideation
- Weight problems

Pediatric

- Problems in school

Key Conceptual Relationships

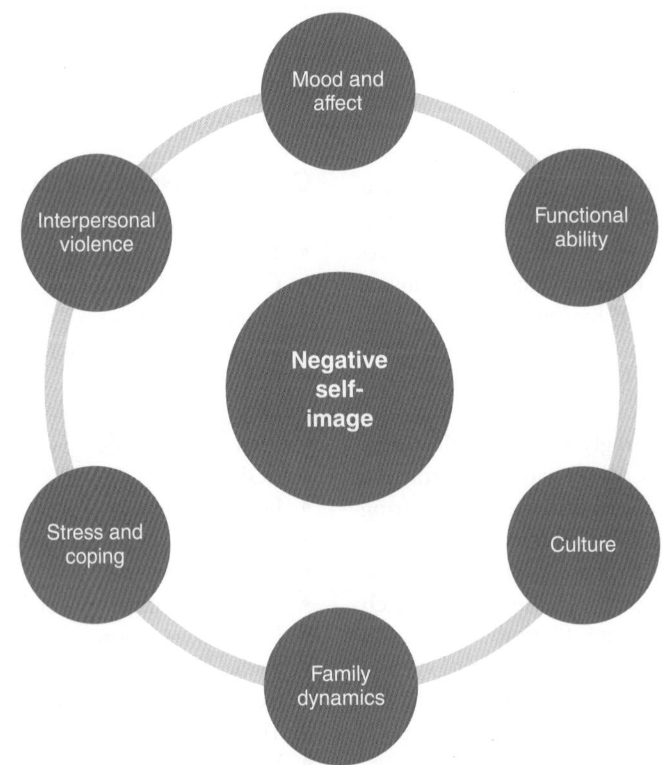

ASSESSMENT OF SELF-IMAGE	RATIONALE
Assess for risk factors that may affect the patient's self-image.	A thorough history can identify conditions or situations that place patients at risk for a problem with self-image.
Use a valid, reliable tool, such as the Rosenberg Self-Esteem Scale (Table 3.1), to screen for a negative self-image.	Identifying a negative self-image allows for early identification and intervention.
Assess the patient's self-image, including: • Self-esteem • Body image • Role performance • Perceived sexuality	Identifying a self-image problem allows for early identification and intervention.
Evaluate for manifestations of a negative self-image	Identifying a self-image problem allows for early identification and intervention.
Assess the patient's support system: • Who they live with • Employment status • Accessible friends and family • Use of community resources	Interest and support from others are an important aspect in the development and maintenance of a positive self-image.
CULTURE: Assess the role of cultural values and social media on the patient's self-image.	Self-image is significantly influenced by cultural values and social media use.

ASSESSMENT OF SELF-IMAGE	RATIONALE
STRESS AND COPING: Assess the current and past use of stress management and coping strategies.	A patient with a negative self-image may be relying on substance use or other negative behaviors as a means of coping.
FUNCTIONAL ABILITY: Perform a psychosocial assessment, evaluating for lifestyle effects, such as problems with social interaction, ability to perform responsibilities, and engage in physical activities.	Problems resulting from a negative self-image can affect all aspects of a person's life.
MOOD AND AFFECT: Assess mental status and screen for coexisting psychological problems.	Persons with a negative self-image may have coexisting depression and other psychological problems.
FAMILY DYNAMICS: Evaluate family dynamics and current level of functioning and observe family interactions.	How family members act and react to the patient affects symptoms and management.
INTERPERSONAL VIOLENCE: Screen the patient at each encounter for interpersonal violence.	Being a victim of interpersonal violence may require action to promote patient safety.
Evaluate the effectiveness of measures used to improve self-image through ongoing monitoring of self-image.	Monitoring the patient's self-image allows for evaluation of therapy effectiveness.

Table 3.1 Rosenberg Self-Esteem Scale

Statement	Strongly Agree	Agree	Disagree	Strongly Disagree
1. I feel that I am a person of worth.				
2. I feel that I have a number of good qualities.				
3. All in all, I am inclined to think that I am a failure.				
4. I am able to do things as well as most other people.				
5. I feel I do not have much to be proud of.				
6. I take a positive attitude toward myself.				
7. On the whole, I am satisfied with myself.				
8. I wish I could have more respect for myself.				
9. I certainly feel useless at times.				
10. At times I think I am no good at all.				

Calculate scores as follows:
For items 1, 2, 4, 6, and *7:* Strongly agree = 3; Agree = 2; Disagree = 1; Strongly disagree = 0
For items 3, 5, 8, 9, and *10:* Strongly agree = 0; Agree = 1; Disagree = 2; Strongly disagree = 3
The scale ranges from 0 to 30. Scores between 15 and 25 are within normal range; scores below 15 suggest low self-esteem.

Expected Outcomes

The patient will:

- make positive statements about self
- use strategies to improve self-image and stop self-negating behavior
- identify positive self-aspects and strengths
- take part in role and self-care responsibilities
- demonstrate acceptance of appearance

INTERVENTIONS TO IMPROVE SELF-IMAGE	RATIONALE
Implement collaborative interventions addressed at treating underlying factor contributing to a negative self-image.	Treatment of underlying causative or risk factors can assist in improving the patient's self-image.
Establish a therapeutic nurse–patient relationship: • Provide privacy and a safe environment. • Use therapeutic touch with patient's consent. • Remain nonjudgmental. • Be attentive and use active listening.	Words and actions that convey sincere acceptance and interest have a positive effect on the patient and help establish trust.

Continued

INTERVENTIONS TO IMPROVE SELF-IMAGE	RATIONALE
Encourage the patient to identify and express feelings about the way they feel about or view themselves.	Self-image can be improved by clarifying thoughts and feelings.
Assist the patient to reframe and redefine negative expressions and identify distortions and misconceptions that contribute to self-image problems.	Reframing may improve image problems by changing negative thoughts and feelings into positive ones.
Discuss changes in body function or physical appearance, particularly if a medical condition is present.	The nurse's help with medically related changes in body image can be the key to helping the patient find support and adapt successfully.
Assist the patient in identifying persons to whom they can express feelings openly.	Self-image may be enhanced through sharing thoughts and feelings.
Encourage the patient to evaluate their own behavior, including their behavior in interactions with others.	By helping understand the relationship between their thoughts and actions, the patient will be able to reflect and work towards building a more positive self-image.
Assist the patient in identifying and reinforcing positive self-aspects and abilities.	The more the patient focuses on positive self-aspects, the less likely the patient will focus on negative aspects.
Discuss media health literacy with the patient and the influence of social media on self-image.	Media literacy interventions can reduce the harmful effects of social media through influencing media-related beliefs and attitudes.
Clarify what life changes and events mean and their effects on self-image.	Positive and negative life events, including successes and failures, influence self-image, as these events are perceived as personal successes or failures.
Have patient verbalize or write positive self-affirmations daily.	Daily positive affirmations help counter negativity.
Praise the patient's acceptance of compliments and encouragement from others.	Compliments and encouragement from others reinforce a positive self-image.
Encourage the patient to accept new challenges through participating in activities in which the patient can succeed.	Activities that allow success raise the patient's confidence level and self-esteem.
Encourage the patient to take part in regular physical activity.	Exercise improves mental health by decreasing feelings of depression and negativity and increasing self-confidence.
SPIRITUALITY: Assist patient in self-examination of spirituality and faith.	Surrendering to faith in a power greater than oneself has given hope to many persons with self-image problems.
STRESS AND COPING: Provide patient with the resources to develop positive stress management and coping behaviors.	Use of positive coping skills equips the patients with multiple skills to manage self-image problems.
FUNCTIONAL ABILITY: Implement measures to promote positive social interaction.	Social interaction can decrease feelings of isolation and promote a more realistic self-appraisal.
MOOD AND AFFECT: Initiate appropriate safety protocols if the patient is at risk for self-harm.	The risk of self-harm necessitates implementing appropriate guidelines to keep the patient safe.
ANXIETY: Implement measures to assist the patient in managing anxiety they may be experiencing.	Patients with anxiety often have concerns related to impaired sexual function.
FUNCTIONAL ABILITY: Help the patient develop strategies to increase participation in activities of daily living.	These strategies address apathy and lack of interest in taking part in activities of daily living that accompany a negative self-image.
FAMILY DYNAMICS: Institute measures to promote optimal family function.	How family members act and react to the patient's negative self-image affects symptoms and management.
INTERPERSONAL VIOLENCE: Provide the patient with adequate referrals or removal from situation when interpersonal violence is present.	Effective interventions can reduce violence, abuse, and physical or mental harm to the patient.
Older Adult	
Discuss perceptions of health problems, including declining socioeconomic status, spousal loss or bereavement, and loss of social support system with retirement.	Specific stressful life events have a great impact on quality of life and image.
Employ reminiscence-based therapy, encouraging storytelling and photograph review.	Reminiscence-based intervention can enhance self-esteem and promote psychological well-being and happiness.

COLLABORATION	RATIONALE
Counseling with cognitive–behavioral therapy	Counseling and cognitive–behavioral therapy may assist the patient in managing self-image problems.
Social work or case management	The social worker can explore community resources available to help the patient obtain access to appropriate health care.
Support groups	Specialty mental health support services are available to assist the patient with managing a negative self-image.
FAMILY DYNAMICS: Family-focused therapy	Family therapy focuses on the cause, symptoms, and treatment of a negative self-image, resulting in improved patient outcomes.
MOOD AND AFFECT: Treatment for coexisting psychological problems, including depressed mood	Treatment of an underlying psychological problem is an important part of addressing a negative self-image.
FUNCTIONAL ABILITY: Social skills training	Assisting the patient in developing social skills will help their maintaining relationships with others.

PATIENT AND CAREGIVER TEACHING

- Factors that may be contributing to negative self-image
- Management of underlying problems contributing to negative self-image
- Manifestations of negative self-image
- Social skills
- Self-image building measures
- Positive coping and stress management strategies
- Community and self-help resources available
- Sources of information and social support
- Anticipatory guidance about situations that may be problematic
- Importance of health promotion behaviors, including nutrition, sleep, exercise
- When to notify the health care provider (HCP)

DOCUMENTATION

Assessment

- Assessments performed
- Manifestations of negative self-image

Interventions

- Discussions with other interprofessional team members
- Notification of the HCP about patient status
- Therapeutic interventions and the patient's response
- Teaching provided
- Referrals initiated

Evaluation

- Patient's status: improved, stable, declined
- Manifestations of negative self-image
- Response to teaching provided
- Response to therapeutic interventions

Parenting Problem 4

Definition

Inability or change in the ability of the parent to provide care that promotes optimal growth and development of the child

A parent is the caregiver of a child. Most often, it is the father or mother, but many persons, such as grandparents or guardians, can act in the caregiver role and parent a child. Attachment, or bonding between the child and parent, is mainly determined by the type of parenting the child receives. Children who are cared for in a consistent, understanding, and responsive way develop secure attachments with their parents. They have better outcomes than children with impaired attachment. Children with impaired attachment are likely to have impaired growth and development and social and emotional problems.

To meet the varied needs of their child, parents must have confidence in their parenting abilities. Education is the cornerstone of managing parenting problems. Parents need to have knowledge of development milestones, positive parenting, methods of discipline, and measures that keep their child safe and healthy. Nurses need to understand growth and development and parenting skills so that they can provide nursing care that promotes an optimal parent–child relationship based on the dyad's specific needs.

Associated Clinical Problems

- Impaired Caregiver Child Attachment: a lack of bonding and security between and caregiver and child
- Parent Role Conflict: conflict resulting from a change in parent role or responsibilities

Common Risk Factors

Parent

- Adolescent parent
- Chronic stress
- Economically disadvantaged
- Family or marital conflict
- Impaired family function
- Inadequate support
- Interpersonal violence, including abuse and domestic violence, in the home
- Lack of knowledge about parenting practices
- Lack of positive family role models
- Low education level
- Poor coping skills
- Poor health
- Psychological problems, including depression, anxiety
- Single parent
- Sleep deprivation
- Social isolation
- Substance use
- Unemployment or job problems
- Unrealistic expectations of child
- Unwanted pregnancy, unwanted child

Child

- Being in foster care or residential care settings
- Congenital and genetic disorders
- Difficult temperament
- Disability
- Impaired growth and development
- Loss of parent
- Multiple changes of primary caregiver

Parent Role Conflict

- Changes in parent role
- Disruption in parenting routine
- Separation from child

Manifestations

Parent

- Anger and hostility toward child or parenting role
- Child abandonment
- Decreased ability to manage or control child
- Frustration with role as parent
- Inappropriate or inconsistent care of child
- Lack of concern for the child and the child's health
- Makes negative statements about the child
- Perpetrator of interpersonal violence, including abuse and neglect
- States perceived or actual inadequacy about parenting
- Unsafe home environment

Child

- Behavior problems
- Decline from prior level of functioning
- Diminished separation anxiety

- Failure to thrive
- Feeding problems
- Frequent illness
- Impaired growth and development
- Inability to participate in age-appropriate activities
- Inappropriate responses to everyday stressors
- Learning disabilities
- Runaway
- School problems
- Sleep problems

Parent Role Conflict
- Anxiety
- Feeling of guilt, frustration
- Not participating or reluctance to participate in normal parenting activities

Key Conceptual Relationships

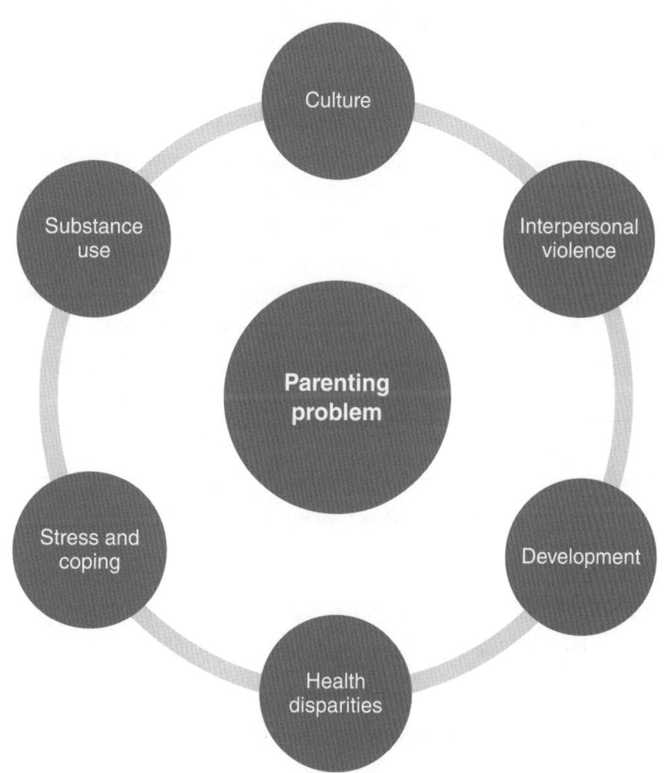

ASSESSMENT OF PARENTING	RATIONALE
Assess for common causes and risk factors that influence parenting and optimal attachment.	A thorough history of all common causes and risk factors that may influence parenting and attachment is essential for early identification of families at risk.
Obtain a demographic profile of the family, including: • Who is in the family? • Who lives in the household? • Has anyone moved out recently? • Have there been any recent changes? • What language is spoken? • What is the family's financial status?	Demographic data provide basic information about the family structure.
Assess the quality of parent–child interaction with each encounter, noting: • Parent and child involvement • Types of interactions • Comfort, affection of child (touching, holding) • Discipline techniques • Support of child's development (play activities, development toys)	Problems in parent–child interaction reflect parenting skills, significantly contribute to attachment problems, and negatively influence the child's development.

Continued

ASSESSMENT OF PARENTING	RATIONALE
Use an appropriate tool, such as the Keys to Interactive Parenting Scale (KIPS) or the Parenting Scale, to formally assess parenting.	Parenting skills influence attachment and child development.
Assess the quality and pattern of parent–child attachment through direct observation and structured parent and child interviews, using attachment assessment tools, such as the CARE Index.	An attachment assessment evaluates the pattern of relatedness between a child and parent, which may be used as a basis for therapy.
Evaluate family dynamics and current level of functioning and observe family interactions.	Family dynamics and parent–child relationships have significant effects on all family members' functioning.
CULTURE: Assess the role of culture on parenting and attachment.	Culture-based expectations exist for parenting and attachment behaviors.
HEALTH DISPARITIES: Explore the availability of social support and resources, including housing, occupational, health care, and financial.	Families without adequate resources face additional hardships that can lead to impaired parenting.
STRESS AND COPING: Assess the parent's strengths and weaknesses and normal coping behaviors.	Parents who use positive coping and stress management strategies deal better with the stress of parenting and changing life situations.
SUBSTANCE USE: Screen the parent for substance use.	Identifying substance use is important for initiating care.
INTERPERSONAL VIOLENCE: Screen the parent at each encounter for interpersonal violence.	Interpersonal violence in the home increases the risk of impaired parenting and may require action to promote personal safety.
MOOD AND AFFECT: Screen the parent for the presence of coexisting psychological problems.	Identifying depression or other psychological problems and initiating treatment can improve the parent–child relationship.
DEVELOPMENT: Assess the child's level of physical and emotional development.	Parenting and attachment behaviors influence a child's development level and health status.
Evaluate the effectiveness of measures used to influence the parenting problem through ongoing assessment.	Ongoing monitoring of the parenting problem allows for evaluation of therapy effectiveness.

Expected Outcomes

The child will:

- meet expected development milestones.
- display age-appropriate behaviors.
- achieve the highest level of function possible.

The parent will:

- demonstrate appropriate parenting skills.
- demonstrate positive attachment behaviors.
- identify and use resources available for parenting assistance.
- state confidence in parenting abilities.
- provide a safe, nurturing environment.

INTERVENTIONS TO ADDRESS A PARENTING PROBLEM	RATIONALE
Establish a therapeutic relationship to explore the parent's understanding of the parenting problem: • Be empathetic. • Remain nonjudgmental. • Use active listening with therapeutic communication skills. • Avoid blaming.	Words and actions that convey sincere acceptance and interest have a positive effect on the parent and help establish trust.
Encourage parents to share their feelings about parenting and problems they may be experiencing.	Information obtained about the problems parents are experiencing is used to tailor parent education and interventions to promote positive parenting.
CULTURE: Encourage the parents to establish their own goals and culturally considerate parenting strategies.	Establishing their own goals and parenting strategies promotes the parents' sense of control and supports agreement about parenting decisions.
Provide positive reinforcement about areas of strength observed during encounters.	Positive reinforcement motivates the parent to continue behavior related to existing strengths.

INTERVENTIONS TO ADDRESS A PARENTING PROBLEM	RATIONALE
Discuss positive parenting techniques, including: • Offering warmth and support • Talking at the child's level • Providing clear expectations • Having realistic expectations • Validating the child's feelings • Being empathetic	Positive parenting promotes positive family interactions and guides the development of appropriate child behavior.
Discuss age-appropriate discipline techniques and role-play disciplining a child.	Successful discipline requires the imposition of clear and consistent rules, perspective taking, and acceptance, rather than rejection of the child.
Promote attachment when separation of parent and child is necessary because of illness, including: • Having parent provide care as able • Encouraging parents to spend time with child • Incorporating information about the child's routines, likes and dislikes, and behavior • Providing frequent updates	Maintaining involvement in decision making and care will reduce feelings of parent role conflict and promote attachment.
Assist the parent in working with school officials to develop an education plan for how the child will be supported in school.	A child with impaired growth and development may have difficulties at school and with peer relationships, which are addressed through an education plan, thus maximizing learning.
Institute measures to address problems with family function as appropriate.	Family functioning and parent–child relationships have significant interacting effects on all family members' functioning.
DEVELOPMENT: Institute measures to promote child growth and development.	Parenting skills and behaviors have a strong influence on a child's growth and development.
Help the parent identify support systems for parents, such as extended family, neighbors, or support groups.	Support systems decrease family stress.
INTERPERSONAL VIOLENCE: Provide the parent with adequate referrals or removal from situation when interpersonal violence is present.	Effective interventions can reduce the negative effects of violence on parenting and family dynamics.
STRESS AND COPING: Assist parent to identify and use positive coping and stress management strategies.	Positive coping and stress management strategies help the parent learn to deal with stress and changing life situations.
SUBSTANCE USE: Implement measures to address any substance use.	Long-term support and assistance to address substance use will improve overall family functioning.
SAFETY: Assist the parent with identifying and implementing measures to promote a safe environment.	Parent must initiate appropriate behaviors to ensure a safe and clean environment for the child.

COLLABORATION	RATIONALE
Behavior parenting therapy	Behavior parenting therapy teaches parents skills to help manage a child's behavior problems, promoting optimal treatment outcomes.
Parent–child interaction therapy	Therapy can help improve communication between children and the parent and teach parenting skills.
Family-centered treatment	Family functioning and parent–child relationships have significant interacting effects on all family members' development.
Support groups	Support groups can provide the parent with ongoing training and peer support that promote parenting.
Parent education classes, as appropriate	Parent education class provide the parent with ongoing training and support that promote positive parenting.
School counselor	A child with impaired attachment often has problems at school and with peer relationships, which are addressed through an education plan, thus maximizing learning.

Continued

COLLABORATION	RATIONALE
HEALTH DISPARITIES: Social work or case management	Meeting the needs of family members for basic resources allows the family to focus on relationships and higher-level needs. They can provide adequate referrals or assist with removal from situation when interpersonal violence is present.
MOOD AND AFFECT: Treatment for coexisting psychological problems	Initiating treatment for depression or coexisting psychological problems may assist with improving parenting.

 PARENT AND CAREGIVER TEACHING

- Normal growth and development
- Anticipatory guidance regarding expected age-related behaviors at each stage of child development
- Factors that may contribute to a parenting problem
- Differences in child temperament
- Influencing and risk factors for parenting problems
- Positive parenting techniques
- Appropriate discipline techniques
- Positive verbal and nonverbal communication skills
- Resources available for assistance with parenting skills
- Coping and stress management strategies
- When to notify the HCP

 DOCUMENTATION

Assessment

- Assessments performed
- Manifestations of a parenting problem

Interventions

- Discussions with other interprofessional team members
- Therapeutic interventions and the response
- Teaching provided
- Referrals initiated

Evaluation

- Family's status: improved, stable, declined
- Manifestations of a parenting problem
- Response to teaching provided
- Response to therapeutic interventions

Impaired Family Function 5

Definition

Inability of the family to meet family members' needs

Family function refers to a family's social and structural properties. These include interactions and relationships within the family, especially levels of conflict and cohesion, adaptability, organization, and communication. The family dynamic is created by how the family lives, interacts with one another, makes decisions affecting the family, and supports one another. That dynamic—whether positive, healthy, and supportive, or negative, dysfunctional, and damaging—changes who people are and influences how they view and interact with the world outside of the family. The dynamic evolves and changes over time and is influenced by many factors. Changes in one family member's behavior affect everyone else in the family unit.

One emphasis in nursing today is providing family-centered care and empowering families to achieve optimal level functioning. Wherever nurses practice, they will work with families and observe family dynamics across the lifespan. No family is 100% functional. A healthy family is able to adapt and adjust to roles that change over time. Healthy families are concerned with all members' needs and encourage positive communication. In times of illness and stress, family interactions may change—sometimes for the better and sometimes for the worse. As nurses interact with families, they must recognize family dynamics that promote health and family dynamics that place families at risk for impaired family function.

Associated Clinical Problems

- Family Conflict: active opposition or disagreement between family members
- Lack of Family Support: lack of social support for maintaining the function of the family as a whole

Common Contributing Factors

- Chronic stress
- Cultural belief conflicts
- Disability
- Disruption in normal family routine
- Family configuration changes, including birth, divorce, death, marriage
- Family member with disability, chronic illness, poor health
- Family values
- Inability of a family member to fulfill usual roles
- Low education level
- Parenting practices
- Poor family support system
- Poverty
- Role change
- Separation from or loss of parent, caregivers, family, significant others
- Significant incident involving a family member, such as crime or jail
- Social isolation
- Socioeconomic status
- Substance use
- Unemployment and unstable work history
- Violence, including abuse, neglect, and domestic violence, in the home
- Work obligations

Manifestations

- Aggression, hostility
- Conflict avoidance
- Impaired role performance
- Inability to communicate effectively
- Inability to meet family members' needs
- Inappropriate roles
- Mood problems, including depression, anxiety
- Negative family interactions, including chaos, conflict, over criticism
- Interpersonal violence, including abuse and neglect, in the home
- Sleep problems
- Social isolation
- Stress-related illnesses
- Substance use

Pediatric

- School problems
- Sibling rivalry

Key Conceptual Relationships

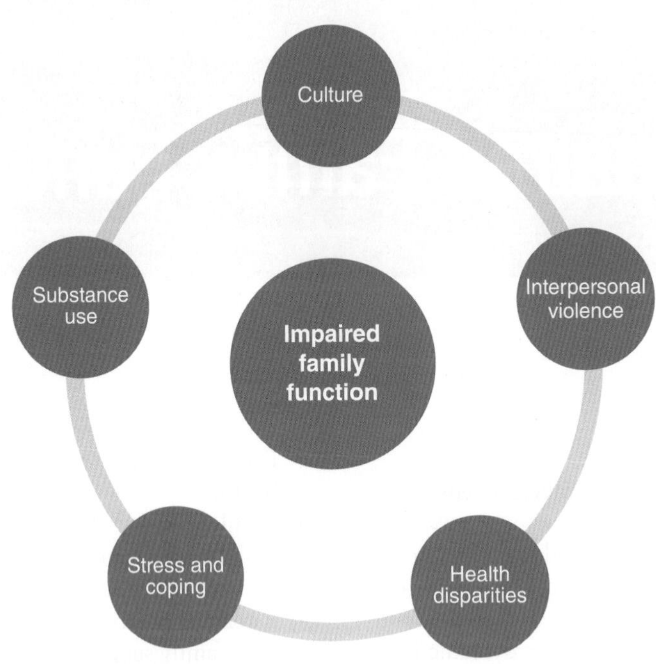

ASSESSMENT OF FAMILY FUNCTION	RATIONALE
Assess for common causes and risk factors that influence family function.	A thorough history of all common causes and risk factors that may influence family function is essential for early identification of families at risk.
Obtain a demographic profile of the family, including: • Who is in the family? • Who lives in the household? • Has anyone moved out recently? • Have there been any recent changes? • What language is spoken? • What is the family's financial status?	Demographic data provide basic information about the family structure.
Perform a functional family assessment.	A functional assessment reveals how the family members behave in relation to one another and assists with developing family interventions.
Assess roles, responsibilities, and expectations of each family member.	Roles and responsibilities vary greatly with families, with changes in the role of one family member often affecting the role of other family members.
Assess boundaries with those outside the family.	Families with limited social support or resources are more likely to have inadequate resources in times of crisis than families with support systems.
Assess the verbal and nonverbal communication among family members: • Is communication effective? • Are all members free to share feelings? • Are there positive interactions? • What types of negative interactions occur? • How are decisions made?	Positive interactions and communications produce cohesion and growth, whereas negative interactions and communications lead to impaired family function.
Assess the quality of parent–child interaction with each encounter, noting: • Parent and child involvement • Types of interactions • Comfort, affection of child (touching, holding) • Discipline techniques • Support of child's development (play activities, development toys)	Problems in parent–child interaction reflect parenting skills, are a significant contributor to attachment problems, and negatively influence the child's development.

ASSESSMENT OF FAMILY FUNCTION	RATIONALE
Assess the availability of resources, including housing, occupational, health care, and financial.	Resources may be available to help the family meet basic needs.
Develop a family genogram.	A genogram helps outline and summarize the family's information.
STRESS AND COPING: Assess how the family members cope with stressors, including how they manage changes in structure and roles.	Positive coping and stress management strategies help family members deal with stress and changing life situations.
CULTURE: Assess the role of culture on family function.	Culture has a strong influence on family roles, communication, values, and expectations.
SUBSTANCE USE: Screen family members for the presence of alcohol, tobacco, and/or other substance use problems.	Identifying substance use among the family is important for initiating care.
INTERPERSONAL VIOLENCE: Screen family members for interpersonal violence in the home.	Interpersonal violence negatively influences family functioning and may require action to promote the safety of family member(s).
SPIRITUALITY: Complete a spiritual assessment.	Spiritual practices are part of the family values system that support the family in daily life and in times of crisis.
HEALTH DISPARITIES: Explore the family's availability of social support and resources, including housing, occupational, health care, and financial.	Families without adequate resources face additional hardships and stress that can lead to impaired family dynamics.
MOOD AND AFFECT: Screen for coexisting psychological problems among family members.	Identifying depression or other psychological problems and initiating treatment can improve family function.
Evaluate the effectiveness of measures used to influence family function through ongoing assessment.	Monitoring family function allows for evaluation of therapy effectiveness.

Expected Outcomes

The family will:

- display positive, healthy, and respectful relationships.
- provide nurturance and assistance to all family members.
- communicate openly and positively with each other.
- meet the needs of all family members.
- have positive social interactions outside the family.
- obtain resources to meet family members' needs.
- use appropriate strategies to resolve family conflict.

INTERVENTIONS TO ENHANCE FAMILY FUNCTION	RATIONALE
Establish a therapeutic relationship: • Be empathetic. • Remain nonjudgmental. • Use active listening with therapeutic communication skills. • Avoid blaming. • Do not take sides in family disagreements.	A nurse's words and actions that convey sincere acceptance and interest have a positive effect on the family and help establish trust.
Encourage problem solving and open communication among family members by: • having them verbalize their own feelings and share those feelings with each other. • having them appraise their current situation. • discussing their concerns and problems. • reviewing each family member's role expectations. • assisting them with developing solutions.	Open communication among family members helps the family to identify problems and find ways to cope with them.
CULTURE: Encourage the family members to establish their own goals and culturally considerate strategies to address family function.	Establishing their own goals and strategies promotes the family's sense of control.

Continued

INTERVENTIONS TO ENHANCE FAMILY FUNCTION	RATIONALE
Provide positive reinforcement about the family's areas of strength.	Positive reinforcement motivates the family to continue behavior related to existing strengths.
Assist the family with appraising situations and behaviors that are impairing family function.	The process of developing insight helps the family members process and understand their problems.
Help the family establish clear family roles: • Clarify what they want and need from each other. • Make sure that everyone understands what is expected of them in their role. • Know that roles may change over time. • During major life changes or crisis, roles may need to be reassigned. • Ensure that roles are appropriate for each person.	Having clearly defined roles provides a way to share responsibilities among members in such a way that it helps ensure healthy family function.
Institute measures to address parenting problems identified.	Positive parenting skills have a significant influence on family functioning and parent–child relationships.
Explore sources of social support for the family and how support systems can influence family function.	Social support networks can positively influence family function by providing information and resources.
STRESS AND COPING: Assist family members to identify and use positive coping and stress management strategies.	Positive coping and stress management strategies help family members deal with stress and changing life situations.
INTERPERSONAL VIOLENCE: Provide the family members with adequate referrals or removal from the situation when interpersonal violence is present.	Effective interventions can reduce the negative effects of violence on family function.
MOOD AND AFFECT: Institute referral and treatment for coexisting psychological problems.	Identifying depression or other coexisting problems and initiating treatment may assist with improving family function.
SUBSTANCE USE: Implement measures to address any substance use.	Provides long-term support and assistance by addressing substance use and improving overall family functioning.
SPIRITUALITY: Assist the family members in implementing measures to address their spiritual state.	Spiritual practices are part of the family values system that supports the family in daily life and in times of crisis.

COLLABORATION	RATIONALE
Individual counseling	Counseling may help individual family members modify their attitudes and behaviors and enhance communication skills.
Structural family therapy, as appropriate	Structured family therapy addresses problems with interactions and communication and can help create a healthier family dynamic.
Parent–child interaction therapy	Therapy can help improve communication between children and parents.
Support groups	Support groups can provide family members with ongoing training and peer support that promotes positive family function.
HEALTH DISPARITIES: Social work or case management	Meeting the needs of family members for basic resources allows the family to focus on relationships and higher-level needs. They can provide adequate referrals or assist with removal from the situation when interpersonal violence is present.
MOOD AND AFFECT: Treatment for coexisting psychological problems	Initiating treatment for a coexisting psychological problem may assist with improving family dynamics.

PATIENT AND CAREGIVER TEACHING

- Factors that may be contributing to impaired family function
- Manifestations of impaired family function
- Measures being used to address impaired family function
- Anticipatory guidance regarding situations that may be problematic
- Positive verbal and nonverbal communication skills
- Community and self-help resources
- Positive coping and stress management strategies
- Conflict resolution strategies
- Role of case management
- When to notify the health care provider (HCP)

DOCUMENTATION

Assessment

- Assessments performed
- Manifestations of impaired family function

Interventions

- Discussions with other interprofessional team members
- Therapeutic interventions and the family's response
- Teaching provided
- Referrals initiated

Evaluation

- Family's status: improved, stable, declined
- Manifestations of impaired family function
- Response to teaching provided
- Response to therapeutic interventions

Impaired Role Performance 6

Definition

Impaired ability to perform normal daily activities required to fulfill usual roles in the family, workplace, and community

A key factor that influences a person's quality of life is their ability to fulfill usual roles in their family, workplace, and community. Roles are the duties and tasks, associated with a particular position or status, that a person is expected to fulfill. We all have multiple roles in life, such as spouse, employee, child, sibling, or parent. The functional capacity of a person to perform a task, activity, or behavior to fulfill their roles is their role ability. *Disability* refers to varying degrees of a person's inability to perform the tasks required to fulfill their roles and complete normal life activities without assistance.

Instrumental activities of daily living (IADLs) include complex skills requiring higher levels of functional ability that are essential to fulfilling roles. Examples of IADLs are managing finances, shopping, cooking, cleaning, computer use, and driving. Adults who are responsible for home maintenance and employment rely on these skills. Thus illness or injury that influences the ability to perform IADLs significantly affects the person's ability to fulfill role responsibilities. Changes in functional ability that impair role performance may be temporary, such as recovering from major surgery, or long term. Those who experience a spinal cord injury or develop a degenerative neuromuscular condition will have permanent changes in functional ability that affect role performance. The family often must adapt to change when role impairment is present. Role reversal is common if an older adult becomes ill, with the child often assuming many of the parent's responsibilities.

Nursing care for the patient with impaired role function includes recognizing the possibility of role-performance alterations, performing a functional assessment, and planning and delivering care specific to the patient's needs. The results of the functional assessment determine the patient's role ability and the level of functional impairment present, thus guiding the nurse in optimizing the patient's independent role function.

Associated Clinical Problems

- Activity Planning Problem: problem with participating in desired or usual activities
  - Diversion Activity Deficit: lack of interest or participation in leisure or recreational activities
  - Impaired Ability to Perform Leisure Activity: loss of ability to participate in leisure activities
  - Lack of Play Activity: lack of participation in activities for enjoyment or self-amusement
- Altered Role Performance: any change in a person's usual duties and responsibilities or the ability to perform those duties and responsibilities
  - Involuntary Role Reversal: two people involuntarily exchange duties and responsibilities so that each now does what the other used to do
  - New Role: assuming new duties and responsibilities
  - Role Change: change in a person's duties and responsibilities
  - Role Loss: loss of a person's usual duties and responsibilities
- Impaired Home Maintenance: loss of the ability to maintain a safe home environment
  - Impaired Ability to Manage Finances: loss of the ability to manage finances
  - Impaired Ability to Prepare Food: loss of the ability to prepare food
  - Impaired Ability to Shop: loss of the ability to shop

Common Risk Factors

- Age
- Arthritis
- Cancer
- Chronic illness, personal or family member
- Degenerative neuromuscular conditions
- Depression
- Disability, personal or family member
- Excessive demands
- Fatigue
- Impaired cognition
- Impaired mobility
- Inadequate resources
- Lack of motivation
- Lengthy, frequent hospitalizations
- Major surgery
- Musculoskeletal problems
- Pain
- Psychological problems
- Sensory deficits
- Spinal cord injury

- Stroke
- Substance use
- Trauma
- Traumatic brain injury
- Unrealistic expectations

Pediatric

- Autism
- Behavior problems
- Communication problems
- Impaired growth and development

Impaired Home Maintenance

- Inadequate support systems
- Lack of knowledge

Role Performance Alteration

- Change in household composition
- Change in others' perception of role
- Death of family member
- Role loss, change, denial, reversal, overload, or dissatisfaction

Manifestations

- Difficulty participating in role responsibilities
- Difficulty performing IADLs
- Negative self-image
- Role changes
- Role reversal

Activity Planning Problem

- Boredom
- Inability to participate in usual activities

Pediatric

- Lack of play activity
- School problems

Impaired Home Maintenance

- Financial problems
- Lack of necessities in the home
- Uncleanliness

Key Conceptual Relationships

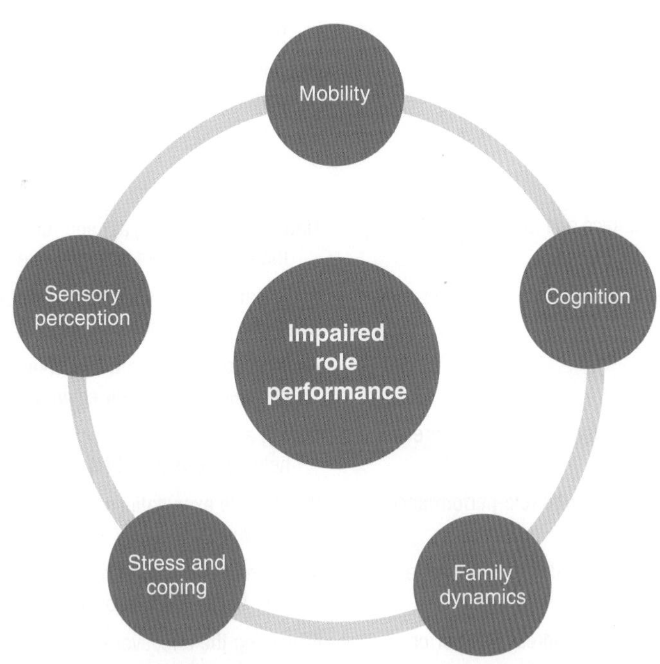

ASSESSMENT OF ROLE PERFORMANCE	RATIONALE
Assess for risk factors that may be influencing role performance.	Identifying factors that place the patient at risk for impaired role performance allows for early intervention.
Evaluate the patient's underlying health status.	Underlying health status has a significant influence on role performance.
Assess the patient's ability to perform personal care:	
• Directly observe the patient performing IADLs.	The results of the functional assessment help determine the patient's ability to fulfill their roles and the type of assistance needed.

Continued

ASSESSMENT OF ROLE PERFORMANCE	RATIONALE
• Assess self-report and caregiver report of role performance ability.	Self-report measures are part of the overall functional assessment but because of potential inaccuracy, they require validation with other measures.
• Use a valid, reliable tool appropriate for the patient's age and cognition to perform a formal assessment of role performance, such as the Lawton Instrumental Activities of Daily Living Scale (Table 6.1).	The results of the functional assessment help determine the patient's ability to fulfill their roles and the type of assistance needed.
Perform a physical assessment and obtain diagnostic tests based on the patient's history, including the following:	
• **COGNITION:** Cognitive and mental status	Cognitive impairments contribute to impaired role performance.
• **PAIN:** Comprehensive pain assessment	Experiencing pain negatively affects the ability to perform usual role responsibilities.
• **MOBILITY:** Mobility and musculoskeletal function	Physical mobility problems have a significant impact on the ability to independently perform role responsibilities.
• **SENSORY PERCEPTION:** Vision and hearing	Sensory deficits may interfere with the ability to independently fulfill role responsibilities.
Obtain a formal occupational therapy evaluation as appropriate.	Occupational therapists assess, plan, and implement interventions that promote a person's ability to fulfill role responsibilities.
Obtain a formal physical therapy evaluation as appropriate.	Physical therapists assess, plan, and implement interventions that promote a person's ability to fulfill role responsibilities.
Determine the expected length of any role impairment.	Knowing the expected length of a role performance problem is vital in planning care and securing resources.
Assess the patient's support system: • Who do they live with? • Are they employed? • Do they have accessible friends and relatives? • Have they used any community resources?	Support from others is an important aspect of managing impaired role performance.
FAMILY DYNAMICS: Evaluate family dynamics and the impact of impaired role function.	How family members act and react to the patient's impaired role performance influences potential role-performance alterations.
Assess current and past hobbies, interests, and activities that the patient enjoys and participates in.	Participating in activities the patient enjoys can provide the patient with a sense of purpose.
Develop an ecomap for the patient.	An ecomap is a diagram that shows the social and personal relationships of a person with their environment.
STRESS AND COPING: Assess the patient's use of coping and stress management strategies.	Coping and stress management strategies can improve quality of life by helping the patient better manage impaired role performance.
CULTURE: Assess the role of culture in the patient's role-performance expectations.	Various role expectations are significantly influenced by cultural norms and values.
Assess caregiver support for families with older adult and child role reversal.	Assessing the caregiver for signs of role strain and alteration is necessary to be able to provide adequate support.
Evaluate the effectiveness of measures used to address role performance through ongoing assessment.	Evaluating the effectiveness of measures to address role performance allows for adjustment of therapy to maximize independence.
Pediatric	
DEVELOPMENT: Assess the child's level of physical and emotional development.	The types of activities in which the child participates depend on the child's age, developmental level, and health status.

Table 6.1 Lawton Instrumental Activities of Daily Living Scale

Ability to Use Telephone	
1. Operates telephone on own initiative; looks up and dials numbers	1
2. Dials a few well-known numbers	1
3. Answers telephone but does not dial	1
4. Does not use telephone at all	0
Shopping	
1. Takes care of all shopping needs independently	1
2. Shops independently for small purchases	0
3. Needs to be accompanied on any shopping trip	0
4. Completely unable to shop	0
Food Preparation	
1. Plans, prepares, and serves adequate meals independently	1
2. Prepares adequate meals if supplied with ingredients	0
3. Heats and serves prepared meals or prepares meals but does not maintain adequate diet	0
4. Needs to have meals prepared and served	0
Housekeeping	
1. Maintains house alone with occasion assistance (heavy work)	1
2. Performs light daily tasks such as dishwashing and bed making	1
3. Performs light daily tasks but cannot maintain acceptable level of cleanliness	1
4. Needs help with all home maintenance tasks	1
5. Does not participate in any housekeeping tasks	0
Laundry	
1. Does personal laundry completely	1
2. Launders small items	1
3. All laundry must be done by others	0
Mode of Transportation	
1. Travels independently on public transportation or drives own car	1
2. Arranges own travel via taxi but does not otherwise use public transportation	1
3. Travels on public transportation when assisted or accompanied by another	1
4. Travel limited to taxi or automobile with assistance of another	0
5. Does not travel at all	0
Responsibility for Own Medications	
1. Is responsible for taking medication in correct dosages at correct time	1
2. Takes responsibility if medication is prepared in advance in separate dosages	0
3. Is not capable of dispensing own medication	0
Ability to Handle Finances	
1. Manages financial matters independently (budgets, writes checks, pays bills)	1
2. Manages day-to-day purchases but needs help with banking and major purchases	1
3. Incapable of handling money	0

Scoring: For each category, circle the item description that most closely resembles the client's highest functional level (either 0 or 1). The higher the score, the greater the person's abilities.

From Hartford Institute for Geriatric Nursing. The Lawton Instrumental Activities of Daily Living (IADL) Scale. https://consultgeri.org/try-this/general-assessment/issue-23.pdf.

Expected Outcomes

The patient will:

- perform role behaviors.
- take part in desired activities of daily living.
- use community resources as needed.
- maintain satisfactory relationships with others.
- identify and implement measures to enhance role performance.
- participate in diversion or play activities.
- maintain ongoing contact with the appropriate community resources.

INTERVENTIONS TO ENHANCE ROLE PERFORMANCE	RATIONALE
Implement collaborative interventions aimed at treating underlying factors contributing to impaired role performance.	Role-performance problems may improve or resolve with the treatment of an underlying contributing factor.
Assist the patient in identifying personal strengths and abilities.	Identifying personal strengths will help the patient integrate those strengths into enhancing role performance.
Encourage the patient to share concerns about their role performance and their experience of impairments in role abilities.	Perceived failures in meeting role expectations can produce a negative self-image.
Help the patient and family outline realistic role responsibilities.	Discussion assists the family in clarifying roles and determining who will perform specific responsibilities.
CULTURE: Encourage the patient to establish their own goals and culturally considerate strategies to address role performance.	Establishing their own goals and strategies promotes the patient's sense of control and respects cultural norms and values.
Encourage the use of adaptive devices for mobility and IADLs.	The use of adaptive devices improves role ability and promotes independence.
Assist with implementing the plan of care developed by occupational therapy.	The occupational therapist's plan of care is designed to promote the performance of IADLs.
Assist with implementing the plan of care developed by physical therapy.	The physical therapist's plan of care is designed to promote optimal mobility and physical function.
CARE COORDINATION: Assist the patient in obtaining necessary adaptive devices and making needed environmental adaptations.	Adaptive devices and environmental modifications can assist the patient in performing personal care independently.
COGNITION: Implement measures to address impaired cognition, if present.	Role performance is directly related to impaired cognitive function.
MOBILITY: Implement measures to address impaired mobility, if present.	Improving the patient's level of mobility may improve role performance.
DEVELOPMENT: Implement measures to assist the patient in maintaining a positive self-image.	Failure to fulfill role expectations can produce a negative self-image.
PAIN: Implement measures to address pain, if applicable.	There is a strong association between role performance and pain; reducing pain may enhance role performance.
Implement measures to address caregiver support for families with older adult and child role reversal.	It may be difficult for the caregiver to ask for or accept help if role changes, role reversal, and new roles occur.
SENSORY PERCEPTION: Implement measures to address sensory deficits, if present.	Addressing sensory deficits may enhance the ability to independently fulfill role responsibilities.
Pediatric	
DEVELOPMENT: Institute measures to promote the child's growth and development.	Providing appropriate activities is necessary for nurturing the child's growth and development.

INTERVENTIONS TO ADDRESS AN ACTIVITY PLANNING PROBLEM	RATIONALE
Discuss the patient's preferred interests and involve them in selecting and planning diversion or play activities.	Participating in activities the patient enjoys can provide the patient with a sense of purpose.
Pediatric Encourage the child to participate in play activities appropriate to age, developmental level, and abilities.	A child's normal role includes participating in play activity.

INTERVENTIONS TO ADDRESS IMPAIRED HOME MAINTENANCE	RATIONALE
Discuss with the patient measures that can address problems, such as: • Meal delivery • Using reminders and lists • Automatic bill payment • Alternative transportation methods	The use of compensatory measures leads to a higher level of role performance.
Obtain necessary adaptive devices to help the patient fulfill roles in the home environment.	Adaptive devices can assist the patient in fulfilling roles in the home environment.
Assist the patient with identifying support persons or caregivers to assist with performing home maintenance.	Helping with home maintenance can help the patient in the home and keep the home orderly.

COLLABORATION	RATIONALE
MOBILITY: Physical therapy	Physical therapists assess, plan, and implement interventions that promote a person's ability to fulfill role responsibilities.
Occupational therapy	Occupational therapy can recommend assistive devices and help with skill development so the patient can fulfill roles in the home.
CARE COORDINATION: Social work or case management	A social worker or case manager can help the patient and caregiver identify community resources to assist with fulfilling role responsibilities.
Community support groups	Support groups can play a key role in promoting adjustment to role changes.

PATIENT AND CAREGIVER TEACHING

- Cause of impaired role performance, if known
- Factors contributing to impaired role performance
- Manifestations of impaired role performance
- Management of underlying condition associated with impaired role performance
- Measures to enhance role performance
- Anticipatory guidance regarding situations that may be problematic
- Role of physical and occupational therapies
- Community and self-help resources
- How to safely use adaptive devices
- Modifications in the living environment to promote safety
- Importance of long-term follow-up
- Role of case management
- When to notify the health care provider (HCP)

DOCUMENTATION

Assessment

- Assessments performed
- Diagnostic and laboratory test results
- Manifestations of impaired role performance
- Screening test results

Interventions

- Discussions with other interprofessional team members
- Environmental modifications made
- Notification of HCP about patient status
- Therapeutic interventions and the patient's response
- Teaching provided
- Referrals initiated

Evaluation

- Patient's status: improved, stable, declined
- Presence of manifestations of impaired role performance
- Response to teaching provided
- Response to therapeutic interventions

Impaired Socialization 7

Definition

Insufficient or ineffective quality of human interaction

A social relationship is one that is initiated for the purpose of friendship, companionship, enjoyment, or accomplishment of a shared task. Mutual needs are met during social interaction. There may be feelings of caring about others, being cared about by others, and belonging to a community. Socially supportive relationships are an important resource for promoting health and managing the demands of illness. Those who are not socially connected have an increased risk for reduced health, depression and negative self-image, and impaired role function.

Cultural beliefs and practices may support or discourage socialization in health and during an illness. Health conditions and the personal perceptions of those conditions may affect the willingness or ability to socialize. Nurses play a key role in identifying the person experiencing social isolation and loneliness. Once identified, nurses can facilitate the development of supportive social interactions with persons and groups.

Associated Clinical Problems

- Housebound: unable to leave the dwelling because of health status or able to leave the dwelling only with extensive support and resources
- Inadequate Social Support: lack of reliable assistance from others
- Relationship Problems: difficulty in maintaining interactions with others over time
- Social Isolation: lack of interaction with others

Common Risk Factors

- Absence of significant others
- Autism
- Caregiving
- Communication barriers
- Dehabilitation
- Disturbance in self-concept
- Disturbance in thought processes
- Environment barriers, such as lack of transportation
- Extreme obesity
- Hospitalization
- Housebound
- Impaired mobility
- Language barriers
- Loss of significant other(s)
- Problems with peer group
- Relocation
- Retirement
- Sociocultural dissonance
- Therapeutic isolation
- Vision and hearing problems

Manifestations

- Discomfort in social situations
- Dissatisfaction with social engagement
- Dysfunctional interactions with others
- Expresses loneliness
- Family report of change in interaction
- Impaired social functioning

Key Conceptual Relationships

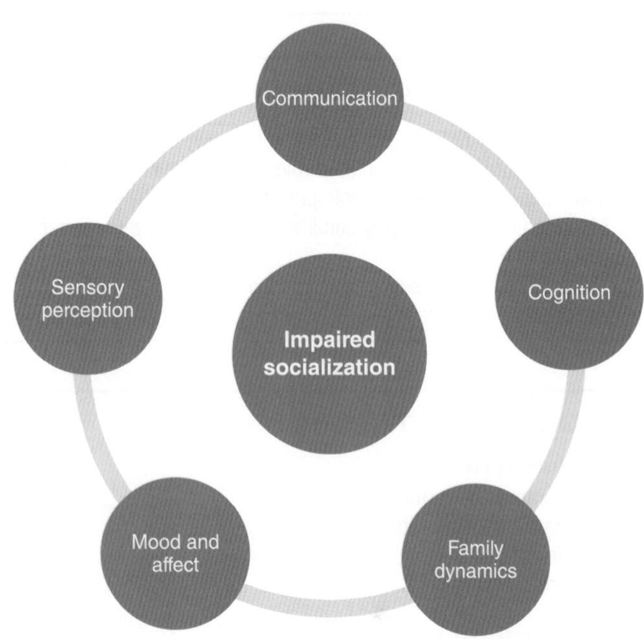

ASSESSMENT OF IMPAIRED SOCIALIZATION	RATIONALE
Assess for risk factors for impaired socialization.	Identifying factors that place the patient at risk for impaired socialization allows for early intervention.
Evaluate the patient's underlying health status.	Underlying health status has a significant influence on the ability to participate in social interaction.
Use tools, such as the Three-Item Loneliness Scale (Table 7.1) or the Lubben Social Network Scale–6 (Table 7.2), to screen the patient for social isolation or loneliness.	Detecting impaired socialization allows for early intervention.
Perform a physical assessment, noting factors that may influence the ability to socialize:	
• **COGNITION:** Mental status and cognitive function	Cognitive decline may limit social interaction.
• **SENSORY PERCEPTION:** Sensory deficits and the use of corrective measures, such as glasses and/or hearing aids	Sensory deficits can be a major barrier to participating in social interaction.
• **MOOD AND AFFECT:** Screen for depression and other psychological problems	Depression may be associated with limited or impaired social interaction.
• **MOBILITY:** Musculoskeletal function and mobility	Physical mobility problems have a significant impact on socialization and may leave the patient homebound.
Assess for health-related and environment barriers to social interaction.	Focus interventions on managing barriers.
Assess for the patient's preferred type and amount of social interaction.	People vary in preferences for size of group and type of interactions.
Assess the patient's support system, including: • Who do they live with? • Are they employed? • Are friends and relatives accessible? • How often do they see friends and family? • Are they members of any clubs or groups?	Support from others is an important aspect of managing social isolation.
FAMILY DYNAMICS: Assess availability of family members and evaluate family dynamics.	Family and significant others are a primary source of support and socialization.
Develop an ecomap for the patient.	Evaluating the social and personal relationships of a person with their environment helps focus interventions.
CULTURE: Assess the role of culture in the patient's socialization.	Cultural norms and values significantly influence socialization.
STRESS AND COPING: Assess the patient's use of coping and stress management strategies in managing social isolation.	Coping and stress management strategies can improve quality of life by helping the patient better manage social isolation.
Assess a caregiver's social interactions outside the caregiving relationship and quality of available social support.	Maintaining social relationships helps the caregiver to avoid social isolation and loneliness.
Evaluate the patient's response to measures to enhance socialization through ongoing assessment.	Identifying the response to measures to enhance socialization allows for evaluation of therapy effectiveness.

Table 7.1 Three-Item Loneliness Scale

For each question, tell me how often you feel that way.

1. First, how often do you feel that you lack companionship: hardly ever, some of the time, or often?
   1 [ ] Hardly ever
   2 [ ] Some of the time
   3 [ ] Often
2. How often do you feel left out: hardly ever, some of the time, or often?
   1 [ ] Hardly ever
   2 [ ] Some of the time
   3 [ ] Often

Continued

Table 7.1 Three-Item Loneliness Scale—cont'd

3. How often do you feel isolated from others: hardly ever, some of the time, or often?
   1 [] Hardly ever
   2 [] Some of the time
   3 [] Often

Scoring:
Sum the total of all items. Higher scores indicate greater degrees of loneliness.

Source: Hughes ME, Waite LJ, Hawkley LC, Cacioppo JT. A short scale for measuring loneliness in large surveys: Results from two population-based studies. *Res Aging.* 2004;26:655.

Table 7.2 Lubben Social Network Scale–6

Family: Considering the people to whom you are related, either by birth or marriage:

1. How many relatives do you see or hear from at least once a month?
   0 [] None
   1 [] One
   2 [] Two
   3 [] Three or four
   4 [] Five through eight
   5 [] Nine or more
2. How many relatives do you feel at ease with and can talk to about private matters?
   0 [] None
   1 [] One
   2 [] Two
   3 [] Three or four
   4 [] Five through eight
   5 [] Nine or more
3. How many relatives do you feel close to such that you could call on them for help?
   0 [] None
   1 [] One
   2 [] Two
   3 [] Three or four
   4 [] Five through eight
   5 [] Nine or more

Friendships: Considering all your friends, including those who live in your neighborhood:

4. How many of your friends do you see or hear from at least once a month?
   0 [] None
   1 [] One
   2 [] Two
   3 [] Three or four
   4 [] Five through eight
   5 [] Nine or more
5. How many friends do you feel at ease with and that you can talk to about private matters?
   0 [] None
   1 [] One
   2 [] Two
   3 [] Three or four
   4 [] Five through eight
   5 [] Nine or more
6. How many friends do you feel close to such that you could call on them for help?
   0 [] None
   1 [] One
   2 [] Two
   3 [] Three or four
   4 [] Five through eight
   5 [] Nine or more

Scoring Instructions: The Lubben Social Network Scale–6 (LSNS-6) total score is an equally weighted sum of these 6 items. Scores range from 0 to 30. The LSNS-6 has a cutoff of 12 as at risk for social isolation.

Source: Lubben J, Blozik E, Gillmann G, et al. Performance of an abbreviated version of the Lubben Social Network Scale among three European community-dwelling older adult populations. *Gerontologist.* 2006;46:503.

Expected Outcomes

The patient will:

- identify barriers to social interactions.
- use successful social interaction behaviors.
- report effective interactions with others.

INTERVENTIONS TO ENHANCE SOCIALIZATION	RATIONALE
Establish a therapeutic relationship with the patient: • Be respectful and courteous. • Build rapport and trust. • Maintain eye contact. • Show genuine interest.	This demonstrates respect for the patient and helps to establish a positive relationship.
Use caring touch, such as on the hand or arm when speaking, and eye contact, if acceptable to the patient.	Touch is a nonverbal indication of regard. Be mindful that personal preferences vary.
Encourage the patient to talk about feelings of loneliness and their causes.	Talking about feelings and concerns helps build rapport and decreases the sense of isolation.
Encourage the development of a support system, or mobilize the patient's family, friends, and neighbors to form one.	Family and significant others, including families of choice, are a primary source of support and socialization.
COMMUNICATION: Incorporate the use of phone and video technology and social media to enhance socialization.	Technology can be useful in overcoming barriers such as distance, lack of mobility, or therapeutic isolation.
Facilitate the patient joining groups with shared interests or concerns, either in person or online.	Groups may provide social interaction and social support.
Help the patient identify barriers to socialization, such as lack of transportation, and explore available options.	Helping the patient overcome real and perceived barriers may enhance socialization.
Encourage the patient to explore ways to dine with others.	Eating in a social setting offers the chance to enhance relationships with others.
Implement measures to develop means of alternate communication if needed.	Impaired communication can be a significant contributor to social isolation.
To enhance the patient's social skills: • Role play social interactions. • Use focused imitation interventions. • Give positive verbal and nonverbal feedback for prosocial behavior.	The development of social skills and improved communication will facilitate positive interactions.
Consider referrals to specialized programs for social training or music/art therapy, theater skills, and animal therapy.	Participating in a specialized program can promote social interaction and engagement.
SENSORY PERCEPTION: Encourage the use of any needed vision and hearing aids.	Audiovisual aids improve the ability to perceive and engage with others.
COGNITION: Implement measures to address impaired cognition, if present.	Addressing impaired cognition may have a positive effect on socialization difficulties related to disorientation.
Encourage participation in volunteer activities.	Volunteering provides an opportunity to extend social networks and maintain social relationships.
STRESS AND COPING: Help the patient cope with impaired socialization by using positive stress management and coping behaviors.	Quality of life for patients and caregivers is related to the stress management and coping strategies they use.
MOBILITY: Encourage physical activity within health limits.	Physical activity promotes opportunities for socialization.
Implement measures to address caregiver role strain if present.	Caregiver role strain negatively affects the ability to maintain social relationships.
Older Adult	
Encourage participation in neighborhood and community groups, activities, and clubs (e.g., senior center, adult classes).	Social interaction supports health promotion.

Continued

INTERVENTIONS TO ENHANCE SOCIALIZATION	RATIONALE
Pediatric	
Provide opportunities for interaction if parents/caregivers have limited mobility.	The parent's health status may limit the child's interactions.

COLLABORATION	RATIONALE
MOOD AND AFFECT: Treatment for coexisting psychological problems, particularly depression	Being unable to socialize can lead to depression and other psychological problems.
HEALTH DISPARITIES: Social work or case management	A social worker or case manager can help the patient and caregiver identify helpful community resources, such as transportation.
STRESS AND COPING: Support groups	Groups of patients who are experiencing the same problem can assist in rehabilitation and decrease social isolation.

PATIENT AND CAREGIVER TEACHING

- Communication skills
- Use of communication technology
- Community and self-help resources available
- Sources of information and social support
- Need for any therapeutic isolation and how long it may last, if known
- Anticipatory guidance about avoiding and managing problematic situations

DOCUMENTATION

Assessment

- Current social interaction
- Desire for social interaction
- Communication skills

Interventions

- Discussions with other interprofessional team members
- Environmental modifications made
- Therapeutic interventions and the patient's response
- Teaching provided
- Referrals initiated
- Use of alternate forms of communication

Evaluation

- Development of interactions
- Response to teaching provided

Personal Care Problem 8

Definition

Impaired ability to adequately perform personal care

Activities of daily living (ADLs), or basic ADLs, include the fundamental self-care abilities needed to manage basic physical needs. These include eating and hygienic and grooming activities such as bathing, mouth care, dressing, and toileting. We usually master ADLs early in life. Physical function is a significant factor in the ability to perform ADLs. When impaired cognitive function is present, the ability to perform personal care usually is present much longer compared with higher-level tasks associated with role performance.

The patient with a personal care disability requires various degrees and types of support. Difficulty completing personal care can lead to a loss of autonomy and a negative self-image. Appropriate interventions can improve quality of life, health outcomes, and independence. Nursing care focuses on functional assessment and planning and delivery of individualized care appropriate to the patient's level of functional ability. Two common strategies are personal assistance, or having someone help do the task, and equipment assistance, or using special aids and devices. Ideally, nurses should identify adaptive techniques that promote the patient's maximum degree of independence.

Associated Clinical Problems

- Impaired Ability to Bathe: impaired ability to cleanse oneself
- Impaired Ability to Dress: impaired ability to dress and groom oneself
- Impaired Ability to Perform Oral Hygiene: impaired ability to perform oral hygiene for oneself
- Impaired Ability to Self-Feed: impaired ability to feed oneself
- Impaired Ability to Toilet: impaired ability to urinate or defecate
- Self-Neglect: inability or unwillingness to attend to one's personal needs or hygiene

Common Risk Factors

- Age
- Arthritis
- Cancer
- Chronic pain
- Degenerative neuromuscular conditions
- Fatigue
- Impaired cognitive function
- Impaired mobility
- Impaired psychological status
- Lack of coordination
- Lack of motivation
- Major surgery
- Mood problems, including depression
- Musculoskeletal problems
- Pain
- Sensory deficits
- Spinal cord injury
- Stroke
- Substance use
- Trauma
- Traumatic brain injury
- Weakness

Manifestations

- Dependence on others to meet personal care needs
- Difficulty in performing or inability to perform personal care activities
- Unwilling to perform personal care activities
- Impaired nutrition
- Insufficient personal hygiene
- Self-report of inability to perform personal care activities

Key Conceptual Relationships

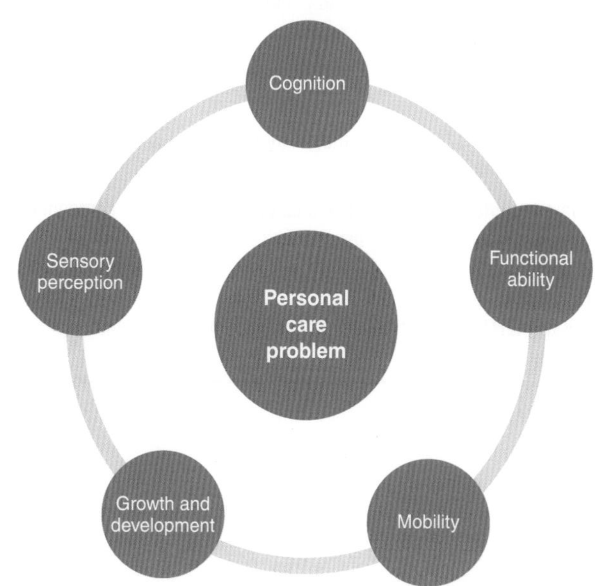

ASSESSMENT OF ABILITY TO PERFORM PERSONAL CARE	RATIONALE
Assess for risk factors that are influencing the ability to perform personal care.	Identifying factors that place the patient at risk for a personal care problem allows for early intervention.
Determine the potential cause of a personal care problem.	Treating the underlying cause may resolve the problem.
Evaluate the patient's underlying health status.	Underlying health status has a significant influence on the ability to perform personal care.
Assess the patient's ability to perform personal care:	
• Directly observe the patient performing personal care.	The results of the functional assessment help determine the patient's ability to perform personal care and determine the types of assistance the patient may need.
• Assess self-report and caregiver reports of personal care ability.	Self-report measures are part of the overall functional assessment, but because of potential inaccuracy, they require validation with other measures.
• Use a valid, reliable tool appropriate for the patient's age and cognition to perform a formal assessment of ability to perform personal care. Examples include the Katz Index of Independence in Activities of Daily Living (Table 8.1).	The results of the functional assessment help determine the patient's ability to perform personal care and determine the types of assistance the patient may need.
Perform a physical assessment and obtain diagnostic tests based on the patient's history, including:	Physical assessment and diagnostic tests evaluate for secondary causes of a personal care problem so that appropriate treatment can be initiated.
• **COGNITION:** Cognitive and mental status	Cognitive impairments contribute to problems performing personal care.
• **MOBILITY:** Mobility and musculoskeletal function	Physical mobility problems have a significant impact on the ability to independently perform personal care.
• **PAIN:** Comprehensive pain assessment	Experiencing pain negatively affects the ability to perform personal care.
• **SENSORY PERCEPTION:** Vision and hearing	Sensory deficits involving sight and hearing may interfere with the ability to independently perform personal care.
Obtain a formal occupational therapy evaluation, if appropriate.	Occupational therapists assess, plan, and implement interventions that promote a person's ability to perform personal care.
Obtain a formal physical therapy evaluation, if appropriate.	Physical therapists assess, plan, and implement interventions that promote a person's ability to perform personal care.
Obtain a formal speech evaluation, if appropriate.	Speech therapists evaluate feeding and swallowing ability and recommend interventions that promote safe self-feeding.
Determine the expected length of the personal care problem.	Knowing the expected length of a personal care problem is vital in planning care and securing resources.
Assess whether the person is simply refusing or unwilling to complete personal care and if so, the reason.	Refusal or unwillingness to participate in personal care is a sign of self-neglect.
CULTURE: Evaluate the role of culture in personal hygiene practices.	Cultural norms related to hygienic practices and the level of assistance provided to those who have difficulty vary widely.
FUNCTIONAL ABILITY: Assess the ability of caregivers to safely provide needed personal care.	The caregiver needs to understand the patient's needs and be able to provide safe, effective care.
Evaluate the effectiveness of measures used to address a personal care problem through ongoing assessment.	Evaluating the effectiveness of measures to address a personal care problem allows for adjustment of therapy to maximize independence.
Pediatric	
DEVELOPMENT: Assess physical and emotional development.	The degree of ability to perform personal care depends on the child's age, developmental level, and health status.

Table 8.1 Katz Index of Independence in Activities of Daily Living

Activities	Independence (1 Point) (No Supervision, Direction, or Personal Assistance)	Dependence (0 Points) (with Supervision, Direction, Personal Assistance, Or Total Care)
BATHING Point: ______	(1 POINT) Bathes self completely or needs help in bathing only a single part of the body, such as the back, genital area, or disabled extremity.	(0 POINTS) Needs help in bathing more than one part of the body and getting out of the tub or shower. Requires total bathing.
DRESSING Point: ______	(1 POINT) Gets clothes from closets and drawers and puts on clothes and other garments, complete with fasteners. May have help tying shoes.	(0 POINTS) Needs help with dressing self or needs to be completely dressed.
TOILETING Point: ______	(1 POINT) Goes to toilet, gets on and off, arranges clothes, cleans genital area without help.	(0 POINTS) Needs help transferring to the toilet, cleaning self, or using bedpan or commode.
TRANSFERRING Point: ______	(1 POINT) Moves in and out of bed or chair unassisted. Mechanical transferring aids are acceptable.	(0 POINTS) Needs help in moving from bed to chair or requires a complete transfer.
CONTINENCE Point: ______	(1 POINT) Exercises complete self-control over urination and defecation.	(0 POINTS) Is partially or totally incontinent of bowel or bladder.
FEEDING Point: ______	(1 POINT) Gets food from plate into mouth without help. Preparation of food may be done by another person.	(0 POINTS) Needs partial or total help with feeding or requires parenteral feeding.
TOTAL POINTS ______	6 = High (patient independent)	0 = Low (patient very dependent)

From Hartford Institute for Geriatric Nursing. Katz Index of Independence in Activities of Daily Living. Retrieved from https://clas.uiowa.edu/socialwork/sites/clas.uiowa.edu.socialwork/files/NursingHomeResource/documents/Katz%20ADL_LawtonIADL.pdf.

Expected Outcomes

The patient will:

- perform personal care to maximum ability.
- take part in desired personal care activities.
- use needed adaptive devices to perform personal care.
- demonstrate optimal hygiene after performing personal care.
- participate in decision making about personal care.

INTERVENTIONS TO ADDRESS A PERSONAL CARE PROBLEM	RATIONALE
Implement collaborative interventions aimed at treating an underlying factor contributing to a personal care problem.	The ability to perform personal care may improve or resolve with the treatment of an underlying contributing factor.
Assist the patient in identifying personal strengths and abilities.	Identifying personal strengths will help the patient integrate those strengths into personal care routines.
CULTURE: Determine what the patient perceives as their personal care needs and mutually establish culturally appropriate care goals.	Overcoming the impaired ability to perform personal care requires effort and commitment on the patient's part.
Encourage the patient to share concerns about their personal care problems.	Difficulty completing personal care can lead to a negative self-image.
Discuss the patient's preferred routines and preferences and develop a personal care routine based on those preferences.	Including the patient's preferences communicates respect.
Encourage the use of adaptive devices for mobility and personal care.	The use of adaptive devices improves the ability to perform personal care and promotes independence.
Implement measures to promote independence with personal care: • Provide a structured environment, minimizing distractions. • Perform personal care when the patient is most likely to participate. • Ensure that everything needed is within reach. • Allow the patient time to complete activities on their own. • Provide assistance when the patient cannot complete the activity. • Gradually withdraw assistance as the patient becomes more independent. • Praise the patient for independent accomplishments.	Providing a structured, consistent environment and routine helps the patient achieve maximum independence.

Continued

INTERVENTIONS TO ADDRESS A PERSONAL CARE PROBLEM	RATIONALE
Implement measures to address impaired ability to bathe: • Provide desired personal products. • Use no-rinse, prepackaged bathing products if needed.	Respecting preferences and providing the appropriate products communicates respect and may increase independence.
Implement measures to address impaired ability to dress: • Encourage the patient to dress in simple clothing that is easy to put on. • Lay clothes out in the order in which the patient will need them.	Simplifying the dressing routine promotes the ability to dress independently.
Implement measures to address impaired ability to self-feed: • Do not serve food the patient dislikes. • Assist with oral hygiene before and after meals. • Provide social interaction while eating. • Place the patient in the most normal eating position they can assume. • Prepare foods as needed, such as cutting food or opening packages.	A pleasant, normalized mealtime increases participation and intake.
Implement measures to address impaired ability to toilet: • Encourage the patient to wear clothing that is easy to remove. • Anticipate when there may be a need to toilet or toilet on a schedule. • Keep the route to the toilet free of obstructions and clutter.	Promoting independence in toileting can reduce the embarrassment and loss of dignity associated with an impaired ability to toilet.
Assist with implementing the plan of care developed by occupational therapy.	Occupational therapy can recommend assistive devices to help the patient perform personal care.
Assist with implementing the plan of care developed by physical therapy.	The physical therapist's plan of care is designed to promote optimal mobility and physical function.
Assist with implementing the plan of care developed by speech therapy.	The speech therapist's plan of care is designed to promote safe self-feeding.
SAFETY: Implement measures to reduce the risk of injury while performing personal care.	Having experienced a fall or previous injury increases the risk of injury associated with performing personal care.
CARE COORDINATION: Assist the patient in obtaining necessary adaptive devices and making environmental adaptations.	Finding the adaptive devices and environment modifications that can assist the patient in performing personal care independently may be difficult and costly.
COGNITION: Implement measures to address impaired cognition, if present.	The ability to perform personal care is impacted by impaired cognitive function.
MOBILITY: Implement measures to address impaired mobility, if present.	Physical function is a significant factor in the ability to perform personal care.
SENSORY PERCEPTION: Implement measures to address any sensory deficits.	Sensory deficits may interfere with the ability to complete personal care independently.
PAIN: Implement measures to manage pain, if present.	Experiencing pain negatively affects the ability to perform personal care.
Assist the patient with identifying support persons or caregivers to assist with performing personal care.	The caregiver needs to understand the patient's needs and be able and willing to provide assistance accordingly.
FUNCTIONAL ABILITY: Implement measures to address any caregiver role strain.	Assessing the caregiver for signs of role strain is necessary to be able to provide adequate support.

COLLABORATION	RATIONALE
MOBILITY: Physical therapy	Physical therapists assess, plan, and implement interventions that promote a person's ability to fulfill role responsibilities.
Occupational therapy	Occupational therapy can recommend assistive devices and assist with skill development to help the patient fulfill roles in the home.
CARE COORDINATION: Social work or case management	A social worker or case manager can help the patient and caregiver identify community resources to assist with fulfilling role responsibilities.

COLLABORATION	RATIONALE
GAS EXCHANGE: Speech therapy	Speech therapists evaluate feeding and swallowing ability and recommend interventions that promote safe self-feeding.
Dental care	Dentists can perform periodic deep cleaning and recommend assistive devices to help the patient perform oral care.
Cognitive–behavior therapy	Cognitive–behavior therapy may assist the patient with self-neglect in promoting performance of personal care.
Adult protective services	Adult protective services advocate for the well-being of older adults who may be in danger and have no one to assist them.

PATIENT AND CAREGIVER TEACHING

- Cause, if known, of a personal care disability
- Factors that may be contributing to a personal care disability
- Manifestations of a personal care disability
- Management of an underlying condition associated with a personal care disability
- Frequency and quality of appropriate personal care
- Measures to manage a personal care disability
- How to safely use adaptive devices
- Role of physical, speech, and occupational therapies
- Importance of encouraging independence, not dependence
- Community and self-help resources
- Modifications in the living environment to promote safety
- Role of case management
- When to notify the HCP

DOCUMENTATION

Assessment

- Assessments performed
- Diagnostic and laboratory test results
- Manifestations of a personal care problem
- Screening test results

Interventions

- Discussions with other members of the interprofessional team
- Environmental modifications made
- Notification of HCP about patient status
- Therapeutic interventions and the patient's response
- Teaching provided
- Referrals initiated

Evaluation

- Patient's status: improved, stable, declined
- Presence of manifestations of a personal care problem
- Response to teaching provided
- Response to therapeutic interventions

Health Maintenance Alteration 9

Definition

Impaired ability to manage health or access help to maintain health.

Self-management refers to the person's ability to manage health and well-being, especially in response to living with a chronic illness. It refers to managing symptoms, medications and treatment regimen, physical and psychosocial consequences, and lifestyle changes. Self-management practices include engaging in health promotion to prevent other conditions, manage current conditions, and reduce risk for complications and comorbid illness.

Chronic diseases have significant consequences for patients regarding symptoms, daily medications, therapy, social and work circumstances, and stress. Effective self-management occurs in collaboration with the family and health care team members as patients and their caregivers become knowledgeable about their disease and treatment, monitor and respond to changes in condition, and communicate important information with health care providers (HCPs).

Even in the absence of illness, self-management of key health behaviors such as diet, activity, sleep, and coping are critical for maintaining good health across the lifespan. Parents or caregivers initially manage the health of children until the children are developmentally able to take over the self-management behaviors. Nurses provide important support that facilitates patient self-management and health maintenance.

Associated Clinical Problems

- Complex Medication Regimen: prescribed set of drugs that require multiple administration times, with a high risk for confusion and medication errors
- Polypharmacy: use of several different drugs, possibly prescribed by different HCPs and filled in different pharmacies, by a patient who may have one or several health problems
- Risk for Polypharmacy: increased risk for the use of several different drugs, possibly prescribed by different HCPs and filled in different pharmacies, by a patient who may have one or several health problems
- Impaired Ability to Manage Regimen: difficulty keeping track of and completing health behaviors and therapies
- Difficulty Managing Dietary Regimen: impaired ability to control healthy dietary intake
- Difficulty Managing Exercise Regimen: impaired ability to complete regular exercise
- Difficulty Managing Incontinence Appliance: impaired ability to clean and apply equipment for incontinence
- Difficulty Managing Medication Regimen: impaired ability to administer drugs as prescribed
- Difficulty Managing Nephrostomy Care: impaired ability to clean and apply nephrostomy equipment
- Difficulty Managing Peritoneal Dialysis: impaired ability to handle fluid exchanges and equipment for peritoneal dialysis
- Difficulty Managing Stoma: impaired ability to care for stoma
- Difficulty Managing Urinary Catheter: impaired ability to clean and insert urinary catheter
- Difficulty Self-Monitoring Disease: impaired ability to recognize changes in condition
- Ineffective Family Therapeutic Regimen Management: impaired ability to regulate and organize health-related behaviors into daily family life

Common Causes and Risk Factors

- Complex treatment regimen
- Cultural or health belief conflicts
- History of not maintaining health
- Impaired cognition
- Impaired decision making
- Impaired family function
- Impaired motor skills
- Impaired sensory perception
- Ineffective communication skills
- Ineffective coping strategies
- Lack of resources
- Low health literacy
- Spiritual problem

Pediatric

- Delayed development

Manifestations

- Disinterest in health-promoting behaviors
- Exacerbations or complications of illness
- Not following treatment regimen
- Inability to complete basic health practices
- Lack of knowledge

- Lack of recognition or action in response to changes in condition
- Self-report of difficulty self-managing health
- Social isolation

Key Conceptual Relationships

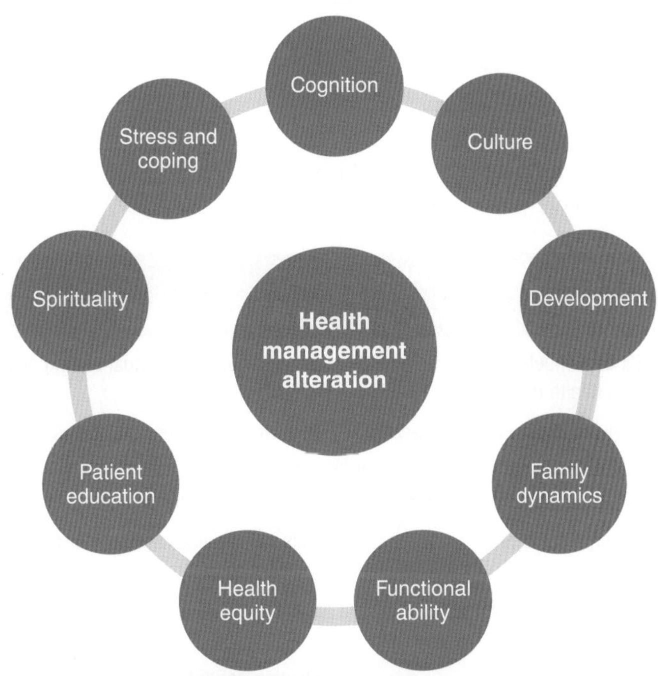

ASSESSMENT OF HEALTH MAINTENANCE	RATIONALE
Assess the patient's current level of following the therapeutic regimen.	Identify any gaps between expected and actual self-care.
Assess feelings, values, and reasons for not following the prescribed plan of care.	Understanding related factors will support specific plans for intervention.
Perform a complete physical assessment and evaluate underlying health status, including sensory deficits, mental status, and cognition.	A sensory deficit or impaired cognition can challenge the ability to manage health or perform self-care.
CULTURE AND SPIRITUALITY: Assess patient priorities in health, including cultural and spiritual aspects.	Respecting individual cultural and spiritual values and beliefs promotes trust.
HEALTH EQUITY: Evaluate the person's access to resources.	An inability to obtain supplies, a lack of finances or transportation, or a lack of other resources may prevent self-care behaviors.
STRESS AND COPING: Assess for the presence of coping strategies that influence health and self-management.	Positive coping strategies support the ability to self-manage health.
MOOD AND AFFECT: Screen for the presence of any coexisting depression or other problems.	The presence of a depressed mood or coexisting psychological problem can impair the ability to self-manage health.
FAMILY DYNAMICS: Evaluate family dynamics and determine the extent of enabling behaviors.	How family members act and react to the patient's health concerns affects the patient's ability to self-manage health.
CULTURE: Assess the patient's support system and availability of caregivers: • Who do they live with? • Are they employed? • Do they have accessible friends and relatives? • Have they used any community resources? • Has anyone served or is anyone able to serve as a caregiver?	Interest and support from others are important aspects of managing health.
FUNCTIONAL ABILITY: Determine the patient's ability to perform basic and instrumental activities of daily living.	The ability to self-manage health is directly related to a person's functional status.

Continued

ASSESSMENT OF HEALTH MAINTENANCE	RATIONALE
Pediatric	
DEVELOPMENT: Assess ability to manage care previously provided by parents/caregivers.	As the child develops, they may be able to assume increased responsibility for self-care.

Expected Outcomes

The patient will:

- set mutual goals with health providers for health maintenance.
- meet goals for health care maintenance.

INTERVENTIONS FOR PROMOTING HEALTH MAINTENANCE	RATIONALE
CULTURE: Set achievable mutual goals for health behaviors and plan culturally considerate strategies to address health maintenance.	Engaging in mutual goal setting and planning clearly communicates intentions.
PATIENT EDUCATION: Include family/caregivers in planning and teaching as preferred by the patient.	Involving caregivers provides social and direct support to the patient.
Reinforce and provide information about disease process and treatments.	Information supports decision making and the implementation of self-care.
Provide suggestions for additional information resources.	This will provide a source for answering future questions or expanding knowledge.
SELF-MANAGEMENT: Assist the patient to prioritize when multiple behavior changes are recommended.	Avoid overwhelming the patient with changes by prioritizing actions.
Use motivational interviewing to initiate behavior change.	Helping patients identify why they would want to make a change and how they might do it is more effective than telling them they should.
Help the patient to schedule complex medication regimens, such as those that must be taken with or without food and those that must be taken at different times than other medications.	Complex, multiple medications can be overwhelming to the patient and caregiver.
Reinforce the patient's positive health management behaviors.	Reinforcement provides motivation to continue healthful activities.
Encourage the use of memory aids and reminders, such as electronic calendars with reminder functions, daily schedules, and text messages from family members.	This will provide assistance with remembering and completing complex regimens.
Help the patient set up simple records for tracking health information, such as weight, blood pressure, and other data.	Data pertinent to treatment will be useful for health provider communication.
Help the patient develop a system for observing their own progress.	Self-monitoring is a key component of a successful change in behavior.
Assist the patient in developing appropriate problem-solving strategies.	Problem-solving skills support the patient in taking actions to manage health.
Encourage the patient to keep a list of questions to ask providers at next visits.	Keeping a list of concerns is a memory aid for addressing health concerns.
Encourage the patient to use health portal resources when available.	Access to laboratory results, visit summaries, and other health information may help the patient to understand the current condition and treatment plan.
Monitor for the ability to maintain self-care and prepare to increase assistance during times of acute illness.	Self-management may be impaired during times of increased stress or acute illness.
CULTURE: Implement measures to promote positive social interaction.	Interest and support from others are important aspects of managing health.
FUNCTIONAL ABILITY: Help the patient develop strategies to help with participation in activities of daily living in the home, at work, and socially.	The ability to self-manage health is directly related to a person's functional status.
STRESS AND COPING: Help the patient develop positive coping and stress management behaviors.	The use of positive coping skills equips the patient with multiple skills, including enhanced self-efficacy.

INTERVENTIONS FOR PROMOTING HEALTH MAINTENANCE	RATIONALE
FAMILY DYNAMICS: Institute measures to promote optimal family function as appropriate.	Impaired family function negatively influences the patient's ability to self-manage health.
COGNITION: Implement measures to promote optimal cognitive function.	Impaired cognition influences the ability to perform self-care.
Pediatric	
DEVELOPMENT: Assist the child in taking over self-care from parents/caregivers as appropriate.	The developing child may be able to assume increased responsibility for self-care.

COLLABORATION	RATIONALE
Support groups	Groups may provide practical advice and emotional support for dealing with chronic illness.
HEALTH EQUITY: Social services or case management	Support may be needed to obtain financial, transportation, or other resources.
Self-care programs	Self-care programs help patients assume the primary role in managing their conditions through education.
Physical therapy	Physical therapists assess, plan, and implement interventions that promote a person's ability to manage health.
Occupational therapy	Occupational therapists can recommend assistive devices and assist with skill development to help the patient manage their health.
SPIRITUALITY: Pastoral care professional or their preferred spiritual or religious leader	The patient may find comfort from their religious leaders as they provide patient support and perform spiritual counseling.
MOOD AND AFFECT: Treatment for any coexisting psychological problems, including depressed mood and emotional problems	The presence of a depressed mood or coexisting psychological problem can impair the ability to self-manage health.

PATIENT AND CAREGIVER TEACHING

- Cause of health conditions, if known
- Manifestations of health conditions
- Measures being used to improve the health condition
- Lifestyle changes recommended
- Scheduling and managing a complex regimen
- Early recognition of problems and how to manage them
- Safe use of medications, including proper use, side effect management, administration, and how they fit into the overall management plan
- Management of any underlying conditions
- Measures to reduce the risk of complications
- Where to find additional information
- Importance of long-term follow-up and communication with the health care team
- When to notify the HCP

DOCUMENTATION

Assessment

- Current management of health behaviors
- Manifestations of condition
- Manifestations of impaired health maintenance
- Diagnostic test results

Interventions

- Discussions with other members of the interprofessional team
- Medications given
- Notification of HCP about diagnostic test results and assessment findings
- Therapeutic interventions and the patient's response
- Teaching provided
- Referrals made

Evaluation

- Progress in managing health
- Diagnostic test results
- Patient's response to therapeutic interventions
- Response to teaching provided
- Presence of continued manifestations

Nonadherence 10

Definition

An intentional choice to omit or an unintentional overlooking of health-promoting actions

Adherence is reflected in a person's persistence in practicing health behaviors, with active participation in the related decisions. Adherence represents three dimensions of thought and attitudes regarding behaviors associated with recommended treatment and therapies: compliance, persistence, and concordance. *Compliance* is the behavior of conforming to treatment for a recommended length of time. *Persistence* is a measure of the continuation of the recommended behavior. *Concordance* reflects the development of an alliance among providers and patients based on realistic expectations and a clear understanding of the options. The range of adherence also includes a person's intentional decision to stop the medication or therapy or to change the dose or frequency of the medication or therapy.

Nonadherence can be considered in terms of degrees of a continuum. Before reaching an optimal level of adherence, people may alternate between periods of adherence and nonadherence. The greatest concern associated with behavior that reflects nonadherence is that it may lead to partially effective or ineffective treatment outcomes. Adherence does not occur if a person is not motivated or able to perform the health behavior. Nurses have a role in helping patients understand and persist with healthy behaviors.

Associated Clinical Problems

- Nonadherence With Diagnostic Testing: intentional choice to omit or unintentional overlooking of scheduling/completing prescribed testing
- Nonadherence With Diet Regimen: intentional choice to omit or unintentional overlooking of recommended nutritional plans
- Nonadherence With Fluid Regimen: intentional choice to omit or unintentional overlooking of fluid intake recommendation
- Nonadherence With Immunization Regimen: intentional choice to omit or unintentional overlooking of recommended immunizations
- Nonadherence With Medication Regimen: intentional choice to omit or unintentional overlooking of prescribed medication dosing and frequency
- Nonadherence With Safety Precautions: intentional choice to omit or unintentional overlooking of recommended precautions to prevent injury or illness
- Nonadherence With Therapeutic Regimen: intentional choice to omit or unintentional overlooking of recommended therapy and follow-up actions
- Nonadherence With Treatment: intentional choice to omit or unintentional overlooking of recommended therapy

Common Risk Factors

- Complicated treatment regimens
- Conflict with cultural or religious beliefs
- Fragmented health care
- Impaired cognition
- Inadequate support
- Lack of information
- Lack of resources to manage therapies

Manifestations

- Adjusting the dose or frequency of therapy or medications
- Exacerbations or complications of illness
- Failure to keep health care appointments
- Intentional omission of therapy or medications
- Self-report of difficulty adhering to therapy
- Unintentionally forgetting to complete therapy or take medications
- Serum drug levels showing the presence and relative amount of prescribed medications

Key Conceptual Relationships

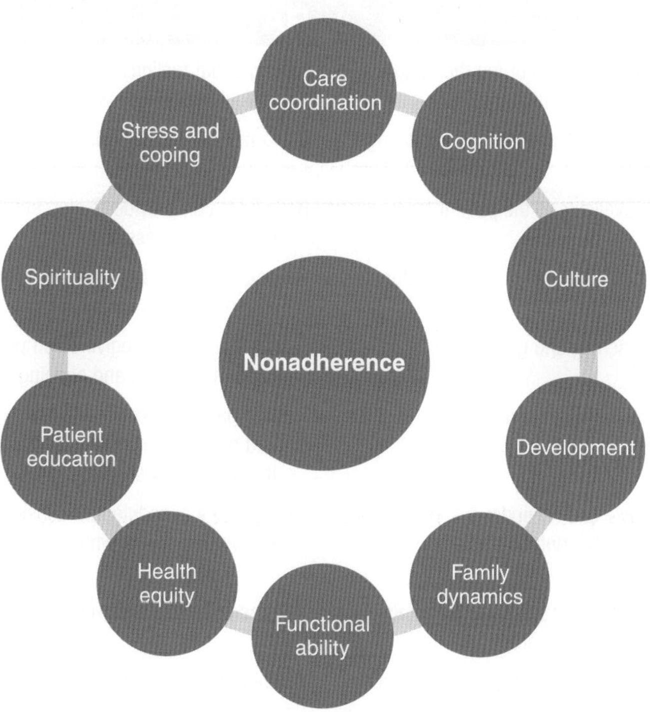

ASSESSMENT OF ADHERENCE	RATIONALE
Assess the patient's current knowledge about the proposed medication or treatment.	Adherence requires understanding what is proposed.
Assess the patient's current adherence to the prescribed therapeutic regimen.	Identify any gaps between expected and actual self-care.
Assess feelings, values, and reasons for not following the prescribed therapeutic regimen.	Understanding related factors will support specific plans for intervention.
HEALTH EQUITY: Assess the patient's ability to carry out the proposed therapy, considering access to care, financial/health insurance resources, and mobility.	Adherence may require physical mobility and coordination, a supportive environment, and other resources, including financial resources, transportation, and access to supplies.
COGNITION: Assess the patient's health literacy and ability to learn new information.	Determine whether omission of medication or treatment may be unintentional and improved with reminders.
CULTURE AND SPIRITUALITY: Assess the patient's values of culture and spirituality that may affect treatment choices.	The patient may be experiencing a conflict with personal beliefs that makes it emotionally difficult to adhere to therapy.
FAMILY DYNAMICS: Evaluate family dynamics and determine the extent of enabling behaviors.	How family members act and react to the patient's health concerns affects the patient's decision to adhere to the therapeutic plan.
FUNCTIONAL ABILITY: Assess the need for physical assistance to carry out recommended therapy.	The patient may be reluctant to request assistance or admit an inability to manage therapy or equipment.
Evaluate the patient's level of adherence on an ongoing basis.	Periodic review of the patient's level of adherence will allow for any necessary adjustments to be made.
Pediatric	
DEVELOPMENT: Help parents/caregivers assess what level of independent action is appropriate for the developmental age of the child.	A child may be able to manage some aspects of therapy with supervision, and the ability to participate may change over time.

Expected Outcome

The patient will:

- follow through on health-promoting behaviors and therapies collaboratively agreed upon by the patient and health care team.

INTERVENTIONS TO PROMOTE ADHERENCE	RATIONALE
Encourage the patient to talk about their perception of the therapeutic regimen and voice any concerns influencing adherence.	Talking about feelings and concerns helps build rapport and assists the patient in deciding whether to adhere.
PATIENT EDUCATION: Provide information to fill in assessed knowledge gaps using multiple methods.	Using multiple teaching/learning methods improves information retention.
Provide teaching resources that will be available to the patient for later reference.	Resources can provide reinforcement or clarification of information after the teaching session.
Include information about why, how, when, and how much/how often.	Patients need multiple types of information to adhere to complex medications or treatments.
Include family members/caregivers in teaching and goal setting.	Family members/caregivers can provide important social and practical support for initial and ongoing adherence.
Use motivational interviewing to promote behavior change.	Helping patients identify why they would want to have better adherence and how they might accomplish that is more effective than telling them that they should.
Assist the patient in developing a schedule and reminder system that allows them to keep appointments, considering commitments such as work and childcare.	Developing a schedule that considers what is important to the patient shows respect for what the patient values.
Implement measures to promote self-health management, including record keeping and systems for monitoring progress.	Self-monitoring is a key component of a successful change in behavior.
Help the patient set up memory aids, such as medication dose reminders and timers.	Where adherence is dependent on remembering tasks over time, automated reminders can be helpful.
Assist the patient to schedule therapies with cues to other daily activities, such as lunch or bedtime.	Connecting new behaviors to existing habits helps cue remembering.
STRESS AND COPING: Provide support to caregivers who are helping the patient with managing therapies.	Support from caregivers and the ability to access needed equipment/skills may be critical to managing therapies.
Pediatric	
Develop routines that integrate therapy into daily habits and schedule, including the school day.	Developing a routine helps with remembering and helps parents/teachers with negotiating the completion of daily therapies.
Assist parents/caregivers to identify and use appropriate motivational aids for children who need to take medication regularly or complete therapy.	Simple aids such as sticker charts can serve as reminders and reinforcement for health behaviors.

COLLABORATION	RATIONALE
Disease or symptom management programs	Disease or symptom management programs help patients understand their treatment regimens and address the complex needs of those with chronic illness.
Physical therapy	Physical therapists assess, plan, and implement interventions that promote a person's ability to complete therapy.
Occupational therapy	Occupational therapists can recommend assistive devices and assist with skill development to help the patient complete therapy or self-administer medication.
HEALTH EQUITY: Social services or case management	Support may be needed to obtain financial, transportation, or other resources.
DEVELOPMENT: Child life specialist	Developmentally appropriate strategies for developing therapy routines may increase adherence and decrease the potential for family conflict.

PATIENT AND CAREGIVER TEACHING

- Cause and manifestations of the health condition, if known
- Management of underlying conditions
- Importance of taking medications as prescribed
- How and why to complete therapeutic exercises or treatments
- Hand hygiene techniques
- Measures being used to improve the health condition
- Measures to reduce the risk of complications
- When to notify the health care provider (HCP)

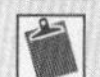

DOCUMENTATION

Assessment

- Manifestations of the health condition
- Assessments performed

Interventions

- Medications given
- Notification of the HCP about patient status
- Therapeutic interventions and the patient's response
- Teaching provided
- Referrals made
- Discussions with other members of the interprofessional team

Evaluation

- Response to therapeutic interventions
- Response to teaching provided
- Presence of any continued manifestations of the health condition

Spiritual Problem 11

Definition

Distress associated with conflicts regarding meaning and purpose in life

Defining spirituality is difficult because we each express our spirituality in unique ways. We are all driven to derive meaning and purpose from life. For some, spirituality is based on religion, principles, a sense that people are part of a larger plan, and a connection with and belief in God/Higher Being. Religiosity is a person's practice of their beliefs or faith. A fundamental function of religion is to help people fulfill their yearning for purpose and meaning. For others, spirituality has no connection to religious beliefs. It is experienced as a connection of mind, body, and spirit.

Spiritual care is defined as actions to meet the spiritual needs of the patient and caregivers. Attending to spiritual needs is an essential part of holistic nursing practice. Spirituality affects a patient's quality of life, physical and psychological health, and health outcomes. Illness and life experiences affect spirituality. During times of stress, some may feel anger that illness has happened to them or a loved one, or that they have done something wrong and deserve to be punished. There may be despair or hopelessness regarding their health and future. Nurses provide spiritual care in an attempt to improve the patient's quality of life. We can help ease the patient's suffering through our understanding and compassion. Thus nurses should address spiritual problems with the same intent and urgency as treatment for any other physical or psychological problem.

Associated Clinical Problems

- Conflicting Religious Belief: conflict between religious beliefs and recommended treatments
- Conflicting Spiritual Belief: inner conflicts or struggles about beliefs
- Despair: complete loss of hope
- Disrupted Spiritual Rituals: inability to exercise usual spiritual rituals
- Hopelessness: having no expectation of a favorable outcome
- Lack of Meaning: believing one's life lacks purpose and worth
- Spiritual Distress: disturbance in a person's belief system
- Risk for Spiritual Distress: increased risk for a disturbance in a person's belief system

Contributing Factors

- Challenges to belief or value system
- Change in marital status
- Crisis events
- Difficulty coping with illness, crisis, or disability
- Failing health
- Fear of the unknown; uncertainty
- Long-term stress
- Loss of a family member or friend
- Loss of abilities to perform role and participate in activities of daily living
- Miscarriage or stillbirth
- Mental health problems, including depression and anxiety
- New family members through birth, adoption, or custody
- Separation from religious ties
- Social isolation
- Substance use
- Terminal illness
- Victim of violence, including abuse and neglect

Disrupted Spiritual Rituals

- Diet restrictions
- Medical regimen

Manifestations

- Anger, bitterness
- Crying, sadness, despair
- Emotional detachment
- Expresses loss of faith or anger at God/Higher Being
- Fear
- Feelings of being punished
- Hopelessness
- Impaired sleep
- Mood problems, including depression and anxiety
- Negative self-image, including low self-esteem
- Not participating in usual activities
- Not practicing spiritual or religious rituals by choice
- Questions meaning of life
- Sense of abandonment by God/Higher Being
- Suicidal ideation

Key Conceptual Relationships

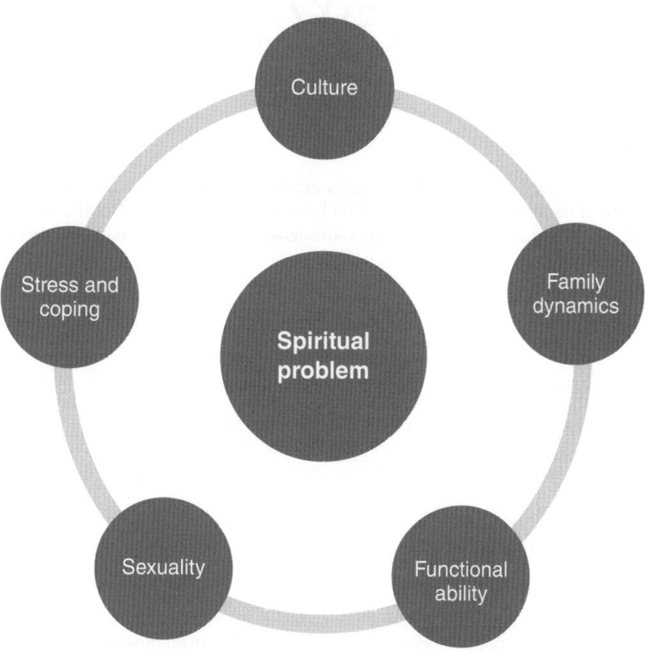

ASSESSMENT OF SPIRITUAL STATE	RATIONALE
Assess for contributing factors that place the patient at risk for a spiritual problem.	Identify conditions or situations that contribute to the risk for a spiritual problem.
Obtain basic spirituality-related information, including: • Religious preference • If the patient would like a chaplain or other person to visit • Whom the patient identifies as their support system	Nonthreatening questions can lead to the opportunity to assess spirituality and the patient's problems more deeply.
Use a valid, reliable tool to assess spirituality, such as the Faith, Importance and Influence, Community, and Address (FICA) Tool for Spiritual Assessment (Fig. 11.1) or the HOPE questions (https://www.aafp.org/afp/2001/0101/p81.html).	A spiritual assessment should be done to identify spiritual and religious beliefs and practices, especially related to health and coping with illness and disability.
Obtain additional information as part of the spiritual assessment, including:	
• Any religious or spiritual practices the patient wishes to participate in	Practicing spiritual or religious rituals can provide the patient with meaning and purpose and be a source of strength.
• Presence of any concerns or conflicts between spiritual or religious beliefs and health care	Modifications in the patient's care may need to be made based on their spiritual or religious beliefs.
• Use of any spiritually related coping strategies	Spiritual coping methods, such as spiritual support, positive religious reframing, and spiritual connectedness, are associated with better mental health and less distress.
CULTURE: Assess the role of culture in the patient's spirituality.	Spirituality is embedded in a person's belief system and strongly influenced by the context of their culture.
FAMILY DYNAMICS: Evaluate family dynamics and current level of functioning and observe family interactions.	Because the family strongly influences a person's belief system and religious practices, disagreements or conflicting spiritual or religious beliefs can lead to impaired family function.
FUNCTIONAL ABILITY: Perform a functional assessment, evaluating for any role-performance effects of a spiritual problem, including the ability to perform work and household duties and engage in physical and social activities.	Despair and hopelessness can adversely affect participation in role performance and activities of daily living.
Evaluate the effectiveness of measures used to address a spiritual problem through ongoing monitoring.	Monitoring the patient for continued manifestations of a spiritual problem allows for evaluation of therapy effectiveness.

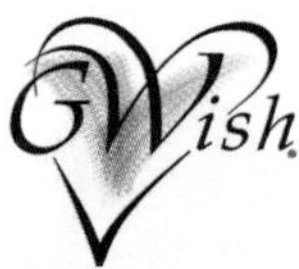

FICA Spiritual History Tool ©™

The FICA Spiritual History Tool was developed by Dr. Puchalski and a group of primary care physicians to help physicians and other healthcare professionals address spiritual issues with patients. Spiritual histories are taken as part of the regular history during an annual exam or new patient visit but can also be taken as part of follow-up visits, as appropriate. The FICA tool serves as a guide for conversations in the clinical setting.

The acronym FICA can help structure questions in taking a spiritual history by healthcare professionals.

F- Faith, Belief, Meaning

"Do you consider yourself spiritual or religious?" or "Is spirituality something important to you" or "Do you have spiritual beliefs that help you cope with stress/ difficult times?" (Contextualize to reason for visit if it is not the routine history.)

If the patient responds "No," the healthcare provider might ask, "What gives your life meaning?" Sometimes patients respond with answers such as family, career, or nature.

(The question of meaning should also be asked even if people answer yes to spirituality.)

I - Importance and Influence

"What importance does your spirituality have in your life? Has your spirituality influenced how you take care of yourself, your health? Does your spirituality influence you in your healthcare decision making? (e.g., advance directives, treatment, etc.)

C - Community

"Are you part of a spiritual community? Communities such as churches, temples, and mosques, or a group of like-minded friends, family, or yoga can serve as strong support systems for some patients. Can explore further: "Is this of support to you and how? Is there a group of people you really love or who are important to you?"

A - Address/Action in Care

"How would you like me, your healthcare provider, to address these issues in your healthcare?" (With the newer models including diagnosis of spiritual distress, A also refers to the "Assessment and Plan" of patient spiritual distress or issues within a treatment or care plan.

Puchalski, C., & Romer, A. L. (2000). Taking a spiritual history allows clinicians to understand patients more fully. *Journal of Palliative Medicine*, *3*(1), 129-137.

GWish, 2600 Virginia Ave, NW, Suite 300, Washington, DC 20037; 202-994-6220; www.gwish.org

FIG. 11.1 The Faith, Importance and Influence, Community, and Address (FICA) Spiritual History Tool. (Copyright C. Puchalski, 1996–2020. Source: Puchalski C, Romer AL. Taking a spiritual history allows clinicians to understand patients more fully. *J Palliat Med.* 2000;3:129-137.)

Expected Outcomes

The patient will:

- discuss beliefs and feelings about spiritual issues.
- reflect on their spiritual values.
- perceive that life has meaning.
- participate in desired spiritual and religious practices.
- express a sense of hope.
- maintain satisfactory relationships with others.
- engage in meaningful activities.

INTERVENTIONS TO ADDRESS SPIRITUAL STATE	RATIONALE
Create time, space, and privacy as needed for the patient to participate in spiritual or religious rituals, such as prayer or meditation.	Practicing spiritual or religious rituals can provide the patient with meaning and purpose and be a source of strength.
Establish a compassionate presence with the patient: • Be empathetic. • Use therapeutic touch, with the patient's consent. • Remain nonjudgmental. • Show sensitivity to the patient's beliefs. • Use active listening with therapeutic communication skills. • Demonstrate commitment to the patient.	Patients may appreciate an interpersonal, trusting relationship with the nurse as a prerequisite to discussing spiritual needs.
Encourage the patient to identify and express their feelings about meaning and purpose.	Engaging in conversation about spirituality conveys willingness to discuss their spiritual and religious beliefs and concerns.
Assist the patient in identifying persons to whom they can express feelings openly.	Persons who show an accepting attitude can serve as strong support systems for some patients with a spiritual problem.
Have the patient share their story of what led to their spiritual distress.	Listening to the patient's story gives the nurse information about what influenced the patient's spiritual distress, hopelessness, and despair.
Give verbal support and encouragement of the patient's spiritual and religious beliefs.	Providing verbal support demonstrates caring and respect for the patient.
Help the patient and family discover their own spiritual and religious resources and how those resources can help them.	Engaging the family demonstrates caring and respect for their specific spiritual and religious traditions and empowers them to arrive at their own answers.
Pray with the patient at the patient's request, if acceptable to the nurse.	Praying with the patient and family conveys a powerful message of sincere concern and genuineness.
Encourage the patient to participate in spiritual support practices, such as meditation, yoga, mindful breathing, and tai chi.	Spiritual support practices assist a person to connect with their inner sources of strength, helping them find meaning and purpose.
NUTRITION: Communicate dietary needs to the dietitian and ensure that the patient's meals follow the prescribed diet and meet any religious restrictions.	A person who follows a specific diet for religious reasons expects us to be respectful and provide meals that meet their dietary and religious needs.
FAMILY DYNAMICS: Institute measures to promote optimal family function, as appropriate.	Spiritual problems may impede a family's ability to manage conflicts and may have a devastating effect on family well-being.
STRESS AND COPING: Help the patient develop positive coping behaviors and stress management strategies.	The use of positive coping skills and stress management strategies equips the patient with multiple skills to manage spiritual problems.
Discuss with the patient options for assistance with decision making if they are struggling with health care–related decisions.	Assistance in the form of educational materials and counseling may help the patient resolve any care-related dilemmas.
Assist the patient with evaluating their situation and developing short-term goals.	Achieving goals that are appropriate for their situation can enhance self-esteem and promote hope.
Implement measures to assist the patient with managing grief, if appropriate.	Loss is often a trigger for a spiritual problem.
SEXUALITY: Implement measures to assist the patient in managing a negative self-image, if present.	Persons with a spiritual problem may have a negative self-image and low self-esteem.
FUNCTIONAL ABILITY: Help the patient develop strategies to help with participation in activities of daily living in the home, at work, and socially.	An increase in role performance and participation in activities of daily living often indicates a reduction in the level of hopelessness and despair.
Pediatric Allow opportunities for the child to participate in play therapy, referring to a play therapy specialist as needed.	Play therapy provides insight into the child's coping and can help them cope with their emotions.

COLLABORATION	RATIONALE
SPIRITUALITY: Pastoral care professional or their preferred spiritual or religious leader	Many derive spiritual comfort from their religious leaders, who provide patient support, perform spiritual counseling, and meet sacramental needs.
Community-based religious organizations	Community-based religious organizations provide the opportunity to participate in religious rituals, supporting coping with spiritual issues.
Faith-based support groups	Faith-based support groups provide support and encouragement in an atmosphere consistent with the patient's belief system.
FAMILY DYNAMICS: Family-focused therapy	Spiritual problems may impede a family's ability to manage conflicts and have a devastating effect on family well-being.

PATIENT AND CAREGIVER TEACHING

- Manifestations of a spiritual problem
- Measures that can help with spiritual problems
- Availability of spiritual resources, such as a chapel or prayer room and a chaplain
- Ways to connect with spiritual and religious beliefs
- Positive coping and stress management strategies
- Sources of community support
- When to talk with the health care provider (HCP)

DOCUMENTATION

Assessment

- Assessments performed
- Manifestations of a spiritual problem
- Screening test results
- Spiritual care preferences

Interventions

- Discussions with other members of the interprofessional team
- Therapeutic interventions and the patient's response
- Teaching provided
- Referrals initiated

Evaluation

- Response to teaching provided
- Response to therapeutic interventions
- Patient's status: improved, stable, declined
- Manifestations of a spiritual problem

Acid–Base Imbalance 12

Definition

Imbalance in the state of equilibrium between the acidity and alkalinity of body fluids

The body normally maintains a steady balance between the acids continually made during normal metabolism and the bases that neutralize and promote acid excretion. Because acids alter the body's internal environment, their regulation is necessary to maintain homeostasis and the acid–base balance. The body relies on multiple mechanisms to regulate the acid–base balance. These include the buffer system, respiratory system, and renal system. Acid–base balance parameters are shown in Table 12.1.

Many health problems can lead to an acid–base imbalance. Patients with diabetes, chronic obstructive pulmonary disease (COPD), or kidney disease often develop an acid–base imbalance. Acid–base imbalances are classified as respiratory or metabolic (Table 12.2). Respiratory imbalances result from changes in carbonic acid concentration. Metabolic imbalances affect the base bicarbonate (HCO_3^-). Acidosis occurs with an increase in carbonic acid (respiratory acidosis) from hypoventilation or a decrease in HCO_3^- (metabolic acidosis). Alkalosis occurs with a decrease in carbonic acid (respiratory alkalosis) from hyperventilation or an increase in HCO_3^- (metabolic alkalosis).

Assessing for an acid–base imbalance and collaborating with the interprofessional team are important nursing roles. The primary treatment involves correcting the underlying cause. Obtain a thorough history and perform a complete physical examination because acid–base problems affect all body systems. Implement fall and seizure precautions for patients at risk. Maintain a safe environment. Administer medications and fluids as ordered. Implement measures to provide respiratory support.

Associated Clinical Problems

- Metabolic Acidosis: base bicarbonate deficit
- Metabolic Alkalosis: base bicarbonate excess
- Respiratory Acidosis: carbonic acid excess
- Respiratory Alkalosis: carbonic acid deficit

Common Causes

Metabolic Acidosis

- Diabetic ketoacidosis
- Diarrhea
- Ethanol ingestion
- Gastrointestinal (GI) fistulas
- Hyperparathyroidism
- Lactic acidosis
- Renal failure
- Renal tubular acidosis
- Rhabdomyolysis
- Salicylate toxicity
- Sepsis
- Shock
- Starvation

Metabolic Alkalosis

- Electrolyte problems: hypokalemia, hypercalcemia, hypomagnesemia
- Excess HCO_3^- intake
- GI suctioning
- Hyperaldosteronism
- Medications: antacids, corticosteroids, loop and thiazide diuretics
- Multiple blood transfusions
- Vomiting

Respiratory Acidosis

- Airway obstruction
  - Atelectasis
  - Chest wall abnormality
  - Chronic respiratory disease: COPD, emphysema, bronchiectasis, asthma
- Degenerative neuromuscular disease
- Mechanical hypoventilation
- Pneumonia
- Pulmonary edema
- Respiratory muscle weakness
- Sedative overdose
- Smoke inhalation

Respiratory Alkalosis

- Hyperventilation from anxiety, exercise, fear, fever, pain
- Liver failure
- Mechanical hyperventilation
- Medications: catecholamines, nicotine, salicylates
- Respiratory center stimulation from brain injury, meningitis, sepsis, stroke

Table 12.1 Acid–Base Balance Parameters

pH	7.35–7.45
$Paco_2$	35–45 mm Hg
Bicarbonate (HCO_3^-)	22–26 mEq/L (mmol/L)
Anion gap	8–12 mmol/L

Table 12.2 Arterial Blood Gas (ABG) Values in Acid–Base Imbalances

	pH	$Paco_2$	HCO_3^-
Metabolic acidosis	↓	Normal-uncompensated ↓ compensated	↓
Metabolic alkalosis	↑	Normal-uncompensated ↑ compensated	↑
Respiratory acidosis	↓	↑	Normal-uncompensated ↑ compensated
Respiratory alkalosis	↑	↓	Normal-uncompensated ↓ compensated

Manifestations

- Dysrhythmias
- Headache
- Impaired cognition
- Muscle weakness
- Nausea and vomiting
- Tachycardia

Metabolic Acidosis

- Abdominal pain
- ↓ Blood pressure (BP)
- Diarrhea
- ↑ Respiratory rate with weak respirations
- Laboratory tests: ↓ sodium, ↓ calcium, ↓ magnesium, and ↓ phosphorus levels; ↓ or ↑ potassium; ↑ lactic acid

Metabolic Alkalosis

- Anorexia
- Hyperreflexia
- Irritability
- Numbness and tingling
- ↓ Respiratory rate
- Tetany, seizures
- Laboratory tests: ↓ potassium, ↑ calcium levels

Respiratory Acidosis

- ↓ BP
- Dizziness
- ↓ Respiratory rate
- Seizures

Respiratory Alkalosis

- Angina
- Dizziness
- Tetany, seizures
- Tingling in fingers and toes
- Tremors
- Laboratory tests: ↓ phosphorus, ↓ potassium levels

Key Conceptual Relationships

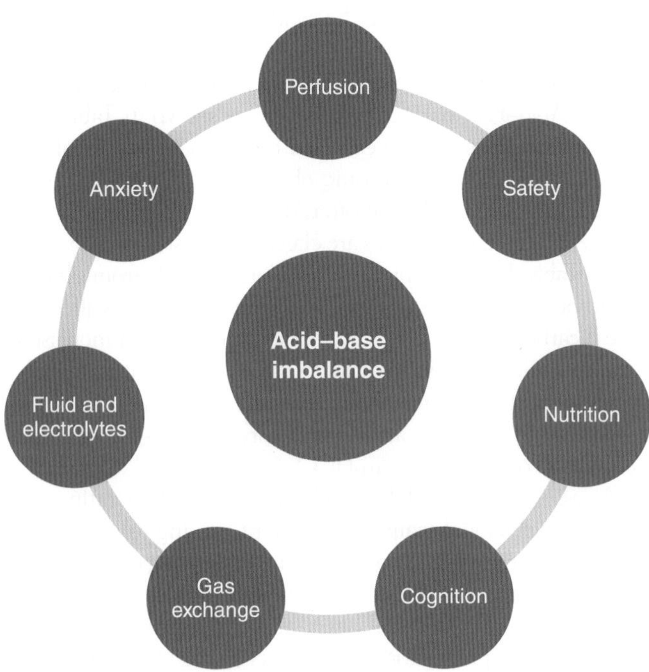

ASSESSMENT OF ACID-BASE BALANCE	RATIONALE
Identify patients in need of emergency management so that they can be immediately stabilized.	Identifying respiratory distress or myocardial dysfunction allows for early intervention.
Assess risk factors for an acid–base imbalance.	Identifying factors that place the patient at risk for an acid–base imbalance allows for early intervention.
Determine the potential cause of an acid–base imbalance.	It is more effective to treat the cause rather than the imbalance.

ASSESSMENT OF ACID–BASE BALANCE	RATIONALE
Determine acid–base status by evaluating ABGs and trends in arterial pH, $Paco_2$, and HCO_3^-.	ABGs can help determine acid–base balance, the type of imbalance, and the body's ability to compensate.
Perform a complete physical assessment and monitor indicators of acid–base balance on an ongoing basis:	
• Manifestations of an acid–base imbalance	Identifying manifestations of an acid–base imbalance allows for early intervention.
• **FLUID AND ELECTROLYTES:** Serum and urine electrolyte levels	Electrolyte imbalances often accompany an acid–base imbalance.
• **PERFUSION:** Cardiac monitoring	An acid–base imbalance influences heart rate and can cause dysrhythmias.
• **COGNITION:** Neurologic status	Acid–base balance affects cerebral perfusion.
• O_2 consumption, such as Svo_2, if available	Tissue oxygenation may be inadequate with an acid–base imbalance.
• Capnography, if available	Capnography gives information about CO_2 production and elimination.
Calculate the anion gap.	The anion gap increases in metabolic acidosis associated with acid gain and is normal in metabolic acidosis caused by bicarbonate loss.
Determine whether compensatory changes are present.	Respiratory or renal compensation or both may occur in response to an acid–base imbalance.
Monitor for the loss of acid- or base-rich fluids, including emesis, nasogastric (NG) output, stool, and urine.	Identifying fluid loss that increases risk for an acid–base imbalance allows for early intervention.
Monitor for manifestations of respiratory failure, such as low Pao_2, increased $Paco_2$ levels, and respiratory muscle fatigue.	Identifying respiratory failure allows for early intervention.
Monitor for complications from correcting an acid–base imbalance.	Identifying complications allows for early intervention.
Evaluate the patient's response to measures to correct acid–base imbalance through ongoing assessment.	Identifying an acid–base imbalance allows for evaluation of therapy effectiveness.

Expected Outcomes

The patient will:

- achieve and maintain acid–base balance.
- be free from complications of an acid–base imbalance.
- have no manifestations of an acid–base imbalance.
- adhere to the prescribed therapeutic regimen.
- recognize factors that may lead to an acid–base imbalance and take preventative action.

INTERVENTIONS TO PROMOTE ACID–BASE BALANCE	RATIONALE
Provide collaborative interventions addressed at treating the underlying cause of the acid–base imbalance.	The acid–base imbalance may resolve with treatment of the underlying cause.
Be prepared to institute resuscitation protocols and respiratory support.	An acid–base imbalance can cause respiratory muscle fatigue, leading to respiratory distress, and myocardial dysfunction, leading to dysrhythmias.
PERFUSION: Treat dysrhythmias according to agency policy.	Addressing changes in cardiac rhythm improves patient outcomes.
GAS EXCHANGE: Administer O_2 therapy, as appropriate.	Oxygen therapy can prevent and correct hypoxia.
Administer medications as prescribed, based on trends in arterial pH, $Paco_2$, HCO_3^-, and serum electrolytes, including:	
• **FLUID AND ELECTROLYTES:** Electrolyte solutions	Overcorrection can lead to poor outcomes.
• **FLUID AND ELECTROLYTES:** IV fluid therapy	Fluids support adequate hydration and restoration of normal fluid volumes.

Continued

INTERVENTIONS TO PROMOTE ACID–BASE BALANCE	RATIONALE
• Sedatives	Sedation with close monitoring may be needed for a patient who is not hypoxemic but is hyperventilating.
• **PAIN:** Analgesics	Analgesia may support improved ventilation.
Administer dialysis, as appropriate, evaluating patient response.	Dialysis may be effective in restoring acid–base balance by removing needed electrolytes and fluids.
Notify the health care provider (HCP) if manifestations of acid–base imbalance persist or worsen.	Achieving an effective treatment plan often requires adjustments in therapy.
SAFETY: Provide a safe environment for the patient with neuromuscular manifestations by initiating fall and seizure precautions.	Changes in cognition and the potential for seizures often accompany an acid–base imbalance.
GAS EXCHANGE: Elevate the head of the bed and encourage deep, slow, or pursed lip breathing as needed and tolerated.	Positioning the patient to improve O_2 delivery and coaching the patient in breathing exercises helps decrease dyspnea and work of breathing.
Promote adequate rest periods, such as 90 minutes of undisturbed sleep, by organizing nursing care and limiting visitors, as appropriate.	Rest interspersed with care activities reduces O_2 consumption.
COGNITION: Implement measures to orient the patient.	Acid–base imbalances may be associated with changes in cognition.
MOBILITY: Aid with range of motion exercises and physical activity, as tolerated.	Participating in activities helps preserve muscle mass and prevent fatigue.
ANXIETY: Provide measures to promote comfort and reduce anxiety, as needed.	These measures reduce O_2 consumption and minimize hyperventilation.
NUTRITION: Institute measures to manage the GI effects of an acid–base imbalance.	Appropriate management of symptoms can increase the patient's comfort level.
Obtain ABGs and laboratory specimens properly.	A test value may be compromised by a specimen that is not been collected, labeled, handled, or stored properly during the testing process.

INTERVENTIONS TO ADDRESS METABOLIC ACIDOSIS	RATIONALE
Administer medications as prescribed, based on trends in arterial pH, $Paco_2$, HCO_3^-, and serum electrolytes, including:	
• Oral or IV HCO_3^- agents	HCO_3^- agents may be given to correct bicarbonate deficit.
• **GLUCOSE REGULATION:** Insulin, IV fluid therapy, and potassium	These agents treat hyperglycemia and hyperkalemia and prevent dysrhythmias.
NUTRITION: Encourage a low-carbohydrate diet, as appropriate.	A low-carbohydrate diet can aid with managing an acid–base imbalance by decreasing CO_2 production.

INTERVENTIONS TO ADDRESS METABOLIC ALKALOSIS	RATIONALE
Administer medications as prescribed, based on trends in arterial pH, $Paco_2$, HCO_3^-, and serum electrolytes, including:	
• Carbonic anhydrase-inhibiting diuretics	Carbonic anhydrase-inhibiting diuretics increase bicarbonate excretion.
• Chloride	Chloride can replace deficient anions.
• **FLUID AND ELECTROLYTES:** IV potassium chloride	Potassium chloride is given to correct underlying hypokalemia.
• Potassium-sparing diuretics	Potassium-sparing diuretics help minimize hypokalemia.
• **NUTRITION:** Antiemetics	Antiemetics aid in reducing the loss of hydrochloric acid in emesis.
• H_2-receptor antagonist	H_2-receptor antagonists block hydrochloride secretion in the stomach.
Avoid giving alkaline substances, such as IV sodium bicarbonate or antacids.	Alkaline substances can increase HCO_3^- levels and worsen alkalosis.

INTERVENTIONS TO ADDRESS RESPIRATORY ACIDOSIS	RATIONALE
GAS EXCHANGE: Apply noninvasive positive-pressure ventilation techniques, such as nasal continuous positive-pressure ventilation or bilevel ventilation.	Noninvasive positive-pressure ventilation techniques reduce hypercapnia.
Administer medication therapy aimed at reversing the effects of sedative drugs, such as naloxone to reverse opioids.	Reversing the effects of certain opiates and sedative drugs on the respiratory center stimulates ventilation.
NUTRITION: Provide a low-carbohydrate, high-fat diet.	A low-carbohydrate, high-fat diet helps reduce CO_2 production and improve respiratory muscle function.

INTERVENTIONS TO ADDRESS RESPIRATORY ALKALOSIS	RATIONALE
GAS EXCHANGE: Apply rebreather mask for a hyperventilating patient, as appropriate.	Increasing CO_2 retention may correct a carbonic acid deficit.
GAS EXCHANGE: Coach the patient to breathe slowly and deeply.	Slow, deep breathing may help calm the patient and aid in reducing the respiratory rate.
GAS EXCHANGE: Reduce excess minute ventilation in mechanically ventilated patients, as appropriate.	Reducing the respiratory rate or tidal volume may correct a carbonic acid deficit.
Administer neuromuscular-blocking agents along with sedation if the patient is hyperventilating while on mechanical ventilation.	Sedation may be needed to decrease anxiety and decrease the respiratory rate when the patient is receiving mechanical ventilation.

COLLABORATION	RATIONALE
NUTRITION: Dietitian	Collaborating with a dietitian offers the patient further information and support for implementing the prescribed diet.
MOBILITY: Physical therapy	Physical therapists assess, plan, and implement interventions that address potential muscle weakness.
GAS EXCHANGE: Respiratory therapy	Respiratory therapists assess, plan, and implement interventions that address potential problems to promote optimal respiratory function.

PATIENT AND CAREGIVER TEACHING

- Cause of the acid–base imbalance, if known, and how long it may last
- Factors that predispose the patient to an acid–base imbalance
- Manifestations of the acid–base imbalance
- Need for ABG monitoring
- Measures being used to treat the acid–base imbalance
- Management of any underlying condition contributing to the acid–base imbalance
- Needed lifestyle changes to control or prevent the acid–base imbalance
- Early recognition of problems and how to manage them
- When to notify the HCP

DOCUMENTATION

Assessment

- Assessments performed
- ABG results
- Manifestations of acid–base imbalance

Interventions

- Discussions with other interprofessional team members
- Environment modifications made
- Medications given
- Notification of the HCP about patient status
- Therapeutic interventions and the patient's response
- Teaching provided
- Safety measures implemented

Evaluation

- Patient's status: improved, stable, declined
- Presence of manifestations of acid–base imbalance
- Response to teaching provided
- Response to therapeutic interventions

Risk for Clotting 13

Definition

Risk of blood clots forming where they are not needed

Clotting is a normal response to injury of a blood vessel. The normal clotting process prevents hemorrhage. Normally, blood clots do not form where they are not needed. However, a clot that prevents oxygen and chemicals from being exchanged with local tissues may lead to cellular injury. Prolonged ischemia leads to infarction and necrosis of tissue. Clots can form in arteries, in the heart chambers, and in veins.

An arterial thrombosis, the development of a clot in an artery, is an emergency. When an artery is blocked, oxygen and nutrients are not delivered to the tissues in that area. Blockage with a clot in a cerebral artery can result in an ischemic stroke. Blockage with a clot in a coronary artery, if not treated rapidly, can result in myocardial infarction. Blockage in a renal artery can result in kidney failure. Peripheral artery blockage with a clot can result in necrosis and gangrene of an extremity.

When cardiac contraction is impaired, blood is not moving effectively through the heart. The blood pooling in one or more cardiac chambers may begin to form clots. Those clots can be dislodged and travel from the right side of the heart to lodge in the pulmonary arteries as pulmonary emboli. Clots that form in the left side of the heart can be dislodged and travel to the brain or peripheral arteries. For example, when a patient experiences atrial fibrillation, the atria do not contract effectively and clots may form in the atria. Later, those clots may travel out of the heart and cause tissue injury by blocking arteries.

Venous thrombosis involves the formation of a thrombus, or blood clot, with vein inflammation. It is the most common disorder of the veins. Superficial vein thrombosis is the formation of a thrombus in a superficial vein, usually the greater or lesser saphenous vein. Deep vein thrombosis (DVT) involves a thrombus in a deep vein, most often the iliac and/or femoral veins. Venous thromboembolism (VTE) is the preferred terminology to represent the spectrum from DVT to pulmonary embolism.

Anticoagulation therapy is commonly used to prevent and treat excessive clotting. When clotting is impaired by a lack of clotting factors or interference with normal clotting mechanisms, bleeding may progress to severe and life-threatening hemorrhage. Nurses have a critical role in the prevention and management of thrombosis and hemorrhage.

Associated Clinical Problems

- Risk for Bleeding: increased risk for hemorrhage
- Risk for VTE: increased risk for clotting leading to VTE, including DVT and pulmonary embolus
- Impaired Peripheral Neurovascular Function: disruption to the circulatory, motor, or sensory function in an extremity
- Impaired Peripheral Tissue Perfusion: inadequate blood circulation to an extremity

Common Causes and Risk Factors

- Advanced age
- Cancer, chemotherapy
- Clotting disorders
- Decreased cardiac contractility
- Diabetes
- Dysrhythmias
- Elevated serum lipids
- Estrogen therapy, including estrogen-based oral contraceptives
- Genetics
- Hypertension
- Local constriction from clothing, devices
- Obesity
- Pregnancy
- Prolonged immobility
- Prolonged standing
- Smoking
- Sedentary lifestyle
- Sex: Males more common than Females
- Trauma
- Vascular disorders, such as arteriosclerosis, sickle cell disease
- Venous stasis

Risk for VTE

- Abdominal or pelvic surgery
- Atrial fibrillation
- Fractures of the pelvis, hip, leg
- Having a peripherally inserted central catheter (PICC) line
- Heart failure
- History of VTE
- Intravenous drug use
- Orthopedic surgery
- Varicose veins

Key Conceptual Relationships

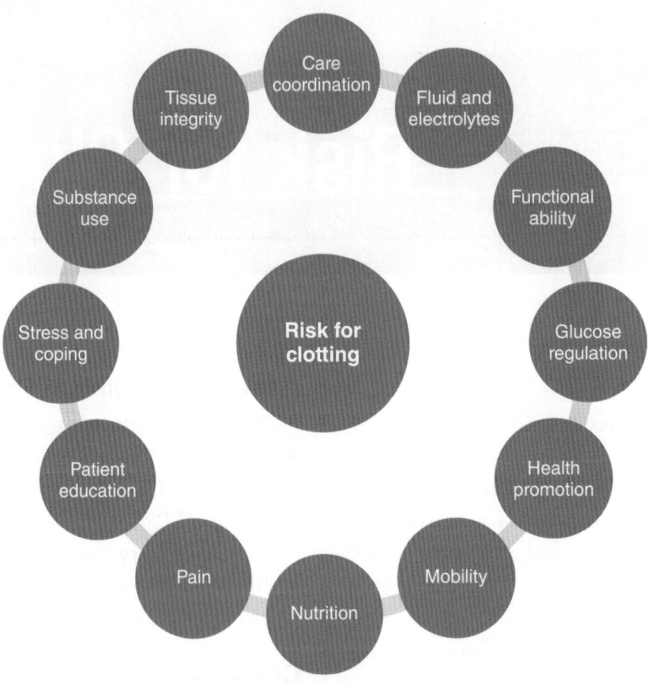

ASSESSMENT OF RISK FOR CLOTTING	RATIONALE
Assess for risk factors for developing blood clots.	Identifying factors that place patients at risk allows for early intervention.
Obtain a complete medication history.	Many drugs increase risk of developing blood clots.
Obtain a thorough history of any symptoms of blood clots, such as acute pain or leg edema, including: • When symptoms started • Onset, sudden or gradual • Frequency • Intensity or severity • Alleviating and aggravating factors • Any pattern to the symptoms • Previous treatment	A thorough history aids in evaluating the problem and helps direct treatment.
Perform a complete physical assessment and monitor indicators of clot development on an ongoing basis:	
• Manifestations of acute arterial thrombosis or VTE	Identifying manifestations allows for early intervention.
• Brachial, radial, dorsalis pedis, posterior tibial, and popliteal pulses bilaterally	Decreases in pulse quality occur with clots that alter perfusion.
• Extremities for color, temperature, capillary refill, sensation, movement, edema	Abnormalities in the peripheral vascular assessment identify changes in perfusion.
• **TISSUE INTEGRITY:** Skin assessment, particularly of the legs and feet	Patient with decreased tissue perfusion are at an increased risk for impaired tissue integrity.
• **PAIN:** Presence of extremity pain, characteristics of that pain	A thorough pain assessment can help differentiate arterial and venous disease and determine the need for analgesia.
Use a Doppler stethoscope for pulses that cannot be found by palpation.	A weak pulse may be found with a Doppler stethoscope.
Calculate the ankle-brachial index unless the patient has recently had percutaneous or surgical intervention on an extremity.	The index indicates relative severity of a tissue perfusion impairment.
Determine if pain, tenderness, swelling in the calf and thigh, or redness are present in the involved extremity.	These are signs of VTE, which would require further attention.

ASSESSMENT OF RISK FOR CLOTTING	RATIONALE
Evaluate the results of diagnostic studies, including ultrasound, arteriography.	Diagnostic tests are performed to evaluate peripheral vascular system function.
FUNCTIONAL ABILITY: Determine the effect of symptoms on the patient's level of fatigue and ability to perform basic and instrumental activities of daily living.	The patient with impaired tissue perfusion may have leg pain with activity and other manifestations that affect functional status.
STRESS AND COPING: Assess the patient's use of coping and stress management strategies.	Coping and stress managements strategies can improve quality of life by helping the patient better manage care.
SUBSTANCE USE: Screen for the presence of tobacco and/or other substance use problems.	Smoking and vaping cause peripheral vasoconstriction, significantly contributing to impaired tissue perfusion.
Evaluate the patient's response to measures to enhance impaired tissue perfusion through ongoing assessment.	Identifying the presence of manifestations of impaired tissue perfusion allows for evaluation of therapy effectiveness.

Expected Outcomes

The patient will:

- prevent or manage thrombosis.
- maintain adequate tissue perfusion.
- be free from complications associated with impaired tissue perfusion.
- adhere to the prescribed therapeutic regimen.
- maintain ongoing contact with the appropriate community resources.
- participate in desired activities of daily living.

INTERVENTIONS TO DECREASE RISK FOR VTE	RATIONALE
Measure for and apply graduated compression stockings or intermittent sequential pneumatic compression (ISPC) leg sleeves as ordered.	Stockings may reduce venous stasis, while graduated compression stockings may be contraindicated in patients with peripheral arterial disease.
MOBILITY: Encourage the patient with venous disease or venous ulcer to avoid prolonged sitting or standing.	Mobility decreases venous stasis.
After therapeutic immobilization or bed rest, encourage movement and assist in physical activity (such as walking) as soon as possible.	Mobility decreases venous stasis.
FLUIDS AND ELECTROLYTES: Encourage adequate daily water and fluid intake.	Dehydration increases the risk of VTE.
Encourage women at high risk for clotting who choose contraception to use a non-hormonal method.	Hormonal contraceptives may increase the risk for clots. The effect is magnified when combined with smoking.
SUBSTANCE USE: Encourage cessation of tobacco and marijuana use.	Smoking and vaping cause peripheral vasoconstriction, significantly contributing to impaired tissue perfusion.
Administer anticoagulant agents as ordered, including:	Anticoagulants are used for VTE prevention and treatment with the regimen depending on the patient's VTE risk.
• Vitamin K antagonists, such as warfarin (Coumadin)	Vitamin K antagonists inhibit activation of the vitamin K–dependent coagulation factors II, VII, IX, and X and the anticoagulant proteins C and S.
• Thrombin inhibitors (both indirect and direct)	Thrombin inhibitors bind to and inhibit the activity of thrombin and therefore prevent blood clot formation.
• Factor Xa inhibitors	Factor Xa inhibitors impede fibrin formation in the coagulation process.

INTERVENTIONS TO DECREASE RISK FOR BLEEDING DURING ANTICOAGULATION THERAPY	RATIONALE
Observe closely for any signs of bleeding, including hypotension, tachycardia, hematuria, melena, hematemesis, petechiae, ecchymosis, and bleeding from trauma site or surgical incision.	New signs of bleeding require intervention to avoid poor patient outcomes.
Monitor the results of appropriate laboratory testing, including international normalized ratio (INR), activated partial thromboplastin time (aPTT), prothrombin time (PT), complete blood count, hemoglobin, hematocrit, platelet levels, and/or liver enzymes.	Laboratory tests are performed to evaluate blood clotting ability and the risk for bleeding.
Monitor for and implement measures to reduce the risk of bleeding, including: • Avoid intramuscular injections. • Minimize venipunctures, using the smallest gauge needle possible. • Apply manual pressure for at least 10 minutes on venipuncture sites. • Use electric razors, not straight razors. • Avoid removing or disrupting established clots. • Use soft toothbrushes or foam swabs for oral care. • Limit tape application, using paper tape as appropriate. • Implement measures to reduce constipation.	These measures reduce the incidence of bleeding due to local tissue injury.
Hold medications and notify the health care provider (HCP) if the patient is taking medications that affect bleeding risk, such as aspirin, nonsteroidal anti inflammatory drugs (NSAIDs), and certain antibiotics, like sulfamethoxazole and trimethoprim (Bactrim).	A number of drugs increase the risk for bleeding, particularly by interacting with medications used to treat impaired perfusion.

COLLABORATION	RATIONALE
Disease or symptom management programs	Disease or symptom management programs help patients understand their treatment regimen and address the complex needs of those with chronic illness.
CARE COORDINATION: Social services or case management	Support may be needed to obtain financial, transportation, or other resources.
Community or online support groups	Many patients with chronic disease find benefit in the support offered by persons with similar concerns.
Physical therapy	Physical therapists can assess the patient and develop a plan of care to maximize exercise capability.

PATIENT AND CAREGIVER TEACHING

- Reason the patient is at risk for clot development
- Manifestations of impaired tissue perfusion
- Management of any underlying condition contributing to increased clotting
- Measures being used to decrease clotting risk
- Diagnostic and laboratory tests used to monitor clotting
- Lifestyle changes to decrease clot risk
- Early recognition of problems and how to manage them
- Safe use of medications, including proper use, side effect management, administration, and how they fit into the overall management plan
- VTE precautions
- Community and self-help resources available
- Sources of information and social support
- Gradual physical activity, managing exercise plan
- Tobacco cessation methods
- Importance of long-term follow-up
- Role of therapy and case management
- When to notify the HCP and when to seek emergency care

DOCUMENTATION

Assessment
- Assessments performed
- Manifestations of clotting
- Diagnostic test results

Interventions
- Medications given
- Notification of HCP about diagnostic test results and assessment findings
- Therapeutic interventions and the patient's response
- Teaching provided
- Referrals initiated
- Precautions implemented
- Discussions with other members of the interprofessional team
- Environmental modifications made
- Safety measures implemented, including VTE precautions

Evaluation
- Patient's status: improved, stable, declined
- Patient's response to teaching provided
- Diagnostic test results
- Patient's response to therapeutic interventions
- Presence of any manifestations of impaired tissue perfusion

Impaired Bowel Elimination 14

Definition

Difficulty with formation and evacuation of stool

The human body eliminates various forms of waste. Two important methods of elimination are bowel elimination and urinary elimination. *Bowel elimination* is the passage of stool (feces) through the intestinal tract and expulsion of the stool by intestinal smooth muscle contraction. The most important function of the intestine is the reabsorption of water and electrolytes. Feces are composed of water (75%), bacteria, unabsorbed minerals, undigested foodstuffs, bile pigments, and desquamated (shed) epithelial cells.

Defecation is a reflex action involving voluntary and involuntary control. The large intestine serves as a reservoir for the fecal mass until defecation. Feces in the rectum stimulate sensory nerve endings that produce the sensation of needing to defecate. The reflex center for defecation is in the spinal cord, producing contraction of the rectum and relaxation of the internal anal sphincter. A person who feels the need to defecate can voluntarily relax the external anal sphincter. Suppressing the urge to defecate over a long time can lead to constipation or fecal impaction.

People may be sensitive to discussing bowel habits or symptoms and may be uncomfortable with bowel management when hospitalized. Bowel incontinence may be an acute or chronic problem, which hampers social or intimate contact and makes it hard to maintain activities at school or work. Be sensitive to the patient's feelings when discussing incontinence. Nurses can provide reassurance and sensitivity to support effective bowel elimination by promoting optimal nutrition.

Associated Clinical Problems

- Bowel Incontinence: inability to control defecation
- Constipation: difficulty in passing stools or incomplete or infrequent passage of hard stools
- Chronic Functional Constipation: difficulty in passing stools, or incomplete or infrequent passage of hard stools, with no identifiable cause
- Perceived Constipation: state in which a person makes a self-diagnosis of constipation and ensures a daily bowel movement through the use of laxatives, enemas, and suppositories
- Risk for Constipation: at risk for difficulty in passing stools or incomplete or infrequent passage of hard stools
- Diarrhea: frequent passage of loose, watery stools
- Risk for Diarrhea: at risk for the frequent passage of loose, watery stools
- Fecal Impaction: accumulation of hardened feces in the rectum or sigmoid colon that the individual is unable to move
- Hemorrhoids: varicosities in the lower rectum or anus caused by venous congestion

Common Causes and Risk Factors

- Cancer
- History of gastrointestinal problems, including inflammatory bowel disease and irritable bowel syndrome

Constipation

- Abdominal muscle weakness
- Depression
- Fluid–volume imbalance, dehydration
- Habitual denying or ignoring of urge to defecate
- Impaired cognition
- Inadequate toileting
- Insufficient fiber intake
- Insufficient fluid intake
- Insufficient physical activity
- Irregular defecation habits
- Laxative overdose
- Medication side effects: antacids, anticholinergics, anticonvulsants, antidepressants, antilipemics, bismuth salts, calcium channel blockers, diuretics, iron salts, nonsteroidal antiinflammatory drugs (NSAIDs), opiates, phenothiazines, sedatives, sympathomimetics
- Neuromuscular disorders
- Obstruction by tumor, rectal prolapse, or enlarged prostate
- Pregnancy
- Rectal abscess or ulcer or rectal anal fissures

Diarrhea

- Alcohol use
- Anxiety
- Chemotherapy
- Enteral feedings
- Infection
- Inflammation
- Laxative abuse
- Malabsorption

- Medication side effects: antacids, antibiotics, antidepressants, proton pump inhibitors
- Parasites
- Toxins
- Travel to specific locations
- Radiation exposure
- Stress

Hemorrhoids
- Ascites
- Constipation
- Diarrhea
- Heavy lifting
- Obesity
- Pregnancy
- Prolonged sitting and standing

Incontinence
- Anorectal injury
- Fecal impaction
- Impaired cognition
- Impaired physical mobility
- Poor anal sphincter control

Manifestations

- Abdominal discomfort
- Anorexia
- Perianal skin problems

Constipation
- Dry, hard formed stools
- Hypoactive bowel sounds
- Infrequent defecation
- Nausea and/or vomiting
- Straining with defecation

Diarrhea
- Bowel urgency
- Hyperactive bowel sounds
- Minimum of three loose liquid stools per day
- Steatorrhea
- Diagnostic tests
  - Imaging may show cause of obstruction
  - Stool culture may be positive for infectious organisms

Hemorrhoids
- Anal burning or itching
- Bleeding with defecation
- Pain
- Protruding mass

Incontinence
- Dribbling of stool
- Inability to delay bowel movements
- Lack of awareness of defecation

Key Conceptual Relationships

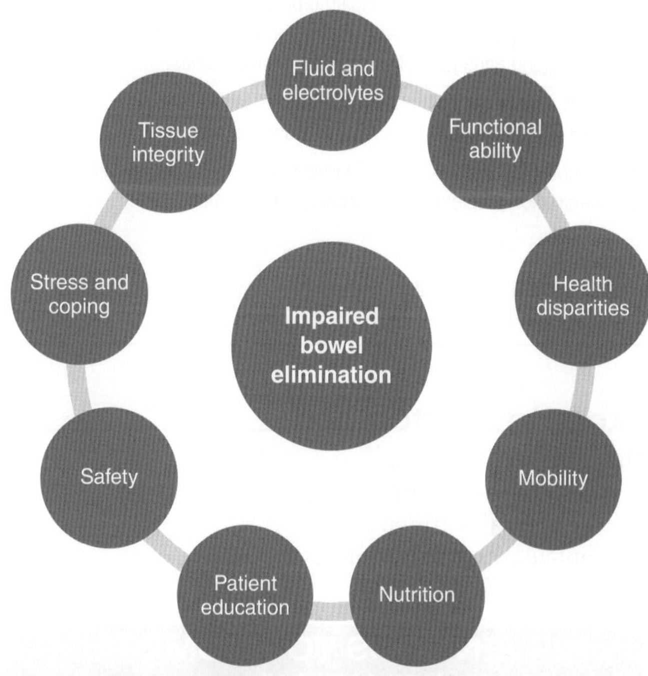

ASSESSMENT OF BOWEL ELIMINATION	RATIONALE
Assess for risk factors and manifestations of impaired bowel elimination.	Identifying factors that place the patient at risk for impaired bowel elimination and early recognition of signs and symptoms allows for prompt intervention.
Determine the potential cause of impaired bowel elimination.	It is more effective to treat the cause rather than the imbalance.
Obtain a thorough history of the patient's bowel habits, including: • Number of stools per day • Characteristics of stool—consistency, shape, volume, color • Occurrence of other symptoms • Onset, sudden or gradual • Duration • Frequency • Alleviating and aggravating factors • How the patient is managing symptoms	The normal frequency of defecation varies widely.

Continued

ASSESSMENT OF BOWEL ELIMINATION	RATIONALE
Perform a complete physical assessment and monitor indicators of bowel elimination on an ongoing basis: • Bowel sounds, noting a pattern of decreasing bowel sounds • Abdomen for distention, tenderness, or masses	Decreased bowel sounds indicate a decrease in peristalsis and motility, which can lead to and be present with constipation. An abdominal assessment can help identify potential causes of altered bowel function.
• **TISSUE INTEGRITY:** Integrity of the perianal tissues	Frequent extended contact with stool may break down tissue, whereas straining may cause fissures and hemorrhoids.
• Weight and intake and output	Monitoring weight and intake and output ensures that the patient has an adequate fluid intake.
• Mobility, dexterity, and functional ability	Assessment of mobility and functional ability partly determines the patient's ability to self-toilet and the need for assistive devices.
Obtain a complete medication history.	A number of medications influence bowel elimination.
Obtain a stool sample culture, as prescribed.	Stool tests provide objective data that may help identify the reason for impaired bowel elimination.
FUNCTIONAL ABILITY: Perform a psychosocial assessment, evaluating for any lifestyle effects of impaired bowel elimination, such as the ability to sleep, interact with others, perform work and household duties, and engage in physical and social activities.	Many bowel elimination problems can negatively affect the person's daily life.
SAFETY: Assess the environment for any obstacles to toileting, such as poor lighting, lack of grab bars, or insecure toilet seat.	Environmental obstacles contribute to bowel incontinence and increase the risk of toileting-related falls.
Evaluate the patient's response to measures to correct a bowel elimination problem through ongoing assessment.	Identifying the presence of manifestations of impaired bowel elimination allows for evaluation of therapy effectiveness.
Pediatric **DEVELOPMENT:** Assess the child's level of physical and emotional development.	The child's ability to control bowel elimination partly depends on the child's age, developmental level, and health status.

Expected Outcomes

The patient will:

- pass soft, formed stool.
- have optimal nutrition status.
- maintain perianal tissue integrity.

INTERVENTIONS TO PROMOTE BOWEL ELIMINATION	RATIONALE
Speak with sensitivity about bowel elimination.	Many people may be uncomfortable sharing information about bowel habits and findings.
Provide privacy for toileting and an odor eliminator.	Discomfort with lack of privacy may prevent patients from defecating.
Assist the patient with developing a bowel schedule:	
• Go first thing in the morning or after the first meal of the day.	This is the best time to toilet because people often have the urge to defecate at this time.
• Respond to the urge to have a bowel movement as soon as possible.	Delaying defecation results in hard stools and a decreased "urge" to defecate.
• Place the patient as close as possible in a position that promotes defecation.	Defecation is easiest when the person is sitting on a commode, with the knees higher than the hips.
FLUID AND ELECTROLYTES: Ensure the patient maintains a minimal fluid intake of 2500 mL/day unless contraindicated.	Adequate hydration helps prevent constipation and provides fluid replacement in case of diarrhea.

INTERVENTIONS TO PROMOTE BOWEL ELIMINATION	RATIONALE
NUTRITION: Encourage the patient to increase high-fiber foods, such as whole-grain breads and cereals and fresh fruits and vegetables, unless contraindicated.	A high-fiber diet stimulates peristalsis and promotes movement of the stool through the colon.
Implement measures to make toileting more efficient for patients, such as: • Call light in reach • Bedside commode • Easy-to-manage clothing • Assistive devices available • Environment free of hazards	Measures that enable the patient to toilet in a timely manner help reduce the risk of incontinence.

INTERVENTIONS TO MANAGE CONSTIPATION	RATIONALE
Administer medications as ordered, including:	
• Bulk-forming laxatives	Bulk-forming laxatives absorb water and increase bulk, thereby stimulating peristalsis.
• Emollients	Emollients lubricate the intestinal tract and soften feces, making hard stools easier to pass.
• Prosecretory agents	Prosecretory drugs increase intestinal fluid secretion through direct action on epithelial cells, speeding colonic transit.
• Saline and osmotic solutions	These solutions cause retention of fluid in the intestinal lumen, reducing stool consistency and increasing volume.
• Stimulants	Stimulants increase peristalsis and speed colonic transit by irritating the colon wall and stimulating enteric nerves.
FUNCTIONAL ABILITY: Implement measures to promote the ability to self-toilet.	Adaptive devices and environmental modifications can assist the patient in performing toileting at the optimal level of independence.
Remove a fecal impaction manually, if necessary.	Impaction is unlikely to resolve without manual removal.
Encourage the patient to drink hot liquids, such as coffee, tea, or lemon water, upon arising in the morning.	Hot drinks can stimulate peristalsis and promote regularity.
MOBILITY: Increase physical activity as tolerated.	Exercise stimulates peristalsis.

INTERVENTIONS TO MANAGE DIARRHEA	RATIONALE
Advance diet gradually from fluids to small meals.	Gradual introduction of fluid and food helps prevent a sudden increase in peristalsis and diarrhea.
NUTRITION: Encourage the patient to avoid foods and fluids known to aggravate diarrhea, including spicy foods, alcohol, coffee, fatty foods, very hot or cold foods, lactose-containing foods, high-fiber foods, and nonabsorbable sugars.	Substances that increase intestinal motility may increase the liquidity of the stool.
Administer antidiarrheal medications as ordered.	Many antidiarrheal medications slow motility and decrease peristalsis, lessening diarrhea.
STRESS AND COPING: Encourage the patient to use positive coping and stress management strategies.	Stress may increase intestinal motility.
MOBILITY: Encourage the patient to rest and limit activity.	Physical activity stimulates peristalsis.
Review safe food preparation with the patient and caregiver.	Food contamination is a common cause of diarrhea.
TISSUE INTEGRITY: Assist the patient with keeping the perianal area clean with soap and water after loose and/or frequent stools.	Stool contents contacting external tissue may cause discomfort and tissue excoriation.

INTERVENTIONS TO RELIEVE HEMORRHOIDS	RATIONALE
Implement measures to prevent constipation.	Conservative therapy is tried first and is effective for many patients.
Instruct the patient to avoid prolonged standing or sitting.	Pressure from gravity or weight on the affected area may increase discomfort.
Administer a sitz bath for 15–20 minutes, 2 or 3 times each day.	Sitz baths may help reduce the discomfort and swelling associated with hemorrhoids.
Apply ointments, creams, suppositories, and impregnated pads that contain antiinflammatory agents or astringents and anesthetics as needed.	These agents help shrink the mucous membranes and relieve discomfort.

INTERVENTIONS TO MANAGE INCONTINENCE	RATIONALE
Use a gentle cleansing preparation for perianal hygiene and apply a moisture barrier cream as needed.	Skin preparations protect the skin from the irritating content of stool.
Keep linens clean and dry.	Excess moisture may lead to macerated tissue.
SAFETY: Implement fall precautions and make environment modifications as needed for safe and efficient toileting.	Environment obstacles contribute to bowel incontinence and increase the risk of toileting-related falls.
Manage the use of rectal tube or fecal collection device, if necessary.	Emptying and changing the device as recommended help maintain tissue integrity.

COLLABORATION	RATIONALE
HEALTH EQUITY: Social work or case management	The social worker can explore resources for access to supplies, such as adult diapers, and making needed environmental modifications.
NUTRITION: Dietitian	Collaborating with a dietitian offers the patient further information and support for implementing the prescribed diet.
MOBILITY: Physical therapy	Physical therapists assess, plan, and implement interventions that address potential muscle weakness.
Support groups	Groups of patients who are experiencing the same problem can assist in rehabilitation and decrease social isolation.
Occupational therapy	Occupational therapy can recommend assistive devices and assist with skill development that promotes the patient's ability to self-toilet.

PATIENT AND CAREGIVER TEACHING

- Cause of impaired bowel elimination, if known, and how long it may last
- Management of any underlying condition causing impaired bowel elimination
- Normal bowel function and measures being used to improve bowel elimination
- Dietary adjustments to be made
- Safe use and administration of bowel medications
- Avoiding misuse of laxatives, enemas, and drugs that affect bowel elimination
- Any needed lifestyle changes to control bowel elimination
- Hygienic care
- Community and self-help resources, additional information available
- When to notify the health care provider (HCP)

DOCUMENTATION

Assessment

- Assessments performed
- Diagnostic and laboratory test results
- Manifestations of impaired bowel elimination
- Diagnostic test results

Interventions

- Discussions with other members of the interprofessional team
- Environmental modifications made
- Medications given
- Notification of the HCP about patient status
- Therapeutic interventions and the patient's response
- Teaching provided
- Referrals initiated
- Diet implemented

Evaluation

- Patient's status: improved, stable, declined
- Frequency and characteristics of stools
- Response to teaching provided
- Response to therapeutic interventions
- Diagnostic test results

Impaired Urinary Elimination 15

Definition

Difficulty with the collection and discharge of urine

Urinary elimination is the passage of urine through the urinary tract. Evacuation of urine is termed *urination*, *micturition*, or *voiding*. On average, 200–250 mL of urine in the bladder causes moderate distention and the urge to urinate, whereas 400–600 mL of urine begins to cause bladder discomfort. Bladder capacity ranges from 600 to 1000 mL.

People may be sensitive to discussing bladder habits or symptoms, including incontinence. An alteration in urinary elimination may cause psychosocial problems, such as social isolation resulting from embarrassment, and physiologic problems, such as fluid imbalance or infection. Nurses can provide reassurance and interventions to support effective urinary elimination.

Associated Clinical Problems

- Abnormal Urination Pattern: voiding either more or less frequently despite a normal urine volume
- Delay When Passing Urine: trouble starting or maintaining a urine stream, also called urinary hesitancy
- Impaired Kidney Function: decreased ability of the kidneys to eliminate wastes
- Impaired Urination: difficulty voiding the urine that has been produced by the kidneys
- Nocturia: frequent need to urinate at night
- Proteinuria: presence in the urine of abnormally large quantities of protein, usually albumin
- Urinary Frequency: urination or urgency quite often, without an increase in the total daily volume of urine
- Urinary Incontinence: inability to control urination or defecation
- Functional: loss of control of urine as a result of cerebral clouding and/or physical factors that make it difficult to get to bathroom facilities in time
- Overflow: occurs when the urinary tract is obstructed or when the detrusor muscle fails to contract as bladder capacity is reached
- Reflex: occurs when there is detrusor hyperreflexia and/or urethral relaxation as a result of neurologic causes, such as spinal cord injury
- Risk for Urge Incontinence: increased risk for the inability to delay voiding after a sensation of bladder fullness is perceived
- Stress: precipitated by coughing, sneezing, or straining
- Total: complete absence of control over urination
- Urge: inability to delay voiding after a sensation of bladder fullness is perceived
- Urinary Retention: condition in which the bladder is full but is not able to be emptied

Common Causes and Risk Factors

- Alcohol or caffeine intake
- Atrophic urethritis or vaginitis
- Bladder outlet obstruction or other urine blockage
- Cancer
- Congenital abnormality
- Decreased bladder capacity
- Diabetes
- Fecal impaction
- High intraabdominal pressure
- High urethral pressure caused by weak detrusor
- Impaired cognition, vision, or mobility
- Infection
- Neuromuscular disorder
- Medication side effects: anticholinergics, antidepressants, calcium channel blockers, decongestants, diuretics
- Pregnancy
- Prostate problems
- Severe pelvic prolapse
- Tissue damage
- Urethral sphincter deficiency
- Weakened supporting pelvic structures

Impaired Kidney Function

- Acute glomerulonephritis
- Aneurysm and aneurysm repair
- Burn injury
- Crush injury
- Heart failure
- Hypotension or shock
- Nephrotoxicity
- Renal artery stenosis or thrombosis

Urinary Retention

- Postoperative status
- Postpartum status

Manifestations

- Absence of urine output
- Bladder distention
- Dribbling of urine
- Dysuria
- Frequent voiding or voiding small amounts
- Hesitancy
- Nocturia
- Residual urine
- Retention
- Sensation of bladder fullness or difficulty urinating
- Urgency
- Diagnostic tests: urodynamic studies may show altered motor or sensory function of the bladder and sphincters.

Impaired Kidney Function

- Anorexia
- Blurred vision
- Fluid imbalance
- Headache
- Malaise
- Thirst

Key Conceptual Relationships

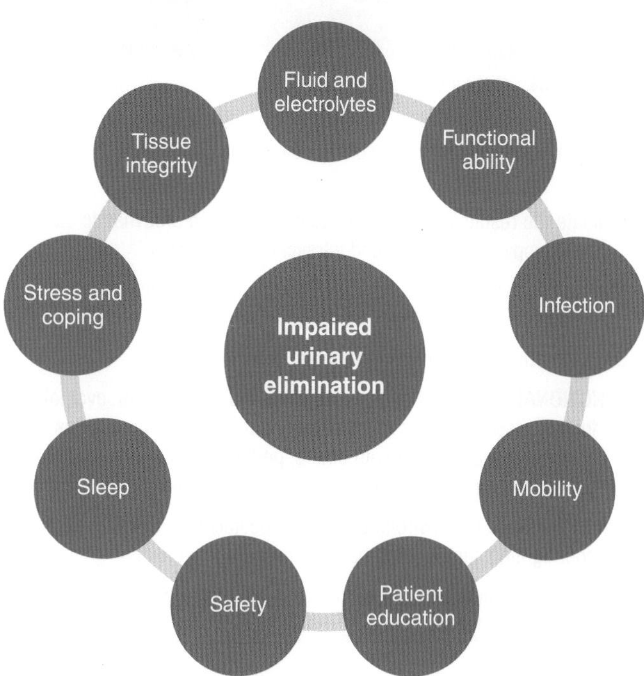

ASSESSMENT OF URINARY ELIMINATION	RATIONALE
Assess risk factors for impaired urinary elimination.	Identifying factors that place the patient at risk for impaired urinary elimination allows for early intervention.
Determine the potential cause of impaired urinary elimination.	It is more effective to treat the cause rather than the imbalance.
Screen for urinary incontinence by asking if the patient has any problems controlling urine or going to the bathroom.	Early recognition allows for prompt intervention.
Assess pattern of fluid intake and urination habits: • Times, types, and amounts of fluid intake • Times and amounts of voluntary and involuntary voiding • Reports of sensation of need to void • Activities preceding incontinence • Frequency of urinary problems (retention, incontinence) • Onset of problems, sudden or gradual • Occurrence of other symptoms • Characteristics of urine • Factors that make symptoms worse • How the patient is managing symptoms	Obtain information to plan individualized interventions.
Perform a complete physical assessment and monitor indicators of urinary elimination on an ongoing basis:	
• Manifestations of impaired urinary elimination	Early recognition of signs and symptoms allows for prompt intervention.
• Abdominal assessment: inspect abdomen; palpate and percuss the bladder and kidneys.	Abdominal assessment provides information about the potential cause of urinary elimination problems.
• **TISSUE INTEGRITY:** Integrity of the perineal tissues	Frequent extended contact with urine may break down tissue.
• **FLUID AND ELECTROLYTES:** Fluid balance indicators, including weight, intake and output, blood urea nitrogen (BUN), and creatinine	Urinary elimination problems may be accompanied by fluid imbalances and caused by alterations in renal function.
• Mobility, functional ability, and dexterity	Assessment of mobility and functional ability partly determines the patient's ability to self-toilet and the need for assistive devices.

Continued

ASSESSMENT OF URINARY ELIMINATION	RATIONALE
• BUN, creatinine, and creatinine clearance	Blood tests are useful in determining whether a kidney impairment is present.
Obtain a urinalysis and urine culture as ordered.	Diagnostic tests provide objective data that may help identify the reason for impaired urinary elimination.
Evaluate the results of diagnostic studies, including urodynamic studies, cystoscopy, radiography, and intravenous pyelogram.	Diagnostic tests are performed to evaluate the process of urine formation and elimination.
Measure postvoid residual volumes through straight catheterization or bladder scan as needed.	Measuring volumes prevents complications related to bladder overdistention.
SAFETY: Obtain a complete medication history.	A number of medications are nephrotoxic and influence urinary elimination.
FUNCTIONAL ABILITY: Perform a psychosocial assessment, evaluating for any lifestyle effects of impaired urinary elimination, such as the ability to sleep, interact with others, perform work and household duties, and engage in physical and social activities.	Many urinary elimination problems can negatively affect the person's daily life.
SAFETY: Assess the environment for any obstacles to toileting, such as poor lighting, lack of grab bars, or insecure toilet seat.	Environment obstacles contribute to urinary incontinence and increase the risk of toileting-related falls.
Evaluate the patient's response to measures to correct a urinary elimination problem through ongoing assessment.	Identifying the presence of manifestations of impaired urinary system function allows for evaluation of therapy effectiveness.
Pediatric	
DEVELOPMENT: Assess the child's level of physical and emotional development.	The child's ability to control urinary elimination partly depends on the child's age, developmental level, and health status.

Expected Outcomes

The patient will:

- void at normal intervals.
- experience continence.

INTERVENTIONS TO PROMOTE URINARY ELIMINATION	RATIONALE
Notify the HCP if manifestations of impaired urinary elimination persist or worsen.	Achievement of an effective treatment plan often requires adjustments in therapy.
SAFETY: Notify the health care provider (HCP) if adverse medication effects, including nephrotoxicity, are suspected.	The presence of adverse medication effects may require an adjustment in medication or dose.
Speak with sensitivity about urinary findings.	Urinary findings may be a source of reticence or embarrassment for the person.
Provide privacy for toileting.	Discomfort with lack of privacy may prevent the person from urinating.
Assist the patient with developing positive urination habits:	
• Offer the opportunity to void and assist to the bathroom every 2 to 4 hours if indicated.	Emptying the bladder before the pressure becomes too great reduces the risk of incontinence.
• Urinate when the urge is first felt.	Chronically suppressing the urge results in a decreased urge to void.
• Allow the patient to assume a functional position for voiding (usually sitting for females and standing for males) unless contraindicated.	A sitting or standing position uses gravity to facilitate bladder emptying.
• Have the patient lean forward and gently press downward on the lower abdomen when attempting to void.	Increased pressure on the bladder can promote voiding.
• If having difficulty voiding, run water, place the patient's hands in warm water, and/or pour warm water over the perineum.	These actions may trigger the reflex to void.

INTERVENTIONS TO PROMOTE URINARY ELIMINATION	RATIONALE
Implement measures to make toileting more efficient for patients who have a short time between the urge and voiding, such as: • Call bell in reach • Bedside commode • Easy-to-manage clothing • Assistive devices available • Environment free of hazards	Measures that enable the patient toilet in a timely manner help reduce the risk of incontinence.
Implement measures to increase pelvic muscle floor strength, including pelvic floor muscle exercises and biofeedback if appropriate.	Pelvic floor muscle exercises help strengthen the pelvic floor muscles and improve the tone of the external urinary sphincter.
SAFETY: Implement fall precautions and make environmental modifications as needed.	Environmental obstacles contribute to urinary incontinence and increase the risk of toileting-related falls.
FUNCTIONAL ABILITY: Implement measures to promote the ability to self-toilet.	Adaptive devices and environmental modifications can assist the patient in performing toileting at the optimal level of independence.
FLUID AND ELECTROLYTES: Have the patient space fluids evenly throughout the day rather than drinking a large quantity at one time.	Drinking a large amount of fluid at one time results in rapid filling of the bladder, which increases pressure in the bladder and the subsequent risk of incontinence.
Limit oral fluid intake late in the evening.	Decreased awareness of bladder filling while asleep may increase the risk of incontinence.
Encourage the patient to avoid drinking alcohol and beverages containing caffeine, such as colas, coffee, and tea.	Alcohol and caffeinated beverages have a mild diuretic effect and are chemically irritating to the bladder.
Administer medications as ordered to increase or decrease bladder tone, including:	
• Anticholinergics	Anticholinergics reduce overactive bladder contractions and improve the storage capacity of bladder.
• Antidepressants	These drugs reduce sensory urgency and overactive bladder contractions.
Perform catheterization as ordered.	For some types of incontinence and urinary retention, catheterization may be a necessary treatment option.
For the patient with an indwelling urinary catheter:	
• Reassess the need for an indwelling catheter daily and discuss removal with HCP when feasible.	Limiting the duration of indwelling catheter use decreases the risk of UTI.
• Implement measures to ensure its patency by keeping the tubing free of kinks and the collection bag below bladder level	Maintaining patency of the indwelling catheter prevents urinary retention.
• **INFECTION:** Provide regular hygiene care and maintain the sterility of the catheter system.	Preventing a catheter-associated urinary tract infection is a key safety measure.

INTERVENTIONS TO MANAGE IMPAIRED KIDNEY FUNCTION	RATIONALE
Maintain prescribed diet and fluid volumes, following any restrictions, such as sodium or protein intake.	Dietary intake influences fluid balance and the accumulation of acidic end products.

INTERVENTIONS TO MANAGE URINARY RETENTION	RATIONALE
Administer medications, such as α-adrenergic blockers, as prescribed.	These drugs relax the smooth muscle of the bladder neck and prostatic urethra and may decrease urethral resistance.

COLLABORATION	RATIONALE
HEALTH EQUITY: Social work or case management	The social worker can explore resources available to help the patient obtain access to appropriate supplies, such as adult diapers, and make needed environmental modifications.
MOBILITY: Physical therapy	Physical therapists assess, plan, and implement interventions that address potential muscle weakness.
Support groups	Groups of patients who are experiencing the same problem can assist in rehabilitation and decrease social isolation.
NUTRITION AND FLUID AND ELECTROLYTES: Dietitian	The dietitian can provide detailed instructions regarding fluid management and the optimal diet to promote optimal kidney function and fluid balance.
Occupational therapy	Occupational therapy can recommend assistive devices and assist with skill development that promotes the patient's ability to self-toilet.

 PATIENT AND CAREGIVER TEACHING

- Cause of impaired urinary elimination, if known, and how long it may last
- Normal urinary function
- Normal age-related variations in urinary elimination
- Management of any underlying condition causing impaired urinary elimination
- Measures being used to improve urinary continence
- Measures to reduce the risk of incontinence
- Importance of adequate fluid intake
- Pelvic floor exercises
- Catheter care
- Any needed lifestyle changes to control urinary elimination
- Hygienic care
- Community and self-help resources available
- Where to find additional information
- When to notify the HCP

DOCUMENTATION

Assessment

- Assessments performed
- Diagnostic and laboratory test results
- Manifestations of a urinary problem

Interventions

- Discussions with other members of the interprofessional team
- Medications given
- Notification of the HCP about patient status
- Therapeutic interventions and the patient's response
- Teaching provided
- Referrals initiated
- Patency of urinary catheter, if present

Evaluation

- Patient's status: improved, stable, declined
- Presence of any manifestations of a urinary problem
- Diagnostic test results
- Response to teaching provided
- Response to therapeutic interventions

Electrolyte Imbalance 16

Definition

Higher- or lower-than-normal concentration of an electrolyte

Electrolytes are substances whose molecules dissociate, or split, into charged particles called *ions* when placed in water. Electrolytes are present in all body fluids and tissues. The body uses many regulatory processes to keep electrolytes within normal limits and maintain homeostasis. The main electrolytes are:

Sodium (Na^+)	136–145 mEq/L (136–145 mmol/L)
Potassium (K^+)	3.5–5.0 mEq/L (3.5–5.0 mmol/L)
Calcium (Ca^+)	9.0–10.5 mg/dL (2.25–2.62 mmol/L)
Magnesium (Mg^+)	1.3–2.1 mEq/L (0.65–1.05 mmol/L)
Phosphorus (P^-)	3.0–4.5 mg/dL (0.97–1.45 mmol/L)

Many conditions and their treatments affect electrolyte balance and lead to an imbalance. There are two types of electrolyte imbalances: low plasma concentrations (hypo-) and high plasma concentrations (hyper-). Conceptually, electrolyte imbalances often affect perfusion, gas exchange, cognition, intracranial regulation, and mobility. Potassium, magnesium, and calcium imbalances can affect perfusion and gas exchange. Most imbalances can cause neuromuscular problems, leading to acute confusion, lethargy, muscle weakness, tremors, and numbness. These problems pose safety concerns and affect functional ability.

Assessing for an electrolyte imbalance and collaborating with the interprofessional team for treatment is an important nursing role. Implement fall and seizure precautions for patients at risk. Maintain a safe environment. Administer medications and fluids as ordered. Assist the patient with implementing the prescribed diet plan.

Common Causes

- Acid–base imbalance
- Cancer
- Changes in intake
- Endocrine problems
- Fluid imbalance
- Gastrointestinal (GI) problems, including vomiting, diarrhea, fistulas, nasogastric suction, ileostomy drainage
- Impaired nutrition
- Liver disease
- Medication side effects
- Renal problems
- Tissue catabolism from fever, crush injury, sepsis, and burns
- Tumor lysis syndrome
- Metastatic bone disease

Manifestations

- Change in bowel patterns
- Changes in reflexes
- Electrocardiogram (ECG) changes with dysrhythmias
- Fatigue
- Impaired cognition
- Manifestations of any corresponding fluid imbalance
- Muscle cramps
- Nausea and vomiting
- Seizures, tetany
- Weakness

Key Conceptual Relationships

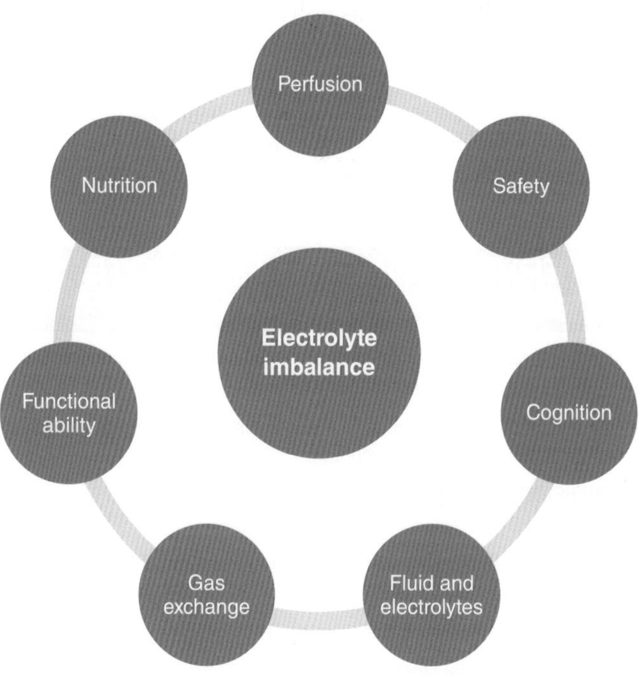

ASSESSMENT OF ELECTROLYTE BALANCE	RATIONALE
Assess for risk factors for an electrolyte imbalance.	Identifying factors that place the patient at risk for an electrolyte imbalance allows for early intervention.
Determine the potential cause of an electrolyte imbalance.	It is often more effective to treat the cause rather than the imbalance.
Identify patients who need emergency management of an electrolyte imbalance so that they can be stabilized.	Identifying an electrolyte imbalance allows for early intervention.
Perform a complete physical assessment and determine the patient's electrolyte status on an ongoing basis:	
• Serum and urine electrolyte levels and trends in levels, as available	Electrolyte levels help evaluate patient status and treatment effectiveness.
• Manifestations of an electrolyte imbalance	Identifying an electrolyte imbalance allows for early intervention.
• **PERFUSION:** Cardiac rhythm with ECG monitoring	Changes in cardiac rhythm are common with calcium, magnesium, potassium, and phosphorus imbalances.
• Fluid balance indicators, including weight, intake and output, blood urea nitrogen, and creatinine	Many electrolyte imbalances are accompanied by fluid imbalances and alterations in renal function.
Estimate the ionized calcium level when only total calcium levels are available.	Serum calcium levels reflect the total level of all forms of plasma calcium. Ionized calcium levels are measured using special laboratory techniques or calculated using a formula.
Monitor for the loss of electrolyte-rich body fluids.	Identifying factors that place the patient at risk for an electrolyte imbalance allows for early intervention.
SAFETY: Monitor for side effects, including nausea, vomiting, and diarrhea, of prescribed supplemental electrolytes.	Identifying side effects of electrolyte therapy allows for early intervention.
Monitor for complications of therapy.	Identifying complications allows for early intervention.
Evaluate the patient's response to measures to correct electrolyte imbalance on an ongoing basis.	Identifying manifestations of an electrolyte imbalance allows for evaluation of therapy effectiveness.

Expected Outcomes

The patient will:

- achieve and maintain electrolyte balance.
- be free from manifestations of an electrolyte imbalance.
- be free from complications of an electrolyte imbalance.
- adhere to the prescribed therapeutic regimen.
- recognize factors that may lead to an electrolyte imbalance and take preventative action.
- appropriately use therapies to achieve and maintain electrolyte balance.

INTERVENTIONS TO PROMOTE ELECTROLYTE BALANCE	RATIONALE
Implement collaborative interventions aimed at treating the underlying cause of an electrolyte imbalance.	The electrolyte imbalance may resolve with treatment of the underlying cause.
GAS EXCHANGE: Be prepared to institute resuscitation protocols and respiratory support, as appropriate.	Some electrolyte imbalances can cause respiratory muscle fatigue, potentially leading to respiratory distress.
PERFUSION: Treat dysrhythmias according to agency policy.	Identifying changes in cardiac rhythm that are common with electrolyte imbalances allows for early intervention.
Notify the health care provider (HCP) if manifestations of an electrolyte imbalance persist or worsen.	Achieving an effective treatment plan often requires adjustments in therapy.
Administer pharmacologic therapies as prescribed, including:	
• Supplemental electrolytes	Supplemental electrolyte therapy may be needed to correct deficiency imbalances.

INTERVENTIONS TO PROMOTE ELECTROLYTE BALANCE	RATIONALE
• Electrolyte binding or excreting agents	Administering electrolyte binding or excreting agents promotes electrolyte excretion.
• Diuretic therapy	Diuretics promote urinary output and the renal excretion of electrolytes.
• Intravenous (IV) fluid therapy	IV hydration promotes the renal excretion of electrolytes.
Administer prescribed IV solutions containing electrolytes at a constant flow rate.	Administering IV replacement electrolytes too rapidly can cause cardiac dysrhythmias.
NUTRITION: Provide the prescribed diet for the specific electrolyte imbalance, such as low sodium or no added salt.	The appropriate diet can assist with the management of an electrolyte imbalance.
Properly obtain laboratory specimens for electrolyte levels.	Test values may be compromised by specimens that have not been collected, labeled, handled, or stored properly before and during the testing process.
Provide the prescribed amount of fluid intake.	Fluid intake affects hemodilution and electrolyte balance.
Administer dialysis as ordered and evaluate patient response.	Dialysis may be effective in restoring electrolyte balance by removing excess electrolytes and fluid.
SAFETY: Provide a safe environment for the patient with neuromuscular manifestations of an electrolyte imbalance by instituting fall and seizure precautions.	Electrolyte imbalances may cause cerebral edema, resulting in changes in cognition that place the patient at risk for falls and seizures.
COGNITION: Implement measures to orient the patient.	Electrolyte imbalances may cause cerebral edema, resulting in changes in cognition.
FUNCTIONAL ABILITY: Help the patient prioritize activities and alternate rest and activity periods.	Limiting activities conserves energy and helps prevent fatigue.
Implement measures to address any nausea and vomiting	Nausea and vomiting can lead to further fluid and electrolyte problems.
GAS EXCHANGE: Position the patient to promote ventilation.	Some electrolyte imbalances can cause respiratory muscle fatigue.
SAFETY: Monitor IV sites carefully for extravasation.	Tissue sloughing and necrosis can occur if IV electrolyte solutions infiltrate.
Implement measures to reduce or eliminate common side effects, including nausea, vomiting, and diarrhea, associated with prescribed supplemental electrolytes.	Appropriate management of side effects can increase the patient's comfort level and adherence to therapy.
For patients with nasogastric tubes:	
• Administer prescribed electrolyte and fluid replacement based on output.	Replacing fluids and electrolytes promotes fluid and electrolyte balance.
• Irrigate tubes with normal saline, per agency policy.	Irrigating with normal saline minimizes the loss of GI tract electrolytes.
• Minimize the amount of ice chips and other oral intake when suction is in use.	Increased oral intake increases the amount of fluid lost with suctioning and contributes to electrolyte loss.
• Provide free water with enteral feedings, per agency policy.	Supplemental water with enteral feedings helps prevent hypernatremia.

COLLABORATION	RATIONALE
NUTRITION: Dietitian	Collaborating with a dietitian offers the patient further information and support for implementing the prescribed diet.
MOBILITY: Physical therapy	Physical therapists assess, plan, and implement interventions that address potential muscle weakness.
GAS EXCHANGE: Respiratory therapy	Respiratory therapists assess, plan, and implement interventions that address potential problems to promote optimal respiratory function.

PATIENT AND CAREGIVER TEACHING

- Cause of the electrolyte imbalance, if known
- Manifestations of electrolyte imbalances
- Factors that predispose the patient to electrolyte imbalances
- Measures being used to treat an electrolyte imbalance and the manifestations
- Importance of monitoring electrolyte levels
- Safe use of medications, including electrolyte replacement therapies
- Diet sources of electrolytes
- Appropriate foods for the diet regimen
- Early recognition of problems and how to manage them
- Needed lifestyle changes to control the electrolyte imbalance
- When to notify the HCP

DOCUMENTATION

Assessment

- Assessments performed
- Diagnostic and laboratory test results
- Manifestations of an electrolyte imbalance

Interventions

- Discussions with other interprofessional team members
- Fluids and medications administered
- Notification of the HCP about patient status
- Therapeutic interventions and the patient's response
- Teaching provided
- Referrals and consults initiated
- Safety measures implemented, including seizure and fall precautions

Evaluation

- Patient's status: improved, stable, declined
- Presence of manifestations of an electrolyte imbalance
- Response to teaching provided
- Response to therapeutic interventions

Fluid Imbalance 17

DEFINITION

Any change in or modification of body fluid balance

Body fluids are in constant motion, transporting nutrients, electrolytes, and oxygen to cells and carrying waste products away from cells. The body uses many regulatory mechanisms to keep the composition and volume of fluids within narrow limits to maintain homeostasis and promote health. Fluid imbalances are usually classified as a volume deficit, hypovolemia, or a volume excess, hypervolemia. The main causes of hypovolemia are inadequate fluid intake and increased fluid losses. Often, fluid–volume imbalances are accompanied by an electrolyte imbalance, particularly changes in the serum sodium level.

Many conditions and their treatments affect fluid balance. Conceptually, fluid imbalances often affect perfusion, gas exchange, mobility, and cognition. The patient is at risk for falls because of orthostatic hypotension, muscle weakness, and changes in level of consciousness. Good skin care is important, because changes in the skin and altered mobility increase the risk for impaired tissue integrity. Infants and older adults are at greater risk for fluid imbalances because of their percentage of body water and impaired regulatory mechanisms.

Monitoring the patient's fluid balance is an important nursing role. Obtain a thorough history and perform a complete physical examination. Fluid imbalances affect all body systems. The primary treatment involves correcting the underlying cause. Administer fluids and medications as ordered. Provide good skin care. Implement fall and seizure precautions, maintaining a safe environment for the patient.

Associated Clinical Problems

- Hypervolemia: extracellular fluid–volume excess
  - Ascites—abnormal accumulation of fluid in the peritoneal cavity
  - Dependent Edema—edema of the lowermost parts of the body relative to the heart, affected by gravity and position
  - Edema—accumulation of fluid in the interstitial space
- Hypovolemia: extracellular fluid–volume deficit
  - Dehydration—fluid–volume deficit characterized by the loss of pure water
  - Thirst—perceived desire for water or other fluid
- Risk for Fluid Imbalance: increased risk for an alteration in fluid volume

Common Causes

Hypervolemia

- Adrenal tumor
- Corticosteroid use
- Cushing syndrome
- Excess isotonic or hypotonic intravenous (IV) fluids
- Excess sodium intake
- Heart failure
- Liver problems
- Primary polydipsia
- Renal failure
- Syndrome of inappropriate antidiuretic hormone (SIADH)

Hypovolemia

- Diabetes insipidus
- Gastrointestinal (GI) losses from vomiting, nasogastric suction, diarrhea, fistula drainage
- Infection, sepsis
- Impaired cognition
- Insensible water loss, including perspiration, fever, heatstroke
- Insufficient fluid intake
- Hemorrhage
- Malnutrition
- Medications: caffeine, diuretics, enemas, laxatives
- Osmotic diuresis
- Third-space fluid shifts, including burns and pancreatitis
- Voluntary restriction of intake

Manifestations

Manifestations of Hypovolemia and Hypervolemia

Manifestation	Hypovolemia	Hypervolemia
Vital signs	• Postural hypotension, ↑ heart rate, ↓ central venous pressure (CVP), ↑ respiratory rate	• Bounding pulse, ↑ blood pressure (BP), ↑ CVP
Cognition/neurologic	• Confusion, restlessness, drowsiness, lethargy, dizziness • Seizures, coma	• Confusion, headache, lethargy • Seizures, coma
General Assessment	• Cold, clammy skin • ↓ Capillary refill • Thirst, dry mucous membranes • Weakness	• Dyspnea, crackles, pulmonary edema • S_3 heart sound • Neck vein distention • Edema, ascites • Muscle spasms
Urine	• ↓ Urine output, concentrated urine	• Polyuria (if normal renal function)
Weight	• Weight loss	• Weight gain
Laboratory tests	• ↑ Specific gravity, ↑ hematocrit, ↑ blood urea nitrogen (BUN)	↓ Specific gravity, ↓ hematocrit, ↓ BUN
Pediatric	• Sunken fontanels	• Bulging fontanels

Key Conceptual Relationships

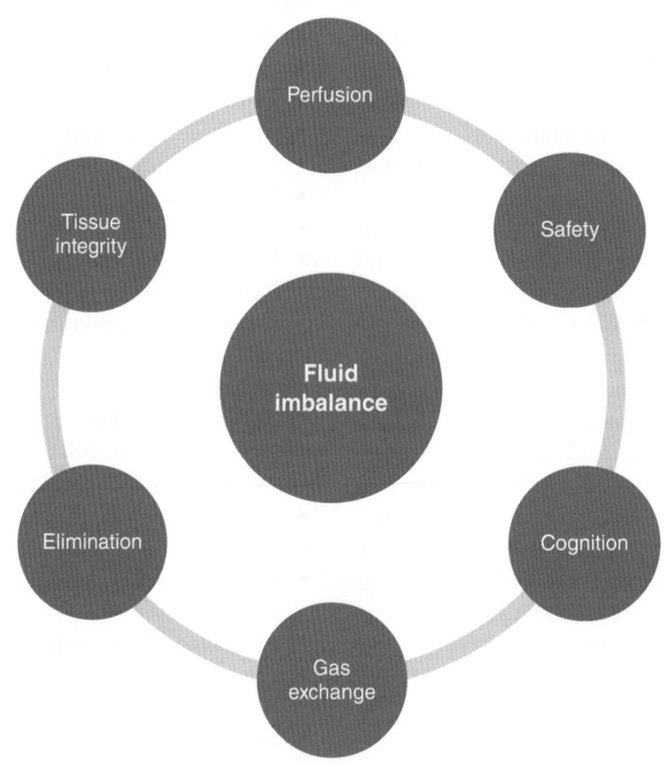

ASSESSMENT OF FLUID BALANCE	RATIONALE
Identify patients who need emergency management of a fluid imbalance so that they can be immediately stabilized.	Identifying an electrolyte imbalance allows for early intervention.
Assess risk factors for a fluid imbalance, including the patient's ability to self-manage hydration.	Identifying factors that place the patient at risk for fluid imbalance allows for early intervention.
Determine the potential cause of a fluid imbalance.	It is more effective to treat the cause rather than the imbalance.

ASSESSMENT OF FLUID BALANCE	RATIONALE
Obtain a history of the amount and type of fluid intake and elimination habits.	A thorough history helps determine contributing factors to fluid imbalance.
Perform a complete physical assessment and monitor indicators on an ongoing basis:	
• Daily weight	Changes in weight correspond with fluid volume changes.
• Urine color, quantity, and specific gravity	Changes in urine output, color, and specific gravity correspond with changes in fluid balance.
• **PERFUSION:** Vital signs, including orthostatic BP	Tachycardia and changes in BP are common signs of fluid imbalance.
• Changes in cardiac rhythm	Dysrhythmias are common with fluid imbalances.
• Peripheral pulses, capillary refill, skin color and temperature	Fluid volume changes can profoundly affect peripheral perfusion.
• Hemodynamic status, such CVP, mean arterial pressure (MAP), pulmonary artery pressure (PAP) levels, if available	Changes in hemodynamic parameters reflect fluid balance and are early indicators of shock.
• **FLUID AND ELECTROLYTE:** Neck vein distention	Neck vein distention may occur with hypervolemia and cardiac decompensation.
• Mucous membranes, skin, and sclera	Fluid volume changes, particularly hypovolemia, manifest as changes in the mucous membranes and skin.
• Edema, noting type, location, and degree	Edema results from fluid accumulation in the interstitial compartment of the extravascular space.
• Lung sounds	Adventitious lung sounds may occur with hypervolemia and signal the potential for impaired gas exchange.
• Thirst	Thirst is an indicator of hypovolemia, whereas diminished thirst contributes to hypovolemia.
• **INTRACRANIAL REGULATION:** Neurologic status	Alterations in fluid balance place the patient at risk for changes in cognition and deep tendon reflexes and seizures.
• Pediatric: Tears, salivation, fontanels	A child with hypovolemia will not produce tears or salivate, and the fontanels may be sunken. Bulging fontanels may occur with hypervolemia.
• Relevant laboratory results, such as hematocrit, BUN, and creatinine	Laboratory levels related to fluid balance assist in determining patient needs and treatment effectiveness.
• Electrolyte levels	Many patients with a fluid imbalance also have an electrolyte imbalance.
Calculate serum osmolality.	Osmolality increases with hypovolemia and decreases with hypervolemia.
Keep an accurate record of intake and output, including oral intake, enteral intake, IV intake, antibiotics, fluids given with medications, nasogastric tubes, drains, emesis, rectal tubes, colostomy drainage, and urine.	Intake and output records help determine fluid balance and evaluate the effectiveness of therapy.
Record incontinence episodes in patients requiring accurate intake and output.	Recording the number of incontinence episodes offers a means of evaluating intake and output.
Count and weigh diapers.	The wet diaper weight in grams minus the weight of the dry diaper equals the milliliters of urine.
Monitor weight change before and after dialysis.	Monitoring weight helps the health care provider (HCP) determine how much fluid needs to be removed with dialysis.
Determine whether the patient has assessment findings that indicate a fluid imbalance.	Identifying a fluid imbalance allows for early intervention.
Monitor for signs and symptoms of worsening hypervolemia or hypovolemia.	Identification of worsening fluid imbalance, such as oliguria, cognitive changes, seizures, and changes in BP, allows for early intervention.
Evaluate response to measures to correct the fluid imbalance.	Identifying manifestations of a fluid imbalance allows for evaluation of therapy effectiveness.

Expected Outcomes

The patient will:

- achieve and maintain fluid balance.
- be free from complications from abnormal or undesired fluid levels.
- be free from manifestations of a fluid imbalance.
- adhere to the prescribed therapeutic regimen.
- recognize factors that can lead to a fluid imbalance and take preventative action.

INTERVENTIONS TO PROMOTE FLUID BALANCE	RATIONALE
Implement collaborative interventions aimed at treating the underlying cause of the fluid imbalance.	The fluid imbalance may resolve with treatment of the underlying cause.
SAFETY: Maintain an appropriate IV infusion, blood transfusion, or enteral flow rate.	Administering IV solutions at a consistent rate prevents administering a fluid bolus.
NUTRITION: Provide a prescribed diet for the specific fluid imbalance, such as a low-sodium or fluid-restricted diet.	The right diet can aid in managing a fluid imbalance.
ADHERENCE: Help patients manage concerns regarding their therapeutic regimen, such as the patient who limits fluid intake for fear of urinary incontinence from diuretic therapy.	Directly addressing patient concerns promotes adherence to the therapeutic regimen.
SAFETY: Provide a safe environment for the patient with neuromuscular manifestations of a fluid imbalance.	Fluid imbalances may cause cerebral edema, resulting in changes in cognition and the potential for seizures, which increase the risk for injury.
TISSUE INTEGRITY: Assist the patient with changing positions frequently.	Patients with a fluid imbalance are at high risk for a pressure injury.
Provide frequent skin and oral care.	Patients with a fluid imbalance are at high risk for altered tissue integrity.
FUNCTIONAL ABILITY: Help the patient as needed with activities of daily living.	A fluid imbalance can result in muscle weakness, fatigue, and postural hypotension that can interfere with the ability to perform activities of daily living.
MOBILITY: Aid with range of motion exercises and physical activity, as needed.	Participating in physical activity helps preserve muscle mass and prevent fatigue.
COGNITION: Implement measures to orient the patient.	Fluid imbalances may cause changes in cognition.
Insert a urinary catheter, if needed.	A catheter can aid in accurately measuring urinary output.
Obtain laboratory specimens properly.	A test value may be compromised by specimens that have not been collected, labeled, handled, or stored properly before and during the testing process.
Notify the HCP if:	
• Manifestations of fluid imbalance persist or worsen.	Early intervention for persistent or worsening fluid imbalance promotes the best patient outcomes.
• ELIMINATION: Urine output is less than 0.5 mL/kg/hr.	A minimal urine output ensures kidney function and adequate hydration.

INTERVENTIONS TO ADDRESS HYPERVOLEMIA	RATIONALE
Restrict fluid intake, as ordered.	Fluid restriction is a safe first-line treatment for hypervolemia.
Distribute fluid intake over 24 hours.	Evenly distributing fluid intake helps relieve thirst and the discomfort associated with dry mucous membranes.
Administer pharmacologic therapies to increase urinary output, as prescribed, including:	
• Diuretic therapy	Diuretics promote urine output and the renal excretion of excess fluids.

INTERVENTIONS TO ADDRESS HYPERVOLEMIA	RATIONALE
• Albumin infusion	Albumin may help maintain intravascular volume and increase urine output in the patient with ascites by increasing plasma colloid oncotic pressure.
Administer dialysis and evaluate patient response.	Dialysis may be effective in restoring fluid balance by removing excess electrolytes and fluids.
PERFUSION: Implement measures to promote venous return in edematous extremities.	Enhancing venous return promotes fluid mobilization.
GAS EXCHANGE: Encourage coughing and deep breathing and maintain a semi-Fowler position.	Fluid in the lungs can impair gas exchange.
DEVELOPMENT: Implement measures to assist with maintaining a positive self-image if the patient is concerned about fluid retention or edema.	A positive body image promotes healthy self-esteem.
Assist the HCP with performing paracentesis for the patient with ascites.	Paracentesis can remove excess fluid associated with severe ascites.

INTERVENTIONS TO ADDRESS HYPOVOLEMIA	RATIONALE
Be prepared to institute resuscitation protocols.	Hypovolemia can lead to the development of shock.
PERFUSION: Administer prescribed fluid replacement, including the following:	
• IV fluids	Fluid administration can improve perfusion.
• Blood products	Blood products may be indicated if hypovolemia is related to blood loss.
Promote oral intake:	
• Offer oral fluids that are the patient's preference, place in easy reach, provide a straw, and provide fresh water.	These measures are often effective in increasing fluid intake.
• Offer a variety of drinks and high-fluid-content foods.	Offering favorite drinks and foods often is effective in increasing fluid intake.
COGNITION: Offer patients with impaired mental status fluids at regular intervals.	Cognitive impairments can interfere with the recognition of thirst.
FUNCTIONAL ABILITY: Aid patients with physical conditions, such as dysphagia, weakness, or paralysis.	Without help, patients with physical conditions may be unable to achieve fluid balance.
Encourage caregivers to help the patient.	Caregiver engagement in patient care can be an effective way to increase oral intake.
Minimize intake of foods and drinks with diuretic or laxative effects, such as caffeine-containing fluids.	Limiting the intake of foods and drinks with diuretic or laxative effects decreases fluid loss.
Pediatric	
Offer appealing fluids (e.g., ice pops, frozen juice bars, snow cones, water, milk).	Appealing fluids may assist in increasing fluid intake.
Use age-appropriate unusual containers (colorful cups, decorative straws), games, charts, rewards, and activities.	Age-appropriate measures are often effective in increasing fluid intake.
Older Adult	
Offer the patient fluid at regular intervals.	A general decrease in thirst puts older adults at risk for not drinking enough fluids to maintain fluid balance.

COLLABORATION	RATIONALE
NUTRITION: Dietitian	Collaborating with a dietitian offers the patient further information and support for implementing the prescribed diet.
FUNCTIONAL ABILITY: Occupational therapy	The occupational therapist's plan of care is designed to promote independent performance of activities of daily living, including the ability to feed oneself.
GAS EXCHANGE: Respiratory therapy	Respiratory therapists assess, plan, and implement interventions that address potential problems to promote optimal respiratory function.

 PATIENT AND CAREGIVER TEACHING

- Cause of the fluid imbalance, if known, and how long it will last
- Normal fluid requirements
- Factors that predispose the patient to a fluid imbalance
- Management of an underlying condition contributing to the fluid imbalance
- Measures being used to treat the fluid imbalance
- Lifestyle changes to control or prevent a fluid imbalance
- Reason for fluid restrictions or hydration measures
- How to monitor intake, output, and daily weight
- Appropriate foods and fluids for the diet regimen
- Early recognition of problems and how to manage them
- Ways to maintain skin integrity
- When to notify the HCP

DOCUMENTATION

Assessment

- Assessments performed
- Diagnostic and laboratory test results
- Intake and output
- Manifestations of a fluid imbalance
- Screening test results

Interventions

- Discussions with other interprofessional team members
- Fluids and medications administered
- Notification of the HCP about patient status
- Therapeutic interventions and the patient's response
- Teaching provided
- Referrals and consults initiated
- Safety measures implemented, including fall precautions

Evaluation

- Patient's status: improved, stable, declined
- Presence of manifestations of a fluid imbalance
- Response to teaching provided
- Response to therapeutic interventions

Impaired Respiratory Function 18

DEFINITION

Inability to ventilate, clear the airway, and/or diffuse oxygen and carbon dioxide

Gas exchange is the process by which oxygen is transported to cells and carbon dioxide is transported from cells. This process requires the work of the neurologic, respiratory, and cardiovascular systems. The three phases of gas exchange are ventilation, transport, and perfusion. *Ventilation* is the process of inhaling oxygen into the lungs and exhaling carbon dioxide from the lungs. Ventilation may be impaired when oxygen is less available, such as at high altitudes, or when air is not moved effectively between the upper airway and the alveoli. *Transport* refers to the availability of hemoglobin to carry oxygen from alveoli to cells for metabolism and to carry carbon dioxide produced by cellular metabolism from cells to alveoli to be eliminated. Altered oxygen transport occurs when an insufficient number or quality of erythrocytes is available to carry oxygen or when the amount of hemoglobin in the blood is low. *Perfusion* refers to the ability of blood to transport oxygen-containing hemoglobin to cells and return carbon dioxide–containing hemoglobin to the alveoli (see Perfusion).

Hypoxemia is reduced oxygenation of arterial blood. *Hypoxia* is insufficient oxygen reaching cells, whereas anoxia is the total lack of oxygen in body tissues. Variations in gas exchange are seen among people across the life span, with multiple causative factors and a wide range of impact and duration. Nurses have a role in identifying problems with respiratory function and gas exchange. Essential nursing care includes monitoring physical assessment parameters, providing treatment, and monitoring the patient's response to treatment. Nurses may intervene in a crisis and help patients manage chronic respiratory conditions.

Associated Clinical Problems

- Abnormal Breath Sounds: unusual sounds heard over the airways and lung fields, such as fine and coarse crackles, wheezes, pleural rubs, and stridor
- Abnormal Sputum: material of an unusual amount, color, or components that is coughed up from the lungs
- Apnea: absence of spontaneous respirations
- Aspiration: inhaling foreign material or acidic vomitus into the lower airway
- Cough: sudden audible expulsion of air from the lungs, usually to clear the respiratory tract from debris
- Dyspnea: distressful subjective sensation of uncomfortable breathing
- Dyspnea at Rest: difficult or uncomfortable breathing without any exertion
- Dyspnea on Exertion: difficult or uncomfortable breathing during physical activity
- Hyperventilation: increased respiration rate and/or an increased tidal volume that exceeds what is needed for normal gas exchange
- Impaired Airway Clearance: difficulty in maintaining patent air passages
- Impaired Breathing: inspiratory and expiratory effort that does not provide adequate ventilation or gas exchange
- Impaired Gas Exchange: difficulty with ventilation, diffusion, or transport of oxygen and/or carbon dioxide
- Impaired Ventilatory Weaning: difficulty in maintaining gas exchange without continued mechanical support
- Posterior Rhinorrhea: discharge of a thin, watery nasal fluid from the sinuses down the back of the throat
- Risk for Apnea: increased risk for an absence of spontaneous respiration
- Risk for Aspiration: increased risk for inhaling foreign material or acidic vomitus
- Risk for Impaired Respiratory Function: increased risk for inability to ventilate, clear the airway, and/or diffuse oxygen and carbon dioxide
- Risk for Suffocation: increased risk for an interruption in breathing with oxygen deprivation, usually caused by an obstruction in the airways
- Wheezing: breath sounds of a high-pitched or low-pitched musical quality, caused by a high-velocity flow of air through a narrowed airway

Common Causes and Risk Factors

- Acute respiratory distress syndrome
- Acute respiratory failure
- Age-related changes, such as stiff chest wall, weak muscles, and decreased alveolar surface area

- Airway spasm
- Anemia
- Anxiety
- Asthma
- Bed rest, immobility
- Bronchoconstriction
- Cancer
- Chest wall deformity or trauma
- Chronic bronchitis
- Chronic obstructive pulmonary disease (COPD)
- Cystic fibrosis
- Decreased level of consciousness
- Excessive mucus
- Fatigue
- Foreign body in airway
- Heart failure
- Immunosuppression
- Infection, including tuberculosis and upper respiratory infection
- Neuromuscular impairment, spinal cord injury
- Obesity
- Obstructive sleep apnea
- Pain
- Pneumonia
- Pulmonary edema
- Pulmonary emboli
- Recent travel to or immigration from certain areas
- Respiratory muscle fatigue
- Smoking

Manifestations

- Absent, chronic, or ineffective cough
- Adventitious or diminished breath sounds
- Altered chest excursion
- Altered respiratory pattern or rate
- Bradypnea
- Central cyanosis
- Confusion
- Diaphoresis
- Difficulty speaking
- Dyspnea, at rest or with exertion
- Excessive sputum
- Headache upon awakening
- Increase in anterior-posterior chest diameter
- Low oxygen saturation
- Nasal flaring
- Orthopnea, use of three-point (tripod) position
- Pursed-lip breathing
- Requires oxygen to prevent hypoxemia
- Restlessness and irritability
- Rhinorrhea
- Somnolence
- Tachycardia
- Tachypnea
- Use of accessory muscles to breathe
- Wide-eyed look
- Diagnostic tests:
  - Arterial blood gases (ABGs) indicate respiratory acidosis, hypoxemia, and/or hypercarbia.
  - Complete blood count (CBC) indicates anemia.
  - Culture positive for infecting organism in sputum.
  - Chest radiography shows foreign bodies and infiltrates.
  - Spirometry shows altered respiratory volumes.

Key Conceptual Relationships

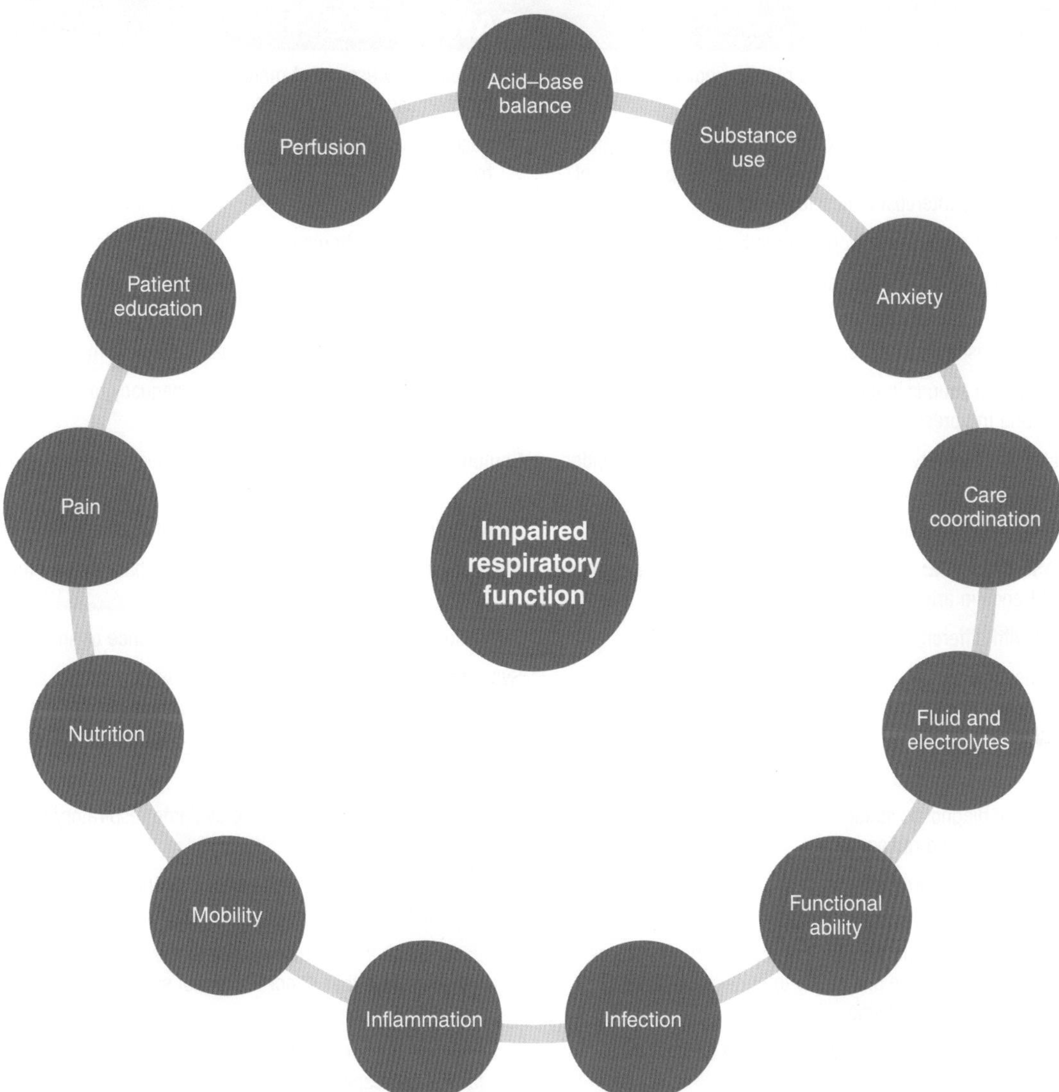

ASSESSMENT OF RESPIRATORY FUNCTION	RATIONALE
Identify patients in need of emergency management of respiratory problems.	Identifying the presence of a respiratory problem allows for the patient to be immediately stabilized.
Assess for risk factors for impaired respiratory function.	Identifying a patient's risk factors for impaired respiratory function allows early intervention.
Determine the potential cause of impaired respiratory function.	It is more effective to treat the cause rather than the imbalance.
Obtain a thorough history of any respiratory symptoms, such as cough or dyspnea, including: • When symptoms started • Onset, sudden or gradual • Frequency • Intensity or severity • Alleviating and aggravating factors • Any pattern to the symptoms	A thorough history aids in evaluating the degree of the patient's respiratory problem and helps direct treatment.
Obtain a complete vaccination history.	The vaccine history helps to identify the patient's risk for specific respiratory infections.

Continued

ASSESSMENT OF RESPIRATORY FUNCTION	RATIONALE
Perform a complete physical assessment and monitor indicators of impaired respiratory function on an ongoing basis.	Identifying the presence of manifestations of impaired respiratory function allows for early intervention.
• Assess the rate, rhythm, depth, and effort of respirations, noting chest symmetry, use of accessory muscles, and the presence of supraclavicular and intercostal muscle retractions.	Increased breathing effort may be an effort to compensate for hypoxemia.
• Monitor breathing pattern and work of breathing.	Altered breathing patterns may indicate neurologic or metabolic conditions.
• Monitor oxygen saturation levels, doing so continuously for patients who are sedated or have risk factors.	Oxygen saturation provides early warning of hypoxemia.
• Monitor for increased restlessness, anxiety, confusion, or air hunger.	Changes in mental status may be early signs of hypoxia.
• Auscultate breath sounds, noting areas of decreased or absent ventilation and the presence of adventitious sounds.	Breath sounds are an indicator of the adequacy of ventilation.
• Note quality and quantity of sputum produced and notify provider of a change to purulent sputum.	Sputum characteristics and changes provide clues to possible infection.
• **PERFUSION:** Heart rate and cardiac monitoring	Tachycardia is a common manifestation of impaired respiratory function.
• **ACID–BASE BALANCE:** Determine acid–base status by evaluating ABGs and trends in arterial pH, $Paco_2$, and HCO_3^-.	ABGs are a means to determine acid–base balance and the effectiveness of gas exchange.
• CBC count with differential	Evaluation of the CBC can confirm the presence of anemia.
• Oxygen consumption, such as Svo_2, if available	Svo_2 monitoring can be used to assess oxygen supply-and-demand balance and guide treatment that supports sufficient tissue oxygenation.
• Capnography, if available	Capnography gives information about carbon dioxide production and elimination.
Evaluate the results of diagnostic studies, including bronchoscopy, pulmonary function tests, and radiographs.	Diagnostic tests are performed to evaluate respiratory system function.
Obtain sputum specimens as ordered.	Sputum cultures determine the type of pathogen present and guide treatment.
FUNCTIONAL ABILITY: Determine the effect of respiratory symptoms on the patient's level of fatigue and ability to perform basic and instrumental activities of daily living.	The patient with a respiratory problem may have fatigue and other manifestations that affect functional status and activity tolerance.
SUBSTANCE USE: Screen for the presence of tobacco and/or other substance use problems.	Smoking and the presence of secondhand smoke are significant risk factors for respiratory problems.
Evaluate the patient's response to measures to correct impaired respiratory function through ongoing assessment.	Identifying the presence of manifestations of impaired respiratory function allows for evaluation of therapy effectiveness.
Pediatric	
Promptly address the presence of bradypnea, dyspnea, nasal flaring, orthopnea, tachypnea, and the use of accessory muscles to breathe.	These signs indicate ineffective breathing in children who may not communicate verbally.
Older Adult	
Assess for changes in the older adult's chest wall anatomy and cough mechanism.	Impaired cough mechanisms may lead to retention of pulmonary secretions, airway plugging, and atelectasis. Changes in the chest wall with aging, such as kyphosis, may restrict ventilation.

Expected Outcomes

The patient will:

- maintain a patent airway.
- report ability to breathe comfortably.
- have normal oxygen and carbon dioxide levels.
- maintain tissue oxygenation.

INTERVENTIONS FOR PROMOTING RESPIRATORY FUNCTION	RATIONALE
Implement collaborative interventions aimed at treating the underlying cause of the respiratory problem.	Respiratory function may improve with treatment of the underlying cause.
Be prepared to institute resuscitation protocols and respiratory support.	Support is needed in emergency situations to preserve life.
Administer oxygen therapy with humidification, as appropriate.	Oxygen therapy is used to prevent and correct hypoxia.
Notify the health care provider (HCP) if impaired respiratory function persists or worsens.	Achievement of an effective treatment plan often requires adjustments in therapy.
Administer medications as prescribed, including bronchodilators, β_2-adrenergic agonists, methylxanthines and derivatives, and anticholinergics.	Bronchodilators open the airways and decrease the risk of breathing difficulties.
• **INFLAMMATION:** Corticosteroids	Corticosteroids reduce inflammation in the respiratory tract.
• Leukotriene receptor antagonists and inhibitors	These drugs suppress leukotriene activity, inhibiting airway edema, bronchoconstriction, mucus production, and inflammation.
• Immunomodulators, including anti–immunoglobulin E (IgE) and anti–interleukin-5 drugs	Immunomodulators inhibit the immune response.
• **INFECTION:** Antimicrobials	The appropriate antimicrobial therapy is given to treat any respiratory infection.
• Antihistamines	Antihistamines block histamine release, relieving acute symptoms of an allergic response.
• Decongestants	Decongestants promote vasoconstriction of superficial vessels in the nose and reduce nasal congestion.
• Mucolytics	Mucolytics help break up tenacious mucus, making it easier to expel by coughing.
• **FLUID AND ELECTROLYTES:** Intravenous (IV) fluid therapy	Liquefying secretions facilitates their removal by coughing.
• Sedatives	Sedation may be needed for a patient who is hyperventilating.
• **PAIN:** Analgesics	Analgesics reduce dyspnea by aiding with pain management.
Implement measures to promote clearance of secretions: have the patient breathe deeply and cough (inhale, hold, cough two or three times) as needed.	Deep breathing and coughing promote the clearance of secretions.
Encourage the use of incentive spirometry as needed.	The visual reinforcement of the spirometer may be useful.
Encourage the patient to splint the painful area with a pillow, towel, or hands with deep breathing and coughing.	Splinting helps minimize localized pain.
Encourage slow, deep breathing; turning; and coughing for patients with limited mobility.	Position changes and coughs help mobilize secretions.
For patients with COPD or an inability to cough normally, teach the huff cough (deep breath, hold, then say "huff, huff").	This alternative cough technique is useful for patients with airway obstructive conditions.
Perform chest physical therapy or teach the patient to use a flutter device as prescribed.	Chest physical therapy may help mobilize secretions.
If the patient is unable to clear secretions, consider secretion removal by suctioning.	Patients too weak to cough forcefully may be unable to clear the airway independently.
MOBILITY: Assist the patient to change positions and or ambulate as able while monitoring for changes in oxygenation related to position.	Position changes help mobilize secretions; oxygenation may vary with positions.
Promote adequate rest periods, such as 90-minute periods of undisturbed sleep, organized nursing care, and limited visitors, as appropriate.	Rest interspersed with care activities reduces oxygen consumption and fatigue.
Position the patient to optimize respiratory function, such as: • Semi-Fowler's, high Fowler's, sitting up in chair while leaning on padded overbed table • Lying with the "good lung down" • Prone positioning	Depending on the patient situation, positioning in a certain manner promotes gas exchange, enhances ventilation, and decreases the work of breathing.
FLUID AND ELECTROLYTES: Ensure adequate fluid intake.	Liquefying secretions facilitates their removal by coughing.

Continued

INTERVENTIONS FOR PROMOTING RESPIRATORY FUNCTION	RATIONALE
INFECTION: Administer vaccinations as needed, according to recommended schedules and patient need.	Vaccinations can be effective in preventing common infections, such as influenza, pertussis, diphtheria, and pneumonia.
SUBSTANCE USE: Implement measures to address substance use, particularly smoking or vaping behaviors, if present.	Smoking and the presence of secondhand smoke are significant risk factors for respiratory problems.
NUTRITION: Ensure adequate nutrition with small, frequent meals and supplements during the acute phase.	Dyspnea may prevent oral intake of adequate calories, and loss of muscle mass may impair respiratory effort.
Assist the patient with developing a regular physical activity plan, considering capabilities, daily routine, and personal preferences.	Regular physical activity is an important part of care for many patients because it builds endurance and maintains the strength of the respiratory muscles.
ANXIETY: Provide measures to promote comfort and reduce anxiety, as appropriate.	These measures reduce oxygen consumption and minimize hyperventilation.
Provide oral hygiene every 4 hours or as needed.	Oral hygiene removes secretions, debris, and plaque, maintaining the integrity of the mucous membranes and reducing the risk of infection.
FUNCTIONAL ABILITY: Help patient with activities of daily living, as needed.	Impaired respiratory function can result in fatigue and other symptoms that can interfere with the ability to complete activities of daily living.
Pediatric	
Use games to encourage deep breathing (blow bubbles with bubble blower, blow on pinwheel, whistle, harmonica, feather).	Engage children in care by adding fun.

INTERVENTIONS TO RELIEVE DYSPNEA	RATIONALE
Ensure airflow in the environment and/or provide a gentle fan in the room.	The sensation of air movement may provide some relief from dyspnea.
Stay in the patient's line of sight when possible and ensure the call bell is within reach if leaving the patient temporarily.	Seeing the caregiver may help avoid panic, which may increase respiratory distress.

INTERVENTIONS TO FACILITATE VENTILATOR WEANING	RATIONALE
Collaborate with members of the health care team to develop and implement a weaning plan.	The use of a weaning protocol decreases ventilator days.
Perform a spontaneous breathing trial (SBT) daily for patients who meet criteria.	An SBT assesses the patient's ability to breathe and be weaned from respiratory assistance.
Implement measures to promote successful weaning: • Choose a time when the patient is comfortable and well rested. • Limit use of medications associated with respiratory depression. • Provide emotional support for the patient. • Allow the patient to rest as needed.	Support measures enhance the patient's ability to be successfully weaned from mechanical ventilation.

INTERVENTIONS TO DECREASE RISK FOR ASPIRATION	RATIONALE
Collaborate with speech and occupational therapists to provide an appropriate patient plan, including diet and use of assistive devices.	Speech and occupational therapists provide in-depth clinical assessment and recommend strategies to treat swallowing problems.
Provide food and fluids of the appropriate consistency, based on the swallowing evaluation.	Modifying the consistency of foods and fluids improves the patient's ability to swallow, with a reduced risk of choking.
Provide an environment to promote swallowing: • Remove distractions. • Have the patient in an upright position, with the head flexed forward. • Keep the patient upright for 30 minutes after eating.	These measures assist with reducing the risk of aspiration associated with a swallowing problem.

COLLABORATION	RATIONALE
Pulmonary rehabilitation	The aim of pulmonary rehabilitation is to build respiratory strength to minimize disease exacerbations.
Respiratory therapy	Respiratory therapists assess, plan, and implement interventions that promote a person's optimal respiratory function.
Dietitian	Collaborating with a dietitian offers the patient further information and support for implementing the prescribed diet.
Disease or symptom management programs	Disease or symptom management programs help patients understand their treatment regimen and address the complex needs of those with chronic illness.
Speech therapy	A swallowing evaluation by a speech therapist can detect changes in swallowing ability that affect the ability to safely consume a nutritionally sound diet.
CARE COORDINATION: Social services or case management	Support may be needed to obtain financial, transportation, or other resources.
Community or online support groups	Many patients with chronic respiratory disease find benefit in the support offered by persons with similar concerns.
Physical therapy	Physical therapists can assess the patient and develop a plan of care to maximize exercise capability.

PATIENT AND CAREGIVER TEACHING

- Cause of impaired respiratory function, if known
- Manifestations of impaired respiratory function
- Management of any underlying condition causing impaired respiratory function
- Measures being used to improve respiratory function and reduce the risk of complications
- Need for monitoring ABG analyses, sputum studies, chest radiographs, and other tests
- Coughing and deep breathing techniques
- Importance of avoiding smoking, vaping, and secondhand smoke
- Safe use of medications, including proper use, side effect management, administration, and how they fit into the overall management plan
- Safe use of oxygen and respiratory equipment
- Use of peak expiratory flow rate (PEFR) meter and when to seek medical attention
- Use of metered-dose inhalers
- Any needed lifestyle changes to promote respiratory function
- Early recognition of problems and how to manage them
- Need to avoid exposure to persons with upper respiratory infections and crowds of people
- Recommended immunizations (influenza, pneumococcus, pertussis, others)
- Hand hygiene techniques
- Community precautions, such as wearing of masks, if needed
- Importance of health promotion behaviors, including nutrition, sleep, and exercise
- Signs and symptoms of infection
- Community and self-help resources, additional information available
- Importance of long-term follow-up if appropriate
- When to notify the HCP and seek additional care

DOCUMENTATION

Assessment
- Manifestations of impaired respiratory function
- Diagnostic test results
- Assessments performed
- ABG results

Interventions
- Medications given
- Notification of HCP about diagnostic test results and assessment findings
- Therapeutic interventions and the patient's response
- Teaching provided
- Referrals made
- Precautions implemented
- Environmental modifications made

Evaluation
- Patient's status: improved, stable, declined
- Diagnostic test results
- Patient's response to therapeutic interventions
- Patient's response to teaching provided
- Presence of any manifestations of altered respiratory function

Altered Blood Glucose Level 19

Definition

Impaired ability to maintain optimal blood glucose levels

The process of maintaining optimal blood glucose levels requires a balance between nutrient intake, hormonal responses, and glucose uptake by the cells. After food is eaten, insulin is released in response to rising glucose levels. Insulin facilitates glucose metabolism by binding to insulin receptors on the cell wall, signaling molecules that facilitate glucose entry into the cell. Insulin suppresses glucagon secretion and facilitates glycogen storage. After glucose enters a cell, the glucose is oxidized through cellular respiration to provide energy.

Glucose metabolism is reflected in circulating blood glucose levels. Normal blood glucose levels range between 70 and 99 mg/dL in the fasting state and 100 and 140 mg/dL in the 2-hour post meal state. Impaired glucose regulation is seen in abnormally high or low blood glucose levels.

Hyperglycemia occurs because of insufficient insulin production or secretion, insulin resistance, or excessive counterregulatory hormones (glucagon, epinephrine, cortisol, and growth hormone). The American Diabetes Association (ADA) recognizes four different classes of diabetes: type 1 and type 2 diabetes, gestational diabetes, and other specific types of diabetes with various causes. Diabetes is a major contributor to heart disease, stroke, and cancer and is the leading cause of adult blindness, end-stage renal disease, and nontraumatic lower-limb amputations. Managing diabetes and keeping blood glucose levels within normal limits require the individual to make daily decisions about food intake, blood glucose monitoring, medication, and exercise.

Glycemic control is assessed using hemoglobin $A1_c$ ($HbA1_c$) values, continuous glucose monitoring, or serial blood glucose monitoring (BGM). An $HbA1_c$ goal for many nonpregnant adults (without significant hypoglycemia) is <7% (53 mmol/mol). Glycemic goals can be individualized to the patient to promote adherence and avoid episodes of hypoglycemia. Hypoglycemia, a cellular deficiency of glucose, typically occurs because of insufficient nutritional intake, an adverse reaction to medications, excessive exercise, or as a consequence of disease states. Glucagon is a hormone released in response to hypoglycemia. Glucagon suppresses insulin and stimulates the liver to break down glycogen, which raises glucose levels.

Successful blood glucose management involves ongoing interaction among the patient, caregiver, and interprofessional team. Nurses play a vital role in promoting the patient's self-management of glucose levels by providing comprehensive patient and caregiver education.

Associated Clinical Problems

- Hyperglycemia: state of elevated blood glucose levels, generally defined as greater than 100 mg/dL in the fasting state or greater than 140 mg/dL 2 hours postprandial
- Hypoglycemia: state of insufficient or low blood glucose levels, defined as less than 70 mg/dL

Common Causes and Risk Factors for Hyperglycemia

- Autoimmune disorder
- Cystic fibrosis
- Endocrine problems, including Cushing syndrome, hyperthyroidism, acromegaly
- Ethnicity, particularly persons who are Black, Asian American, Hispanic, Native Hawaiian or other Pacific Islanders, or Native American
- Family history of type 2 diabetes, obesity, or metabolic syndrome
- Having a large-for-gestational-age infant
- Hemochromatosis
- Medications: angiotensin-converting enzyme (ACE) inhibitors, antibiotics, antipsychotics, β-blockers, bronchodilators, corticosteroids, estrogen, phenytoin, potassium-depleting diuretics
- Metabolic syndrome
- Neonate of mother with diabetes
- Obesity
- Parenteral nutrition
- Pregnancy
- Recurrent pancreatitis

Common Causes and Risk Factors for Hypoglycemia

- Alcohol use without food intake
- Delayed, omitted, or inadequate food intake
- Insulin or oral hypoglycemic agents taken at wrong time or at too large of a dose
- Too much exercise without adequate food intake

Common Causes and Risk Factors for the Patient With Known Diabetes

- Change in eating, insulin, or exercise plan

- Inadequate treatment of diabetes
- Lack of knowledge about diabetes management
- Nonadherence to diabetes management plan
- Recent trauma, infection, or illness

Manifestations

Key Conceptual Relationships

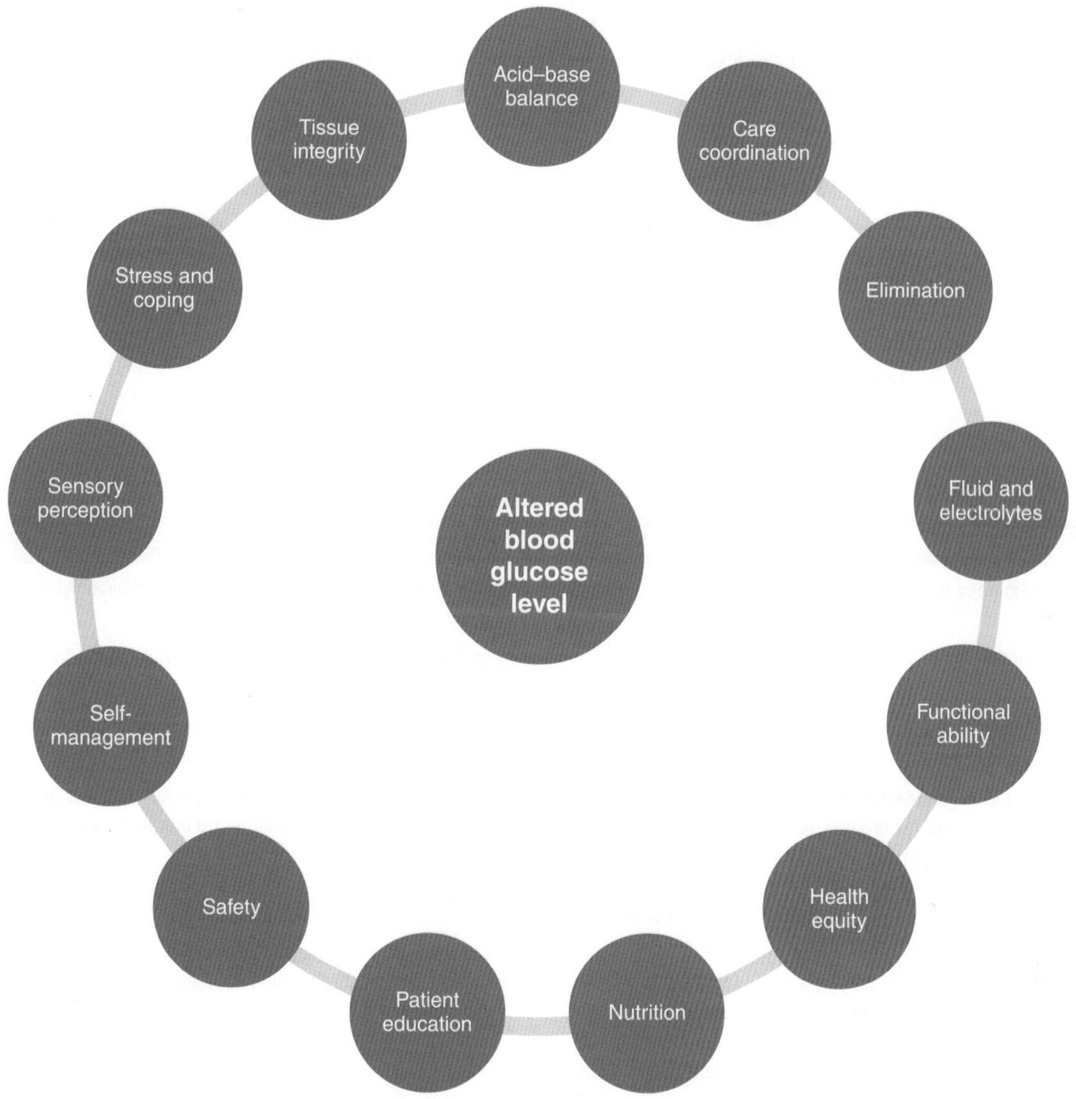

Comparing Manifestations of Hyperglycemia and Hypoglycemia

Type of Manifestation	Hyperglycemia	Hypoglycemia
Cardiovascular	Tachycardia if dehydrated	Tachycardia
Cognition/mood	Impaired cognition Coma if untreated ketoacidosis	Anxiety Behavior changes Difficulty concentrating Dizziness, faintness Impaired cognition Irritability, nervousness Seizures, coma
Gastrointestinal	Abdominal cramps Nausea, vomiting	

Continued

Comparing Manifestations of Hyperglycemia and Hypoglycemia

Type of Manifestation	Hyperglycemia	Hypoglycemia
General	Fatigue, malaise Impaired wound healing	Tremors Unsteady gait, slurred speech
Laboratory studies	Elevated blood glucose, glycosylated hemoglobin ($HbA1_c$) >6.5%, acidosis, abnormal potassium levels	Blood glucose <70 mg/dL (3.9 mmol/L)
Respiratory	Deep, rapid respirations Acetone odor to breath	
Sensory	Blurred vision Excessive hunger Excessive thirst Peripheral neuropathy	Headache Hunger Vision changes Numbness of fingers, toes, or mouth
Skin	Warm, moist skin	Cold, clammy skin Diaphoresis Pallor
Urinary	Nocturia, polyuria Ketonuria, glycosuria Bladder infections	

ASSESSMENT OF BLOOD GLUCOSE	RATIONALE
Identify patients who need emergency management of an altered blood glucose level.	Identifying the presence of hyperglycemia or hypoglycemia allows for early intervention.
Determine the potential cause of an altered blood glucose level.	It may be necessary to treat the cause while also addressing the altered blood glucose level.
Perform a complete physical assessment and monitor indicators of an altered blood glucose level on an ongoing basis.	Identifying manifestations of an altered blood glucose level allows for early intervention and prevention of complications
NUTRITION: Obtain blood glucose levels as needed: • When hypoglycemia or hyperglycemia is suspected • Before meals and snacks • At bedtime • Every 4–6 hours in the patient not receiving nutrition or receiving continuous enteral or parenteral nutrition	Knowing the blood glucose level allows adjustments to be made and appropriate doses of insulin to be administered as needed.
Elicit history from the patient and/or caregiver about factors that preceded a specific episode about hypoglycemia or hyperglycemia, including: • Time of last food intake and what was eaten • Recent medications taken, noting time and any antiglycemic drugs • Recent blood glucose levels • Onset of symptoms • Symptoms experienced • Time of last exercise and duration • Last alcohol intake, if any	Many times, a specific episode is precipitated by a known cause, such as management of diet, activity, or medications, or an acute illness.
Evaluate blood glucose levels in ill or hospitalized patients before administering oral hypoglycemic agents or insulin.	Blood glucose levels may be more variable in illness and when off the patient's usual schedule.
SELF-MANAGEMENT: Assess recent $HbA1_c$ level and compare to patient's trend over time.	This evaluates glucose control over the previous 3 months.
SELF-MANAGEMENT: Assess the patient's self-management of hypoglycemia and hyperglycemia: • How episodes of hypoglycemia and hyperglycemia are being managed • Adherence to the medication regimen and whether the patient is adjusting insulin doses • Adjustments made for exercise or illness • Customary dietary intake and relationship to taking medications	An assessment will identify any deviations from the plan of care that may cause hypoglycemia or hyperglycemia.

ASSESSMENT OF BLOOD GLUCOSE	RATIONALE
FUNCTIONAL ABILITY: Assess the patient and caregiver's ability to perform blood glucose monitoring and administer injections.	Assistive devices or referrals for assistance may be needed for the patient and/or caregiver to safely perform actions that contribute to blood glucose management goals.
Obtain a complete medication history, noting medications known to affect blood glucose levels or associated with drug interactions with antiglycemic drugs.	Numerous drugs can cause fluctuations in blood glucose levels or interact with antiglycemic drugs, altering their effectiveness.

ASSESSMENT OF HYPERGLYCEMIA	RATIONALE
ACID–BASE BALANCE: Determine acid–base status by evaluating arterial blood gas values (ABGs) and trends in arterial pH, $Paco_2$, and HCO_3^-.	ABGs can determine the presence of metabolic acidosis, a common occurrence with hyperglycemia.
SENSORY PERCEPTION: Assess for complications of hyperglycemia, including peripheral neuropathy and vision impairment.	Hyperglycemia is associated with microvascular and macrovascular complications.
ELIMINATION: Review laboratory results to evaluate kidney function.	Hyperglycemia may cause nephropathy over time.

Expected Outcomes

The patient will:

- maintain blood glucose in the normal range.
- maintain $HbA1_c$ <7%.
- be free from complications of long-term hyperglycemia.
- recognize factors that may lead to altered blood glucose levels and take preventive action.
- engage in self-management of diabetes.

INTERVENTIONS TO STABILIZE BLOOD GLUCOSE LEVELS	RATIONALE
SELF-MANAGEMENT: Reinforce and teach blood glucose self-monitoring and recording.	Self-management helps with control of glucose levels.
Encourage regular exercise five times per week, reviewing the need for glucose testing and adjustment of food intake and activity based on glucose level.	Regular exercise helps with glucose control.
PATIENT EDUCATION: Periodically evaluate the accuracy of glucose self-monitoring and insulin dosing.	Changes in vision and development of peripheral neuropathy may create challenges with physical skills.
SAFETY: Provide a safe environment for the patient with neurologic or neuromuscular manifestations by initiating fall and seizure precautions.	Changes in cognition and the potential for seizures often accompany altered blood glucose levels.
Stress the importance of carrying identification stating the patient has diabetes.	Identification allows health care personnel to properly care for the patient who is unable to communicate.
SELF-MANAGEMENT: Implement measures to assist the patient with adhering to the therapeutic plan, such as setting up memory aids and automated reminders and using diabetes management apps.	Reminders to check glucose levels and tracking diabetes information through management tools can be helpful in adherence by improving the patient's decision-making abilities.
FUNCTIONAL ABILITY: Assist the patient in obtaining any needed adaptive devices (e.g., insulin syringe magnifiers).	Adaptive devices can assist the patient in being able to self-manage their diabetes adequately.
Properly obtain blood glucose, ABG, and laboratory specimens.	A test value may be compromised by specimens that have not been properly collected, labeled, handled, or stored prior to and during the testing process.
Notify the health care provider (HCP) if manifestations of altered blood glucose levels persist or worsen.	Achievement of an effective treatment plan often requires adjustments in therapy.

INTERVENTIONS TO MANAGE HYPERGLYCEMIA	RATIONALE
Institute emergency protocols according to agency policy when the patient is experiencing hyperglycemia:	
• Titrate intravenous (IV) insulin drip based on frequent blood glucose testing.	IV insulin can cause rapid changes in blood glucose levels.
• **SAFETY:** If administering an IV insulin drip, monitor blood glucose every 30 minutes to 2 hours.	IV insulin can cause rapid changes in blood glucose levels.
• Ensure patent airway and apply oxygen via nasal cannula or nonrebreather mask as needed.	Oxygen therapy is used to prevent and correct any hypoxia.
FLUID AND ELECTROLYTES: Administer prescribed IV fluids.	Fluids support adequate hydration and restoration of normal fluid volumes.
Test urine for ketones during acute illness, trauma, surgery, or stress.	Stress may precipitate ketoacidosis.
Administer antiglycemic drugs as ordered, based on blood glucose level.	Antiglycemic drugs lower elevated blood glucose levels.

INTERVENTIONS TO MANAGE HYPOGLYCEMIA	RATIONALE
Institute emergency protocols according to agency policy when the patient is experiencing hypoglycemia: *Conscious Patient* • Have the patient eat or drink 15 g of quick-acting carbohydrates (e.g., 4–6 oz of regular soda, 5–8 hard candies, 1 tablespoon syrup or honey, 4 teaspoons jelly, 4–6 oz orange juice, commercial dextrose products). • Wait 15 minutes. Recheck glucose. • If blood glucose is still <70 mg/dL, have patient repeat treatment of 15 g of carbohydrate. • Once the glucose level is stable, give the patient additional food of carbohydrates plus protein or fat (e.g., crackers with peanut butter or cheese) if the next meal is more than 1 hour away or the patient is engaged in physical activity. • Immediately notify the HCP or emergency service (if patient is outside the hospital) if symptoms do not subside after two or three doses of quick-acting carbohydrates. *Worsening Symptoms or Unconscious Patient* • Administer subcutaneous or intramuscular (IM) injection of 1 mg glucagon or 20–50 mL of 50% glucose IV.	Restoring glucose level to normal levels through glucose administration helps prevent injury.
Remind the patient not to drive or perform dangerous activities when hypoglycemic symptoms are noted.	Falls or other injuries may result when hypoglycemic.
Ensure that the patient always has ready access to emergency supplies, including candy, sugar paste, and glucagon.	Access to emergency supplies is needed to treat episodes of hypoglycemia quickly.
Ensure that caregivers can test glucose and administer glucose and glucagon.	The patient may not be able to provide self-care when experiencing hypoglycemia.

COLLABORATION	RATIONALE
Diabetes educator	Diabetes educators focus on teaching people with diabetes how to self-manage to achieve optimal blood glucose management.
NUTRITION: Dietitian	A dietitian offers the patient further information and support in implementing the prescribed diet for managing glucose levels and maintaining weight goals.
Support groups	Diabetes support groups can help the patient with resolving challenges they may encounter in managing diabetes.

COLLABORATION	RATIONALE
SELF-MANAGEMENT: Diabetes self-management program	Disease or symptom management programs help patients understand their treatment regimen and address the complex needs of those with chronic illness.
HEALTH EQUITY, CARE COORDINATION: Social work or case management	Social workers and case managers can explore resources for access to appropriate health care to manage diabetes and maintain continuity of care.
School nurse, counselor, social worker, or school psychologist	These individuals can provide the services necessary to ensure the needs of a child with diabetes are met at school.
DEVELOPMENTAL: Child-life specialist	Experts can assist the child with coping strategies for the stress of chronic illness.
SENSORY PERCEPTION: Ophthalmologist	An annual eye examination by an ophthalmologist can detect and manage retinopathy associated with hyperglycemia.

PATIENT AND CAREGIVER TEACHING

- The causes and effects of diabetes
- How hyperglycemia and hypoglycemia occur
- Recognizing and treating hypoglycemia and hyperglycemia
- Blood glucose self-monitoring and recording
- Safe administration of oral antiglycemic drugs and/or insulin
- How to adjust insulin based on blood glucose levels
- Eating patterns, stressing effects on blood glucose and timing with medications
- Proper use and disposal of needles and syringes if applicable
- Treatment options, such as continuous glucose monitoring and insulin pumps
- Sick day management
- Effect of regular exercise on managing blood glucose and how to adjust medications and food intake for exercise
- Effect of stress on blood glucose
- Effect of alcohol use on glucose levels and monitoring needed with alcohol intake
- Management of any underlying condition causing altered glucose regulation
- Measures to reduce the risk of complications
- Foot care and the need to inspect the feet daily
- Lifestyle changes to help control blood glucose levels
- Anticipatory guidance for problem situations, such as time-zone travel, shift work
- When to notify the HCP

DOCUMENTATION

Assessment

- Assessments performed
- Manifestations of hypoglycemia or hyperglycemia
- Diagnostic and laboratory test results
- Home blood glucose testing results

Interventions

- Discussions with other members of the interprofessional team
- Medications given
- Notification of the HCP about patient status
- Therapeutic interventions and the patient's response
- Teaching provided
- Referrals initiated
- Precautions implemented

Evaluation

- Patient's status: improved, stable, declined
- Patient's response to teaching provided
- Diagnostic test results
- Patient's response to therapeutic interventions
- Presence of any complications

Impaired Endocrine Function 20

Definition

A problem involving the mechanisms that regulate the secretion and action of hormones of the endocrine system

The glands and organs of the endocrine system are involved in the synthesis and secretion of hormones that affect all body systems. Many problems can lead to hormone imbalance. Endocrine problems can result from too much or too little of a specific hormone. Glands and hormone actions are influenced by the aging process, particularly during adolescence and among older adults. The severity of a problem varies widely. Subtle or vague symptoms are often attributed to other physiologic or psychologic causes, especially in the older adult. Other patients present with life-threatening symptoms that demand immediate intervention.

Your careful assessment may reveal early and subtle changes in the patient suspected of having impaired endocrine system function. Because of the wide range of actions of hormones, endocrine problems are associated with changes that can affect many aspects of a person's life and lead to a decreased quality of life. You may see adverse effects on perfusion, metabolism, and nutrition. Regulating fluid and electrolyte balance, skin integrity, and temperature may be difficult. The patient may have problems with growth and reproductive processes because these are hormone dependent. There may be a wide range of psychologic responses, including anxiety and depression. Patient teaching focusing on the long-term management of problems is important.

Common Risk Factors

- Advancing age
- Autoimmune condition
- Cancer, history of cancer treatment
- Chronic medical condition
- Family history of an endocrine problem
- Hypothalamic–pituitary disease
- Medications: hormone therapy, corticosteroids
- Multiple endocrine neoplasia
- Obesity
- Pregnancy
- Sedentary lifestyle
- Stress
- Trauma

Manifestations

- Behavior changes
- Changes in bowel habits
- Electrolyte imbalance
- Fatigue
- Fluid imbalance
- Headache
- Menstrual changes
- Mood problems, including anxiety, irritability, depression
- Muscle weakness
- Skin, hair, and nail changes
- Sleep problems
- Weight changes

Key Conceptual Relationships

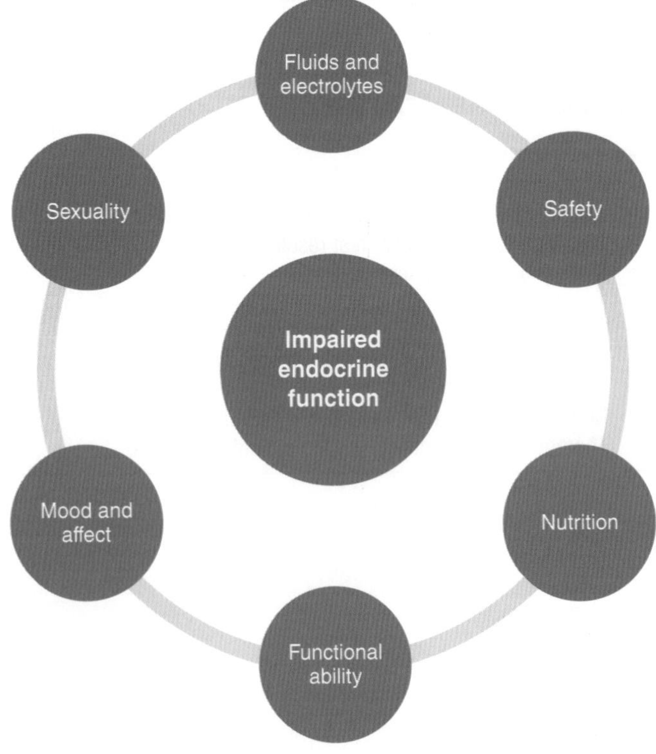

ASSESSMENT OF ENDOCRINE FUNCTION	RATIONALE
Identify patients who need emergency management for an endocrine problem so that they can be stabilized.	Identifying an acute endocrine-related emergency allows for early intervention.
Assess risk factors for an endocrine problem.	Identifying factors that place the patient at risk for an endocrine problem allows for early intervention.
Determine the potential cause of an endocrine problem.	It is more effective to treat the cause of the endocrine problem rather than the hormone imbalance.
Ask about the use of all medications, herbs, and diet supplements, including the reason for taking the drug, the dosage, and the length of time the drug has been taken.	Drug–drug interactions and adverse medication effects can contribute to endocrine problems.
Perform a complete physical assessment and monitor indicators of endocrine function on an ongoing basis:	
• Vital signs	Variations in temperature, heart rate, and blood pressure can occur with an endocrine problem.
• **NUTRITION:** Height and weight, calculation of body mass index (BMI)	These measures help determine the degree of body fat and an optimal weight.
• Color, pigmentation, and texture of the skin, hair, and nails	Changes in skin pigmentation, skin texture and moisture, and hair distribution can occur with an endocrine problem.
• Manifestations of a specific endocrine problem	Identifying manifestations of an endocrine problem allows for early intervention.
• **MOOD AND AFFECT:** Mental status and screening for coexisting psychologic problems	Many patients with an endocrine problem have depression, anxiety, or other psychologic problems.
• Serum and urine hormone levels	One of the best ways to assess hormone function is a direct measure of the hormone level in the blood or urine.
• Stimulation and suppression testing	These tests evaluate hormone secretion and inhibition.
• **FLUID AND ELECTROLYTES:** Indicators of electrolyte and fluid balance, including electrolyte levels, intake and output, and weight changes	Many endocrine problems are accompanied by fluid and electrolyte imbalances.
NUTRITION: Obtain a detailed weight history, noting changes in weight, whether the changes are unintentional, or if there are changes in appetite.	Changes in appetite and weight are common indicators of an endocrine problem.
SEXUALITY: Obtain a detailed history of menstruation.	Menstrual problems can occur with disorders of the ovaries and the pituitary, thyroid, and the adrenal glands.
FUNCTIONAL ABILITY: Perform a psychosocial assessment, evaluating for lifestyle effects of a hormone imbalance, such as on the ability to sleep, interact with others, perform work and household duties, and engage in physical and social activities.	Hormone imbalance may affect many aspects of life.
SAFETY: Monitor for side effects of prescribed hormone replacement or suppression therapies.	Identifying side effects of hormone replacement or suppression therapy allows for early intervention.
Monitor for complications associated with an endocrine problem.	Identifying complications allows for early intervention.
Evaluate response to measures to correct an endocrine problem.	Identifying manifestations of hormone imbalance allows for evaluation of therapy effectiveness.
Pediatric	
Screen newborn infants for congenital hypothyroidism as part of the uniform screening panel.	Thyroid screening in infants allows for early intervention.
DEVELOPMENT: Assess the child's growth patterns and stages of physical and emotional development.	Endocrine problems can cause growth, physical, and emotional development problems that require early intervention.

Expected Outcomes

The patient will:

- achieve and maintain hormone balance.
- be free of manifestations of an endocrine problem.

- be free of complications from altered hormone levels.
- adhere to the prescribed therapeutic regimen.
- appropriately use pharmacologic therapies to achieve hormone balance.
- maintain nutrition balance.

INTERVENTIONS TO PROMOTE ENDOCRINE SYSTEM FUNCTION	RATIONALE
Implement collaborative interventions aimed at treating the underlying cause of an endocrine problem.	Hormone imbalance may resolve with treatment of the underlying cause.
Institute resuscitation protocols according to agency policy when the patient is experiencing an endocrine emergency.	The goal of emergency management is to prevent life-threatening complications that occur because of hypersecretion or deficiency of hormones.
Notify the health care provider (HCP) if manifestations of an endocrine problem persist or worsen.	Achieving an effective treatment plan often requires adjustments in therapy.
Administer prescribed medication therapy for the specific endocrine problem.	Medication therapies are used to control hormone synthesis, replace hormones, and manage the effects of altered hormone levels.
Emphasize the importance of adhering to the drug plan.	Abruptly stopping drug therapy can result in an exacerbation of an endocrine problem.
FLUID AND ELECTROLYTES: Implement measures to address any fluid and electrolyte imbalance.	Therapy may be needed to correct fluid and electrolyte imbalances that accompany many endocrine problems.
Administer IV fluid therapy as prescribed.	IV fluid therapy is administered to achieve and maintain fluid balance.
NUTRITION: Provide prescribed diet for the patient's weight and specific endocrine problem, such as a low-sodium or no added salt diet.	The appropriate diet can assist with the management of hormone imbalance.
Institute measures to manage the GI effects of an endocrine problem.	Appropriate management of adverse GI effects can increase the patient's comfort level and promote optimal nutrition.
SEXUALITY: Implement measures to address any impaired sexual function the patient may be experiencing.	Endocrine problems are frequently associated with impaired sexual function, including decreased libido and erectile dysfunction.
DEVELOPMENT: Implement measures to address any body image concerns the patient is experiencing.	Persons with an endocrine problem may have a negative self-image with low self-esteem.
THERMOREGULATION: Implement measures to maintain normothermia.	Variations in temperature can occur with many endocrine problems.
Properly obtain laboratory specimens for hormone levels.	Test values may be compromised by specimens that have not been properly collected, labeled, handled, or stored prior to and during the testing process.
FUNCTIONAL ABILITY: Help the patient prioritize activities and alternate rest and activity periods.	Hormone imbalance can result in muscle weakness, fatigue, and other manifestations that can interfere with activities of daily living.
SAFETY: Provide a safe environment for the patient with neuromuscular manifestations by initiating fall and seizure precautions.	Changes in cognition and the potential for seizures may accompany a hormone imbalance.
FUNCTIONAL ABILITY: Help the patient develop strategies to assist with participation in activities of daily living in the home, at work, and socially.	Facilitating participation in activities of daily living will improve patients' functional ability.
MOOD AND AFFECT: Ensure treatment for coexisting psychologic problems.	Treating an underlying psychologic problem is important to enhancing quality of life.
STRESS AND COPING: Help the patient develop positive coping behaviors.	Enhanced coping skills equip patients for improved self-management of an endocrine problem.
FUNCTIONAL ABILITY: Implement measures to promote positive social interaction.	Social interaction can decrease the isolation associated with fatigue and decreased functional ability.

COLLABORATION	RATIONALE
STRESS AND COPING: Counseling	Hormone imbalances can affect self-confidence, so patients may benefit from counseling to promote effective coping.
Support groups	Hormone imbalances can affect interpersonal relationships, so patients may benefit from peer support groups to promote effective coping.
NUTRITION: Dietitian	Collaborating with a dietitian offers the patient further information and support for implementing the prescribed diet.

PATIENT AND CAREGIVER TEACHING

- Cause of the endocrine problem, if known
- Manifestations of the endocrine problem
- Factors contributing to the endocrine problem
- Role of the endocrine system in maintaining health
- Measures being used to treat the endocrine problem
- Continued laboratory monitoring
- Lifestyle changes to control the endocrine problem
- Safe use of medications, including hormone replacement therapies, and how they fit into the overall management plan
- Appropriate foods and fluids for the diet regimen
- Early recognition of problems and how to manage them
- Importance of long-term follow-up
- When to notify the HCP

DOCUMENTATION

Assessment

- Assessments performed
- Diagnostic and laboratory test results
- Manifestations of an endocrine problem

Interventions

- Discussions with other interprofessional team members
- Medications given
- Notification of the HCP about patient status
- Therapeutic interventions and the patient's response
- Teaching provided
- Referrals initiated

Evaluation

- Patient's status: improved, stable, declined
- Presence of manifestations of an endocrine problem
- Response to teaching provided
- Response to therapeutic interventions

Increased Intracranial Pressure 21

Definition

A potentially life-threatening situation that results from an increase in brain tissue, blood, and/or CSF within the skull

The brain, part of the central nervous system, is the primary structure associated with intracranial regulation. Normal intracranial regulation involves interaction among brain structures through a complex communication system. Neurons are cells in the nervous system that transmit information within the brain and throughout the body.

Brain function depends on a consistent supply of blood that delivers oxygen and nutrients. The body has various ways to regulate the intracranial space and promote optimal brain function. Acute intracranial problems can disrupt these processes, leading to increased intracranial pressure (ICP), reduced blood flow to the brain, and brain tissue damage. Head injuries, brain tumors, cerebral infections, and inflammatory disorders are common problems that disrupt intracranial regulation.

Normal ICP is 5 to 15 mm Hg; pressures over 20 mm Hg are treated aggressively. Increased ICP is a potentially life-threatening situation that results from an increase in any or all of the three components (brain tissue, blood, cerebrospinal fluid [CSF]) within the closed skull structure. Increased ICP is clinically significant because it decreases cerebral perfusion pressure (CPP), increases risks for brain ischemia and infarction, and is associated with a poor prognosis.

It is critical to maintain cerebral blood flow to preserve tissue and minimize secondary injury to the brain tissue. Prolonged increases in ICP cause brainstem compression and herniation. Herniation occurs as the brain tissue is forced from the compartment of greater pressure to a compartment of lesser pressure. The compression of the brainstem and cranial nerves caused by herniation may be fatal.

Autoregulation of cerebral blood flow is preserved with a minimum mean arterial pressure (MAP) of 70 mm Hg. Below this level, cerebral blood flow decreases and symptoms of cerebral ischemia, such as syncope and blurred vision, occur. The CPP is the pressure needed to ensure blood flow to the brain. The calculation for cerebral perfusion pressure is CPP = MAP – ICP. Normal CPP is 60 to 100 mm Hg. A CPP of less than 50 mm Hg is associated with ischemia and neuronal death. Nurses have a role in monitoring CPP and preventing secondary brain injury.

Common Causes and Risk Factors

- Anoxic or ischemic episodes
- Brain abscess or tumor
- Brain surgery
- Cerebral infarction, thrombotic or embolic
- Encephalitis
- Head injuries: contusion, hematoma
- Hemorrhage
- Hepatic encephalopathy
- Lead or arsenic intoxication
- Meningitis
- Posttraumatic brain swelling
- Uremia
- Venous sinus thrombosis

Manifestations

Early

- Change in level of consciousness
- Headache, progressing in frequency or severity
- Vomiting, usually not preceded by nausea, may be projectile
- Infants
  - Bulging fontanel
  - Flat affect, lethargy
  - Irritability
  - Poor feeding

Late

- Blurred or double vision
- Change in body temperature
- Changes in extraocular eye movements
- Cushing triad (systolic hypertension, bradycardia, irregular respirations)
- Dilated, sluggish, or unresponsive pupil(s)
- Papilledema
- Hemiplegia or hemiparesis
- Posturing, decorticate (flexor) or decerebrate (extensor)
- Diagnostic tests
  - Brain imaging shows mass, edema, or ventricular shift
  - Continuous ICP monitoring, ICP >20 mm Hg

Key Conceptual Relationships

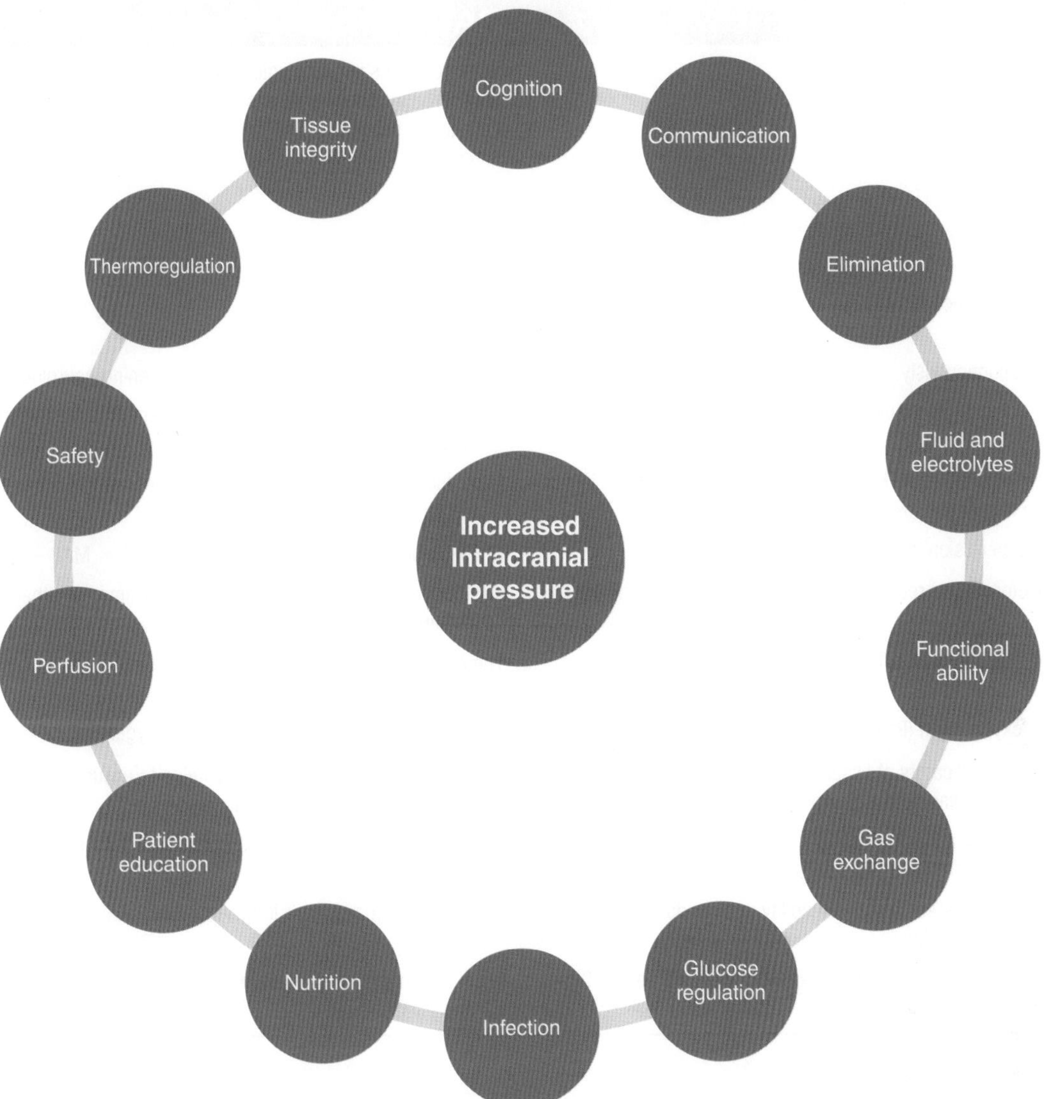

ASSESSMENT OF INTRACRANIAL PRESSURE	RATIONALE
Assess risk factors for increased ICP.	Identifying factors that place the patient at risk for increased ICP allows for early intervention.
Determine the potential cause of increased ICP.	It is more effective to treat the cause rather than the imbalance.
Identify patients who need emergency management for increased ICP.	Identify increased ICP for early intervention and prevention of complications.
Perform a complete physical assessment and monitor indicators and trends of ICP on an ongoing basis:	
• Manifestations of increased ICP	Identifying the presence of manifestations of increased ICP allows for early intervention.
• Respiratory function	Increased ICP may impair the respiratory center.

Continued

ASSESSMENT OF INTRACRANIAL PRESSURE	RATIONALE
• Neurologic status: • General appearance and behavior • Level of consciousness • Orientation • Sensation • Movement • Cranial nerve function • Response to stimuli, including verbal, tactile, motor • Mood and affect • Reflexes	Subtle changes in neurologic status are an early sign of increased ICP. Thorough and diligent assessment is key to early identification and intervention.
• Vital signs, continuously	Changes in vital signs may indicate worsening neurologic status.
• Glasgow Coma Scale (Table 22.1) score, with trends	This standardized tool promotes consistent documentation and communication.
• **FLUID AND ELECTROLYTES:** Fluid and electrolyte balance, including intake and output, osmolality, and weight	Fluid and electrolyte imbalances are associated with cerebral edema and seizures.
Calculate cerebral perfusion pressure.	CPP is equal to the MAP minus the ICP (CPP = MAP − ICP).
Analyze ICP waveforms and record ICP pressure readings, if available.	ICP monitoring provides trending and real-time data that may require intervention.
Monitor amount, rate, and characteristics of CSF drainage.	The quality and quantity of CSF drainage may indicate a need for further intervention.
Monitor cerebral oxygenation ($Pbto_2$, $Sjvo_2$) if needed.	These invasive measures assess brain oxygen levels.
PERFUSION: Monitor indicators of tissue oxygen delivery, including $Paco_2$, Sao_2, and cardiac output, if available.	Monitoring tissue oxygen delivery helps to ensure adequate oxygenation to support cerebral metabolic needs.
Evaluate the results of diagnostic studies, including imaging studies, electroencephalography (EEG), and angiography.	Diagnostic tests are performed to evaluate for a cause of increased ICP.
FUNCTIONAL ABILITY: Assess functional ability and needs for assistance with activities of daily living.	Increased ICP may impair long-term functional outcomes.
Evaluate the patient's response to measures to address increased ICP through ongoing reassessment.	Identifying manifestations of increased ICP allows for evaluation of therapy effectiveness.

Expected Outcomes

The patient will:

- maintain an adequate CPP.
- be free from complications associated with increased ICP.
- achieve or maintain baseline neurologic functioning.

INTERVENTIONS FOR NORMALIZING INTRACRANIAL PRESSURE	RATIONALE
Implement collaborative interventions aimed at treating the underlying cause of increased ICP.	Increased ICP may resolve with treatment of the underlying cause.
Be prepared to institute resuscitation protocols and respiratory support.	Support is needed in emergency situations to preserve life.
Monitor neurologic status and notify the health care provider (HCP) if neurologic status changes or manifestations of increased ICP persist or worsen.	Rapid detection of changes allows for early intervention and potential preservation of brain tissue and function.
Monitor ICP continuously and respond rapidly to intervene for ICP >20 mm Hg or sustained periods at >15 mm Hg.	Elevated ICP requires rapid intervention to preserve brain tissue.
COMMUNICATION: Speak to the patient calmly and explain what is happening, even if the patient is not visibly responsive.	This demonstrates respect for the patient who may be able to hear but not respond and may be anxious or frightened.

INTERVENTIONS FOR NORMALIZING INTRACRANIAL PRESSURE	RATIONALE
Assess neurologic status with oncoming staff at shift change and when assuming care.	Neurologic examination findings may have subjective and subtle variations.
Implement measures to reduce cerebral edema:	
• Position patient in a neutral position of the head, neck, and spine.	Avoiding jugular vein compression and limiting hip flexion enhances venous drainage from the head. Ensure no contraindications to head of the bed restrictions prior to positioning.
• Maintain the head of the bed elevated at 30 degrees.	Elevation decreases ICP; ensure there are no contraindications to doing so prior to positioning.
• If intubated, suction only when necessary and not routinely.	Suctioning increases ICP by increasing intrathoracic pressure.
• Decrease stimuli in the patient's environment.	Excess environmental stimuli can contribute to increased ICP.
• Space activities with rest periods to avoid prolonged periods of stimulation.	Prevent long periods of time with increased ICP.
• Remind staff and family to avoid stimulating the patient unnecessarily if the patient responds with signs of increasing ICP.	While stimulation is necessary for neurologic checks and some care activities, it should be avoided when not necessary because it increases ICP.
THERMOREGULATION: Maintain normothermia with antipyretics, cooling blankets, or ice packs.	Elevated core body temperature may increase ICP by increasing metabolic demand.
FLUID AND ELECTROLYTES: Maintain fluid balance and assess osmolality.	Electrolyte disturbances, most often sodium, can cause cerebral edema and worsening elevation in ICP.
INFECTION: If the patient requires invasive ICP monitoring, manage the system aseptically.	Maintain invasive ICP monitoring catheters aseptically to reduce the risk of ventriculitis or an abscess.
Drain CSF from an intraventricular catheter system as ordered.	Inadequate drainage of CSF may contribute to sustained elevations in ICP; however, excessive CSF drainage poses risks for intracranial injury.
Administer medications as prescribed, including:	
• Sedation	Sedation decreases the response to stimulation and limits neurologic assessment. Sedation may be minimized unless ICP monitoring system is in place.
• Antiseizure drugs	Seizures are a possible complication of increased ICP.
• Hypertonic saline, mannitol	These medications decrease cerebral edema.
• **COGNITION:** High-dose barbiturates	Barbiturates reduce cerebral metabolism and are used to manage severely increased ICP that is refractory to other interventions.
• **ELIMINATION:** Stool softeners, laxatives	Straining with bowel elimination increases ICP because it increases intrathoracic pressure and decreases venous return.
GAS EXCHANGE: Monitor and maintain adequate oxygenation using supplemental oxygen and/or mechanical ventilation if needed.	Avoid cerebral hypoxia, which could worsen cerebral edema and extend brain injury.
PERFUSION: Maintain systolic arterial pressure between 100 and 160 mm Hg.	Hypertension may impair autoregulation, whereas hypotension may impair cerebral perfusion.
Maintain CPP $>$60 mm Hg.	A CPP of 60 mm Hg is the minimal level for adequate brain perfusion.
SAFETY: Provide a safe environment for the patient with neurologic or neuromuscular manifestations by initiating fall and seizure precautions.	Changes in cognition and a potential for seizures often accompany increased ICP and may place the patient at an increased risk of injury.
GLUCOSE REGULATION: Monitor blood glucose levels regularly and maintain a stable level.	Avoid hypoglycemia because glucose is needed for brain metabolism.
FUNCTIONAL ABILITY: Help the patient with activities of daily living as needed.	The patient may require assistance to complete activities of daily living if increased ICP impairs functional ability.
TISSUE INTEGRITY: Monitor skin integrity and implement measures to prevent changes.	Immobility and sensory alterations place the patient at high risk for skin breakdown.

COLLABORATION	RATIONALE
MOBILITY: Physical therapy	Physical therapists can provide assistance with performing range of motion and mobilization.
NUTRITION: Dietitian	It is recommended that nutrition be initiated early to promote cellular support and healing. The patient may receive nutrition via the enteral or parenteral route.
Occupational therapy	Occupational therapists can provide assistance with devices to maintain functional alignment of the hands and feet.

PATIENT AND CAREGIVER TEACHING

- Cause of increased ICP, if known
- Manifestations of increased ICP
- Management of any underlying condition causing increased ICP
- Measures being used to improve ICP and reduce the risk of complications
- Interacting with the patient while avoiding increases in ICP
- Need for ICP monitoring and frequent neurologic checks

DOCUMENTATION

Assessment

- Manifestations of increased ICP
- Continuous ICP monitoring, if available
- Diagnostic test results

Interventions

- Medications given
- Notification of the HCP about diagnostic test results and assessment findings
- Therapeutic interventions and the patient's response
- Teaching provided
- Referrals initiated
- Safety measures implemented, including seizure and fall precautions

Evaluation

- Patient's status: improved, stable, declined
- Diagnostic test results
- Patient's response to therapeutic interventions
- Presence of any manifestations of increased ICP

Neurologic Problem 22

Definition

Impaired cognitive, motor, sensory, and/or regulatory functions of the central or peripheral nervous system

There are many types of neurologic conditions. This section focuses on the care of persons with clinical problems caused by conditions that include headache, stroke, seizures, degenerative nerve diseases, and spinal cord injuries. Headache is the most common type of pain reported. Most headaches are functional types, such as migraine or tension-type headaches. Organic headaches are those caused by intracranial or extracranial disease.

A stroke occurs when there is (1) ischemia (inadequate blood flow) to a part of the brain, or (2) hemorrhage (bleeding) into the brain that results in the death of brain cells. In a stroke, functions such as movement, sensation, thinking, and talking, as well as emotions controlled by the affected area of the brain, are lost or impaired. The severity of the loss of function varies according to the location and extent of the brain damage.

A seizure is a sudden, abnormal, excessive electrical discharge of neurons in the brain. Multiple neurons firing at a faster rate than normal cause involuntary movements, sensory phenomena, emotional expression, and unusual behaviors. Seizures may accompany a variety of disorders or occur without an apparent cause. Children may have seizures with high fever. *Seizure disorder*, or *epilepsy*, is a group of neurologic diseases marked by recurring seizures.

Degenerative nerve diseases are those that lead to worsening nerve damage as the disease progresses. Degenerative nerve diseases include multiple sclerosis, Parkinson disease, myasthenia gravis, amyotrophic lateral sclerosis, and Huntington disease. These conditions affect many activities, including balance, movement, and speech, and may affect cardiopulmonary function. Patients must deal with the disease and its impact on their quality of life. Many patients have concerns regarding safety, mobility, self-care, and coping. Patients and their caregivers often need our psychosocial support, especially if the disease progresses and disability worsens. Most degenerative neurologic problems have no cure. Treatment aims to reduce symptoms and help the patient maintain optimal function.

Cervical and lumbar injuries are the most common types of spinal cord injuries because these areas are associated with the greatest flexibility and movement. The degree of spinal cord involvement may be either complete or incomplete (partial). Spinal cord injury above the level of T6 creates a potential risk for autonomic dysreflexia. Autonomic dysreflexia is the result of impaired function of the autonomic nervous system caused by simultaneous sympathetic and parasympathetic activity, such as may occur with bowel or bladder distention pain or a pressure injury. It is usually a medical emergency. Stimuli such as bowel or bladder distention or skin irritation cause hyperactive reflexes and inappropriate autonomic responses that can lead to an extreme sympathetic nervous system reaction and complications such as stroke.

Associated Clinical Problems

- Apraxia: impaired ability to perform purposeful acts or to manipulate objects without any loss of strength, sensation, or coordination
- Autonomic Dysreflexia: syndrome affecting persons with a spinal cord lesion above the T6 thoracic level that is characterized by hypertension, bradycardia, severe headaches, pallor below and flushing above the cord lesions, and convulsions
- Coma: prolonged unconsciousness
- Decreased Coordination: impaired ability to complete motor tasks smoothly
- Dizziness: sensation of faintness and whirling or an inability to maintain normal balance in a standing or seated position
- Impaired Kinesthesia: diminished ability to perceive one's own body parts, weight, and movement
- Impaired Psychomotor Activity: diminished ability or strength to move muscles in a coordinated way
- Seizure: hyperexcitation of neurons in the brain leading to abnormal electric activity that causes a sudden, violent, involuntary series of contractions of a group of muscles
- Risk for Impaired Neurologic Function: increased risk for impairment of cognitive, motor, sensory, and/or regulatory functions of the central or peripheral nervous system
- Unilateral Neglect: disturbed perceptual abilities leading to ignoring one-half of the body

Common Causes

- Amyotrophic lateral sclerosis (ALS)
- Alzheimer disease
- Bell palsy
- Birth defects of the brain and spinal cord
- Brain aneurysm

- Brain injury
- Brain tumor
- Cerebral palsy
- Chiari malformation
- Chronic fatigue syndrome
- Concussion
- Craniofacial abnormalities
- Craniosynostosis
- Dementia
- Developmental disorders
- Disk disease of the neck and lower back
- Dizziness
- Encephalopathy
- Gait/walking disorders
- Gilles de la Tourette syndrome
- Guillain-Barré syndrome
- Headaches (cluster, tension, or migraine)
- Hydrocephalus
- Hypotonia
- Metabolic problems
- Movement disorders
- Myelomeningocele (spina bifida)
- Multiple sclerosis
- Muscular dystrophy
- Neuralgia
- Neuropathy
- Neuromuscular and related diseases
- Parkinson disease
- Psychiatric conditions, such as severe depression and obsessive-compulsive disorder
- Scoliosis
- Seizure disorder
- Spasticity
- Spinal cord, nerve, and muscle diseases
- Spinal deformity
- Spinal disorder, such as subacute combined degeneration
- Spine tumor
- Stroke
- Traumatic spinal cord injury
- Vertigo

Autonomic Dysreflexia

- High-level spinal cord injury (above thoracic level 6)

Manifestations

- Altered gait
- Aphasia (expressive and/or receptive)
- Back pain
- Changes in balance
- Changes in recent or remote memory
- Dysphagia
- Headache
- Impaired cognition; confusion
- Impaired development
- Loss of bowel or urinary control
- Loss of consciousness
- Muscle weakness
- Numbness, tingling, and neuralgia
- Paralysis
- Seizure activity
- Sensory deficits, including vision and hearing
- Syncope
- Tremor or other motion disturbances
- Vertigo and dizziness
- Vomiting
- *Diagnostic Tests*
  - Imaging may show structural changes in the brain or spinal cord.
  - Electroencephalography (EEG) and other electrographic studies may show seizure activity and abnormal nerve impulse transmission.
  - Angiography may reveal aneurysms and tumors.
  - Lumbar puncture with CSF fluid analysis can show infection.

Autonomic Dysreflexia

- Blurred vision
- Bradycardia
- Chest pain
- Chills without fever
- Diaphoresis above the level of injury
- Facial flushing
- Headache
- Hypertension
- Tachycardia

Key Conceptual Relationships

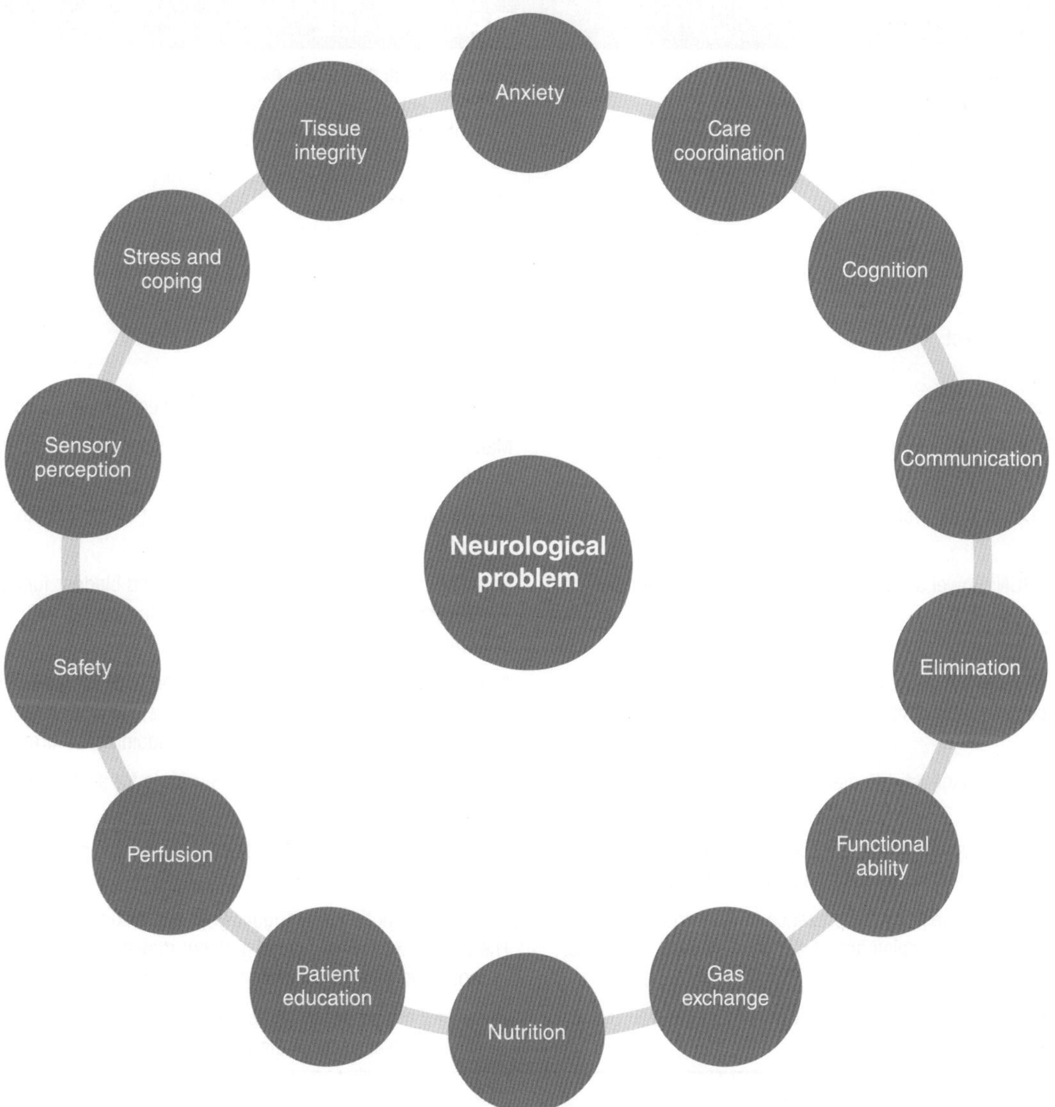

ASSESSMENT OF NEUROLOGIC FUNCTION	RATIONALE
Assess risk factors for a neurologic problem.	Identifying factors that place the patient at risk for a neurologic problem allows for early intervention.
Determine the potential cause of a neurologic problem.	It is more effective to treat the cause rather than the imbalance.
Identify patients in need of emergency management for a neurologic problem so that they can be immediately stabilized.	Identifying a neurologic problem allows for early intervention and may minimize long-term consequences and poor outcomes.
Perform a complete physical assessment and monitor indicators and trends of the neurologic problem on an ongoing basis.	
• Manifestations of the specific neurologic condition	There is a wide range of neurologic problems and each requires specific assessment.
• **GAS EXCHANGE:** Respiratory function	Many neurologic problems impair respiratory efforts.

Continued

ASSESSMENT OF NEUROLOGIC FUNCTION	RATIONALE
• Neurologic status: • General appearance and behavior • Level of consciousness • Orientation • Sensation • Movement • Cranial nerve function • Response to stimuli, including verbal, tactile, and motor • Cognition • Mood and affect • Reflexes	Changes in the neurologic exam may be subtle but clinically significant. Serial neurologic assessment is imperative to identifying early problems requiring intervention.
• Vital signs as needed	Changes in vital signs may indicate worsening neurologic status.
• **NUTRITION:** Ability to swallow safely	Many neurologic problems can alter swallowing, placing the patient at high risk for aspiration.
• Glasgow Coma Scale (Table 22.1) score, noting trends	This standardized tool promotes consistent documentation and communication of neurologic function.
• **ELIMINATION:** Bowel and bladder continence and retention	Neurologic conditions may impair bowel and bladder function. Special considerations may need to be taken in patients with spinal cord injuries.
• **TISSUE INTEGRITY:** Skin integrity, particularly in areas of decreased sensation or mobility	An inability to sense or move areas of the body increases the risk for skin and tissue damage from pressure, shear, and other forces. Patients may need assistance in offloading pressure points.
Evaluate the results of diagnostic studies, including imaging studies, EEG, lumbar puncture, CSF analysis, and angiography.	Diagnostic tests are performed to evaluate for a cause of a neurologic problem.
FUNCTIONAL ABILITY: Assess the patient's functional ability and determine whether the patient needs assistance with activities of daily living.	Neurologic conditions may impair functional ability.
STRESS AND COPING: Assess for the presence of grief and anxiety. Assess the patient's use of coping and stress management strategies.	The loss of function may trigger grief and anxiety. The patient with a neurologic problem may experience increased stress and have difficulty coping with the neurologic problem.
Evaluate the patient's response to measures to address the neurologic problem through ongoing assessment.	Identifying the presence of manifestations of the neurologic problem allows for evaluation of therapy effectiveness.

Table 22.1 Glasgow Coma Scale

Appropriate Stimulus	Response	Score
Eyes Open		
• Approach to bedside • Verbal command • Pain	Spontaneous response	4
	Opening of eyes to name or command	3
	Lack of opening of eyes to previous stimuli but opening to pain	2
	Lack of opening of eyes to any stimulus	1
	Untestable[a]	U
Best Verbal Response		
• Verbal questioning with maximum arousal	Appropriate orientation; conversant; correct identification of self, place, year, and month	5
	Confusion; conversant, but disorientation in one or more spheres	4
	Inappropriate or disorganized use of words (e.g., cursing), lack of sustained conversation	3
	Incomprehensible words, sounds (e.g., moaning)	2

Table 22.1 Glasgow Coma Scale—cont'd

Appropriate Stimulus	Response	Score
	Lack of sound, even with painful stimuli	1
	Untestable[a]	U
Best Motor Response • Verbal command (e.g., "raise your arm," "hold up two fingers") • Pain (pressure on proximal nail bed)	Obedience of command	6
	Localization of pain, lack of obedience but presence of attempts to remove offending stimulus	5
	Flexion withdrawal,[a] flexion of arm in response to pain without abnormal flexion posture	4
	Abnormal flexion, flexing of arm at elbow and pronation, making a fist	3
	Abnormal extension, extension of arm at elbow, usually with adduction and internal rotation of arm at shoulder	2
	Lack of response	1
	Untestable[a]	U

[a]Added to the original scale by some centers.

ASSESSMENT OF AUTONOMIC DYSREFLEXIA	RATIONALE
Monitor for complications of dysreflexia, including cerebral hemorrhage, myocardial infarction, seizures, and ocular hemorrhage.	Early identification of complications allows for rapid treatment and reduces the risk of prolonged disability.

Expected Outcomes

The patient will:
- maintain or improve neurologic function.
- be free from any neurologic complications.
- maintain ongoing contact with the appropriate community resources.
- take part in desired activities of daily living.

INTERVENTIONS TO PROMOTE NEUROLOGIC FUNCTION	RATIONALE
Implement collaborative interventions aimed at treating the underlying cause of a neurologic problem.	The neurologic problem may resolve with treatment of the underlying cause.
Be prepared to institute resuscitation protocols and respiratory support.	Support is needed in emergency situations to preserve life.
Notify the health care provider (HCP) if neurologic status changes or manifestations of the problem persist or worsen.	Rapid detection of changes allows for early intervention.
COMMUNICATION: Speak to the patient respectfully and often, even if there is no apparent response.	The patient may be able to hear but not respond.
Encourage family members to speak calmly and interact with the patient.	Family members may need reassurance to interact if the patient is unconscious or confused.
COGNITION: Implement measures to address impaired cognition, if present.	Reorienting may be necessary in reminding the patient of what is happening.
STRESS AND COPING: Provide emotional support to the patient and family regarding changing neurologic status.	Changes such as paresis, seizures, and others may be highly upsetting to the patient and family.
TISSUE INTEGRITY: Position the patient to avoid injury and reposition often.	Measures are needed to prevent skin and tissue damage from pressure if the patient is partially or completely immobile.
Position by careful logrolling if the vertebral column is unstable.	Logrolling the patient with an unstable vertebral column prevents pain and further injury while protecting the spine.

Continued

INTERVENTIONS TO PROMOTE NEUROLOGIC FUNCTION	RATIONALE
SAFETY: Provide eye care and moisture if the eye does not close and/or the patient does not blink.	Proper eye care with drops or lubricant reduces the risk of corneal injury.
Provide or assist with regular oral care.	Good oral hygiene helps prevent dental caries and stomatitis and reduces the risk of ventilator-associated pneumonia.
Provide a safe environment for the patient by initiating fall and seizure precautions.	Changes in cognition and a potential for seizures often accompany neurologic problems.
FUNCTIONAL ABILITY: If the patient is able to eat without aspirating, assist as needed to cut/prepare food, feed, and use assistive devices.	The patient may be able to eat with physical assistance or the use of assistive devices.
ELIMINATION: Assist with bladder and bowel regimen or training as needed.	Bowel and bladder retraining regimens promote continence and regular elimination function.
SENSORY PERCEPTION: Implement measures to address sensory deficits, if present.	Accurate sensory input may improve cognition and neurologic symptoms.
Assist the patient with developing a regular physical activity plan, considering capabilities, daily routine, and personal preferences.	Regular physical activity is an important part of care for many patients because it builds endurance and maintains muscle strength.
STRESS AND COPING: Encourage the use of positive coping and stress management strategies.	Coping and stress management strategies can improve quality of life by helping the patient better manage a neurologic problem.
CARE COORDINATION: Assist the patient in obtaining any necessary adaptive devices and making any needed environment adaptations.	Adaptive devices and environment modifications can assist the patient in performing personal care independently.
GRIEF AND ANXIETY: Implement measures to address any grief and anxiety that the patient may be experiencing.	The loss of function may trigger grief and anxiety.
CAREGIVING: Implement measures to address caregiver role strain, if present.	Assessing the caregiver for signs of role strain is necessary to be able to provide adequate support.

INTERVENTIONS TO ADDRESS AUTONOMIC DYSREFLEXIA	RATIONALE
ELIMINATION AND TISSUE INTEGRITY: Ensure regular bladder drainage or patency of urinary catheter and regular bowel care, and maintain skin integrity.	Identifying and avoiding provoking stimuli is an important measure to prevent episodes of autonomic dysreflexia.
Identify and rapidly treat possible causes of dysreflexia, such as bladder distention, bowel distention, and skin irritation.	A fast response is needed to prevent cerebral injury or myocardial infarction.
Place the patient in the high Fowler position and loosen restrictive clothing or binders while checking for a cause.	These measures decrease cerebral pressure and reduce the risk of cerebral injury.
Use local anesthetic gels if inserting a urinary catheter or disimpacting the bowel while the patient is symptomatic.	Anesthetic gel can prevent worsening of symptoms.
PERFUSION: Monitor blood pressure every 3 to 5 minutes during the acute phase and every 15 to 30 minutes after.	This can identify dangerous levels of hypertension that can cause cerebral injury or myocardial infarction.
Administer antihypertensive agents intravenously as ordered.	A rapid reduction in blood pressure may be necessary.
If the cause is eliminated after an antihypertensive is given, monitor for hypotension.	Rebound hypotension is possible.
Be mindful that menstruation may trigger dysreflexia.	Vigilance is needed during the menstrual cycle.
Help the patient establish an emergency plan with medications and interventions for use at home and with the use of standing orders in an agency.	Having an emergency plan facilitates a rapid response for treatment.

INTERVENTIONS TO MANAGE A SEIZURE	RATIONALE
Encourage the patient to immediately call for help if a seizure aura occurs.	This allows time for safety precautions to be implemented.
SAFETY: Promote a safe environment: • Keep bed height in the lowest position. • Keep suction, oral or nasopharyngeal airway, and Ambu bag at the bedside. • Pad the side rails of the bed. • Remove sharp or fragile objects from the environment.	These measures reduce the risk of injury should a seizure occur.
Administer antiseizure medications and monitor patient adherence with medications.	Antiseizure medications prevent seizure occurrence in many patients.
Obtain serum drug levels as needed.	Some antiseizure medications have a narrow range of safety and require monitoring.
Encourage the patient to carry a medication alert card and/or wear identifying jewelry.	The patient has the responsibility to make their condition known to all HCPs.
Have the patient keep a list of medications with emergency information.	This information is important for providing rapid, safe care.
SAFETY: Discuss with the patient restrictions regarding driving and operating dangerous machinery.	Restrictions may be necessary to prevent injury or a motor vehicle crash.
Provide care during a seizure: • Maintain the airway, using chin lift or oral/nasal airway placement, if needed. • Position lying on the side. • Remain with the patient. • Loosen restrictive clothing. • Apply oxygen, if needed.	These measures help keep the airway patent for oxygenation and promote patient safety.
Observe seizure characteristics, including the type of movement, progression, and length of episode. Observe for incontinence.	The characteristics of the seizure can help determine the type of seizure.
Establish intravenous (IV) access if needed and administer anticonvulsants as ordered.	Extended or frequent seizures may be treated with IV anticonvulsants.
Provide care after a seizure: • Monitor postictal period duration and characteristics. • Calmly reassure and reorient the patient during the seizure and upon awakening. • Assess for, report, and treat for injury.	The patient may be upset or disoriented, and with vigorous seizure activity, the patient may have a physical injury.

COLLABORATION	RATIONALE
FUNCTIONAL ABILITY: Physical therapy	Physical therapists assess, plan, and implement interventions that promote a person's ability to fulfil role responsibilities.
Occupational therapy	Occupational therapists can recommend assistive devices and assist with skill development to help the patient fulfil roles in the home.
Support groups	Support groups can play a major role in promoting adjustment to role changes and managing problems common to neurologic conditions.
Home health agency	A home health agency may be able to provide assistance with the patient's care and household maintenance.
GAS EXCHANGE: Speech therapy	A swallowing evaluation by a speech therapist can detect changes in swallowing ability that increase the risk of aspiration.

Continued

COLLABORATION	RATIONALE
NUTRITION: Dietitian	The patient may receive enteral or parenteral nutrition to maintain muscle mass and support adequate nutrition.
CARE COORDINATION: Social work or case management	A social worker or case manager can help the patient and caregiver identify community resources to assist with fulfilling role responsibilities.
Disease or symptom management programs	Disease or symptom management programs help patients understand their treatment regimen and address the complex needs of those with chronic illness.

PATIENT AND CAREGIVER TEACHING

- Cause of the neurologic problem, if known
- Manifestations of the condition
- Management of any underlying conditions
- Measures being used to improve the neurologic problem and reduce the risk of complications
- Diagnostic and laboratory tests needed
- Safe use of medications, including proper use, side effect management, administration, and how they fit into the overall management plan
- Seizure and postseizure care
- Prevention and treatment of autonomic dysreflexia
- Role of physical and occupational therapies
- Modifications in the living environment to promote safety
- Community and self-help resources available
- Sources of information and social support
- Positive coping and stress management strategies
- How to safely use any adaptive devices
- Community and home precautions
- Early recognition of problems and how to manage them
- Any needed lifestyle changes to control the neurologic problem
- Importance of long-term follow-up
- When to notify the HCP and seek emergency care

DOCUMENTATION

Assessment

- Neurologic status
- Respiratory status
- Functional ability
- Manifestations of the specific neurologic condition
- Diagnostic and laboratory test results

Interventions

- Discussions with other members of the interprofessional team
- Environmental modifications made
- Medications given
- Notification of the HCP about patient status
- Therapeutic interventions and the patient's response
- Teaching provided
- Referrals initiated
- Prevention of complications
- Safety measures implemented, including seizure and fall precautions

Evaluation

- Patient's status: improved, stable, declined
- Diagnostic test results
- Patient's response to therapeutic interventions
- Presence of any manifestations of the specific neurologic condition

Body Weight Problem 23

Definition

Being overweight or underweight

Having a body weight problem is defined as being either overweight or underweight. Being overweight is an increase in body weight beyond the body's physical requirements. This results in an abnormal increase and accumulation of fat cells. Being underweight is often associated with insufficient calorie intake and malnutrition. Both pose multiple health risks, with consequences that extend beyond the physical changes. Social stigma can take an emotional toll on psychologic well-being. Many have problems related to negative self-image and depression and withdraw from social interaction. Those who are obese may experience biases and discrimination resulting from attitudes about obesity.

Exploring a person's motivation for achieving weight goals is essential. You can help patients understand their desire to achieve weight goals and help them gain confidence in their ability to do so. Achieving and maintaining an optimal body weight requires a comprehensive approach, combining multiple strategies. These strategies should include nutrition therapy, exercise, and behavior modification. Some persons may need drug therapy. Surgery may be an option for some who are obese. While teaching patients, stress healthy eating habits and adequate physical activity as lifestyle patterns to develop and maintain.

Associated Clinical Problems

- Overweight: having increased body weight with a body mass index (BMI) > 25
- Underweight: having decreased body weight with a BMI < 18.5

Common Risk Factors

Overweight

- Alcohol use
- Changes in metabolic rate
- Dysfunctional eating pattern
- Environment: eating high-fat, high-calorie convenience foods; large portions; frequent snacking; eating out often
- Endocrine problems: Cushing disease, diabetes, hypothyroidism
- Excess intake in relation to metabolic needs
- Genetic variations in metabolism, body fat distribution, appetite regulation
- Lesion in the hypothalamus
- Medications: antipsychotics, corticosteroids
- Psychologic factors: mindless eating, using food as a coping mechanism
- Sedentary lifestyle

Pediatric

- Maternal diabetes
- Parental smoking
- Rapid weight gain during infancy
- Solid foods as major food source at < 5 months of age

Underweight

- Altered sense of smell and taste
- Decreased food intake in relation to metabolic needs
- Eating disorder: anorexia nervosa, bulimia nervosa
- Hyperthyroidism
- Inability to absorb nutrients
- Inability to ingest food: vomiting, dysphagia, inability to feed self
- Increased metabolic rate
- Psychologic factors: agitation, forgetfulness, impaired judgment

Manifestations

- Dysfunctional eating patterns
- Laboratory test results: abnormal lipid panel; electrolyte values; prealbumin, albumin, and protein values; ↓ iron levels

Overweight

- Weight
  - Adult: BMI > 25
  - Child under 2 years: weight-for length > 95th percentile
  - Child 2–18 years: BMI > 85th but < 95th percentile
- Sedentary lifestyle
- Triceps skinfold > 15 mm in men or > 25 mm in women
- Use of food as a reward or comfort measure

Underweight

- Weight
  - Adult: < 18.5 BMI
  - Child under 3 years: weight-for length under the 10th percentile
  - Child 3–18 years: BMI < 5th percentile
- Manifestations of electrolyte imbalance, vitamin and protein deficits
- Manifestations of malnutrition

Key Conceptual Relationships

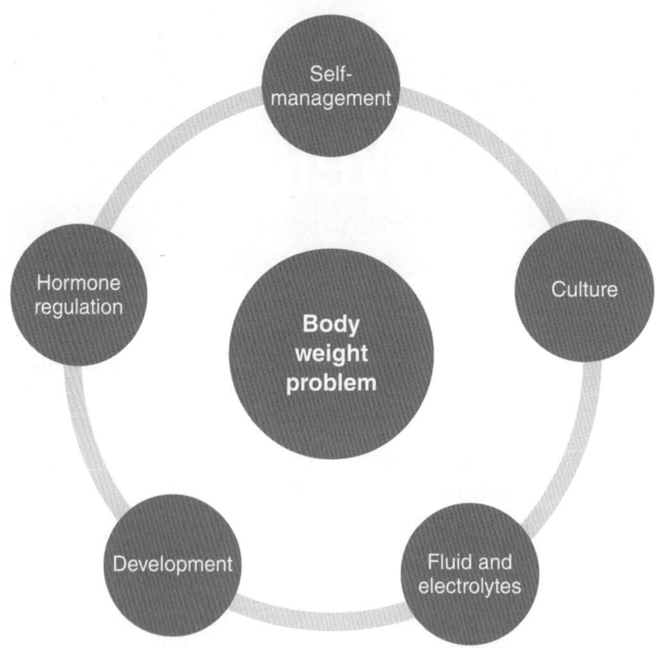

ASSESSMENT OF BODY WEIGHT	RATIONALE
Determine whether conditions that may be causing or contributing to a body weight problem are present.	This helps determine the plan of care and choice of interventions.
Assess for comorbid conditions associated with a body weight problem.	Complications associated with a body weight problem require individualized treatment.
Screen the patient for an eating disorder.	Early treatment is important for those with or at risk of an eating disorder.
Obtain a detailed weight history, including: • Weight pattern over the patient's lifetime • Weight loss or gain within the past 6–12 months • Whether weight changes were intentional • Perceived barriers to attaining weight goals • Diets and strategies they have used • Support or sabotage from significant others in weight reduction efforts	A loss of > 5% of usual body weight over 6 months (whether intentional or unintentional) is a critical indicator for further assessment.
Obtain a diet history, including: • Usual daily caloric intake • Types of foods eaten • Types of beverages and amounts	A history can identify strengths and weaknesses in the diet program and aid in determining the treatment plan.
Evaluate the patient's food environment, including: • Access to food • Food preparation • Housing situation • Socioeconomic status	The food environment influences diet history and diet plan.
Perform a complete physical assessment and monitor indicators of weight and nutrition status on an ongoing basis:	
• Anthropometric measurements: Height, weight, BMI, waist-to-hip ratio, waist and midarm circumference, body fat percent, body shape	These measures are used to determine the degree of body fat and an optimal weight.
• Serum levels and trends in levels as available:	
• Lipid panel (triglyceride level, low- and high-density lipoprotein cholesterol levels)	Being overweight is often associated with hyperlipidemia.
• **HORMONE REGULATION:** Endocrine function, including thyroid panel	Hormone imbalances may be associated with weight problems.

ASSESSMENT OF BODY WEIGHT	RATIONALE
• Prealbumin, albumin, and total protein	Prealbumin, albumin, and total protein are indicators of nutrition status and guide diet selection.
• **FLUID AND ELECTROLYTES:** Electrolytes	Electrolyte imbalances may be present with weight problems.
• Complete blood cell (CBC) count with hemoglobin, hematocrit	The red blood cell (RBC) count and hemoglobin level may show anemia.
• Iron	Iron deficiency is common due to consuming a diet low in iron-rich foods.
• Manifestations of impaired nutrition	Identifying impaired nutrition allows for early intervention.
• Daily food diary with calorie count	Calorie count and a food diary help identify intake patterns and provide a base on which to tailor the diet program.
Assess exercise activity.	Nutrition intake needs to be adjusted to meet energy expenditure.
SELF-MANAGEMENT: Assess the patient's motivation for starting a weight management plan.	Focusing on the reasons for wanting to achieve a goal weight can help in developing an effective weight management plan.
CULTURE: Assess the role of culture on the patient's weight.	Culture influences eating habits and attitudes toward food and body weight.
DEVELOPMENT: Assess the patient's view of self.	Family and cultural practices influence self-view about food and body image.
Monitor the patient's dental health periodically, including fit and condition of any dentures.	Oral health and dentition affect intake.
Weigh on a regular basis at the same time of day and in similar clothing.	Consistent weight monitoring evaluates nutrition and effectiveness of interventions.
MOOD AND AFFECT: Assess mental status and screen for coexisting psychologic problems.	Depression, anxiety, and other psychologic disorders influence food intake and body weight.
Evaluate patient's response to measures to achieve goal weight on an ongoing basis.	Identifying the response to therapeutic measures allows for evaluation of therapy effectiveness.
Reassess caloric requirements every 2–4 weeks.	Changes in weight and exercise require changes in the plan.

Expected Outcomes

The patient will:

- achieve and maintain optimal weight.
- have a nutritionally balanced diet.
- change eating patterns to attain and maintain optimal weight.
- take part in an appropriate exercise program.
- achieve and maintain balanced nutrition.
- be free from complications resulting from a body weight problem.
- use needed community resources.

INTERVENTIONS TO ACHIEVE OPTIMAL WEIGHT	RATIONALE
Use motivational interviewing to initiate behavior change.	Helping patients identify why they would want to make a change and how they might do it promotes behavior change.
Mutually establish a realistic, safe weight goal and plan that considers amount of weight change desired, duration of program, cost, nutrition, and compatibility with lifestyle.	Trying to lose or gain weight too fast may result in a sense of frustration for the patient. Slow changes in weight generally reflect a change in eating habits.
Set up a rewards system for achieving short- and long-term weight change goals.	Earning rewards are useful incentives for achieving weight goals.
Have the patient chart weight progress.	Attaining goals and positive reinforcement promote continued adherence to weight plan.

Continued

INTERVENTIONS TO ACHIEVE OPTIMAL WEIGHT	RATIONALE
SELF-MANAGEMENT: Provide positive reinforcement for achieving nutrition and weight goals.	Positive reinforcement promotes the patient's confidence in continuing behaviors that promote optimal nutrition.
Provide a prescribed diet for weight goals.	The appropriate diet is a critical part of achieving an optimal weight.
Encourage patient to maintain a food diary, including: • What was eaten • How much was eaten • When and where eating occurs • Circumstances around which the food was eaten, such as persons present	A diary provides a means to determine nutrition adequacy and focuses attention on behavior factors that patient can control or change.
Offer and provide assistance with menu selection and diet planning.	Aiding with food selection promotes selection of appropriate foods and assessment of the patient's food choices.
Develop a stimulus control plan with the patient that addresses environment factors (such as avoiding food while watching television, only eating in the kitchen, eating out at work).	Stimulus control is aimed at environment cues that affect eating.
Discuss with the patient how to relate to family and friends who do not share their weight concerns.	Preparing the patient to cope with challenging situations will help them follow their weight management plan.
Administer medications as prescribed, including:	
• Electrolyte supplements	Electrolyte supplements may be needed to correct deficiencies.
• Vitamin and mineral supplements	Vitamin and mineral supplements may be needed to correct deficiencies.
Implement collaborative interventions addressed at treating underlying factors contributing to the weight problem.	Treatment of underlying factors may help the patient achieve weight goals.
Provide additional support when plateaus occur.	Changes in metabolism can result in plateaus, during which patients often need additional support.
Discuss any setbacks that occur.	Discussing setbacks helps the patient overcome challenges and achieve weight goals.
DEVELOPMENT: Implement measures to assist the patient in developing a positive self-image.	Persons with a body weight problem may have a negative self-image.
Mutually establish expectations and behavior contracts for appropriate eating behaviors, food intake, and exercise with the patient who has a dysfunctional eating pattern.	Including the patient in establishing expectations provides the patient with a sense of control that can promote adherence to the plan of care.
Pediatric	
Encourage the support of caregivers, teachers, and peers.	Being positive and supportive throughout treatment can help a child achieve an optimal weight.
Encourage caregivers to be positive role models and involve the entire family in exercise and consuming a healthy diet.	Involving the entire family encourages healthy eating habits and promotes wellness of the child and family.
Limit time with the computer, television, cell phone, and other devices to 2 hours a day.	Limiting device use encourages physical or play activity and other outings.

INTERVENTIONS TO ADDRESS BEING OVERWEIGHT	RATIONALE
Discourage the patient from following restrictive fad diets.	Fad diets often lack adequate nutrients and are hard to maintain on a long-term basis.
Work with interprofessional team members when the patient is prescribed a very-low-calorie diet plan that limits calories to a total of 800 or less per day.	Persons on very-low-calorie diets need frequent monitoring because the severe energy restriction increases the risk for multiple health complications.
Plan an exercise program tailored to the patient's physical condition, goals, and choice.	Exercise, along with diet, are the cornerstones of a permanent weight loss program.

INTERVENTIONS TO ADDRESS BEING OVERWEIGHT	RATIONALE
Administer medications as prescribed, including appetite suppressants and lipase inhibitors.	Medication for obesity is prescribed with comprehensive lifestyle interventions.
Discourage the patient from buying over-the-counter diet aids unless recommended by the health care provider (HCP).	No over-the-counter diet aid has been proven to be both safe and effective.
Assist with preparing the patient for bariatric surgical interventions.	Surgical intervention may be needed to help the patient achieve weight loss goals.

INTERVENTIONS TO ADDRESS BEING UNDERWEIGHT	RATIONALES
Create a pleasant eating environment, serving favorite foods in an attractive manner.	Offering favorite drinks and foods often is effective in increasing intake.
Provide a variety of high-calorie nutritious foods from which to select.	Offering food preferred by the patient enhances intake.
Administer medications as prescribed, including:	
• Nutrition supplements	Nutrition supplements provide extra calories, proteins, fluids, and nutrients.
• Appetite stimulants	Some patients may benefit from appetite stimulants, such as megestrol acetate, to improve intake.
Implement measures to address malnutrition	Many patients who are underweight have an increased risk for being malnourished.
FUNCTIONAL ABILITY: Assist with eating or feeding as needed.	Without help, patients with physical conditions may be unable to achieve an optimal weight.
If needed, accompany patient to bathroom after meals and limit time spent in bathroom during periods when not under observation.	Observation can prevent patients from causing harm to themselves through purging or self-harming.

COLLABORATION	RATIONALE
Dietitian	Collaborating with a dietitian offers the patient further information and support for implementing the prescribed diet.
Community or online support groups	Many patients find benefit in the support offered by persons with similar concerns about weight.
Counseling	Patients who are in a therapy program are more successful in maintaining weight over an extended time.
MOBILITY: Physical therapy	Physical therapists assess, plan, and implement exercise plans that are appropriate for weight goals.
CARE COORDINATION: Social work	Social workers can assist the patient with locating community resources that can be excellent sources for acquiring healthy food.
Dental care	Maintaining oral health and good dentition enhance intake.

PATIENT AND CAREGIVER TEACHING

- Factors that may be contributing to a body weight problem
- Risks associated with a body weight problem
- Classification of weight status
- Management of underlying conditions contributing to a weight problem
- How exercise, diet, habits, customs, and motivation affect weight
- Practical ways to adjust caloric intake
- Appropriate foods for the diet regimen, including portion sizes, calories, nutrition value
- How to maintain and evaluate a food diary
- How to monitor weight
- Life style changes to address a body weight problem
- Community and self-help resources available
- Sources of information and social support
- Safe use of medications and how they fit into the overall weight plan
- Importance of long-term follow up
- When to notify the HCP

DOCUMENTATION

Assessment
- Anthropometric measurements
- Assessments performed
- Diagnostic and laboratory test results
- Manifestations of a body weight problem
- Diet and weight history

Interventions
- Discussions with other interprofessional team members
- Medications and supplements given
- Notification of HCP about patient status
- Therapeutic interventions and the patient's response
- Teaching provided
- Referrals initiated
- Safety measures implemented

Evaluation
- Patient's status: improved, stable, declined
- Manifestations of a body weight problem
- Response to teaching provided
- Response to therapeutic interventions

Impaired Gastrointestinal Function 24

Definition

Impaired ability of the gastrointestinal (GI) system to ingest, absorb, and/or digest food

The main function of the GI system is to supply nutrients to body's cells. Any problem that changes the GI system's physiologic processes affects a person's ability to maintain nutrition status. Many factors influence GI function. A problem can affect the ability to ingest, absorb, and digest food. Medication effects can lead to a decrease in appetite and cause nausea. Caries and periodontal disease can lead to loss of teeth and make consuming adequate nutrition difficult. Diet, alcohol use, smoking, and obesity affect GI organs. Inflammation can make it difficult to attain optimal nutrition despite an appropriate diet or enteral nutrition.

Conceptually, many patients with a GI problem have an increased risk for fluid and electrolyte imbalance and experience pain and symptoms that disrupt activities of daily living. You need to have a basic understanding of the common conditions that impair GI function. A key nursing role is to be able to identify the patient who is at high risk and implement care aimed at relieving symptoms, including pain and nausea, and achieving optimal nutrition intake. Teaching should focus on risk factors and the importance of maintaining good oral hygiene and diet habits.

Associated Clinical Problems

- Heartburn: burning, tight sensation felt intermittently beneath the lower sternum and spreading to the throat or jaw
- Hyperemesis: extreme, persistent nausea and vomiting during pregnancy
- Impaired Dentition: disruption in development, eruption patterns, or structural integrity of the teeth
- Indigestion: group of GI symptoms that occur together, including pain, a burning feeling, or discomfort in the upper abdomen; feeling full too soon while eating; and feeling uncomfortably full after eating
- Nausea: feeling of discomfort with the conscious desire to vomit
- Swallowing Problem: problem with moving fluids and food from the mouth to the stomach
- Vomiting: forceful ejection of stomach contents through the mouth

Common Causes and Risk Factors

- Alcohol use
- Diet
- Food or drugs that decrease lower esophageal sphincter pressure or irritate the esophageal mucosa
- Gallbladder disease
- Gastroesophageal reflux disease (GERD)
- GI cancer
- Infection
- Irritable bowel syndrome
- Malabsorption syndromes
- Medication side effect
- Peptic ulcer disease
- Pregnancy
- Smoking
- Stress

Impaired Dentition

- Bruxism
- Chronic vomiting
- Excess fluoride intake
- Facial trauma
- Impaired self-care
- Ineffective oral hygiene
- Lack of access to dental care
- Nutrition problems

Indigestion

- Consuming coffee, caffeine, carbonated beverages
- Gastritis
- Medications: antibiotics, nonsteroidal antiinflammatory drugs (NSAIDs)

Nausea and Vomiting

- Addison disease
- Brain tumor
- Conditions where the GI tract becomes overly irritated, excited, or distended
- Diabetes

- Impaired cardiac function
- Medications: anesthesia, chemotherapy, opioids, iron
- Meningitis
- Motion sickness
- Renal failure

Swallowing Problem
- Achalasia
- Decreased salivation
- Esophageal stricture
- Neurologic problems: stroke, multiple sclerosis, Parkinson disease

Manifestations
- Anorexia
- Heartburn
- Weight loss
- Laboratory tests: abnormal electrolyte, albumin, prealbumin

Hyperemesis
- Persistent nausea and vomiting

Impaired Dentition
- Caries
- Halitosis
- Lack of or improper fitting dentures
- Malocclusion
- Sensitivity to heat or cold
- Tooth problems: discoloration, erosion, loss, looseness
- Toothache

Indigestion
- Bloating
- Feeling uncomfortably full, or full too soon when eating
- Frequent burping
- Loud growling or gurgling in the stomach
- Nausea
- Pain, burning feeling, or discomfort in the upper abdomen

Nausea and Vomiting
- Electrolyte imbalance
- Hypovolemia
- Increased salivation
- Metabolic acidosis or alkalosis
- "Sick to the stomach"

Swallowing Problem
- Coughing
- Drooling
- Hoarseness
- Pain with swallowing
- Regurgitation
- Sensation of food getting stuck in the throat or chest
- Diagnostic tests: abnormal swallowing evaluation

Key Conceptual Relationships

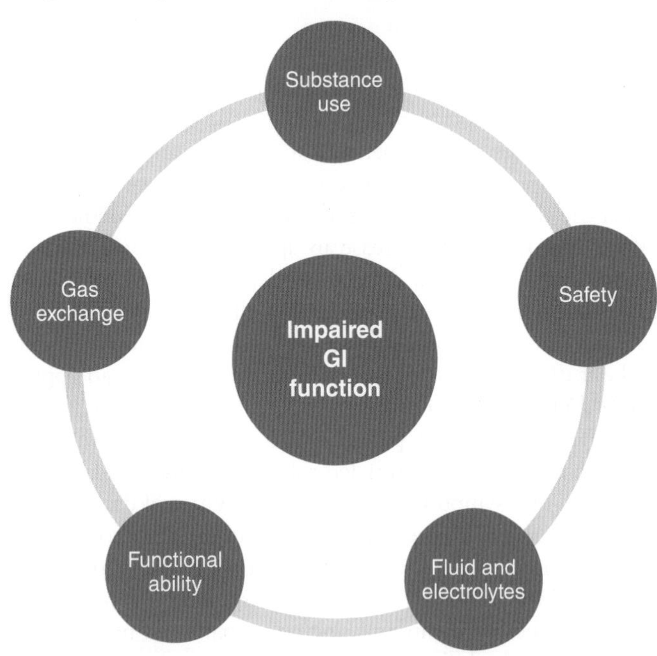

ASSESSMENT OF GI FUNCTION	RATIONALE
Determine whether conditions are present that may be causing or contributing to impaired GI function.	This information aids in determining plan of care and choice of interventions.
Assess for comorbid diseases associated with impaired GI function.	Complications associated with impaired GI function require individualized treatment.
SAFETY: Review medication profile for potential effects on GI function.	Many medications have GI side effects.
Obtain a detailed weight history, including: • Weight pattern over the patient's lifetime • Weight loss or gain within the past 6–12 months • Whether weight changes were intentional • Perceived barriers to attaining weight goals • Following special diets	A loss of > 5% of usual body weight over 6 months (whether intentional or unintentional) is a critical indicator for further assessment.
Obtain a diet history, including: • Usual daily caloric intake • Types of foods eaten • Types of beverages and amounts	A history can identify current strengths and weaknesses in diet intake and aid in determining a treatment plan.

ASSESSMENT OF GI FUNCTION	RATIONALE
Evaluate the patient's food environment, including: • Access to food • Food preparation • Housing situation • Socioeconomic status	The food environment influences diet history and diet plan.
Obtain history of amount and type of fluid intake and elimination habits.	A thorough history helps determine potential contributing factors to GI function.
Perform a complete physical assessment and monitor indicators of GI function on an ongoing basis:	
• Anthropometric measurements	These measures are used to determine the degree of body fat and an optimal weight.
• Oral cavity, noting condition of teeth, gums, mucosa, and salivary glands	Problems with oral health and hygiene can lead to health problems and negatively influence nutrition status.
• Serum levels and trends in levels, as available	
• **FLUID AND ELECTROLYTES:** Electrolytes	Serum electrolyte levels reflect changes taking place between the intracellular and extracellular spaces with nutrition compromise.
• Albumin and prealbumin	Albumin and prealbumin often decrease with impaired nutrition and decreased diet protein intake.
• Manifestations of impaired GI function	Identifying impaired GI function allows for early intervention.
• Daily food diary with calorie count and timing of symptoms	A food diary can help identify patterns that assist with symptom management and help tailor the diet program.
• **FLUID AND ELECTROLYTES:** Fluid balance, including weight, intake and output	Identifying a fluid imbalance that may accompany a GI problem allows for early intervention.
• **GAS EXCHANGE:** Swallowing evaluation	Changes in swallowing affect ability to safely consume a nutritionally sound diet.
Review the assessment for manifestations of impaired nutrition.	Identifying impaired nutrition that may accompany a GI problem allows for early intervention.
FUNCTIONAL ABILITY: Determine the patient's ability to perform basic and instrumental activities of daily living.	Malnutrition affects functional status and functional status affects the ability to obtain and prepare food.
Monitor patient's oral and dental health.	Oral health and dentition affect ability to intake food and fluids. Regular and oral and dental hygiene reduces oral infections and inflammation.
SUBSTANCE USE: Assess for substance use.	Tobacco and alcohol use increase acid production and may cause or worsen problems with GI function.
Weigh patient on a regular basis—preferably at the same time of day and in similar clothing.	Consistent weight monitoring evaluates nutrition state and effectiveness of interventions.
Evaluate patient's response to measures to improve GI function on an ongoing basis.	Identifying the response to therapeutic measures allows for evaluation of therapy effectiveness.

Expected Outcomes

The patient will:

- be free of manifestations of impaired GI function.
- achieve and maintain fluid and electrolyte balance.
- be free of complications from impaired GI function.
- adhere to a prescribed therapeutic regimen.
- recognize factors that can lead to impaired GI function and take preventive action.
- achieve and maintain balanced nutrition.
- achieve and maintain an optimal weight.
- consume a balanced diet.
- demonstrate effective oral hygiene.

INTERVENTIONS TO PROMOTE GI FUNCTION	RATIONALE
Implement collaborative interventions addressed at treating the underlying cause of impaired GI function.	The problem may resolve with treatment of the underlying cause.
Collaborate with the health care provider (HCP) and dietitian to implement interventions that meet the patient's nutrition needs.	The appropriate diet is a key part of resolving impaired nutrition that may accompany a GI problem.
Provide prescribed diet for nutrition goals.	An appropriate diet is a key part of resolving impaired nutrition that may accompany a GI problem.
Offer and provide assistance with menu selection.	Aiding with menu selection promotes selection of appropriate foods and allows an opportunity to determine the patient's understanding of food choices.
FLUID AND ELECTROLYTES: Implement measures, including fluid and electrolyte replacement, to promote proper fluid and electrolyte balance.	Replacement fluid and electrolytes reduce the risk for fluid and electrolyte imbalances.
Notify the HCP if signs and symptoms of impaired GI function persist or worsen.	Achievement of an effective treatment plan often requires adjustments in therapy.
SAFETY: If you suspect a medication is a contributing factor, notify the HCP at once.	The HCP can change the drug dose or prescribe a new drug.
Administer medications as prescribed, including:	
• Antacids	Antacids neutralize acids in the stomach
• Antibiotics	Antibiotics are used to treat *Helicobacter pylori* or other infections.
• H_2 blockers	H_2 blockers decrease the amount of acid the stomach produces.
• Proton pump inhibitors	Proton pump inhibitors decrease the amount of acid the stomach produces.
• Antiemetics	Antiemetics can alleviate nausea and vomiting.
• Cytoprotective agents	Cytoprotective agents protect the gastric mucosa.
SUBSTANCE USE: Promote tobacco and alcohol cessation interventions.	Tobacco and alcohol use increase acid production and may cause or worsen problems with GI function.
GAS EXCHANGE: Implement measures to reduce the risk of aspiration.	The risk of pulmonary aspiration is a concern in patients with impaired swallowing.
Assist with making lifestyle changes needed, such as: • Avoiding exercise right after eating • Chewing food completely • Acheiving a healthy weight • Not eating late-night snacks • Reducing stress • Staying upright 2–3 hours after eating	Implementing lifestyle changes may help relieve some GI symptoms.

INTERVENTIONS TO ADDRESS NAUSEA AND VOMITING	RATIONALE
Maintain nothing by mouth (NPO) status, as appropriate.	Limiting food and fluid intake in certain situations allows the GI tract to rest and reduces the risk of aspiration.
Maintain a quiet, odor-free environment: • Provide oral hygiene between episodes. • Cleanse the face and hands with a cool washcloth. • Help the patient to a comfortable position. • Eliminate noxious odors and sights, such as bedpans and urinals. • Avoid sudden position changes.	These measures make the environment conducive to eating and are often effective in reducing nausea and vomiting.
Encourage the use of relaxation techniques, frequent rest periods, pain management strategies, and diversion.	These measures may help relieve symptoms by reducing factors known to contribute to nausea and vomiting.

INTERVENTIONS TO ADDRESS NAUSEA AND VOMITING	RATIONALE
Explore with the patient the use of appropriate alternative therapies.	Acupressure or acupuncture at specific points, or herbs, such as ginger and peppermint oil, may be effective in reducing nausea and vomiting.
Insert a nasogastric (NG) tube, if prescribed.	The patient may need an NG connected to suction to decompress the stomach.

INTERVENTIONS TO ADDRESS SWALLOWING PROBLEMS	RATIONALE
GAS EXCHANGE: Collaborate with the speech and occupational therapist to provide appropriate interventions, including diet and use of assistive devices.	Speech and occupational therapists provide in-depth clinical assessment and recommend strategies to treat swallowing problems.
Provide food and fluids of the proper consistency based on the swallowing evaluation.	Modifying the consistency of foods and fluids improves the patient's ability to swallow and reduces the risk of aspiration.
Provide an environment to promote swallowing: • Remove distractions. • Have the patient in an upright position with head flexed forward. • Keep the patient upright for 30 minutes after eating.	These measures assist with reducing the risk of aspiration associated with a swallowing problem.

COLLABORATION	RATIONALE
GAS EXCHANGE: Speech therapy	A swallowing evaluation by a speech therapist can detect changes in swallowing ability that affect the ability to safely consume a nutritionally sound diet.
Dietitian	Collaborating with a dietitian offers the patient further information and support for implementing the prescribed diet.
FUNCTIONAL ABILITY: Occupational therapy	The occupational therapist's plan of care is designed to promote performance of activities of daily living.
CARE COORDINATION: Social work	Social workers can assist the patient with locating resources for acquiring healthy food and obtaining dental care.
Dental care	Appropriate care from a dental provider offers the best potential for maintaining dentition and oral health.

PATIENT AND CAREGIVER TEACHING

- Cause of impaired GI function, if known
- Factors that may be contributing to impaired GI function
- Management of conditions contributing to impaired GI function
- Role of GI system and nutrition in maintaining health
- Measures being used to improve GI function
- How to monitor intake, output, and weight
- Ways to maintain fluid and nutrition intake
- Appropriate foods for the diet regimen
- How to care for and maintain teeth and gums
- Safe use of medications, including proper use, side effect management, and how they fit into the overall management plan
- Lifestyle changes to improve GI function
- Early recognition of problems and how to manage them
- Importance of long-term follow-up
- When to notify the HCP or dental provider

DOCUMENTATION

Assessment

- Assessments performed
- Diagnostic and laboratory test results
- Manifestations of impaired GI function
- Screening test results
- Diet and weight history

Interventions

- Discussions with other interprofessional team members
- Medications and supplements given
- Notification of HCP about patient status
- Therapeutic interventions and the patient's response
- Teaching provided
- Referrals initiated

Evaluation

- Patient's status: improved, stable, declined
- Manifestations of impaired GI function
- Response to teaching provided
- Response to therapeutic interventions

Infant Feeding Problem 25

Definition

Difficulty with feeding an infant effectively

Infants require human milk or formula during the first year of life to receive the nutrition necessary for proper growth and development. Exclusive breastfeeding is recommended for the first 6 months of life, with continued breastfeeding and the inclusion of complementary foods until at least 12 months. Breastmilk contains adequate nutrients and vitamins for the first 6 months of life. Solid foods should not be introduced until an infant is 6 months of age.

Feeding issues and problems are relatively common among infants. Not addressing early nutrition compromise is linked to long-term problems in growth, development, and health. Most feeding problems can be managed with outpatient care or care in the community. Nurses play a vital role in supporting parents and infants in implementing good feeding practices and helping them overcome problems.

Associated Clinical Problems

- Breastfeeding Problem: diminished ability to breastfeed
- Lactation Problem: problem with the production and secretion of breastmilk
- Breast Engorgement: excess breast fullness with milk in the postpartum period

Common Risk Factors

Infant

- Being a multiple sibling
- Cleft lip, palate
- Impaired ability to ingest or tolerate feedings
- Infant illness or surgery
- Infant inability to latch on or suck
- Insufficient opportunity to suckle
- Low birth weight
- Neurologic problem
- Poor sucking reflex
- Prematurity
- Receiving supplemental feedings
- Rejection of breast
- Separation of mother and infant
- Small for gestational age
- Weight-for-length or weight-for-height < 5th percentile

Maternal/Parental

- Anxiety
- Breast engorgement
- Cesarean section
- Embarrassment
- Fatigue
- Illness
- Inadequate fluid intake
- Lack of knowledge
- Lack of support
- Malnutrition
- Perceived or inadequate breastmilk supply
- Substance use
- Work schedule

Manifestations

Infant

- Constipation
- Decreased voiding, stools
- Dehydration
- Failure to thrive
- Impaired growth and development
- Infant behaviors
  - Arching or crying at the breast
  - Fussing and/or crying within the first hour after breastfeeding
  - Inability to or resisting latching on correctly
  - Unresponsive to comfort measures
- Slow weight gain, weight loss

Maternal

- Breast engorgement
- Breast tenderness
- Expressed dissatisfaction with breastfeeding
- Inadequate or perceived inadequate milk supply
- Insufficient emptying of breast

Key Conceptual Relationships

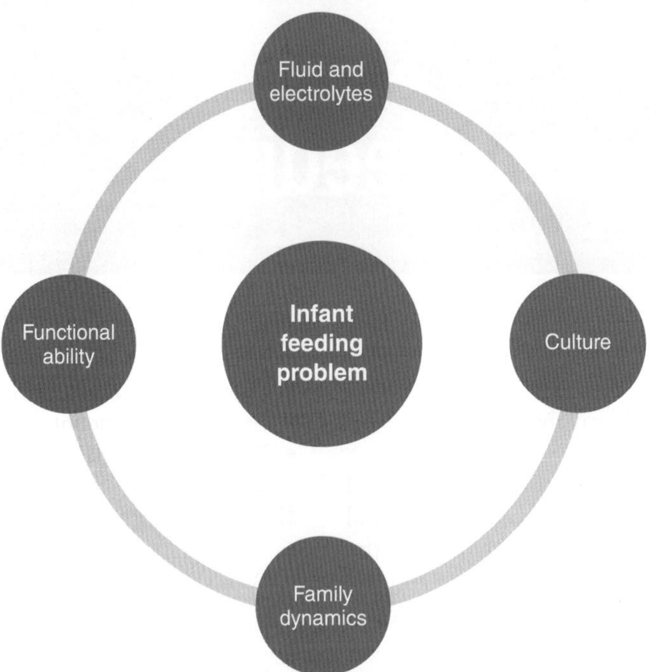

ASSESSMENT OF INFANT FEEDING	RATIONALE
Determine whether infant or maternal physical problems are present that may cause or contribute to an infant feeding problem.	This information aids in determining plan of care and choice of interventions.
Obtain a history of prior breast and formula feeding and review the parent's knowledge base about infant feeding.	This allows the nurse to tailor teaching that is essential to feeding success.
Perform a physical assessment of the infant and monitor indicators of nutrition on an ongoing basis:	
• Growth chart	Analyzing the infant's growth chart for trends can identify areas of concern.
• **FLUID AND ELECTROLYTES:** Number of wet diapers and bowel movements	Evaluating output helps determine the infant's intake, hydration, and nutrition status.
Assess the infant's ability to breastfeed and observe the infant at the breast, noting behavior, position, latch-on, and sucking technique.	An effective sucking technique is important in establishing and maintaining breastfeeding.
Obtain a history of the infant's feeding pattern.	The history of feeding will help determine the adequacy of the infant's source of nutrition and fluid intake.
FAMILY DYNAMICS: Evaluate family dynamics and current level of functioning, and assess parent–child attachment.	Breastfeeding problems and other feeding problems may originate with attachment issues.
Maternal	
Assess the availability of support persons for the parents.	The assistance of support persons helps cope with the challenges of providing infant feeding.
CULTURE: Assess beliefs about infant feeding and breastfeeding, including familial and cultural influences.	Family and cultural practices influence views about infant feeding practices.
Assess the mother's desire and motivation to breastfeed.	Successful breastfeeding depends on the mother's willingness and motivation to breastfeed.
Obtain a maternal diet history, including usual fluid and caloric intake, diet choices, and use of nutrition support.	An adequate fluid intake and appropriate nutrition is necessary to establish and maintain milk supply.
Assess the breast and nipples, noting engorgement, changes in tissue integrity, and pain.	Pain, engorgement, and other problems can interfere with effective infant feeding.
Follow up regularly to reassess status and monitor response to interventions.	Identifying the response to therapeutic measures allows for evaluation of therapy effectiveness.

Expected Outcomes

The infant will:

- have signs of adequate intake: appropriate weight gain, elimination patterns.
- be free from signs of dehydration.
- be free from signs of nutritional compromise.
- have regular, sustained suckling.
- be content after feeding.

The mother will:

- demonstrate effective breastfeeding.
- report satisfaction with the breastfeeding process.
- recognize factors that can lead to ineffective breastfeeding and take preventative action.
- be free of breast problems.

INTERVENTIONS TO PROMOTE INFANT FEEDING	RATIONALE
Determine the most appropriate feeding schedule for the infant.	An infant's feeding schedule depends on age and type of feeding provided.
Include caregivers and support persons when providing teaching and support on infant feeding.	Success with breastfeeding is strongly influenced by family support, values, and beliefs.
Encourage expression of questions and concerns about infant feeding.	Information helps to promote parental self-efficacy and promote an infant feeding pattern appropriate to age.
CULTURE: Tailor education to the parents' cultural beliefs.	Culturally appropriat teaching promotes breastfeeding success.
FUNCTIONAL ABILITY: Encourage the parents to identify support systems to assist with meeting physical and psychosocial needs at home.	Support systems are important in providing optimal infant feeding.
Use measures to promote successful breastfeeding:	
• Assist with correct techniques when performing the first feedings.	Success depends on understanding the basic, correct techniques for breastfeeding.
• Allow for uninterrupted, private breastfeeding periods.	This is an effective strategy to promote exclusive, effective breastfeeding.
• Encourage breastfeeding at least every 2–3 hours initially to establish milk supply, then feed according to infant demand.	Newborns need frequent feeding to satisfy their hunger and establish feeding patterns.
• Encourage the mother to drink at least 2000 mL of fluids daily.	Adequate fluid intake is necessary to maintain breastmilk supply.
• Encourage the mother to follow an appropriate diet.	Increasing caloric intake helps maintain breastmilk supply.
• Assist the mother in planning a day's activities.	Spacing activities helps ensure that the mother gets ample rest.
• To initiate or maintain lactation when the mother cannot breastfeed the infant, have the mother express breastmilk either manually or by using a pump at least every 3 hours.	This assists in establishing and maintaining breastmilk supply.
• Have the mother with engorgement express some breastmilk manually or with a pump.	Expressing breastmilk softens the areola enough to allow the infant to latch on.
Discuss the need to consult the health care provider (HCP) or lactation consultant before taking medications.	Many medications may be delivered to the infant through breastmilk or adversely influence breastmilk supply.
Encourage advanced planning for the mother who intends to continue to breastfeed after returning to work.	This helps the mother establish a breastfeeding schedule that is beneficial for both the mother and infant.
FAMILY DYNAMICS: Institute measures to promote parent–child attachment, as needed.	Breastfeeding problems and other feeding problems may originate with attachment issues in the maternal–child dyad.
Employ measures to promote successful bottle feeding:	
• Assist with correct techniques when providing the first feedings.	This is an opportunity to review basic techniques for bottle feeding.
• Control formula intake by assisting with the choice of bottle size and nipple type.	Bottle and nipple selection need to be appropriate to the infant's sucking style and feeding pattern.
Encourage nonnutritive sucking at the breast or providing a pacifier after feedings if infant shows continued need to suck.	Nonnutritive sucking is comforting and may encourage the development of sucking behavior and improve digestion of a feeding.

COLLABORATION	RATIONALE
Lactation specialist	Collaborating with a lactation specialist offers further information and support for assistance with breastfeeding.
Breastfeeding class	Classes help mothers learn the basics of breastfeeding so they can successfully breastfeed the infant.
Breastfeeding support group	Many mothers find benefit in the support offered by other mothers.

 PATIENT AND CAREGIVER TEACHING

- Cause of an infant feeding problem
- Factors that may be contributing to an infant feeding problem
- What constitutes appropriate infant nutrition
- Appropriate infant feeding schedules
- How to monitor infant's intake, output, weight
- Measures to promote infant sucking
- Use of nonnutritive sucking
- Infant feeding cues
- How to store breastmilk or formula
- Community and self-help resources available
- Anticipatory guidance about common problems
- When to notify the HCP or lactation consultant

Breastfeeding

- Benefits of breastfeeding
- Factors that promote effective breastfeeding
- Importance of proper maternal nutrition
- Effective breastfeeding techniques
- Nipple care
- Ways to reduce or avoid breast engorgement and discomfort
- How to optimize milk supply
- Appropriate diet and hydration for the mother
- Options for milk expression, including use of a breast pump, milk storage

Bottle Feeding

- Effective bottle-feeding techniques
- Appropriate preparation and handling of formula
- How to clean feeding equipment

DOCUMENTATION

Assessment

- Assessments performed
- Growth chart
- Intake and output
- Manifestations of an infant feeding problem

Interventions

- Discussions with other interprofessional team members
- Notification of HCP about patient status
- Therapeutic interventions and the patient's response
- Teaching provided
- Referrals initiated
- Feeding and supplements provided

Evaluation

- Patient's status: improved, stable, declined
- Manifestations of an infant feeding problem
- Response to teaching provided
- Response to therapeutic interventions

Nutritionally Compromised 26

Definition

Poor nutrition due to unbalanced intake or insufficient nutrients

A healthy diet is essential for good nutrition and health. Any change in nutrient intake can result in a person becoming nutritionally compromised. Many problems result in nutritional compromise by changing the way a person ingests, absorbs, digests, and metabolizes nutrients. A patient's nutrition status may be affected by disease or injury state, such as trauma, cancer; physical factors like poor dentition; social factors, including lack of access to food; or psychological factors, such as mental illness. These changes can lead to malnutrition, which impacts health and affects functional status and quality of life.

Nutrition problems occur in all ages, cultures, ethnic groups, and socioeconomic classes and across all education levels. It is important that nurses incorporate assessment and interventions aimed at promoting optimal nutrition. You are responsible for nutrition screening across care settings to identify those who are nutritionally compromised. Collaborate with the health care provider (HCP) and dietitian to implement interventions to meet the patient's nutrition needs. Teach the patient about healthy eating habits and the need for monitoring weights and intake. Explore with them sources for acquiring nourishing food.

Associated Clinical Problems

- Insufficient Fluid Intake: inadequate levels of fluid intake to meet recommended needs
- Loss of Appetite: loss of desire to satisfy bodily need for nutrients or particular types of food
- Poor Response to Enteral Nutrition: no improvement in nutrition status while receiving enteral nutrition
- Risk for Nutrition Problem: increased risk for a deficiency in the quantity and quality of nutrients taken into the body

Common Causes and Risk Factors

- Alcohol use
- Anorexia
- Blood loss
- Burns
- Cancer
- Chronic kidney disease
- Chronic modified diet
- Dementia
- Depression
- Diabetes
- Eating disorder
- Endocrine problems: hyperthyroidism, hyperparathyroidism
- Excess dieting to lose weight
- GI surgeries: gastrectomy, bariatric surgery
- Impaired dentition
- Impaired mobility
- Increased metabolic requirements: fever, infection, trauma
- Involuntary loss or gain of a significant amount of weight (> 10% of usual body weight in 6 months, > 5% in 1 month), even if weight achieved by loss or gain is appropriate for height
- Liver disease
- Malabsorption syndromes
- Medications: antacids, chemotherapy, corticosteroids, H2 receptor antagonists
- Neurologic impairment
- No oral intake and/or receiving standard intravenous solutions for 10 days (adults) or for 5 days (older adults)
- Nutrient losses from malabsorption, dialysis, diarrhea, wounds
- Oral problems: ↓ salivation, impaired mucosal integrity
- Sensory deficits: taste, smell
- Socioeconomic status
- Swallowing problems

Pediatric

- Impaired ability to ingest or tolerate oral feedings
- Low birth weight
- Small for gestational age
- Weight-for-length or weight-for-height < 5th percentile or > 95th percentile

Manifestations

- Anemia
- Anorexia
- Bleeding problems
- Change in bowel habits
- Decreased functional status
- Dizziness
- Dry and scaly skin, brittle nails, rashes
- Edema

- Fatigue
- Frequent infections
- Hair loss; dull, dry, brittle hair
- Hepatomegaly
- Jaundice
- Loss of subcutaneous tissue
- Mental status changes, such as confusion, irritability
- Muscle weakness, ↓ muscle mass
- Nausea
- Neuropathy
- Oral crusting and ulceration, changes in tongue
- Poor wound healing
- Pressure injuries
- Weight loss
- Laboratory studies: abnormal electrolyte levels, ↑ liver enzymes, ↓ hemoglobin and hematocrit, ↓ serum vitamin levels, abnormal CBC, ↓ iron levels

Pediatric

- Impaired growth and development
- Inadequate weight gain or significant ↓ in growth percentile

Key Conceptual Relationships

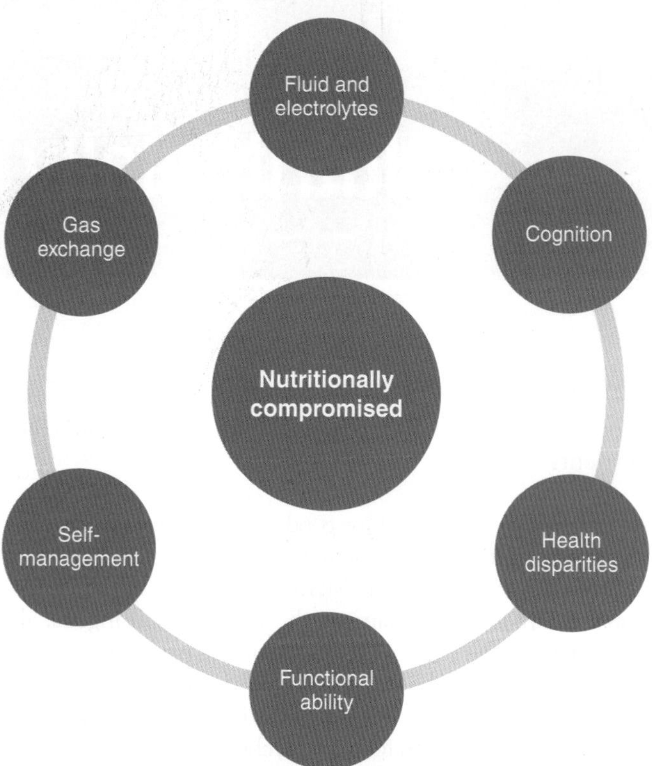

ASSESSMENT OF NUTRITION STATUS	RATIONALE
Determine whether conditions are present that may be causing or contributing to nutritional compromise.	This information aids in determining the plan of care and choice of interventions.
Use a patient-appropriate method to perform a nutrition screening (Table 26.1).	Nutrition risk screening is an integral part of the comprehensive assessment.
Assess for comorbid problems associated with nutritional compromise.	Complications associated with nutritional compromise require individualized treatment.
Obtain a detailed weight history, including: • Weight pattern over the patient's lifetime • Weight loss or gain within the past 6–12 months • Whether weight changes were intentional • Perceived barriers to attaining weight goals • Following specific diets	A loss of $>$ 5% of usual body weight over 6 months (whether intentional or unintentional) is a critical indicator for further assessment.
Obtain a diet history, including: • Usual daily caloric intake • Types of foods eaten • Types of beverages and amounts	A history can identify strengths and weaknesses in the diet and aid in determining a treatment plan.
Evaluate the patient's food environment, including: • Access to food • Food preparation • Housing situation • Socioeconomic status	The food environment influences diet history and diet plan.
Screen the patient for an eating disorder.	Early treatment is important for those with or at risk of an eating disorder.
SAFETY: Review the medication regimen for potential effects on nutrition.	Many drug–nutrient interactions affect the use of nutrients in the body.
IMMUNITY: Assess for food allergies.	A thorough history helps identify food allergies and guides intervention.

ASSESSMENT OF NUTRITION STATUS	RATIONALE
Perform a physical assessment and monitor indicators of nutrition status on an ongoing basis.	
• Anthropometric measurements: height, weight, BMI, waist:hip ratio, waist and midarm circumference, body fat percent, body shape	These measures are used to determine the degree of body fat and optimal weight.
• Serum levels and trends, as available:	
• Vitamin levels	Vitamin levels are often decreased with nutritional compromise.
• Prealbumin, albumin, total protein	Prealbumin, albumin, and total protein are indicators of nutrition stores and guide diet selection.
• Electrolytes	Serum electrolyte levels reflect changes taking place between the intracellular and extracellular spaces with malnutrition.
• CBC with hemoglobin, hematocrit	The RBC count and hemoglobin level may show the presence and degree of anemia. The total lymphocyte count decreases in malnutrition.
• Liver function studies	Liver enzyme levels may be increased with malnutrition.
• Glucose	Glucose reflects carbohydrate metabolism.
• Iron	Iron deficiency is common due to consuming a diet low in iron-rich foods.
• Manifestations of a nutrition imbalance	Identifying an accompanying nutrition imbalance allows for early identification and intervention.
• Daily food diary with calorie count	Calorie count and a food diary help identify patterns requiring change and provide a base on which to tailor the diet program.
Calculate nitrogen balance.	Nitrogen balance is a common proxy measure of protein balance.
SELF-MANAGEMENT: Assess the patient's exercise activity.	Nutrition intake may need adjustments to meet energy expenditure.
Monitor patient's dental health, including fit and condition of dentures.	Oral health and dentition affect ability to intake food and fluids.
FUNCTIONAL ABILITY: Assess the patient's ability to perform basic and instrumental activities of daily living.	Malnutrition affects functional status and functional status affects the ability to obtain and prepare food.
CULTURE: Assess the role of culture on the patient's diet.	Culture influences eating habits and attitudes toward food and body weight.
Weigh on a regular basis—preferably, same time of day and in similar clothing.	Consistent weight monitoring evaluates nutrition and effectiveness of interventions.
Follow up regularly to reassess status and monitor response to interventions.	Identifying the response to therapeutic measures allows for evaluation of therapy effectiveness.
Pediatric	
Determine the ability of the parent/caregiver to provide the diet plan.	The parent/caregiver is the person responsible for providing care needs.

Table 26.1 Mini Nutrition Assessment

A Has food intake declined over the past 3 months due to loss of appetite, digestive problems, chewing or swallowing difficulties?
0 = severe decrease in food intake
1 = moderate decrease in food intake
2 = no decrease in food intake
☐

B Weight loss during the last 3 months
0 = weight loss greater than 3 kg (6.6 lbs)
1 = does not know
2 = weight loss between 1 and 3 kg (2.2 and 6.6 lbs)
3 = no weight loss
☐

C Mobility
0 = bed or chair bound
1 = able to get out of bed/chair but does not go out
2 = goes out
☐

D Has suffered psychological stress or acute disease in the past 3 months?
0 = yes 2 = no
☐

E Neuropsychological problems
0 = severe dementia or depression
1 = mild dementia
2 = no psychological problems
☐

F1 Body Mass Index (BMI) (weight in kg)/(height in m)^2 ☐
0 = BMI less than 19
1 = BMI 19 to less than 21
2 = BMI 21 to less than 23
3 = BMI 23 or greater
☐

F2 Calf circumference (CC) in cm
0 = CC less than 31
3 = CC 31 or greater
☐

Screening score
(max. 14 points) ☐☐

12–14 points: ☐ Normal nutritional status
8–11 points: ☐ At risk of malnutrition
0–7 points: ☐ Malnourished

Save
Print
Reset

Source: Nestle Nutrition Institute. MNA Mini Nutritional Assessment. Retrieved from: https://www.mna-elderly.com/default.html.

Recommendations for Interventions

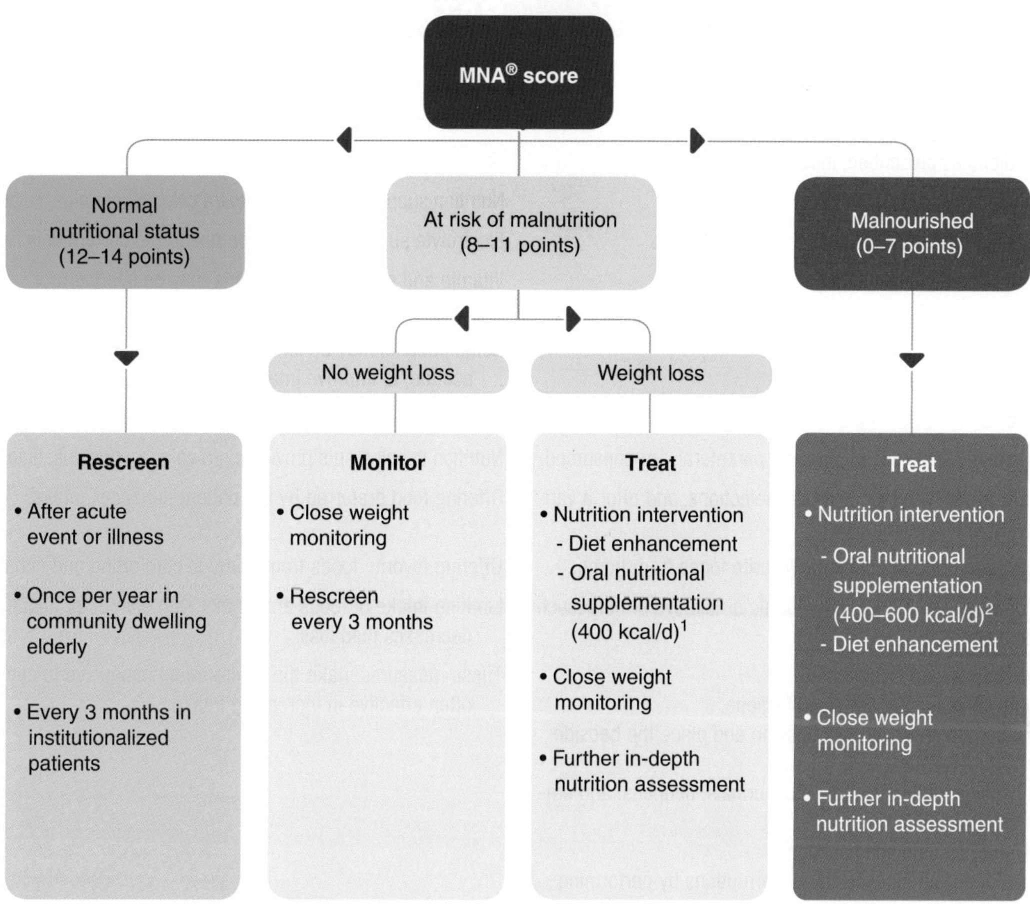

Expected Outcomes

The patient will:

- achieve and maintain balanced nutrition.
- achieve and maintain an optimal weight.
- be free of complications from being nutritionally compromised.
- adhere to a prescribed therapeutic regimen.
- recognize factors that can lead to compromised nutrition and take preventative action.
- consume a balanced diet.
- make food choices appropriate to the diet plan.
- maintain optimal physical functioning.

INTERVENTIONS TO ACHIEVE BALANCED NUTRITION	RATIONALE
Be sensitive and nonjudgmental in asking specific, leading questions about weight, diet, and exercise.	This allows you to obtain information and helps the patient understand the reason for questions asked about weight or diet habits.
Collaborate with the HCP and dietitian to implement interventions to meet the patient's nutrition needs.	Collaborating with a dietitian offers the patient further information and support.
Provide a prescribed diet for nutrition goals.	The appropriate diet is a critical part of achieving balanced nutrition.
Encourage the patient to maintain a food diary, including when and where eating takes place and the circumstances around which the food was eaten.	A diary provides a means to determine nutrition adequacy and focuses attention on behavior factors that the patient can control or change.

Continued

INTERVENTIONS TO ACHIEVE BALANCED NUTRITION	RATIONALE
Offer and provide needed assistance with menu selection.	Aiding with menu selection promotes selection of appropriate foods and allows an opportunity to determine the patient's understanding of food choices.
Administer medications as prescribed, including:	
• Nutrition supplements	Nutrition supplements provide extra calories, proteins, fluids, and nutrients.
• **FLUID AND ELECTROLYTES:** Electrolyte supplements	Electrolyte supplements may be needed to correct deficiencies.
• Vitamin and mineral supplements	Vitamin and mineral supplements may be needed to correct deficiencies.
• Appetite stimulants	Some patients may benefit from appetite stimulants, such as megestrol acetate, to improve intake.
• Antiemetics	Nausea can interfere with the intake of an appropriate diet.
Ensure that supplements, including enteral and parenteral, are consumed.	Nutrition supplements provide extra calories, proteins, fluids, and nutrients.
Allow the patient to assist with food and fluid selections, and offer a variety of appropriate drinks and foods.	Offering food preferred by the patient enhances intake.
Encourage the family to bring the patient's favorite foods from home.	Offering favorite foods from home is comforting and enhances intake.
Minimize intake of foods and drinks with diuretic or laxative effects (such as tea, coffee, prunes).	Limiting intake of foods and drinks with diuretic or laxative effects decreases fluid loss.
Provide a positive meal experience: • Offer oral hygiene and provide hand hygiene. • Help the patient to a comfortable position and place the bedside table at the right height. • Clear the bedside table of clutter. Place urinals, bedpans, and emesis basins out of sight. • If needed, open cartons and packages. • Protect mealtime from unnecessary interruptions by performing non urgent care before or after mealtime.	These measures make the environment conducive to eating and are often effective in increasing intake.
FUNCTIONAL ABILITY: Promote oral intake for those who need assistance.	Without assistance, patients with impaired functional ability may be unable to achieve balanced nutrition.
COGNITION: Offer fluids and food at regular intervals to patients with impaired cognition.	Cognitive impairments can interfere with recognition of thirst and hunger.
IMMUNITY: Institute measures, including an avoidance diet, to address food allergies.	Measures to reduce the risk of food allergies include an avoidance diet.
Assist patients with physical conditions such as reduced physical strength or coordination with eating.	Without assistance, patients with physical conditions may be unable to achieve balanced nutrition.
Assist with implementing the plan of care developed by occupational therapy.	The occupational therapist's plan of care is designed to promote optimal performance of activities of daily living.
Encourage family and significant others to assist the patient, as appropriate.	Involving family and significant others in the patient's care has a positive effect on patient outcomes.
SELF-MANAGEMENT: Provide positive reinforcement for achieving nutrition goals.	Positive reinforcement promotes the patient's confidence in continuing behaviors that promote optimal nutrition.
Pediatric	
Offer appealing fluids (ice pops, frozen juice bars, snow cones, water, milk).	Appealing fluids may help increase fluid intake.
Use age-appropriate fun containers (colorful cups, decorative straws), games, charts, rewards, and activities.	Age-appropriate measures are often effective in increasing oral intake.

COLLABORATION	RATIONALE
GAS EXCHANGE: Speech therapy	A swallowing evaluation by a speech therapist can detect changes in swallowing that affect the to safely consume a sound diet.
Dietitian	Collaborating with a dietitian offers the patient further information and support for implementing the prescribed diet.
FUNCTIONAL ABILITY: Occupational therapy	The occupational therapist's plan of care is designed to promote performance of activities of daily living.
CARE COORDINATION: Social work	Social workers can assist the patient with locating resources for acquiring healthy food and obtaining dental care.
Dental care	Appropriate care from a dental provider offers the best potential for maintaining dentition and oral health.
HEALTH DISPARITIES: Community agencies	Community resources can be an excellent source of acquiring food.

PATIENT AND CAREGIVER TEACHING

- Cause of the patient being nutritionally compromised, if known
- Factors that contribute to nutritional compromise
- Role of diet and nutrition in maintaining health
- Risks associated with nutritional compromise
- Measures being used to achieve nutrition balance
- How long it will take to achieve nutrition balance
- How to monitor intake, output, weight
- Appropriate foods and fluids for the diet plan
- Safe use of medications, including supplements, and how they fit into the overall management plan
- Lifestyle changes to help achieve nutrition balance
- Ways to maintain skin integrity
- Community and self-help resources available
- Importance of long-term follow-up
- When to notify the HCP

DOCUMENTATION

Assessment

- Anthropometric measurements
- Assessments performed
- Diagnostic and laboratory test results
- Manifestations of nutritional compromise
- Screening test results
- Diet and weight history

Interventions

- Discussions with other interprofessional team members
- Medications and supplements given
- Notification of HCP about patient status
- Therapeutic interventions and the patient's response
- Teaching provided
- Referrals initiated
- Safety measures implemented

Evaluation

- Patient's status: improved, stable, declined
- Manifestations of nutritional compromise
- Response to teaching provided
- Response to therapeutic interventions

Impaired Cardiac Function 27

Definition

Inadequate blood pumped from the heart to meet the body's needs

The cells of the body need oxygen and nutrients and a way to discard waste. *Perfusion* is a process of the heart pumping blood through arteries and capillaries to deliver nutrients and oxygen to cells while removing the waste products of metabolism. Adequate cardiac function, patent arteries and veins, and sufficient oxygen and nutrient-rich blood volume are needed to ensure perfusion. Brain function requires an adequate perfusion pressure that can be maintained despite postural changes.

When blood supply to an area is decreased, the term *ischemia* is used. Cells in some areas of the body, such as the brain and heart, are very sensitive to blood flow and become ischemic in minutes without oxygen and glucose. Other tissues can survive periods of little or no blood flow for a longer time. The extent of tissue damage from poor perfusion depends on the size and location of the blood vessel and whether the blood supply is reduced or completely interrupted. Prolonged ischemia eventually leads to infarction and necrosis of tissue.

Maintaining perfusion requires sufficient cardiac output. Normal cardiac output ranges from 4 to 6 L/minute in the adult. The variables that contribute to cardiac output are stroke volume (the amount of blood ejected with each contraction) and heart rate. Stroke volume depends on *preload* (the end-diastolic volume in the heart) and *afterload* (the amount of resistance within the vasculature that the heart must pump against). If central perfusion is impaired, the entire body is affected. Shock occurs when blood supply to tissues is impaired because of inadequate cardiac output, significant blood loss, or systemic vasodilation.

Associated Clinical Problems

- Altered Cardiac Output: volume of blood pumped by the heart outside the normal range
- Angina: paroxysmal thoracic pain caused most often by myocardial anoxia from atherosclerosis or spasm of the coronary arteries
- Bradycardia: slow heart rate, <60/min for an adult
- Impaired Cardiac Output: inadequate blood pumped from the heart to meet the body's needs
- Irregular Heart Rhythm: cardiac electrical activity occurring at uneven intervals
- Risk for Bradycardia: risk for a slowed heart rate
- Risk for Impaired Cardiac Output: risk for inadequate blood pumped from the heart to meet the body's needs
- Tachycardia: rapid heart rate, >100/min for an adult

Common Causes and Risk Factors

- Anaphylaxis
- Burns
- Cardiac tamponade
- Cardiogenic shock
- Cardiomyopathy
- Chest trauma
- Congenital heart defects
- Coronary artery disease
- Dysrhythmias
- Electrolyte imbalance
- Fluid imbalance, including hypovolemia and dehydration
- Heart failure
- Hypertension
- Inflammatory heart disorders, such as infective endocarditis and pericarditis
- Left ventricular hypertrophy
- Myocardial infarction and ischemia
- Neurologic injury
- Rheumatic heart disease
- Septic shock
- Valvular heart disease

Manifestations

- Angina
- Anxiety, restlessness
- Confusion
- Cool, clammy skin ranging from pale to cyanotic
- Crackles
- Decreased peripheral pulses
- Dizziness and fainting
- Dyspnea
- Dysrhythmias and changes in heart rate, including bradycardia and tachycardia
- Fatigue
- Frothy, blood-tinged sputum
- Hypertension
- Hypotension
- Jugular venous distention

- Murmur
- Oliguria
- Orthopnea
- Palpitations
- Paroxysmal nocturnal dyspnea
- Pericardial friction rub
- Peripheral edema
- Pulsus alternans (alternating weak and strong heartbeats)
- S3 and S4 heart sounds
- Sleep apnea
- Tachypnea
- Diagnostic tests
  - Troponin elevations or other elevations in cardiac biomarkers may indicate myocardial injury.
  - A 12-lead electrocardiogram (ECG) may detect myocardial ischemia and infarction.
  - A cardiac stress test may indicate coronary artery disease.
  - A complete blood count may indicate anemia and decreased oxygen-carrying capacity.

Key Conceptual Relationships

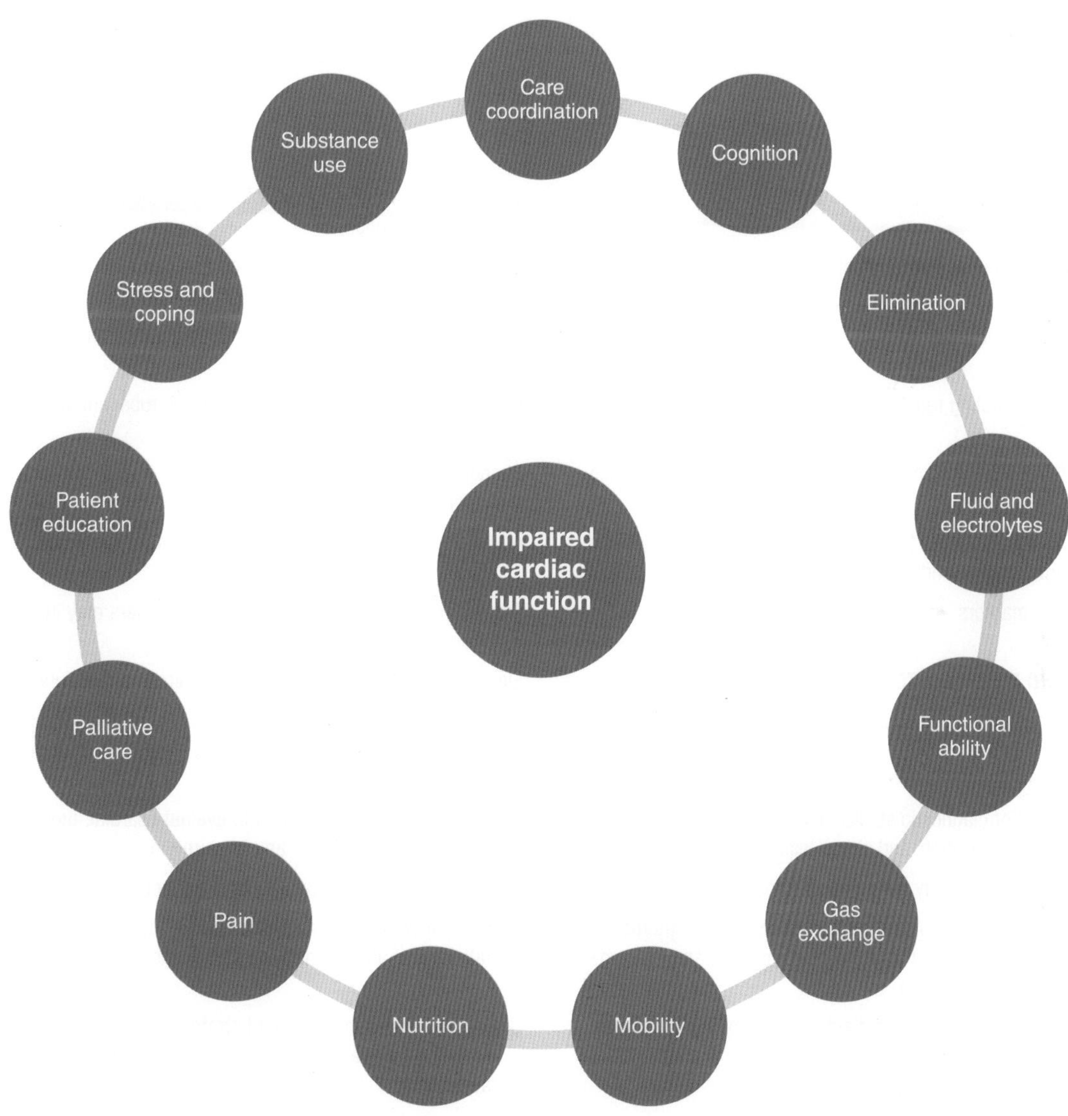

ASSESSMENT OF CARDIAC FUNCTION	RATIONALE
Identify patients who need emergency management of cardiac problems.	Identifying a cardiac problem allows for the patient to be stabilized immediately.
Assess risk factors for impaired cardiac function.	Identifying factors that place the patient at risk for impaired cardiac function allows for early intervention.
Determine the potential cause of impaired cardiac function.	Treating the cause is part of the overall management plan.
Obtain a thorough history of any cardiac symptoms, such as angina or palpitations, including: • When symptoms started • Onset, sudden or gradual • Frequency • Intensity or severity • Alleviating and aggravating factors • Any pattern to the symptoms • Therapy tried and its effectiveness	A thorough history aids in evaluating the degree of the patient's cardiac problem and helps direct treatment.
Perform a complete physical assessment and monitor indicators of cardiac function on an ongoing basis:	
• Manifestations of impaired cardiac function	Identifying the manifestations of impaired cardiac function allows for early intervention.
• Vital signs, including pulse oximetry and orthostatic blood pressure (BP)	Vital signs provide a measure of central perfusion and with oximetry, the oxygen available.
• Continuous cardiac monitoring	Dysrhythmias are a common manifestation and cause of impaired cardiac function.
• Heart sounds, noting regularity and presence of adventitious sounds	Additional heart sounds, including S3, S4, rubs, and murmurs, may occur with various cardiac problems.
• **COGNITION:** Mental status, including orientation to time, place, person, and situation	Changes in cognition and level of consciousness may indicate ↓ perfusion.
• **FLUID AND ELECTROLYTES:** Fluid status, including daily weights, hourly urine output, and intake and output	Adequate fluid volume is needed for adequate perfusion.
• Cardiac biomarkers	Troponin elevations or other cardiac biomarkers may indicate myocardial injury.
• **FLUID AND ELECTROLYTES:** Serum electrolyte levels	Electrolyte imbalances may cause impaired cardiac function.
• Oxygen consumption, such as Svo_2, if available	Svo_2 monitoring can be used to assess the balance of oxygen supply and demand, and guide treatment that supports sufficient tissue perfusion and oxygenation.
Evaluate the results of diagnostic studies, including ECGs, echocardiography, cardiac catheterization, and stress testing.	Diagnostic tests are performed to evaluate cardiac function and help determine the cause of any impairment.
Monitor vital signs continuously during acute impairment.	Continuous monitoring can identify changes in perfusion.
FUNCTIONAL ABILITY: Determine the effect of cardiac symptoms on the patient's level of fatigue and ability to perform basic and instrumental activities of daily living (ADLs).	The patient with a cardiac problem may have fatigue and other manifestations that affect functional status and activity tolerance.
STRESS AND COPING: Assess the patient's use of coping and stress management strategies.	Coping and stress management strategies can improve quality of life by reducing fatigue and helping the patient better manage cardiac symptoms.
SUBSTANCE USE: Screen for tobacco and/or other substance use.	Smoking, vaping, and intravenous (IV) drug use are significant risk factors for cardiac problems.
Evaluate the patient's response to measures to correct impaired cardiac function through ongoing assessment.	Identifying the presence of manifestations of impaired cardiac function allows for evaluation of therapy effectiveness.

Expected Outcomes

The patient will:

- maintain adequate general perfusion.
- be free from complications associated with impaired cardiac function.
- adhere to the prescribed therapeutic regimen.
- maintain ongoing contact with the appropriate community resources.
- participate in desired ADLs.

INTERVENTIONS TO PROMOTE CARDIAC FUNCTION	RATIONALE
Initiate emergency protocols if manifestations of inadequate coronary artery perfusion, such as chest pain or discomfort, ST changes on ECG, and elevated cardiac biomarkers, occur.	Cardiac ischemia may be a cause or a result of impaired cardiac function.
GAS EXCHANGE: Institute measures to enhance optimal tissue oxygenation: • Provide supplemental oxygen if needed. • Administer continuous positive airway pressure (CPAP) or appropriate respiratory support. • Position the patient to optimize respiratory function.	These measures combat hypoxia, which worsens cardiac function.
Monitor hemoglobin level and administer blood products if needed.	Hemoglobin is needed for oxygen transport.
Notify the health care provider (HCP) if manifestations of impaired cardiac function persist or worsen.	The patient may require emergency support and adjustments in the plan of care.
Prepare the patient for urgent cardiac revascularization if needed.	Percutaneous coronary intervention or coronary artery bypass graft may be required to save ischemic cardiac muscle.
STRESS AND COPING: Offer emotional support to the patient and family.	Emotional support can reduce or prevent anxiety, which may worsen cardiac status.
PAIN: Implement measures to relieve pain, if present.	Pain increases anxiety and oxygen demand.
STRESS AND COPING: Respond to patient and family in a calm tone and explain procedures.	Reduce stress to decrease oxygen demand.
Administer medications and fluids as prescribed, including the following:	
• **FLUID AND ELECTROLYTES:** IV fluids and blood products	IV fluids and blood products are given to maintain an optimal fluid volume.
• Antiarrhythmics	Dysrhythmias can result in a dramatic decrease in stroke volume and cardiac output.
• Diuretics	Diuretics decrease blood volume and venous pressure, which decreases preload, stroke volume, and cardiac output, lowering BP.
• Inotropes	Inotropes optimize cardiac function through their influence on heart rate and the strength of cardiac contractions.
• Vasoactive drugs	Vasoactive drugs increase BP through vasoconstriction.
• Antiplatelet agents, thrombolytics, and anticoagulants	These drugs are given to restore or maintain blood flow to the cardiac tissue.
If continuous vasoactive drugs are used, titrate based on continuous BP and maintain continuous cardiac monitoring.	Careful titration of vasoactive drugs is needed for safe administration.
MOBILITY: Maintain bed rest during acute impairment.	Bed rest minimizes oxygen demands.
FUNCTIONAL STATUS: Encourage activity level according to available cardiac output and the patient's abilities.	Regular physical activity builds endurance and maintains muscle strength.
Prepare the patient for ultrafiltration or continuous renal replacement therapy (CRRT) if needed.	Ultrafiltration or CRRT may be used to remove excess fluid volume.
NUTRITION: If the patient is able to eat, provide small meals with limited sodium and saturated fat.	A low-sodium diet avoids fluid overload, which decreases cardiac oxygen demand.
ELIMINATION: Implement measures to address constipation, if needed, including administering stool softeners.	Straining at stools with constipation increases oxygen demand.
SUBSTANCE USE: Encourage tobacco cessation.	Smoking and vaping are serious risk factors for coronary artery disease.

COLLABORATION	RATIONALE
Cardiac rehabilitation	The aim of cardiac rehabilitation is to provide education and monitored exercise to support achieving an optimal level of function.
GAS EXCHANGE: Respiratory therapy	Respiratory therapists assess, plan, and implement interventions that promote a person's optimal oxygenation.
NUTRITION: Dietitian	Collaborating with a dietitian offers the patient further information and support for implementing the prescribed diet.
Disease or symptom management programs	Disease or symptom management programs help patients understand their treatment regimen and address the complex needs of those with chronic illness.
CARE COORDINATION: Social services or case management	Support may be needed to obtain financial, transportation, or other resources.
Community or online support groups	Many patients with chronic cardiac disease find benefit in the support offered by persons with similar concerns.
PALLIATIVE CARE: Palliative care	Palliative care can increase comfort and quality of life and improve care coordination for those with serious chronic heart problems.
Physical therapy	Physical therapists can assess the patient and develop a plan of care to maximize exercise capability.

PATIENT AND CAREGIVER TEACHING

- Cause of impaired cardiac function, if known, and how long it may last
- Normal cardiac function
- Reason the patient is at risk for impaired cardiac function
- Manifestations of impaired cardiac function
- Management of any underlying condition contributing to the impaired cardiac function
- Measures being used to improve impaired cardiac function
- Diagnostic and laboratory tests used to monitor cardiac function
- Any needed lifestyle changes to improve cardiac function
- Early recognition of problems and how to manage them
- Safe use of medications, including proper use, side effect management, administration, and how they fit into the overall management plan
- Low-sodium, low-saturated-fat diet
- Positive coping and stress management strategies
- How to monitor and the importance of daily weights and BP
- Community and self-help resources available
- Sources of information and social support
- Gradual physical activity and exercise plan
- Tobacco cessation methods
- Importance of long-term follow-up
- Role of therapy and case management
- When to notify the HCP and when to seek emergency care

DOCUMENTATION

Assessment

- Assessments performed
- Manifestations of impaired cardiac function
- Diagnostic and laboratory test results

Interventions

- Medications given
- Notification of HCP about diagnostic test results and assessment findings
- Therapeutic interventions and the patient's response
- Teaching provided
- Referrals initiated
- Precautions implemented
- Discussions with other members of the interprofessional team
- Environmental modifications made
- Safety measures implemented, including venous thromboembolism (VTE) precautions

Evaluation

- Patient's status: improved, stable, declined
- Diagnostic test results
- Patient's response to therapeutic interventions
- Presence of any manifestations of impaired cardiac function
- Patient's response to teaching provided

Impaired Tissue Perfusion 28

Definition

Inadequate blood circulation to a particular area of the body

Tissue perfusion refers to the volume of blood that flows through target tissues. This perfusion is supplied by blood flowing from arteries to capillaries and back to veins. Inadequate tissue perfusion can result from a lack of cardiac output or from a local obstruction, such as a blocked blood vessel. The decrease in perfusion can cause ischemia and eventually tissue necrosis.

Patients with impaired tissue perfusion often have pain and difficulties with mobility and taking part in activities of daily living. Education is a key part of management. Nurses can provide support through health promotion regarding proper nutrition, smoking cessation, and exercise. Nurses help patients manage acute and chronic problems of tissue perfusion.

Associated Clinical Problems

- Anemia: inadequate supply of red blood cells or hemoglobin to carry oxygen to the tissues
- Impaired Circulatory System Function: inadequate transportation of nutrients and wastes through the body
- Risk for Impaired Peripheral Neurovascular Function: at risk for disruption to the circulatory, motor, or sensory function in an extremity
- Risk for Ineffective Tissue Perfusion: at risk for inadequate blood circulation
- Risk for Shock: at risk for inadequate oxygen delivery to the body tissues

Common Causes and Risk Factors

- Advanced age
- Cancer, chemotherapy
- Clotting disorders
- Diabetes
- Elevated serum lipids
- Estrogen therapy, including estrogen-based oral contraceptives
- Genetics
- Hypertension
- Local constriction from clothing, devices
- Obesity
- Pregnancy
- Prolong immobility
- Prolonged standing
- Smoking, vaping
- Sedentary lifestyle
- Sex: more common in males than females
- Trauma
- Vascular disorders, such as arteriosclerosis, sickle cell disease
- Venous stasis
- Diagnostic tests: ultrasound showing the presence of a clot

Key Conceptual Relationships

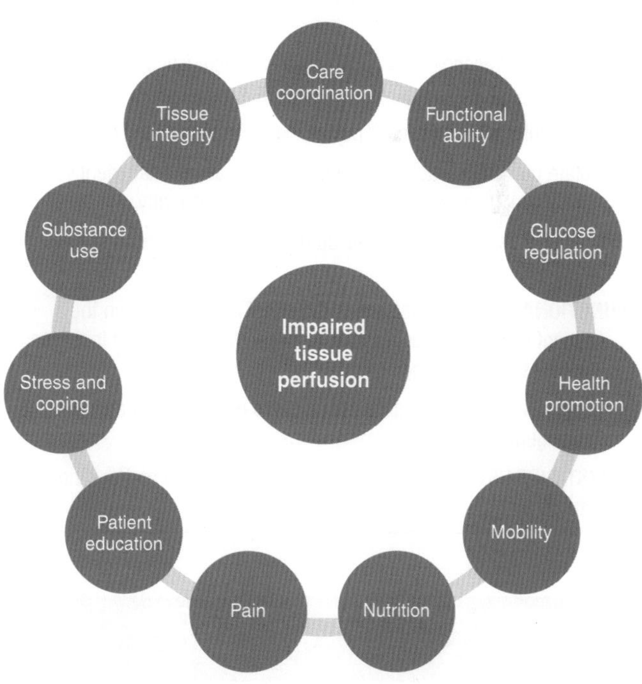

ASSESSMENT OF TISSUE PERFUSION	RATIONALE
Identify patients needing emergency management of a tissue perfusion problem.	Identifying a tissue perfusion problem allows for the patient to be immediately stabilized.
Assess risk factors for impaired tissue perfusion.	Identifying factors that place patients at risk for impaired tissue perfusion allows for early intervention.
Determine the potential cause of impaired tissue perfusion.	Treating the cause is part of the overall management plan.
Obtain a complete medication history.	A number of drugs directly influence perfusion or interact with the medication therapies used to treat impaired perfusion.
Obtain a thorough history of any symptoms of impaired tissue perfusion, such as pain with activity or leg edema, including: • When symptoms started • Onset—sudden or gradual • Frequency • Intensity or severity • Alleviating and aggravating factors • Any pattern to the symptoms • Therapy tried and its effectiveness	A thorough history aids in evaluating the degree of the patient's tissue perfusion problem and helps direct treatment.
Perform a complete physical assessment and monitor indicators of tissue perfusion on an ongoing basis:	
• Manifestations of generalized impairment of tissue perfusion	Identifying impaired cardiac function allows for intervention that may improve general tissue perfusion.
• Brachial, radial, dorsalis pedis, posterior tibial, and popliteal pulses bilaterally	Decreases in pulse quality occur with altered perfusion.
• Extremities for color, temperature, capillary refill, sensation, movement, edema	Abnormalities in the peripheral vascular assessment identify changes in perfusion.
• **TISSUE INTEGRITY:** Skin assessment, particularly of the legs and feet	Patients with decreased tissue perfusion are at an increased risk for impaired tissue integrity.
• **PAIN:** Presence of extremity pain, characteristics of that pain	A thorough pain assessment can help differentiate arterial and venous disease and determine the need for analgesia.
Use a Doppler stethoscope for pulses that cannot be found by palpation.	A weak pulse may be found with a Doppler stethoscope.
Calculate the ankle-brachial index unless the patient has recently had a percutaneous or surgical intervention on an extremity.	The index indicates the relative severity of a tissue perfusion impairment.
Evaluate the results of diagnostic studies, including ultrasound and arteriography.	Diagnostic tests are performed to evaluate peripheral vascular system function.
FUNCTIONAL ABILITY: Determine the effect of symptoms on the patient's level of fatigue and ability to perform basic and instrumental activities of daily living.	The patient with impaired tissue perfusion may have leg pain with activity and other manifestations that affect functional status.
STRESS AND COPING: Assess the patient's use of coping and stress management strategies.	Coping and stress management strategies can improve self-care management and quality of life.
SUBSTANCE USE: Screen for the presence of tobacco and/or other substance use.	Smoking and vaping cause peripheral vasoconstriction, significantly contributing to impaired tissue perfusion.

ASSESSMENT OF RISK FOR BLEEDING	RATIONALE
Observe closely for signs of bleeding, including hypotension, tachycardia, hematuria, melena, hematemesis, petechiae, ecchymosis, or bleeding from trauma site or surgical incision.	New signs of bleeding require intervention to avoid poor patient outcomes.
Monitor the results of appropriate laboratory testing, including INR, aPTT, PT, complete blood count, hemoglobin, hematocrit, platelet levels, and/or liver enzymes.	Laboratory tests are performed to evaluate blood clotting ability and the risk of bleeding.

Expected Outcomes

The patient will:

- maintain adequate tissue perfusion.
- be free from complications associated with impaired tissue perfusion.
- adhere to the prescribed therapeutic regimen.
- maintain ongoing contact with the appropriate community resources.
- participate in desired activities of daily living.

INTERVENTIONS FOR PROMOTING TISSUE PERFUSION	RATIONALE
Notify the health care provider (HCP) immediately if there is a loss of pulse with a cold extremity.	Loss of perfusion requires immediate treatment to preserve the limb.
Administer medications as ordered, including:	
• Antiplatelet agents, such as aspirin or clopidogrel (Plavix)	Antiplatelet agents reduce the risk of arterial and venous thrombosis.
• Antilipemic agents, such as atorvastatin (Lipitor)	Antilipemic agents are used to lower blood cholesterol profiles in peripheral vascular disease.
• Ramipril (Altace)	Ramipril, an ACE inhibitor, is effective in reducing symptoms of intermittent claudication in some patients with peripheral arterial disease.
• Cilostazol, pentoxifylline	These agents may be effective in reducing symptoms of intermittent claudication.
MOBILITY: Encourage patients with intermittent claudication to continue walking to the point of pain.	Mobility promotes the development of collateral circulation.
Position the patient for optimal perfusion, including:	Positioning may vary with arterial and venous conditions.
• Avoid elevating the legs of the patient with arterial disease above the heart level.	Elevation decreases arterial blood flow.
• Elevate the legs above the heart level for the patient with venous disease.	Elevation improves venous return and decreases edema.
Implement measures to protect the tissues from injury: • Use heel protectors and other devices to minimize pressure. • Provide careful foot care. • Do not apply thermal therapies directly to the skin. • Have the patient wear soft, roomy, protective footwear.	Patients with impaired tissue perfusion are at high risk for tissue injury from pressure, heat, or shearing forces.
PAIN: Implement measures to relieve pain, if present.	Tissue ischemia can cause severe pain.
NUTRITION: Encourage the patient to follow the DASH (Dietary Approaches to Stop Hypertension) eating plan and lower overall sodium intake.	The DASH eating plan, which lowers blood pressure and reduces cholesterol, emphasizes fruits, vegetables, fat-free or low-fat milk and milk products, whole grains, fish, poultry, beans, seeds, and nuts.
NUTRITION: Implement measures to assist the patient with losing weight, if needed.	Obesity increases the risk of venous thrombus.
ADDICTION: Encourage tobacco cessation.	Smoking or vaping cause vasoconstriction and are serious risk factors for vascular disease.
GLUCOSE REGULATION: Implement measures to reduce hyperglycemia if needed.	Hyperglycemia is associated with reduced tissue perfusion and accelerated atherosclerosis.
TISSUE INTEGRITY: Implement measures to promote healing if a wound is present and monitor for signs of cellulitis, such as redness and increased swelling.	Peripheral vascular disease increases the risk for wound infection.
Assist the patient with developing a regular physical activity plan, considering capabilities, daily routine, and personal preferences.	Regular physical activity builds endurance and maintains muscle strength.
HEALTH PROMOTION: Encourage the patient to manage hyperlipidemia.	Managing hyperlipidemia slows the progress of atherosclerosis.

Table 28.1 Manifestations of Peripheral Arterial Disease and Peripheral Venous Disease

Characteristic	Peripheral Artery Disease	Peripheral Venous Disease
Ankle-brachial index	≤0.90	>0.90
Capillary refill	>3 sec	<3 sec
Dermatitis	Rare	Often occurs
Edema	Absent unless leg constantly in dependent position	Lower leg edema
Hair	Loss of hair on legs, feet, toes	Hair may be present or absent
Nails	Thickened, brittle	Normal or thickened
Pain	Intermittent claudication or rest pain in foot Ulcer may or may not be painful	Dull ache or heaviness in calf or thigh Ulcer often painful
Peripheral pulses	Decreased or absent	Present, may be hard to palpate with edema
Pruritus	Rare	Often occurs
Skin color	Dependent rubor, elevation pallor	Bronze-brown pigmentation Varicose veins may be visible
Skin temperature	Cool, temperature gradient down the leg	Warm, no temperature gradient
Skin texture	Thin, shiny, taut	Skin thick, hardened, indurated
Ulcer		
Location	Tips of toes, foot, or lateral malleolus	Near medial malleolus
Margin	Rounded, smooth, looks “punched out”	Irregularly shaped
Drainage	Minimal	Moderate to large amount
Tissue	Black eschar or pale pink granulation	Yellow slough or dark red, “ruddy” granulation

Source: Harding M, Kwong J, Hagler D, Reinisch C, eds. *Lewis' medical-surgical nursing: Assessment and management of clinical problems.* 12th ed. Elsevier; 2023.

COLLABORATION	RATIONALE
Cardiac rehabilitation	The aim of cardiac rehabilitation is to provide education and monitored exercise to support achieving an optimal level of function.
Podiatry	The podiatrist assesses and intervenes to maintain optimal skin integrity in the feet.
NUTRITION: Dietitian	Collaborating with a dietitian offers the patient further information and support for implementing the prescribed diet.
Disease or symptom management programs	Disease or symptom management programs help patients understand their treatment regimen and address the complex needs of those with chronic illness.
CARE COORDINATION: Social services or case management	Support may be needed to obtain financial, transportation, or other resources.
Community or online support groups	Many patients with chronic cardiovascular disease find benefit in the support offered by persons with similar concerns.
Physical therapy	Physical therapists can assess the patient and develop a plan of care to maximize exercise capability.

 PATIENT AND CAREGIVER TEACHING

- Cause of impaired tissue perfusion, if known, and how long it may last
- Reason the patient is at risk for impaired tissue perfusion
- Manifestations of impaired tissue perfusion
- Management of any underlying condition contributing to the impaired tissue perfusion
- Measures being used to improve impaired tissue perfusion
- Diagnostic and laboratory tests used to monitor tissue perfusion
- Any needed lifestyle changes to improve tissue perfusion
- Early recognition of problems and how to manage them
- Safe use of medications, including proper use, side effect management, administration, how they fit into the overall management plan
- Low-sodium, low-saturated-fat diet
- Foot care
- Hand hygiene techniques
- Positive coping and stress management strategies
- Community and self-help resources available
- Sources of information and social support
- Where to find additional information
- Gradual physical activity, managing exercise plan
- Tobacco cessation methods
- Signs and symptoms of infection
- How to monitor temperature
- Community and home isolation precautions, if needed
- Importance of long-term follow-up
- Role of therapy and case management
- When to notify the HCP and when to seek emergency care

 DOCUMENTATION

Assessment

- Assessments performed
- Manifestations of impaired tissue perfusion
- Diagnostic test results

Interventions

- Medications given
- Notification of HCP about diagnostic test results and assessment findings
- Therapeutic interventions and the patient's response
- Teaching provided
- Referrals initiated
- Precautions implemented
- Discussions with other members of the interprofessional team
- Environmental modifications made

Evaluation

- Patient's status: improved, stable, declined
- Patient's response to teaching provided
- Diagnostic test results
- Patient's response to therapeutic interventions
- Presence of any manifestations of impaired tissue perfusion

Altered Blood Pressure 29

Definition

Force propelling blood through the body at a level inadequate for perfusion

Blood pressure (BP) is regulated by the homeostatic mechanisms of the body: the volume of the blood, the lumen of the arteries and arterioles, and the force of cardiac contraction. Upon standing, gravity causes more blood to move toward the feet, but reflex arteriolar and venous constriction, ↑ heart rate, and other mechanisms compensate for the change in position. If these compensatory mechanisms are inadequate or impaired, blood pools in the legs and normal arterial pressure cannot be maintained. In that case, the person may experience orthostatic hypotension.

Hypertension, or high BP, is one of the most important modifiable risk factors that can lead to the development of cardiovascular disease. As BP increases, so does the risk of myocardial infarction, heart failure, stroke, and renal disease. Hypertension-induced retinopathy can impair vision. Nursing care focuses on the priorities of maintaining BP at a level that decreases complications and supporting the patient to manage lifestyle changes and a drug regimen with many potential side effects. Patient education is key to hypertension self-management. Proper nutrition and exercise are important health-promotion behaviors.

Associated Clinical Problems

- Low Blood Pressure: inadequate BP for tissue perfusion
- Orthostatic Hypotension: decrease of 20 mm Hg or more in systolic BP, a decrease of 10 mm Hg or more in diastolic BP, and/or an increase in the heart rate of 20 beats/minute upon arising to a standing position

Common Causes and Risk Factors

- Aging
- Congenital heart defects
- Endocrine problems
- Fluid imbalance
- Pregnancy

High Blood Pressure

- Alcohol use
- Diabetes
- Elevated serum lipids
- Ethnicity
- Excess dietary sodium
- Genetics
- Kidney disease
- Medications: corticosteroids, estrogen therapy, NSAIDs, sympathetic stimulants
- Obesity
- Pheochromocytoma
- Sedentary lifestyle
- Smoking
- Stress
- Diagnostic tests
  - An ECG may show ischemic heart disease, dysrhythmias, and left ventricular hypertrophy.
  - An echocardiogram may show structural heart disease and left ventricular hypertrophy.

Low Blood Pressure

- Medications: diuretics, antihypertensives
- Spinal anesthesia
- Spinal cord injury
- Trauma

Related Concepts and Clinical Problems

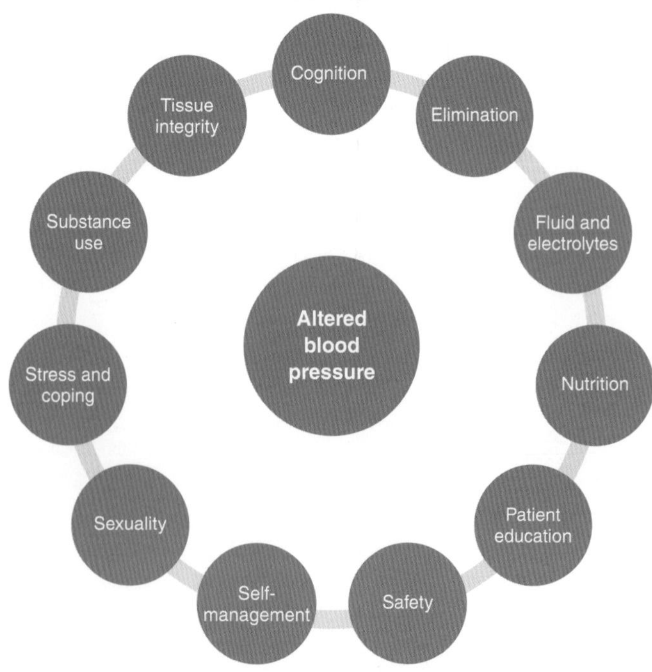

ASSESSMENT OF ALTERED BLOOD PRESSURE	RATIONALE
Identify patients in need of emergency BP management.	Identifying an altered BP allows for the patient to be stabilized immediately.
Assess risk factors for an altered BP.	Identifying factors that place the patient at risk for altered BP allows for early intervention.
Determine the potential cause of an altered BP.	Treating the cause is part of the overall management plan.
Obtain a thorough history of any BP problems, including: • When problems started • Onset, sudden or gradual • Frequency of symptoms • Intensity or severity • Alleviating and aggravating factors • Any pattern to the symptoms • Therapy tried and its effectiveness	A thorough history aids in evaluating the degree of the patient's BP problem and helps direct treatment.
Perform a complete physical assessment and monitor BP indicators on an ongoing basis:	
• Manifestations of altered BP	Identifying manifestations of an altered BP allows for early intervention.
• Regular BP monitoring	The patient needs frequent monitoring to determine whether adjustments to medications or fluids are needed.
• Assess for orthostatic changes in BP and heart rate by measuring serial BP and heart rate with the patient in the supine, sitting, and standing positions.	A normal response is for the systolic BP to decrease less than 10 mm Hg on standing, whereas the diastolic BP and pulse increase slightly; an excessive drop in BP or an increase in heart rate indicates orthostatic hypotension.
• Heart sounds, noting regularity and presence of adventitious sounds	Additional heart sounds, including S3, S4, rubs, and murmurs, may occur with various cardiac problems.
• **COGNITION:** Cognitive and mental status, including orientation to time, place, person, and situation	Changes in level of consciousness may indicate ↓ BP.
• **FLUID AND ELECTROLYTES:** Fluid status, including daily weights, hourly urine output, and intake and output	An appropriate fluid volume is needed to maintain BP.
• Serum electrolytes, glucose level, lipid profile, and metabolic panel	Various tests are done to identify causes of secondary hypertension, evaluate target organ disease, and evaluate cardiovascular risk.
• **ELIMINATION:** Routine urinalysis, blood urea nitrogen (BUN), serum creatinine level, and creatinine clearance	Kidney function tests provide baseline information about kidney injury and the glomerular filtration rate.
If the BP is elevated, determine the patient's BP classification (Table 29.2).	The patient's hypertension classification guides treatment recommendations.
Evaluate the results of diagnostic studies, including 12-lead ECG and echocardiogram.	Diagnostic tests are performed to evaluate cardiovascular system function.
SUBSTANCE USE: Screen for the presence of tobacco use, alcohol use, and/or other substance use problems.	Smoking or vaping cause peripheral vasoconstriction, significantly contributing to hypertension.
NUTRITION: Obtain a diet history, including usual daily caloric intake, dietary choices, and use of nutritional support.	A diet high in sodium intake and saturated fat contributes to the development of high BP.
STRESS AND COPING: Assess the patient's stress level and the use of coping and stress management strategies.	People with high stress may be more likely to develop hypertension.
Assess the patient's participation in exercise activity.	A sedentary lifestyle is a contributing factor to hypertension.
Evaluate the patient's response to measures to normalize the BP through ongoing assessment.	Identifying the manifestations of altered blood pressure allows for the evaluation of therapy effectiveness.

Table 29.1 Manifestations of Altered Blood Pressure

Low Blood Pressure	High Blood Pressure
• Activity intolerance • Dizziness, light headedness • Falling • Changes in mental status • Orthostatic changes in BP and heart rate • Syncope • Tachycardia • Weak peripheral pulses	• Angina • Bounding peripheral pulses • Dyspnea • Erectile dysfunction • Fatigue • Heart failure • Kidney disease • Neuropathy • Palpitations • Retinopathy

Table 29.2 Classification of Hypertension

Category	Systolic BP (mm Hg)		Diastolic BP (mm Hg)
Normal	<120	and	<80
Elevated	120–129	and	<80
Hypertension, stage 1	130–139	or	80–89
Hypertension, stage 2	≥140	or	≥90

From Whelton PK, Carey RM, Aronow WS, et al. 2017 ACC/AHA/AAPA/ABC/ACPM/AGS/APhA/ASH/ASPC/NMA/PCNA guideline for the prevention, detection, evaluation, and management of high blood pressure in adults: a report of the American College of Cardiology/AHA Task Force on Clinical Practice Guidelines. *Hypertension.* 2017;71(6):1269-1324. Source: Harding M, Kwong J, Hagler D, Reinisch C, eds. *Lewis' medical-surgical nursing: Assessment and management of clinical problems.* 12th ed. Elsevier; 2023.

Expected Outcomes

The patient will:

- maintain an adequate BP to support perfusion.
- be free from complications associated with an altered BP.
- adhere to the prescribed therapeutic regimen.
- maintain ongoing contact with the appropriate community resources.
- participate in desired ADLs.
- have minimal side effects from therapy.
- avoid fall injury from postural hypotension.

INTERVENTIONS TO PROMOTE STABLE BLOOD PRESSURE	RATIONALE
Implement collaborative interventions aimed at treating the underlying cause of the altered BP.	The BP alteration may resolve with treatment of the underlying cause.
Be prepared to institute resuscitation protocols and respiratory support.	An altered BP can cause alterations in perfusion that require rapid intervention.
Notify the HCP if the altered BP persists or worsens.	Achievement of an effective treatment plan often requires adjustments in therapy.
Administer medications and fluids as prescribed, including the following:	
• **FLUID AND ELECTROLYTES:** IV fluids	IV fluids are given to replace fluid losses and maintain an optimal fluid volume.
• Adrenergic-inhibiting agents, such as doxazosin (Cardura)	These agents decrease the nervous system effects that increase BP by inhibiting norepinephrine release or blocking the adrenergic receptors on blood vessels.
• Angiotensin II receptor blockers (ARBs), such as losartan (Cozaar) and valsartan (Diovan)	These agents prevent angiotensin II from binding to its receptors in the walls of the blood vessels.
• β-Blockers, including propranolol (Inderal) and atenolol (Tenormin)	β-Blockers reduce BP by blocking β-adrenergic effects in the heart and peripheral vessels.
• Calcium channel blockers, such as diltiazem (Cardizem) and nifedipine (Procardia)	These increase sodium excretion and cause arteriolar vasodilation by preventing the movement of extracellular calcium into cells.

INTERVENTIONS TO PROMOTE STABLE BLOOD PRESSURE	RATIONALE
• Direct vasodilator drugs, such as hydralazine (Apresoline)	Direct vasodilators decrease BP by relaxing the vascular smooth muscle and reducing systemic vascular resistance.
• Diuretics	Diuretics promote sodium and water excretion, reduce plasma volume, and reduce the vascular response to catecholamines.
Notify the HCP if adverse medication effects occur.	The presence of some adverse effects, including extrapyramidal symptoms and liver problems, may require an adjustment in medication or dose.
SAFETY: Assist the patient with managing any side effects that occur from antihypertensive therapy.	Assisting with side effect management will decrease the chance that the patient will stop taking medications as prescribed because of the side effects.
Identify patients at risk for falls and initiate fall precautions.	Fall precautions help reduce the incidence of injury from falls.
SELF-MANAGEMENT: Develop a plan with the patient and caregiver to improve adherence to the therapeutic regimen.	A significant problem in the long-term management of the patient with hypertension is poor adherence to the treatment plan.
Assist the patient with developing a regular physical activity plan, considering capabilities, daily routine, and personal preferences.	Regular physical activity builds endurance and maintains muscle strength.
NUTRITION: Encourage the patient to follow the DASH eating plan and lower overall sodium intake.	The DASH eating plan, which lowers BP and reduces cholesterol, emphasizes fruits, vegetables, fat-free or low-fat milk and milk products, whole grains, fish, poultry, beans, seeds, and nuts.
Implement measures to assist the patient with losing weight, if needed.	Weight reduction has a significant effect on lowering BP in many people.
SUBSTANCE USE: Review the patient's alcohol intake and encourage moderation or cessation.	Excess alcohol intake (drinking three or more drinks per day) is strongly associated with hypertension.
Encourage tobacco cessation.	Smoking or vaping cause vasoconstriction and are serious risk factors for hypertension.
STRESS AND COPING: Encourage the use of positive coping and stress management strategies.	Coping and stress management promote the patient's sense of control by providing a concrete plan for responding to stressful situations.
SEXUALITY: Encourage the patient to discuss any sexual problems and institute measures to address these problems, if present.	Sexual problems may occur with many antihypertensive drugs or may be a direct result of having hypertension.

INTERVENTIONS TO MANAGE LOW BLOOD PRESSURE	RATIONALE
SAFETY: Instruct patient not to stand up without help.	Upright position may cause dizziness or syncope, leading to a potential for fall and injury.
Administer IV fluids and medications as needed for severe hypotension:	
• Vasoconstrictors, such as norepinephrine and dopamine	These drugs bind to α- or β–adrenergic receptors, causing peripheral vasoconstriction and an increase in systemic vascular resistance.
• Volume expanders	Therapy with volume expanders is done to maintain perfusion.
FLUIDS AND ELECTROLYTES: Encourage adequate fluid intake or administer IV fluids with increases in hot weather or for excess losses, such as with fever, vomiting, or diarrhea.	Fluid administration can prevent dehydration by maintaining normal fluid volume.

INTERVENTIONS TO MANAGE ORTHOSTATIC HYPOTENSION	RATIONALE
Have the patient make slow changes in position when arising, such as sitting on the edge of the bed before standing.	Slow position changes help reduce the occurrence of orthostatic hypotension.
SAFETY: Help the patient sit back down or lie down and call for help with ambulation if they experience symptoms when arising.	Ambulating with help reduces the rate of injury from falls.

COLLABORATION	RATIONALE
NUTRITION: Dietitian	Collaborating with a dietitian offers the patient further information and support for implementing the prescribed diet.
Disease or symptom management programs	Disease or symptom management programs help patients understand their treatment regimen and address the complex needs of those with chronic illness.
CARE COORDINATION: Social services or case management	Support may be needed to obtain financial, transportation, or other resources.
Community or online support groups	Many patients with chronic cardiac disease find benefit in the support offered by persons with similar concerns.
Physical therapy	Physical therapists can assess the patient and develop a plan of care to maximize exercise capability.

PATIENT AND CAREGIVER TEACHING

- What BP is and how the body maintains BP
- Factors normally affecting BP and the cause of the altered BP, if known
- Manifestations of the BP alteration
- Management of any underlying condition contributing to the altered BP
- Screening examinations and surveillance for kidney and vision problems
- Measures being used to treat the BP problem
- How to monitor BP—daily weight, pulse, and BP
- Any needed lifestyle changes to help control BP
- Early recognition of problems and how to manage them
- Safe use of medications, including proper use, side effect management, administration, and how they fit into the overall management plan
- Importance of participating in an exercise plan
- Dietary plan and appropriate foods for that plan
- Tobacco cessation measures
- Measures to reduce the risk of falls, such as slow changes in position
- Available community and self-help resources
- Sources of information and social support
- Positive coping and stress management strategies
- Importance of long-term follow-up
- When to notify the HCP and seek emergency care

DOCUMENTATION

Assessment

- Assessments performed
- Manifestations of an altered BP
- BP measurements
- Diagnostic test results

Interventions

- Medications given
- Notification of HCP about diagnostic test results and assessment findings
- Therapeutic interventions and the patient's response
- Teaching provided
- Referrals initiated
- Precautions implemented
- Discussions with other members of the interprofessional team
- Environmental modifications made
- Safety measures implemented, including fall precautions

Evaluation

- Patient's status: improved, stable, declined
- Patient's response to teaching provided
- Diagnostic test results
- Patient's response to therapeutic interventions
- Presence of any manifestations of impaired tissue perfusion

Impaired Sleep 30

Definition

Not obtaining adequate sleep

Sleep is a state in which a person lacks conscious awareness of their surroundings but can be easily aroused. Sleep is essential. The reduced consciousness during sleep provides the time our body needs for essential repair and renewal. Adequate sleep is defined as the amount of sleep one needs to be fully awake and alert the next day. Normal variations associated with age relate mainly to the amount of total sleep needed and the amount of time spent in each stage of sleep. Most adults need 7 to 8 hours of sleep within a 24-hour period. Sufficient quality of sleep is required to decrease the risk of chronic illnesses that affect the respiratory, cardiovascular, metabolic, and endocrine systems.

Sleep adequacy affects physical, psychological, and social functioning. Some functions affected by sleep are memory, hormone secretion, glucose metabolism, immune function, and body temperature. Insufficient sleep quality places people at risk for depression, impaired daytime functioning, social isolation, and overall reduction in quality of life. Sleep problems may exacerbate symptoms of other diseases or impair the ability to cope with the symptoms of other diseases. Impaired sleep has considerable safety and economic consequences. Accidents and injuries can occur because of impaired sleep.

Nurses are in a key position to assess sleep problems. Sleep assessment is important in helping identify personal habits and factors that contribute to impaired sleep. People with sleep problems will benefit from nurses' promoting the use of sleep hygiene practices. For inpatients, nurses play a key role in creating an environment conducive to sleep. This includes scheduling of medications and procedures and reducing light and noise levels to promote opportunities for sleep.

Associated Clinical Problems

- Insomnia: difficulty falling asleep or staying asleep
- Nightmare: recurrent awakening with recall of a frightful or disturbing dream
- Sleep Deprivation: prolonged periods of time without sleep

Contributing Factors

- Alcohol use
- Alzheimer disease
- Bed partner disturbances, such as snoring
- Caregiving responsibilities, such as parenting infants
- Circadian sleep disorder
- Environment: noise, excess light, unfamiliar setting
- Fever
- Frequent napping
- Travel across time zones
- Gastroesophageal reflux disease
- Hospitalization
- Medications: antihistamines, antihypertensives, corticosteroids, diuretics, selective serotonin reuptake inhibitors (SSRIs), thyroid hormone
- Menopause
- Narcolepsy
- Nausea
- Pain
- Parasomnias, including sleepwalking
- Pregnancy
- Psychological problems: anxiety, depression, stress, grief, loneliness
- Respiratory problems
- Shift work, irregular sleep patterns
- Sleep-related breathing disorders, including obstructive sleep apnea
- Sleep-related movement disorders, including restless leg syndrome
- Smoking and the use of nicotine-containing products
- Travel across time zones

Pediatric

- Enuresis
- Fear of the dark
- Inconsistent sleep rituals

Manifestations

- Altered mood
- Anorexia
- Daytime sleepiness
- Difficulty concentrating
- Drawn appearance, such as dark circles under the eyes
- Fatigue
- Forgetfulness
- Hand tremors
- Irritability
- Malaise
- Nystagmus

- Restlessness
- Sleep-related reports of:
  - Awakening feeling unrefreshed
  - Awakening too early and not being able to fall back to sleep
  - Difficulty falling asleep and staying asleep
  - Dissatisfaction with sleep
  - Frequent awakenings
  - Prolonged night awakenings
- Work and school related: poor performance, decreased productivity, absenteeism
- Yawning
- Diagnostic test results: positive findings from actigraphy or polysomnogram

Key Conceptual Relationships

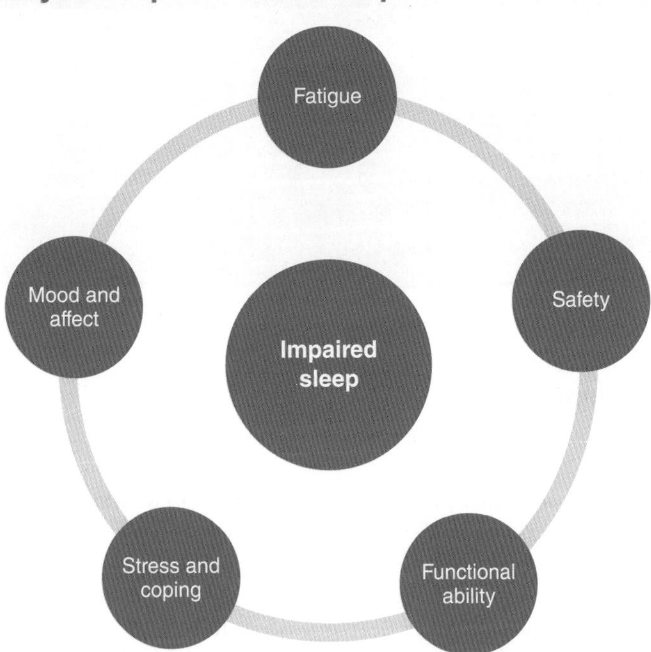

ASSESSMENT OF SLEEP	RATIONALE
Assess risk factors for impaired sleep.	Identifying factors that place the patient at risk for impaired sleep allows for early intervention.
Determine the potential cause of impaired sleep.	Sleep problems often develop as a result or complication of an identifiable problem.
Obtain a comprehensive sleep history: • How the patient feels upon awakening and throughout the day • Duration of sleep problems • Frequency of sleep problems • Typical bedtime routine • Normal bedtime and awakening • Sleep environment • Bed partner's habits • Awakening at night and difficulty falling back asleep • Napping habits • Presence of nightmares, sleep terrors, sleepwalking • Use of medication or other agents to promote sleep	A thorough sleep assessment aids in finding the cause of impaired sleep, helps patients identify habits and environment factors that contribute to impaired sleep, and guides treatment.
Obtain a history of fluid intake, diet intake, and elimination habits.	Assessment can assist with identifying the intake of foods and beverages that promote or interfere with sleep.
Use a formal scale appropriate for the patient's age and cognition as part of the sleep assessment, such as the Pittsburgh Sleep Quality Index (https://www.sleep.pitt.edu/instruments/), Epworth Sleepiness Scale (https://epworthsleepinessscale.com/about-the-ess/), or the Insomnia Severity Index (https://www.ons.org/sites/default/files/InsomniaSeverityIndex_ISI.pdf).	Sleep scales can objectively assess sleep quality and daytime symptoms related to insomnia.
Have the patient keep a sleep diary or log for 1–2 weeks, noting bedtime, awakening time, difficulty getting to sleep, number of awakenings, and reason for awakening (Table 30.1, Figure 30.1).	The determination that impaired sleep is present is often made based on symptom self-report and on an evaluation of a 1- or 2-week sleep log or diary.
Evaluate the results of sleep tests, including: • Polysomnogram	Polysomnograms can evaluate a variety of sleep disorders, including difficulty falling asleep, difficulty staying awake, and sleep-related breathing disorders.

ASSESSMENT OF SLEEP	RATIONALE
• Actigraphy	Actigraphy monitors the time spent in awake and sleeping states and is useful for confirming the patient's sleep self-reports and monitoring the effects of treatments.
FUNCTIONAL ABILITY: Assess for lifestyle effects of impaired sleep, such as impaired ability to perform work and household duties and engage in physical and social activities.	Sleep can adversely influence mood, behavior, and cognitive functioning, which can impair role performance.
MOOD AND AFFECT: Assess mental status and screen for coexisting psychological problems.	Many patients with depression, anxiety, or other psychological problems have impaired sleep.
Evaluate the effectiveness of measures used to promote sleep through ongoing assessment.	Ongoing sleep assessment allows for the evaluation of therapy effectiveness.
Pediatric	
Obtain a sleep history from the caregivers: • Night feedings • Frequency and duration of awakenings • Parental response to awakenings • Nap and bedtime rituals • Sleeping arrangements • Sleeping position • Perceived sleeping problems	A thorough sleep assessment can determine the cause and factors that contribute to impaired sleep and direct interventions.
Women's Health	
CULTURE: Assess sleeping arrangements of caregivers with infants, being sensitive to cultural diversity and family sleeping habits.	Experts discourage cosleeping because of safety concerns.

Table 30.1 Sample Sleep Log

Complete the following questions every morning.

Date:		Day 1	Day 2	Day 3	Day 4	Day 5	Day 6	Day 7
1.	I went to bed last night at:							
2.	I woke up this morning at:							
3.	I get out of bed this morning at:							
4.	I woke up during the night:							
	# of times							
	# of minutes							
5.	How long I slept altogether:							
6.	These things interrupted my sleep:							
7.	When I woke up this morning, I felt:							
	The overall quality of my sleep was:	1 (Poor)	2	3	4	5 (Good)		

Expected Outcomes

The patient will:

- express having obtained adequate sleep.
- express feeling rested.
- follow sleep routines that promote sleep.
- change behaviors that contribute to impaired sleep.
- maintain role performance and take part in desired activities of daily living.

INTERVENTIONS TO PROMOTE SLEEP	RATIONALE
Implement collaborative interventions aimed at treating the underlying cause of impaired sleep.	A sleep problem may be resolved with treatment of the underlying cause.
Notify the HCP if sleep problems are present and persist or worsen.	Notifying the HCP allows for early intervention.
Help the patient choose a sleep diary (Table 30.1, Fig. 30.1) or sleep diary smartphone application that tracks information about sleep.	A sleep diary can help the patient and health care team identify sleep problems.
Assist the patient with developing a bedtime routine by encouraging the patient to: • Go to bed only when sleepy. • Get out of bed and do a nonstimulating activity if still awake after 20 minutes and return to bed only when sleepy. • Adopt a regular bedtime and awakening. • Keep the bedroom dark and a little bit cool. • Keep noise to a minimum. • Use soft music, a fan, or a sound machine to mask noise, if necessary. • Do not read, work, watch TV, talk on the phone, or use technology in bed. • Avoid excess sleep on weekends or holidays.	A bedtime routine prepares the mind, body, and spirit for rest.
Implement diet adjustments to promote sleep, including:	
• Avoid caffeine, nicotine, and alcohol at least 4–6 hours before bedtime.	Caffeine, nicotine, and alcohol are stimulants that interfere with sleep.
• Avoid eating a heavy meal late at night.	Heavy meals cause gastric stimulation, which interferes with sleep.
• Encourage a light, high-carbohydrate snack, along with a beverage such as warm milk or herbal tea.	A light snack can alleviate hunger, which interferes with normal sleep.
Administer medications as prescribed, including:	
• Benzodiazepines, including triazolam and temazepam (Restoril)	These agents are effective for improving sleep in the short term but are not first-line therapies.
• Benzodiazepine-receptor–like drugs, including zaleplon (Sonata), zolpidem (Ambien), eszopiclone (Lunesta)	These agents are the first-line drug treatment for insomnia.
• Orexin-receptor antagonists, including suvorexant (Belsomra) and lemborexant (Dayvigo)	Suvorexant can be used to treat problems with sleep maintenance.
• Melatonin-receptor agonist (ramelteon [Rozerem])	Ramelteon can be used to treat insomnia.
• Antidepressants (e.g., doxepin, trazodone)	Certain antidepressants may be used to treat sleep problems because of their side effect of sedation.
Adjust the medication schedule or encourage the patient to take medications that may interfere with sleep, such as diuretics, early in the day.	Taking medications that may interfere with sleep early in the day helps minimize disrupted sleep.
PAIN: Implement measures to address any pain the patient is experiencing.	Appropriate pain control can relieve pain that interferes with sleep.
Implement measures in the agency environment to ensure the patient has at least 4 or 5 periods of at least 90 minutes each of uninterrupted sleep every 24 hours:	
• Control environment factors that influence sleep, including lighting and noise.	Reducing light and noise levels enhances the patient's ability to sleep.
• Cluster activities.	Clustering activities limits unnecessary disruptions.
• Close the door to the room and limit traffic into the room.	Reducing foot traffic and noise levels enhances the patient's ability to sleep.
• Place the patient in a preferred sleeping position, if able	The preferred sleeping position promotes comfort and follows the patient's usual routine.
• Avoid unnecessary procedures when the patient is sleeping.	Procedures can be a deterrent to sleep.
Help the patient develop an appropriate exercise schedule, avoiding strenuous exercise within 6 hours of bedtime.	Exercise promotes normal daytime fatigue and facilitates normal sleep patterns.

INTERVENTIONS TO PROMOTE SLEEP	RATIONALE
SAFETY: Stress to the patient with impaired sleep that driving, operating heavy machinery, or taking part in some activities may be risky.	Impaired sleep may alter the usual cognitive ability, which increases the chance of accidental injury.
STRESS AND COPING: Help the patient practice stress management techniques, such as relaxation breathing and imagery.	Stress management activities promote relaxation and decrease sympathetic nervous system stimulation, which can help the patient sleep.
Discourage long periods of daytime napping unless absolutely necessary.	Daytime sleep and napping can interrupt circadian rhythms and lead to poor sleep at night.
FATIGUE: Institute measures to assist the patient with managing fatigue.	Impaired sleep is a known cause of fatigue.
Assist the patient who performs shift work to enhance sleep by recommending to: • Take brief periods of on-site napping if available. • Maintain a consistent sleep–wake schedule, even on days off. • Schedule a sleep period just before going to work.	Specific strategies may help reduce sleep problems associated with rotating shift work.
Older Adult Avoid the use of medications for sleep if possible.	Older adults have an increased risk for dependence and excess drowsiness when using sleep medications.
Pediatric Give a warm bath 30 minutes to 1 hour before scheduled bedtime.	A warm bath promotes relaxation and provides quiet time as a part of the bedtime routine.
Read a calm, quiet story to the child immediately after being put to bed.	Reading is a passive, meaningful activity that promotes relaxation.
Feed the child formula or a snack of protein and simple carbohydrates 15 to 30 minutes before bedtime.	A sense of fullness and satiety promotes sleep in young children.
Place child in their own bed while awake.	When children fall asleep somewhere else and then are moved to their own bed, they awaken in unfamiliar surroundings and may not be able to fall asleep until the routine is repeated.
Provide a favorite stuffed animal or blanket.	Favorite items promote security, which enhances the ability to sleep.
For night awakenings after 6 to 12 months, enter the room to check on the child while keeping reassurances brief.	The purpose of the visit is to check on the child and reassure them that they are fine while allowing them to return to sleep on their own.
Women's Health Discuss reasons for sleeping difficulties during pregnancy, such as backache and fetal movements, and review sleeping positions that promote sleep.	Positioning that reduces discomfort associated with pregnancy can promote sleep.
Assist the mother in adapting to the infant's sleep–wake cycle by resting when the infant sleeps and scheduling rest breaks throughout the day.	Proper planning can help reduce fatigue associated with being an infant's caregiver.
Discuss ways to promote nighttime sleep for an infant's parents, such as taking turns during the night to get the baby (the partner can bring the baby to the mother for breastfeeding).	Planning can help reduce fatigue associated with being an infant's caregiver.
Discuss the safety risks associated with cosleeping.	Experts discourage infant/parent cosleeping arrangements because of infant safety concerns.

COLLABORATION	RATIONALE
Cognitive–behavioral therapy for insomnia	Cognitive–behavioral therapy for insomnia includes focused teaching and coaching on how to effectively use sleep hygiene practices, and should be delivered by a qualified HCP.
Sleep medicine specialist	A sleep medicine specialist can determine the most likely cause of a sleep problem and outline an appropriate plan of care.
MOOD AND AFFECT: Treatment for coexisting psychological problems, including depressed mood and emotional problems	Many patients with depression, anxiety, or other psychological problems have impaired sleep.

TWO WEEK SLEEP DIARY

INSTRUCTIONS:

1. Write the date, day of the week, and type of day: Work, School, Day Off, or Vacation.
2. Put the letter "C" in the box when you have ooffee, cola or tea. Put "M" when you take any medicine. Put "A" when you drink alcohol. Put "E" when you exercise.
3. Put a line (I) to show when you go to bed. Shade in the box that shows when you think you fell asleep.
4. Shade in all the boxes that show when you are asleep at night or when you take a nap during the day.
5. Leave boxes unshaded to show when you wake up at night and when you are awake during the day.

SAMPLE ENTRY BELOW: On a Monday when I worked, I jogged on my lunch break at 1 PM, had a glass of wine with dinner at 6 PM, fell asleep watching TV from 7 to 8 PM, went to bed at 10:30 PM, fell asleep around Midnight, woke up and couldn't got back to sleep at about 4 AM, went back to sleep from 5 to 7 AM, and had coffee and medicine at 7:00 in the morning.

Today's Date	Day of the week	Type of Day Work, School OFF, Vacation	Noon	1PM	2	3	4	5	6PM	7	8	9	10	11PM	Midnight	1AM	2	3	4	5	6AM	7	8	9	10	11AM	
sample	Mon	Work		E					A													C M					
																											week 1
																											week 2

Used with permission from the American Academy of Sleep Medicine, Darien, Illinois.

FIG. 30.1 Sample sleep diary. The patient records their daily schedule, including work and medications. (Source: Goldman L, Schafer AI. *Goldman-Cecil Medicine*, ed 26. St. Louis: Elsevier; 2019.)

PATIENT AND CAREGIVER TEACHING

- Cause of impaired sleep, if known
- Normal sleep patterns and age-related variations
- Importance of adequate sleep
- Manifestations of impaired sleep
- Management of underlying conditions associated with impaired sleep
- Measures and bedtime routines to promote sleep
- Lifestyle changes to address impaired sleep
- Safe use of medications, including proper use and how they fit into the overall management plan
- Importance of health-promotion behaviors, including nutrition and exercise
- Where to find more information
- When to notify the HCP

DOCUMENTATION

Assessment

- Assessments performed
- Diagnostic test results
- Manifestations of impaired sleep
- Screening test results
- Sleep history

Interventions

- Discussions with other interprofessional team members
- Medications given
- Notification of the HCP about patient status
- Therapeutic interventions and the patient's response
- Teaching provided
- Referrals initiated

Evaluation

- Amount of uninterrupted sleep each shift
- Patient's status: improved, stable, declined
- Manifestations of impaired sleep
- Response to teaching provided
- Response to therapeutic interventions

Altered Temperature 31

Definition

Inability to maintain core body temperature from 36.2°C to 37.6°C (97.0°F to 100°F)

Thermoregulation occurs through processes controlled by the hypothalamus to balance heat loss and gain. The hypothalamic set point for core body temperature is 37°C (98.6°F). Compensatory and regulatory actions maintain a normal core temperature ranging from 36.2°C to 37.6°C (97.0°F to 100°F), or an average of 37°C (98.6°F). Temperature fluctuation may indicate a disease process, strenuous activity, or extreme environmental exposure.

Body heat is produced through chemical reactions in the cells. The greatest amount of heat is made by muscle contraction and through metabolic activity in the liver. Food consumption, physical activity, and hormone levels affect the amount of heat produced. Chemical thermogenesis occurs as a result of epinephrine release, which increases the metabolic rate. The body conserves heat through peripheral vasoconstriction, which shunts warm blood away from the superficial tissues, and increased muscle tone and shivering.

Heat loss occurs through radiation, conduction, convection, vasodilation, evaporation, reduced muscle activity, and increased respiration. Heat loss by *radiation* occurs as heat is emitted from skin surfaces to the air. *Conduction* is a transfer of heat through direct contact. Loss of heat by air currents from wind or a fan moving across the body surface is referred to as *convection*. Heat loss also can occur through other physiologic compensatory mechanisms. Heat loss can be increased through peripheral *vasodilation*, which brings a greater volume of blood to the body surface. Perspiration promotes heat loss through the *evaporation* of moisture from the skin surface. This provides a significant source of heat reduction and normally accounts for 600 mL of water loss per day. In extreme heat, a person can lose as much as 4 L of fluids in an hour, so replacement of fluids and electrolytes is essential to prevent dehydration. Heat is also lost during the process of respiration as warmed and humidified air is exhaled.

Older adults and children have decreased ability to adapt to extreme temperatures. The child's relatively smaller body surface area, body fluid volume, and amount of protective body fat and less-developed temperature control mechanisms limit the ability to maintain normal body temperature. Children are also at risk for hyperthermia and heatstroke because of their undeveloped temperature regulation. Both young children and frail older adults may develop hyperthermia due to the inability to move away from heat or obtain their own fluids to drink. Surgical patients are at risk for hypothermia during long operations with extensive body exposure. Nurses can plan care to prevent and manage extreme variations in patient body temperature.

Temperature variations can be the result of infectious or inflammatory processes. See also Infection and Inflammation.

Associated Clinical Problems

- Chronic Fever: elevated body temperature lasting more than 10 to 14 days
- Hyperthermia: elevated body temperature
- Hypothermia: core body temperature below 95°F (35°C)
- Risk for Hyperthermia: at risk for increased body temperature
- Risk for Hypothermia: at risk for decreased body temperature
- Risk for Perioperative Hypothermia: at risk for decreased body temperature during a surgical procedure and recovery period

Common Causes and Risk Factors

- Central nervous system (CNS) injuries or tumors
- Change in metabolic rate or ability to perspire
- Diabetes
- Extreme environment temperatures, high humidity
- Inappropriate clothing for the weather
- Peripheral vascular disease
- Substance use

Hyperthermia

- Autoimmune conditions, impaired immune system function
- Cancer
- Dehydration
- Hyperthyroidism
- Infection or inflammation
- Malignant hyperthermia
- Medications: amphetamines, anticholinergics, antidepressants, antihistamines, antipsychotics, barbiturates, diuretics, salicylates
- Pheochromocytoma
- Sickle cell disease
- Transfusion reaction

Hypothermia
- Age
- Anorexia or malnutrition
- Burn injury
- Decreased metabolic rate
- Hypothalamic injury
- Hypothyroidism
- Medically induced
- Prematurity or preterm birth

Risk for Perioperative Hypothermia
- Epidural or spinal anesthesia
- Great amount of exposed skin
- Hypotension
- Long surgical procedures
- Open-cavity procedures
- Prolonged anesthesia administration
- Use of cold irrigants, skin preparations, and unwarmed inhaled gases

Manifestations of Hyperthermia
- Confusion, delirium
- Decreased urinary output
- Diaphoresis or dry flushed skin
- Dry or sticky mucous membranes
- Increased body temperature
- Muscle cramps
- Seizures
- Skin warm or hot to touch
- Thirst
- Tachycardia
- Seizures
- Visual disturbances

Key Conceptual Relationships

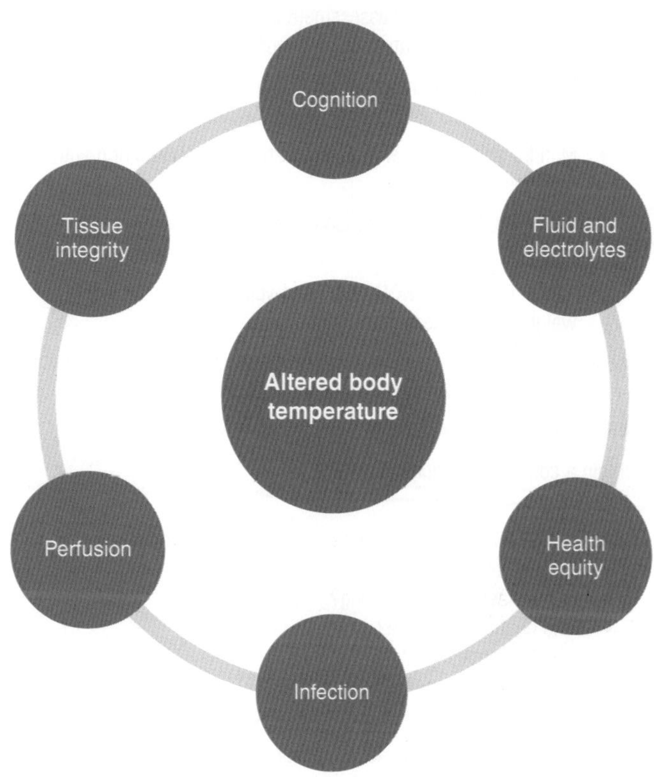

Table 31.1 Manifestations of Hyperthermia

Mild Hypothermia: Temperature < 35°C (95°F)	Moderate Hypothermia: Temperature < 32°C (90°F)	Severe Hypothermia: Temperature < 28°C (82°F)
Confusion	Decreased capillary refill	Cardiovascular collapse
Cool skin	Dysrhythmias	Coma
Fatigue	Lack of shivering	
Poor coordination	Hallucinations	
Shivering	Pallor or cyanosis	
Slurred speech	Stupor	

Source: Harding M, Kwong J, Hagler D, Reinisch C, eds. *Lewis' medical-surgical nursing: Assessment and management of clinical problems.* 12th ed. Elsevier; 2023.

ASSESSMENT OF THERMOREGULATION	RATIONALE
Assess for risk factors and the underlying cause of an altered temperature.	Identifying factors that place the patient at risk for an altered temperature allows for early intervention.
Identify patients in need of emergency management for extreme temperature variation.	Identifying the presence of an emergency state allows for early intervention.
Obtain a detailed history, noting when symptoms started and the symptoms experienced.	Changes in body temperature may indicate a new or ongoing health problem.

ASSESSMENT OF THERMOREGULATION	RATIONALE
Evaluate the patient's underlying health status.	Underlying health status has a significant influence on the ability to regulate temperature.
Perform a complete physical assessment and monitor indicators of ineffective thermoregulation on an ongoing basis:	
• Manifestations of hyperthermia and hypothermia	Identifying manifestations of hyperthermia or hypothermia allows for early identification and intervention.
• Monitor and record temperature at regular intervals and with changes in status.	Monitoring provides a baseline value and record of any changes.
• **PERFUSION:** Initiate continuous cardiac monitoring.	The myocardium is extremely irritable at altered temperatures, making it vulnerable to dysrhythmias.
• **FLUID AND ELECTROLYTES:** Fluid-volume status, including weight and intake/output	Hyperthermia may cause increased evaporation of body water, leading to hypovolemia.
Use a consistent route for monitoring temperature. Oral, rectal, temporal artery, tympanic, and axillary routes are the most common.	Consistency supports analysis of the trend over time.
INFECTION: Assess for signs and symptoms of infection.	The new onset of hyperthermia may indicate a new or ongoing infection.
Obtain a complete medication history.	Certain medications may be associated with a change in body temperature.
HEALTH DISPARITIES: Assess the patient's home environment: • Where do they live? • Do they have air conditioning? • Is the heating adequate? • Is the home well insulated? • Are any rooms closed off? • Have they used any community resources?	Hypothermia or hyperthermia can occur if the home environment does not support a tolerable ambient temperature.
Evaluate the patient's response to measures to correct hyperthermia or hypothermia through ongoing assessment of temperature and manifestations.	Identifying hyperthermia or hypothermia allows for evaluation of therapy effectiveness.
Older Adult Assess for the new onset of changes in cognition or functional status.	Changes in functional status or cognition may signal infection in an older adult, because an older adult can have a significant infection without an elevation in temperature.

Expected Outcomes

The patient will:

- achieve normothermia.
- identify risk factors for an altered temperature and take preventive action.
- be free from complications of an altered temperature.

INTERVENTIONS TO ACHIEVE NORMOTHERMIA	RATIONALE
Implement collaborative interventions aimed at treating the underlying cause of an altered temperature.	Changes in temperature may resolve with treatment of the underlying cause.
GAS EXCHANGE: Administer oxygen therapy and provide appropriate respiratory support.	Changes in temperature influence the respiratory system and oxygen demands.
COGNITION: Provide a quiet, nonstimulating, well-lit environment.	High levels of sensory stimuli can increase confusion for a patient with altered temperature.
Encourage the patient at risk to avoid the use of alcohol or caffeinated beverages.	These beverages increase heat loss, which can exacerbate hypothermia. In the patient with hyperthermia, they promote fluid loss and dehydration.

INTERVENTIONS TO MANAGE HYPERTHERMIA	RATIONALE
Notify the health care provider (HCP) of a temperature greater than 38.3°C (101°F).	Collaborative interventions for hyperthermia may be needed.
Monitor the patient with a temperature up to 38.9°C (102°F) without trying to lower it.	A fever may be a normal and useful response to an inflammatory process, such as infection, allergy, trauma, illness, or surgery.
Focus interventions on patient comfort rather than lowering temperature unless the temperature is greater than 38.9°C (102°F).	This allows the body to progress through the natural course of a fever, which is a useful response in fighting infection.
Administer medications as prescribed:	
• Antipyretics	Antipyretics lower temperature by inhibiting prostaglandin synthesis.
• **INFECTION:** Antibiotics	Antibiotics are administered for a suspected or diagnosed infection.
• **FLUID AND ELECTROLYTES:** Administer intravenous (IV) fluid therapy as prescribed.	Replacement fluids facilitate adequate hydration, avoiding or correcting dehydration.
Implement measures to decrease temperature if temperature is 40°C (102°F) or higher, such as: • Applying cooling blankets • Providing a tepid bath • Applying cold packs • Using a fan to cool the environment	The excessive metabolic demands of hyperpyrexia may be harmful.
Provide clean, dry linens and clothing as often as needed with diaphoresis.	Keeping linens and clothing dry promotes patient comfort, reduces shivering, and protects tissues from maceration.
SAFETY: Provide a safe environment for the patient with neurologic or neuromuscular manifestations by initiating fall and seizure precautions.	Changes in cognition and the potential for seizures may accompany a fever.
FLUID AND ELECTROLYTES: Ensure fluid intake is adequate and that oral fluids can be readily reached.	Provide oral fluids to maintain adequate fluid volume and prevent dehydration.
TISSUE INTEGRITY: Change position often and provide optimal skin and oral care.	Patients with hyperthermia are at increased risk for tissue injury due to dehydration and dry mucous membranes.
PERFUSION: Use measures to treat hyperthermia aggressively in the presence of severe cardiopulmonary disease.	Because hyperthermia increases metabolic demand, those with limited reserves may not be able to supply tissues with adequate oxygen.

INTERVENTIONS TO MANAGE HYPOTHERMIA	RATIONALE
Notify the HCP if the temperature is below 95°F (35°C).	Collaborative interventions for hypothermia may be needed.
Institute measures to promote rewarming, including: • Applying warm, dry clothing • Increasing the room temperature • Keeping the head covered • Using warming blankets • Administering warmed IV fluids if ordered • Applying warm air, externally or inhaled	Rewarming measures are needed to achieve normothermia.
Institute safety measures during rewarming.	
• Monitor for signs of worsening hypothermia.	Patient status may change if initial warming measures allow cold peripheral blood to circulate to the body core.
• Monitor vital signs frequently.	Vasodilation with rewarming may cause a decrease in blood pressure.
When bathing the patient, only expose small sections of the body, and immediately dry and cover the area.	This reduces heat loss from evaporation and convection.
Provide blankets during procedures, transport, and diagnostic testing.	Keep the patient warm while in areas or rooms of the hospital that are intentionally cool.

INTERVENTIONS TO MANAGE HYPOTHERMIA	RATIONALE
Pediatric When caring for the newborn: • Dry the new infant thoroughly and cover with blanket. • Keep the infant covered with a blanket or placed under a radiant heat source. • Bathe and dry the infant in a warm environment. • Keep the head covered. • Provide blankets during procedures, transport, and diagnostic testing.	These measures prevent heat loss in the infant and reduce the incidence of hypothermia.
Older Adult Ensure the patient is always covered during procedures, transport, and diagnostic testing.	These measures help keep the older adult warm while in areas/rooms of the hospital that are intentionally cool.
Suggest keeping room at home warm throughout the day, at least 68°F. Encourage wearing layers of clothing at home, along with socks and slippers.	These measures prevent excessive heat loss for vulnerable older adults.

RISK FOR PERIOPERATIVE HYPOTHERMIA	RATIONALE
During surgery, encourage the team, if able, to: • Apply a forced-air warming blanket. • Limit exposed skin areas. • Warm IV fluids and irrigants.	These measures reduce the risk of heat loss and perioperative hypothermia.

COLLABORATION	RATIONALE
HEALTH EQUITY: Social worker or case manager	A social worker or case manager can help the patient obtain information on emergency shelters, clothing, and financial assistance if cooling and heating the home is financially difficult.

PATIENT AND CAREGIVER TEACHING

- Common causes of hypothermia or hyperthermia
- Measures being used to restore normothermia
- How to measure temperature reliably
- Dressing for the weather and the environment
- Fever management, including when to treat and how
- Comfort measures to employ when experiencing a fever
- Proper use of antipyretic medications
- Maintaining an appropriate temperature in the home
- When to notify HCP and seek emergency care

DOCUMENTATION

Assessment
- Vital signs and physiologic changes
- Comfort level

Interventions
- Measures to promote normothermia
- Measures to provide comfort

Evaluation
- Ongoing comfort
- Temperature

Impaired Fertility 32

Definition

Impaired ability to conceive and bear children

Fertility is the ability to conceive and bear children. It depends on normal reproductive function in each partner and interaction between the partners. Infertility is the inability to conceive after at least 1 year of regular unprotected intercourse. There are two kinds of infertility: primary and secondary. *Primary infertility* means conception has never occurred. Primary infertility is more common. With secondary infertility, conception has occurred before, but either it has not happened again or there is inability to sustain a pregnancy to a live birth.

Infertility is one of the biggest major crises a couple may face. Nurses can provide information about infertility evaluation and treatments and offer valuable psychological support. Many couples experience emotional difficulties. Infertility is often associated with anger, sadness, anxiety, and grief, particularly if treatment options are not successful. Stress increases the more procedures that are done and the longer pregnancy does not occur. The consequences can be debilitating to the couple as they exhaust financial and emotional resources. Infertility may compel them to consider a different future than they imagined.

Associated Clinical Problems

- Reproductive Risk: presence of risk factors that could affect reproductive ability
- Risk for Infertility: increased risk of not being able to conceive after 1 year of regular unprotected intercourse

Common Risk Factors

- Abnormal hormone levels
- Aging
- Cancer and cancer treatment
- Decreased libido
- Endocrine problems
- Exposure to radiation and environmental toxins
- Genetic conditions, including Turner syndrome and Klinefelter syndrome
- Hormone problems or changes
- Malnutrition
- Obesity
- Reproductive tract anomalies
- Sexually transmitted infections (STIs)
- Substance use

Female

- Abnormal menstrual cycles
- Adhesions
- Amenorrhea after discontinuing oral contraceptive agents
- Anemia
- Eating disorders
- Ectopic pregnancy
- Endometriosis
- Inadequate cervical mucus
- Medications: nonsteroidal antiinflammatory drugs (NSAIDs), selective serotonin reuptake inhibitors (SSRIs), spironolactone, steroids
- Pelvic inflammatory disease
- Polycystic ovarian disease
- Premature ovarian failure
- Tubal inflammation and adhesions
- Uterine adhesions and scar tissue
- Uterine displacement
- Uterine prolapse, cystocele, or rectocele

Male

- Anabolic steroid use
- Antisperm antibodies
- Castration
- Cystic fibrosis
- Ejaculatory problems, including premature ejaculation and retrograde ejaculation
- Erectile dysfunction
- Exposure of the scrotum to high temperatures
- Hydrocele
- Hypospadias
- Sperm problems: low count, poor motility, abnormal morphology
- Testicular damage by mumps
- Testosterone replacement therapy
- Torsion
- Undescended testicles
- Varicocele

Manifestations

- Inability to conceive after at least 1 year of regular unprotected intercourse
- Inability to maintain a pregnancy to viability or a live birth
- Diagnostic test results: positive findings from endoscopy, ultrasound, endometrial biopsy, or hysterosalpingogram; abnormal semen analysis

Key Conceptual Relationships

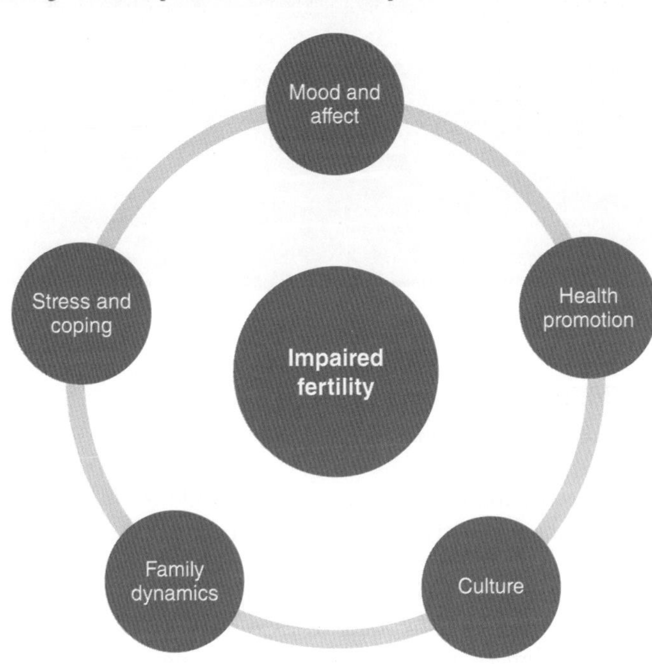

ASSESSMENT OF FERTILITY	RATIONALE
Assess risk factors that influence fertility.	A thorough history can identify factors that influence fertility.
Evaluate the patient's underlying health status.	Underlying health status may have a significant influence on fertility.
Obtain a comprehensive sexual history: • Number and gender of sexual partners • Frequency of intercourse • Sexual behaviors, including types of sexual practices • Sexual response • Safe sex knowledge and practices • Contraceptive history: methods used and reason if discontinued • Measures used to protect against STIs • History of STIs • Age of menarche and menstrual patterns • Obstetric history: Number, living children, multiple births, miscarriages, abortions, duration of pregnancy, each type of delivery, and any complications during any pregnancy or postpartum period	A thorough sexual history aids in determining fertility risks, helps identify factors that influence treatment, and guides treatment.
Obtain a complete vaccination history.	The vaccine history helps to identify protection against STIs and diseases, such as mumps and rubella, which affect fertility.
Perform a physical examination, noting any findings that may influence fertility.	Findings from the physical assessment can identify factors influencing fertility.
Determine each patient's Tanner stage.	Tanner staging estimates sexual development based on primary and secondary sex characteristics.
Obtain ordered culture specimens (vaginal, throat, penile, lesions, urine).	Cultures determine whether a pathogen is present and guide needed treatment.
Evaluate the results of diagnostic testing, including:	
• Endometrial biopsy	An endometrial biopsy is used to determine whether an infection is present, confirm ovulation, and assess whether the endometrium can support implantation.

ASSESSMENT OF FERTILITY	RATIONALE
• Hormone levels	Hormone levels can reveal problems with ovulatory hormones or thyroid and pituitary hormones that control reproductive processes.
• Hysterosalpingogram	A hysterosalpingogram is used to determine fallopian tubes patency, and whether the uterine cavity is normal.
• Semen analysis	A semen analysis measures the quantity and quality of semen, volume of sperm cells, sperm motility, and sperm density.
• Ultrasound (pelvic, transvaginal, testicular, prostate)	Ultrasound can detect structural abnormalities in the reproductive tracts.
• Colposcopy, culdoscopy, laparoscopy, hysteroscopy	Endoscopy is used to assess for reproductive tract structural abnormalities.
• Genetic testing	Genetic testing helps determine whether a genetic condition could contribute to or cause infertility.
STRESS AND COPING: Screen for any distress or coexisting psychological problem.	Those with fertility concerns often struggle with grief, depression, and other problems because of the stress of infertility.
FAMILY DYNAMICS: Evaluate the effects of fertility problems on the couple's relationship and how each is coping with any stress.	Many couples with fertility problems experience significant stress that can affect their relationship.
FUNCTIONAL ABILITY: Ask about support systems: • Do others know that they are trying to conceive? • Are family members and friends supportive? • Are they being asked invasive questions such as, "Why have you not had a baby yet?"	Couples with fertility problems may not have supportive relationships, leading to social isolation.
CULTURE: Assess the role of culture and religion in the experience of having a fertility problem.	Culture and religion strongly influence views on fertility and may affect treatment options.
Evaluate the effectiveness of measures used to influence fertility through ongoing assessment.	Monitoring fertility allows for the evaluation of therapy effectiveness.

Expected Outcomes

The couple will:

- identify factors that influence fertility.
- achieve pregnancy.
- use appropriate coping and stress management strategies.
- express their feelings about the infertility experience.

INTERVENTIONS THAT INFLUENCE FERTILITY	RATIONALE
Implement collaborative interventions aimed at treating any underlying cause influencing fertility.	Treatment of underlying causative or risk factors can influence fertility status.
Administer hormonal agents as prescribed:	
• Follicle-stimulating hormone (FSH) agonists	FSH hormone agonists induce ovulation and sperm production by mimicking natural FSH.
• Gonadotropin-releasing hormone (GnRH) agonists, such as leuprolide	GnRH agonists suppress the release of FSH and luteinizing hormone (LH), increasing the number of eggs retrieved with assisted reproductive technologies.
• GnRH antagonists, such as cetrorelix (Cetrotide)	GnRH antagonists prevent premature LH surges and spontaneous ovulation.
• Chorionic gonadotropin (HCG, Pregnyl)	These agents stimulate the release of eggs from follicles, resulting in ovulation.
• Menotropin	Menotropin promotes the development of multiple eggs in preparation for in vitro fertilization.
• Selective estrogen receptor modulators (SERMs), such as clomiphene	SERMs stimulate the release of FSH and LH, promoting ovulation and sperm production.

Continued

INTERVENTIONS THAT INFLUENCE FERTILITY	RATIONALE
Provide resources for determining ovulation through basal body temperature, changes in vaginal secretions, and ovulation testing.	Ovulation testing assists in affirming if ovulation occurs, guides the timing of certain diagnostic tests, and helps determine the optimal time for coitus.
Assist with a referral to an infertility specialist or fertility preservation specialist for further evaluation and treatment.	Infertility concerns are usually managed by a reproductive endocrinologist or obstetrician who specializes in infertility.
SEXUALITY: Encourage the couple to identify and express feelings about their sexuality, self-image, and fertility.	Expressing thoughts and feelings can improve psychological problems that often accompany a fertility issue.
Discuss general measures that enhance fertility: • Use only water-soluble lubricants during intercourse. • Avoid high scrotal temperatures by avoiding hot tub bathing or sauna use. • Consider wearing boxer shorts instead of briefs. • Avoid douching. • Have intercourse every other night around the time of ovulation.	These general measures are thought to enhance fertility and increase the chances of conception.
HEALTH PROMOTION: Encourage lifestyle measures that promote overall health: • Eat a well-balanced diet. • Exercise regularly. • Decrease alcohol and caffeine intake. • Stop smoking or vaping. • Avoid substance use. • Maintain appropriate weight; lose weight if needed.	These interventions may increase the chances of pregnancy and improve psychological and physical health.
STRESS AND COPING: Encourage the expression of feelings and implement measures to assist in managing any distress present.	Persons with fertility concerns often struggle with grief, depression, and other problems because of the stress of infertility.
IMMUNITY: Administer needed vaccinations according to recommended schedules.	Vaccinations are given to decrease the risk of acquiring an infection that may affect fertility.
STRESS AND COPING: Encourage the use of positive coping behaviors and stress management strategies.	Stress from life issues, including the infertility experience, may have a further negative impact on fertility.
Discuss alternative pathways to parenthood, if appropriate, such as adoption and surrogacy.	Support from the health care team is important when exploring and making decisions about alternative options.

COLLABORATION	RATIONALE
STRESS AND COPING: Counseling	Couples with infertility often struggle with grief, depression, and other problems because of the stress of infertility.
FAMILY DYNAMICS: Support group	A support group focusing on experiencing infertility can help each person and the couple address distress.
Social services, case management	Social workers and case managers can assist with exploring available assistance because the financial costs of addressing a fertility problem can cause catastrophic hardship.
Preconception counseling	Preconception counseling for persons at reproductive risk evaluates the risk for infertility and detects possible genetic conditions.

PATIENT AND CAREGIVER TEACHING

- Normal reproductive system function
- Cause of infertility, if known
- Factors that may be affecting fertility
- Management of any underlying condition related to fertility risk
- Diagnostic and laboratory tests used to evaluate fertility
- Measures to address fertility risk
- Safe use of medications and how they fit into the overall management plan
- Clarification of any myths about sexual function and fertility
- Importance of health promotion behaviors, including nutrition, sleep, and exercise
- Anticipatory guidance about grief and distress and how to deal with each
- Community and self-help resources available
- Sources of information and social support
- Positive coping and stress management strategies
- When to notify the health care provider (HCP)

DOCUMENTATION

Assessment

- Assessments performed
- Diagnostic and laboratory test results
- Manifestations of impaired fertility

Interventions

- Discussions with other interprofessional team members
- Medications given
- Notification of HCP about patient status
- Therapeutic interventions and the patient's response
- Teaching provided
- Referrals initiated

Evaluation

- Patient's status: presence of pregnancy
- Manifestations of impaired fertility
- Response to teaching provided
- Response to therapeutic interventions

Risk for Perinatal Problems 33

Definition

Increased risk for problems during the perinatal period

Pregnancy is the time in which a female has at least one fetus developing in her body. Pregnancy begins at conception and continues until birth or the premature cessation of the pregnancy. The gestation period, or how long a female is pregnant, is usually 38 to 41 weeks. There are various definitions of what is considered the accompanying perinatal period, with a starting range between the 20th to 28th weeks of gestation and ending between 7 and 28 days after birth.

Providing nursing care that addresses risks during the perinatal period is essential for optimal maternal and newborn outcomes. Comprehensive perinatal care includes assessing the health of the fetus and the mother, providing education and counseling, and performing screening to detect risks and complications. Collaborative interventions address the management and treatment of perinatal risks and problems. Equipping expectant mothers with knowledge of the childbirth process and perinatal care enables them to understand what to expect, recognize changes, and be able to take part in making decisions about their health care needs.

Associated Clinical Problems

- Risk for Delivery Problems: at risk for complications during the delivery period
- Risk for Labor Problems: at risk for complications during labor
- Risk for Postpartum Problems: at risk for complications during the postpartum period
- Risk for Problems During Pregnancy: at risk for complications during pregnancy

Common Risk Factors

- ABO incompatibility
- Abruptio placenta
- Age
- Caffeine intake
- Coagulation problems
- Ethnicity
- Fetal congenital and chromosomal conditions
- Gestational diabetes
- Impaired cardiac function
- Impaired immunity
- Impaired nutrition, including malnutrition, dieting, anemia, abnormal weight gain
- Inadequate prenatal care
- Infection
- Lack of social support
- Mood problems, including anxiety, depression
- Multifetal pregnancy
- Obesity
- Placenta previa
- Preeclampsia
- Preterm labor
- Radiation exposure
- Rh incompatibility
- Smoking
- Socioeconomic status
- Stressful life events during the perinatal period
- Substance use
- Trauma
- Victim of interpersonal violence
- Laboratory testing: abnormal complete blood count (CBC), human chorionic gonadotropin (hCG) levels, urinalysis, glucose tolerance test, rubella titers
- Diagnostic testing: abnormal findings with ultrasound and amniocentesis

Labor and Delivery

- Abnormal fetal presentation
- Electronic fetal or uterine pressure monitoring
- Fetopelvic disproportion
- Opioid analgesia administration
- Postterm pregnancy
- Premature rupture of membranes
- Restricted or no ambulation

Postpartum

- Anesthesia complications
- Hemorrhage during labor and delivery
- Large or multiple fetuses
- Prolonged labor and oxytocin-induced labor
- Prolonged rupture of membranes
- Retained placenta
- Trauma during labor and delivery, including third- and fourth-degree lacerations, cesarean birth, forceps-assisted birth
- Uterine problems: rupture, atony, inversion

Key Conceptual Relationships

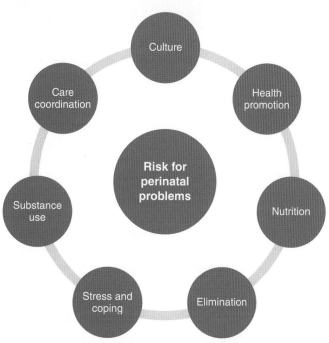

ASSESSMENT FOR PERINATAL PROBLEMS	RATIONALE
Assess for factors that influence risk for perinatal problems.	A thorough history can identify patients at risk for perinatal problems.
Assess the quality and quantity of support offered by the partner, family, friends, and other support persons.	Quality support from a partner, family, friends, or other support persons contributes to positive perinatal outcomes.
Obtain a complete vaccination history, including human papillomavirus (HPV), hepatitis B, rubella, and tetanus, for the mother and those who will be caregivers of the newborn.	The vaccine history helps to identify protection against STIs and diseases, such as rubella, that may cause perinatal problems.
Assess the mother's expectations, concerns, and preferences about pregnancy, childbirth, and perinatal care.	Recognizing the unique expectations, concerns, and preferences each mother has about pregnancy and childbirth fosters empowerment.
Obtain a comprehensive sexual history: • Number and gender of sexual partners • Frequency of intercourse • Sexual behaviors, including types of sexual practices • Sexual response • Safe-sex knowledge and practices • Contraceptive history • History of STIs • Age of menarche • Obstetric history: number, living children, multiple births, miscarriages, abortions, duration of pregnancy, each type of delivery, and any complications during any pregnancy or postpartum period or with the newborn	A thorough sexual history helps determine risk for perinatal problems, identify factors that influence perinatal outcomes, and guide treatment.
MOOD AND AFFECT: Screen for coexisting psychological problems at each encounter.	Identifying depression or other psychological problems and initiating treatment can improve perinatal outcomes.
INTERPERSONAL VIOLENCE: Screen for intimate partner violence at each encounter.	Intimate partner violence during pregnancy is associated with an increased risk for adverse perinatal outcomes.
Evaluate the results of diagnostic testing, including:	Based on the mother's history and needs, routine laboratory tests and diagnostic procedures are done at specific times during pregnancy.
• hCG levels	hCG tests can confirm pregnancy; determine the approximate fetal age; and assist in diagnosing problems.

Continued

ASSESSMENT FOR PERINATAL PROBLEMS	RATIONALE
• Glucose tolerance test	A glucose tolerance test screens for gestational diabetes.
• Amniocentesis	Analysis of amniotic fluid obtained from an amniocentesis gives information about genetic conditions, neural closure defects, fetal distress, and fetal maturity.
• Urinalysis	Glucose, ketones, protein, or bacteria in the urine during pregnancy can indicate complications requiring treatment.
• Ultrasound	Ultrasound is used to estimate fetal age, measure fetal growth, and assess the amniotic sac, placenta, and ovaries.
• CBC	A CBC can detect anemia, infection, or other problems.
• Blood type and Rh factor	Knowing if Rh incompatibility is present allows for interventions to reduce the risk of fetal complications.
• Rubella titer	A mother who contracts rubella is at risk for miscarriage and stillbirth, and the fetus is at risk for severe birth defects.
Obtain ordered culture specimens and tests for gonorrhea, chlamydia, syphilis, HPV, and human immunodeficiency virus (HIV).	Diagnosis of an STI allows for treatment that can prevent or reduce complications.
CULTURE: Assess the role of culture in the pregnancy and childbirth experience.	Culture and ethnicity strongly influence views on perinatal care, pregnancy, and childbirth.
SUBSTANCE USE: Screen for substance use at each encounter.	The newborn at risk for problems associated with maternal substance use will need early intervention.
Assess for the presumptive signs of pregnancy, including: • Breast fullness, tenderness, enlargement • Darkening of the nipples and areola • Fetal movements, or quickening • Nausea and vomiting • Urinary frequency	Presumptive signs of pregnancy are those signs perceived by the mother.
Assess for the probable signs of pregnancy: • Softening of the cervical tip • A violet-blue vaginal mucosa and cervix at 6 weeks • Softening and compression of the lower uterine segment • Uterine enlargement • Braxton-Hicks contractions	The health care provider (HCP) can observe probable signs of pregnancy.
Determine fetal gestational age and date of delivery based on menstrual history and date of last menstrual period, date of pregnancy test result, ultrasound, results, uterine size, and when fetal heart tones first heard.	An accurate gestational age is important in timing perinatal care, performing prenatal tests, evaluating fetal growth, and planning care if preterm birth occurs.
Perform a general physical assessment, focusing on maternal–fetal well-being with each encounter:	The physical assessment may detect problems that increase the risk for perinatal problems.
• Vital signs	Changes in vital signs may cause or occur with a perinatal problem.
• Weight	Weight gain is expected to be within normal limits, depending on prepregnancy body mass index, nutrition status, and pregnancy.
• Fetal heart rate and movements	Fetal heart tones and movements are an indicator of fetal well-being.
• Fundal height	Fundal height is an indicator of fetal growth.

ASSESSMENT DURING LABOR AND DELIVERY	RATIONALE
Complete an admission history, including: • Fetal gestation age and estimated date of delivery • Signs of labor and the time of onset • Parity and gravida status • Childbirth experiences • Characteristics of contractions • Appearance of any vaginal show • Membrane status (ruptured or intact) • Pregnancy history • Prenatal care and education	A complete admission assessment is important so that interventions can be started to address perinatal risk and promote positive birth outcomes.
Perform an initial assessment, including in addition to the general assessment: • Fundal height • Uterine activity, including frequency, duration, and intensity of contraction • Degree of cervical dilatation and effacement • Fetal status, including heart rate, position, and station • Membrane status (ruptured or intact)	The information obtained from the initial assessment forms a baseline against which assessment throughout labor is compared.
Perform ongoing monitoring throughout the labor and delivery process: • Vital signs, including pain level • Fetal heart rate, including response to contractions and recovery time • Uterine activity and general progress of labor • Cervical dilation and effacement • Fetal descent and presentation	Monitoring maternal and fetal well-being allows for early intervention when complications occur.
Perform additional maternal assessment immediately after delivery: • Placental separation • Perianal trauma • Fundal height, position, and firmness • Vaginal discharge	Performing an assessment immediately after delivery allows for early intervention when complications occur.
Perform an initial newborn assessment, including: • Obtain Apgar scores. • Observe for respiratory distress. • Auscultate lungs, heart, and abdomen. • Test reflexes. • Measure head, chest, and length. • Obtain vital signs. • Brief assessment for major anomalies.	Performing an initial newborn assessment allows for early interventions when complications occur.

ASSESSMENT DURING POSTPARTUM	RATIONALE
Evaluate maternal well-being through ongoing assessment, including: • Vital signs • Amount and type of lochia • Fundal height, position, and firmness • Pain level • Wound healing • Breast changes • Intake and output	Monitoring maternal well-being allows for early intervention when complications occur.

Continued

ASSESSMENT DURING POSTPARTUM	RATIONALE
Evaluate newborn well-being through a complete initial assessment and ongoing assessments, including: • Passage of meconium stool • Jaundice • Vital signs • Feeding; intake and output	Monitoring newborn well-being allows for early intervention when complications occur.

Expected Outcomes

The mother will:

- have a positive birth outcome.
- be free from complications during the perinatal period.
- take part in appropriate prenatal and postnatal care.
- adhere to prescribed therapeutic regimen if problems occur.
- identify and use available support systems.

INTERVENTIONS TO ADDRESS PERINATAL RISK	RATIONALE
Notify the HCP if any manifestations of perinatal problems are present.	Reporting any manifestations of perinatal problems allows for early intervention.
Implement collaborative interventions aimed at treating any underlying factor that may contribute to perinatal risk.	Treatment of underlying causative or risk factors can assist in reducing perinatal risk.
Administer needed vaccinations according to recommended schedules and mother and caregiver need.	Vaccinations decrease the risk of acquiring maternal and newborn infections.
Administer medications as prescribed:	
• Prenatal vitamin and mineral supplement	A prenatal supplement is given to ensure the intake of vitamins and minerals essential to maternal–fetal health.
• Iron	Iron supplementation decreases the risk of iron-deficiency anemia.
• Folic acid	Folic acid intake and supplementation decrease the risk of neural tube defects.
Respect the mother's wishes regarding modesty.	Respecting wishes regarding modesty can reduce feelings of embarrassment and enhance dignity.
CULTURE: Provide care that respects the mother's beliefs, traditions, and culture.	Culturally competent care promotes positive patient outcomes.
HEALTH PROMOTION: Encourage 30 minutes of moderate physical activity every day, if able.	Physical activity promotes maternal well-being, improves circulation, and maintains stamina.
ELIMINATION: Institute measures to promote normal bowel function: • Stool softener or osmotic laxative as needed • Adequate fluid intake • Increased diet fiber • Fiber supplement	Constipation and fecal incontinence are common in pregnancy and the postpartum period and cause significant distress.
INTERPERSONAL VIOLENCE: Provide the mother with adequate referrals or removal from the situation when interpersonal violence is present.	Effective interventions can reduce the incidence of violence, abuse, and physical or mental harm.
SUBSTANCE USE: Discourage smoking and substance use and encourage abstinence.	Cessation promotes maternal and fetal well-being.
MOOD AND AFFECT: Institute referral and treatment for coexisting psychological problems.	Identifying depression or other psychological problems and initiating treatment can improve perinatal outcomes.
Offer additional support to the mother experiencing an unplanned or unwanted pregnancy.	A mother with a pregnancy that is unwanted or unplanned is less likely to receive prenatal care and has a higher risk for adverse pregnancy outcomes.

INTERVENTIONS TO ADDRESS PERINATAL RISK	RATIONALE
Encourage the mother to follow appropriate safety precautions: • Proper seat belt use • Avoiding hot tubs and saunas • Using good body mechanics • Avoiding jarring, such as during amusement park rides	Following safety precautions can reduce the risk of miscarriage and injuries.
NUTRITION: Encourage the mother to follow general diet recommendations, including: • Eat nutrient-dense foods. • Increase protein and calcium intake. • Eat small, frequent meals.	Proper nutrition during pregnancy helps promote optimal maternal and newborn outcomes.

INTERVENTIONS DURING LABOR AND DELIVERY	RATIONALE
Recognize fetal heart rate problems and institute corrective measures.	Fetal heart rate problems signal the potential for serious complications which, if addressed, could improve fetal outcomes.
Administer prescribed oxytocic medications.	Oxytocic medications stimulate and strengthen uterine contractions.
Implement measures to reduce the risk of infection, including: • Monitor temperature every 2 hours. • Assess any discharge and amniotic fluid. • Provide frequent perineal care. • Administer prescribed antibiotics. • Change bed linens and gowns as needed. • Provide skin cleansing immediately before cesarean section.	Bacterial infections are among the leading causes of maternal and newborn mortality.
FLUID AND ELECTROLYTES: Ensure adequate intake to meet hydration needs.	Adequate hydration reduces the risk of complications during labor, delivery, and the postpartum period.
Provide continuous emotional support and encouragement during labor.	Continuous labor support promotes positive birth outcomes through lowered risk for cesarean births and less use of pain medication.
PAIN: Institute measures to assist with managing pain.	Pain management strategies can reduce anxiety and improve the mother's ability to cope with contractions.
Encourage the use of various positions and activities.	Activity and changing positions can increase comfort, promote an optimal fetal heart rate pattern, and promote delivery.
ELIMINATION: Encourage voiding at least every 2 hours.	Frequent voiding prevents acute bladder distension.
SAFETY: Institute safety measures for the mother who has received anesthesia or opioid analgesia.	The expected and side effects of anesthesia and analgesia increase the risk of injury.
Institute agency protocol for the proper identification of the mother and newborn.	These measures reduce the risk of newborn abduction or switched newborns.
GAS EXCHANGE: Ensure the newborn's airway passage is clear and be prepared to use suctioning, stimulation, O_2 administration, or resuscitation.	Respiratory problems are common in newborns because the fluid-filled fetal lungs must transition to the extrauterine environment.
THERMOREGULATION: Institute measures to protect the newborn against heat loss: • Immediately after birth, wrap the newborn in a warm blanket and dry off amniotic fluid. • Provide for skin-to-skin contact with the mother while covering the newborn with a warm blanket. • If not providing skin-to-skin contact, wrap the newborn in warm blankets for the mother to hold the newborn. • Place a blanket or cap on the newborn to decrease the loss of heat by evaporation from the newborn's head. • Use a warm, padded surface under a radiant heater during the initial assessment. • Avoid any unnecessary procedures until body temperature is stable.	Because newborns are often unable to keep themselves warm, especially if the environmental temperature is low, measures to prevent heat loss reduce the risk of hypothermia.

Continued

INTERVENTIONS DURING LABOR AND DELIVERY	RATIONALE
Administer prescribed prophylactic medications:	
• Vitamin K	Vitamin K helps protect against neonatal hemorrhagic disease caused by a lack of vitamin K.
• Ophthalmic erythromycin ointment	Erythromycin eye ointment provides protection against ophthalmia neonatorum, a type of conjunctivitis.

INTERVENTIONS DURING POSTPARTUM	RATIONALE
Promote maternal–newborn bonding: • Provide time for skin-to-skin contact. • Encourage rooming- in. • Encourage breastfeeding.	These measures promote maternal affectionate and attachment behaviors and are a standard of care in the newborn period.
PAIN: Institute measures to assist with pain management.	The pain experience varies during the postpartum period depending on the labor and delivery experience and requires a patient-specific approach to pain management.
Encourage perineal care, including: • Applying cold packs to the perineum • Sitz baths • Using a perineal bottle with each pad change and after voiding	Proper perineal care after birth promotes comfort and wound healing and helps prevent infection.
Institute measures to promote newborn attachment.	An emotional and physical attachment provides the newborn with a sense of security.
INFANT FEEDING: Implement measures to promote newborn feeding.	Proper nutrition is essential to optimal health, growth, and development.
Encourage early ambulation with resumption of physical activity, as recommended by the HCP.	Postpartum physical activity can improve mood, maintain cardiorespiratory fitness, promote weight loss, and promote urinary and bowel function.
ELIMINATION: Provide bladder care. • Monitor for bladder distension. • Encourage voiding every 2 hours. • Note urine output and characteristics of urine. • Review how to perform Kegel exercises.	Bladder overdistention can cause permanent bladder damage.

COLLABORATION	RATIONALE
NUTRITION: Dietitian	A dietitian can offer a detailed nutrition plan, especially for those with gestational diabetes, impaired nutrition, a body weight problem, or who are breastfeeding.
CARE COORDINATION: Social work or case management	The social worker can assist with access to the available community health care resources.
Counseling, as needed	Counseling may assist a mother in managing pregnancy-related distress, such as with an unplanned pregnancy or fetal problem.
MOOD AND AFFECT: Treatment for coexisting psychological problems, including depressed mood	Treatment of psychological problems is an important part of promoting positive birth outcomes.

PATIENT AND CAREGIVER TEACHING

- Expected physiologic and psychological changes associated with pregnancy and postpartum
- Fetal development milestones
- Management of underlying conditions contributing to perinatal risk
- Anticipatory guidance about expected discomforts and common problems associated with pregnancy
- Meeting nutrition and hydration needs
- Appropriate weight gain
- Safe use of medications and how they fit into the management plan
- Importance of recommended prenatal and postnatal care
- Importance of proper balance of rest and exercise
- Safety precautions to follow during pregnancy
- Diagnostic and laboratory tests used to monitor pregnancy
- Process of labor and delivery
- Breastfeeding basics
- Newborn care
- What to expect during postpartum
- Community and self-help resources available
- Sources of information and social support
- When to notify the HCP

DOCUMENTATION

Assessment

- Assessments performed
- Diagnostic and laboratory test results
- Manifestations of perinatal problems
- Screening test results

Interventions

- Discussions with other interprofessional team members
- Medications given
- Notification of HCP about patient status
- Therapeutic interventions and the patient's response
- Teaching provided
- Referrals initiated

Evaluation

- Patient's status: improved, stable, declined
- Presence of perinatal problems
- Response to teaching provided
- Response to therapeutic interventions

Impaired Sexual Function 34

Definition

Presence of a problem with sexual function that prevents the person from experiencing satisfaction from sexual activity

Sexual functioning is a complex biological, psychological, and social process, coordinated by the neurologic, vascular, and endocrine systems. A sexually healthy person has intimate relationships, has a positive body image, and accepts sexuality as normal and natural. Impaired sexual function is common: a person may express concern about their sexuality or have a change in sexual function that is viewed as unsatisfying, unrewarding, or inadequate. Impaired sexual function includes concerns about sexual behaviors, communication of feelings and attitudes about sexuality, sexual health, and sexual function.

A number of factors can lead to impaired sexual function, including physiologic, psychologic, social, and environment factors. The significance of impaired sexual function depends on the person's interest in sexual activity and/or reproduction and whether the underlying problem is temporary or chronic (also see Reproduction). Cultural and religious beliefs have a strong influence on sexuality and the interpretation of sexual roles and behaviors.

Impaired sexual function is associated with a negative self-image and lower quality of life. Relationship problems can occur, especially if the sexual activity between a couple has changed. Problems with body image and self-image contribute to sexual problems. The person may develop anxiety and depression.

Nurses play a key role in identifying the presence of impaired sexual function and in providing interventions to promote sexual health. Anticipate that the patient may feel embarrassed, and acknowledge that it can be uncomfortable to talk about sexual health. Avoid making assumptions about the type of sexual activities or partners that an individual may choose. Your efforts to ensure the patient's privacy and increase their comfort promote open communication.

Associated Clinical Problems

- Abnormal Vaginal Bleeding: any vaginal bleeding not related to normal menstruation
- Altered Sexuality Pattern: perceived change in sexuality
- Difficulty Expressing Intimacy: difficulty expressing feelings within close relationships
- Dissatisfied With Sexual Relationship: expresses that negative aspects are present in the sexual relationship
- Problematic Sexual Behavior: sexual behavior that is considered unacceptable by society
- Excess Vaginal Discharge: increase in the amount of vaginal discharge

Common Risk Factors

- Acute illness
- Age
- Anxiety
- Cancer
- Cardiovascular disease
- Cystocele
- Degenerative neuromuscular diseases
- Dementia
- Diabetes
- Ejaculatory problems or erectile dysfunction
- High-risk sexual behavior
- Impaired endocrine system function
- Intimate partner violence
- Lesbian, gay, bisexual, transgender, queer, questioning sexual identity, intersex, asexual, agender
- Medications: anticonvulsants, antidepressants, antihypertensives, diuretics, opioids
- Negative self-image
- Neuropathy
- Pain or discomfort
- Personal conflicts with religion and culture
- Pregnancy
- Rectocele
- Reproductive health concerns
- Sexually transmitted infections (STIs)
- Social isolation or lack of social skills
- Stress
- Substance use
- Surgery, including radical and genitourinary procedures
- Unpartnered

Manifestations

- Abnormal vaginal bleeding
- Avoiding sexual contact
- Changes in urine elimination
- Decreased libido
- Decreased vaginal lubrication
- Ejaculatory or erectile dysfunction

- Expresses concern about sexuality or sexual function
- Excess vaginal discharge
- Genital lesions, pain or tenderness
- Impaired fertility
- Pain with intercourse
- Pelvic pain
- Penile discharge
- Change in achieving sexual satisfaction
- Scrotal pain or swelling
- Self-report of a sexual problem
- Unfulfilled sexual desires
- Urinary problems
- Vaginal discharge
- Vulvar redness
- Diagnostic test results: positive findings from endoscopy and ultrasound
- Laboratory test results: abnormal hormone levels, fluid culture, semen analysis, urinalysis

Key Conceptual Relationships

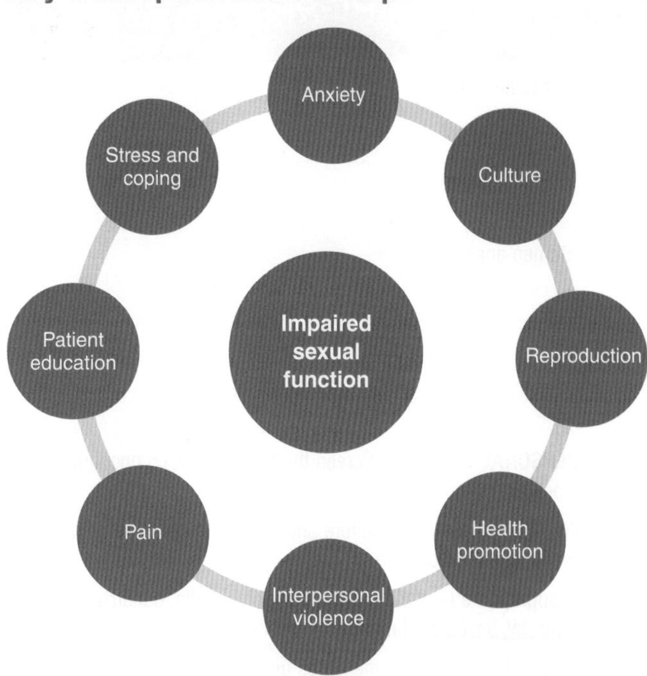

HEALTH AND ILLNESS CONCEPTS

ASSESSMENT OF SEXUAL FUNCTION	RATIONALE
Assess factors that increase the patient's risk for impaired sexual function.	A thorough history can identify patients at risk for impaired sexual function.
Obtain a comprehensive sexual history: • Number and gender of the patient's sexual partners • Frequency of intercourse • Sexual behaviors, including types of sexual practices • Sexual response • Safe sex knowledge and practices • Methods to prevent pregnancy, if desired • Measures used to protect against STIs • History of STIs • Patient's perception of risk for STIs • Age of menarche and menopause, menstrual patterns, and obstetric and gynecologic history	A thorough sexual history aids in determining the cause of impaired sexual function, helps identify factors that contribute to impaired sexual function, and guides treatment.
Obtain a complete vaccination history.	The vaccine history helps to identify protection against the risk of some STIs and diseases, such as mumps and rubella, that affect sexual function.
Ask about self-examination practices and health screenings.	Cervical Pap tests and breast exams are integral to the health of females, whereas males are at risk for testicular and prostate cancer.
Perform a complete physical assessment.	The physical examination is guided by the sexual history and the patient's age, gender, and needs.
Determine the patient's Tanner stage.	Tanner staging estimates sexual development based on the observed changes in primary and secondary sex characteristics.
Obtain culture specimens (eg, vaginal, throat, penile, lesions, urine) as prescribed.	Cultures determine whether a pathogen is present and guide treatment.
Evaluate the results of diagnostic testing, including:	Based on the patient's history and exam, a number of laboratory tests and diagnostic procedures may be indicated.
• Cancer screening and biopsies (cervical, endometrial ovarian, prostate, anal)	Screening and biopsies are used to determine whether an infection or other pathology is present.

Continued

ASSESSMENT OF SEXUAL FUNCTION	RATIONALE
• Hormone levels	Assessing hormone levels can reveal whether there are problems with ovulatory hormones or thyroid and pituitary hormones that control reproductive processes.
• Hysterosalpingogram	A hysterosalpingogram is used to determine whether the fallopian tubes are patent and the uterine cavity is normal.
• Semen analysis	A semen analysis measures the quantity and quality of semen, volume of sperm cells, sperm motility, and sperm density.
• Ultrasound (pelvic, transvaginal, testicular, prostate)	Ultrasound is used to assess for the presence of structural abnormalities in the male and female reproductive tracts.
• Colposcopy, culdoscopy, laparoscopy, and hysteroscopy	Endoscopy is used to assess for the presence of structural abnormalities of the female reproductive tract.
INTERPERSONAL VIOLENCE: Screen the patient at each encounter for interpersonal violence.	Experiencing interpersonal violence related to sexuality may require action to promote patient safety.
CULTURE: Assess the role of culture and religion in the experience of sexuality and reproduction.	Culture and religion strongly influence views on sexuality and may affect treatment options.
Perform appropriate periodic screening for chlamydia, gonorrhea, syphilis, and HIV, based on the patient's level of risk.	Periodic screening for STIs is based on the patient's level of risk, with the goal of reducing morbidity, mortality, and spread of STIs in the community.
Evaluate the effectiveness of measures used to improve sexual function through ongoing assessment.	Monitoring sexual function allows for the evaluation of therapy effectiveness.
Pediatric	
Perform the first genital exam at birth, including an inspection of the external genitalia, evaluation of the patency of the urethra and anus, and, in males, the location of the urinary meatus and any deviation.	The first genital exam should occur at birth to verify the presence of elimination routes and provide baseline data for physical examinations throughout childhood.

Expected Outcomes

The patient will:

- express satisfaction with sexual relationships.
- identify and implement safer sex practices.
- participate in healthy sexual activities.

INTERVENTIONS TO IMPROVE SEXUAL FUNCTION	RATIONALE
Implement collaborative interventions aimed at treating any underlying cause of impaired sexual function.	Treatment of underlying causative or risk factors can assist in improving the patient's sexual function.
Administer vaccinations according to recommended schedules and patient needs.	Vaccinations are given to decrease the risk of acquiring an infection.
Administer medications as prescribed:	
• Antibiotics	Widely ranging antibacterial, antiviral, and antiprotozoal agents are used in the treatment of STIs, depending on the microorganism involved.
• Hormone replacement therapy	Hormone replacement therapy may be used to treat the symptoms of menopause.
• Phosphodiesterase-5 (PDE5) inhibitors	PDE5 drugs are the first-line treatment for erectile dysfunction.
Encourage the patient to identify and express feelings, especially about their sexuality and sexual function.	Expressing thoughts and feelings can improve the problems with self-image that often accompany a sexual problem.
Talk with the patient and partner about alternative ways to attain sexual satisfaction and express sexuality, such as hugging, touching, kissing, masturbation, hand holding, and sexual aids.	An intimate relationship includes multiple expressions of affection and sexuality.

INTERVENTIONS TO IMPROVE SEXUAL FUNCTION	RATIONALE
If dyspareunia is present, have the patient use adequate amounts of water-soluble lubricant.	Water-soluble lubricants increase comfort during coitus and reduce tissue trauma.
Encourage the patient to implement specific measures that can facilitate sexual functioning, such as changes in coital positions and timing at medication peak or when least fatigued.	Specific suggestions can improve comfort during coitus and mitigate the effects of physical limitations.
HEALTH PROMOTION: Discuss safe sex practices and how to decrease the risk of STIs.	Following safe sex practices can decrease the risk of acquiring an STI.
PAIN: Implement measures to manage any pain the patient is experiencing.	The presence of pain is a barrier to healthy sexual expression and contributes to impaired sexual function.
Notify the health care provider (HCP) if signs and symptoms of impaired sexual function persist or worsen.	Achievement of an effective treatment plan often requires adjustments in therapy.
INTERPERSONAL VIOLENCE: Provide the patient with referrals or means of removal from the situation when interpersonal violence is present.	Effective interventions can reduce violence, abuse, and physical or mental harm for partners.
ANXIETY: Implement measures to assist the patient in managing any anxiety they may be experiencing.	Patients with anxiety often have concerns related to impaired sexual function.
STRESS AND COPING: Encourage the use of positive coping and stress management strategies.	Stress from life issues may have a negative impact on sexual function.

COLLABORATION	RATIONALE
Sexual counseling with cognitive–behavioral therapy	Sexual counseling and cognitive–behavioral therapy may be effective in treating sexual problems with psychological origins, especially erectile dysfunction.
Social work or case management	The social worker can explore community resources available to help the patient obtain access to appropriate health care.
Support groups	Specialty support services are available to assist the patient with managing sexual problems.

PATIENT AND CAREGIVER TEACHING

- Healthy human sexuality and sexual function
- Physical changes and changes in sexual function associated with puberty, pregnancy, and aging, including menopause and andropause
- Factors that may be contributing to impaired sexual function
- Management of any underlying condition causing impaired sexual function
- Measures to improve sexual function
- Recommended health screenings and immunizations
- Safe use of medications and how they fit into the overall management plan
- Measures to avoid pregnancy, if desired
- Risk of exposure to STIs and safer sex practices
- Clarification of any myths about sexual function
- Community and self-help resources, additional information available
- When to notify the HCP

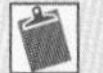

DOCUMENTATION

Assessment

- Assessments performed
- Diagnostic and laboratory test results
- Manifestations of impaired sexual function
- Screening test results

Interventions

- Discussions with other members of the interprofessional team
- Medications given
- Notification of HCP about patient status
- Therapeutic interventions and the patient's response
- Teaching provided
- Referrals initiated

Evaluation

- Patient's status: improved, stable, declined
- Presence of any manifestations of impaired sexual function
- Response to teaching provided
- Response to therapeutic interventions

HEALTH AND ILLNESS CONCEPTS

Fatigue 35

Definition

Lack of physical and/or mental energy that interferes with usual and desired activities

Fatigue is a common symptom reported by many people. Everyone has fatigue at some point. Healthy people can become fatigued from overexertion, added stress, or inadequate sleep. Fatigue in these instances is usually temporary and signals that we need to rest. For others, fatigue is associated with a health problem or related to a person's habits or routines. Depending on the cause, we describe fatigue as acute or chronic. Chronic fatigue lasts longer than 6 months. Many people with chronic illness report fatigue.

Fatigue can cause significant changes in school or work performance and impair the ability to care for oneself. Family and social relationships can be disrupted. The person may experience a negative self-image because others sometimes label the person as lazy. Fatigue resulting from treatment may decrease adherence. The patient with fatigue requires various degrees and types of support. Nurses can play a key role in assessing for fatigue and initiating interventions that alleviate its effects.

Common Risk Factors

- Age
- Alcohol use
- Anemia
- Autoimmune disorders
- Cancer and cancer treatment
- Caregiving, caring for an infant
- Chronic fatigue syndrome
- Chronic obstructive pulmonary disease (COPD)
- Chronic pain
- Degenerative neuromuscular problems
- Depression
- Diabetes
- End-stage kidney disease, hemodialysis
- Excess exercise
- Excess or overwhelming role demands
- Impaired nutrition
- Impaired sleep
- Infection
- Liver disease
- Medications: antianxiety medications, antidepressants, antihypertensives, β-blockers, muscle relaxants
- Pregnancy
- Substance use
- Thyroid problems
- Working shift work

Pediatric

- Congenital heart disease

Manifestations

- Decreased libido
- Decreased motivation
- Difficulty concentrating
- Difficulty participating in role responsibilities and activities of daily living
- Drowsiness
- Impaired judgment
- Impaired memory
- Lack of energy
- Lethargy, listlessness
- Reports fatigue, tiredness, weakness

Pediatric

- Avoiding play and other activities
- School problems

Key Conceptual Relationships

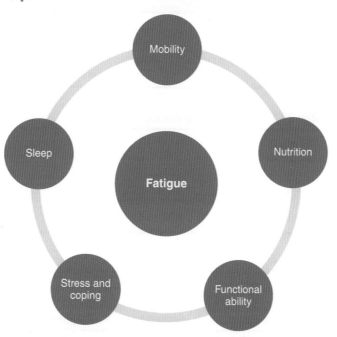

ASSESSMENT OF FATIGUE	RATIONALE
Assess risk factors that may contribute to fatigue.	Identifying factors that place the patient at risk for fatigue allows for early intervention.
Evaluate the patient's underlying health status.	Underlying health status has a considerable influence on fatigue.
Obtain a history of the patient's fatigue experience, including: • Onset, sudden or gradual • Duration • Frequency of fatigue • Intensity or severity • Alleviating and aggravating factors	The history aids in evaluating the fatigue experience and helps direct treatment.
Use a valid, reliable tool appropriate for the patient's age and cognition to perform a formal fatigue assessment, such as the Fatigue Visual Analog Scale (Table 35.1) or the Fatigue Assessment Scale (FAS) (Table 35.2).	The consistent use of fatigue rating scales identifies the intensity of fatigue and helps evaluate the effectiveness of interventions.
Perform a physical assessment and obtain diagnostic tests based on the patient's history.	Physical assessment and diagnostic tests can identify secondary causes of fatigue so that treatment can be initiated.
• **SLEEP:** Sleep and rest patterns, including the effects of rest periods, such as naps, weekends, and vacations.	Impaired sleep is a significant contributing factor to fatigue.
• **PAIN:** Comprehensive pain assessment	There is a strong association between fatigue and pain, with people experiencing pain reporting a high rate of fatigue.
Assess the impact of fatigue on daily life, including the ability to perform work and household duties and engage in physical, mental, and social activities.	The severity and frequency of fatigue directly influence functional ability.
Assess the patient's support system: • Who do they live with? • Are they employed? • Are friends and relatives accessible? • Are they using any community resources?	Support from others is important in managing fatigue.
NUTRITION: Obtain a diet history, including usual daily caloric intake, diet choices, and use of nutrition support.	People with impaired nutrition are at risk for fatigue because of inadequate energy sources.
MOOD AND AFFECT: Screen for coexisting psychological problems.	Most people with depression report fatigue.
STRESS AND COPING: Assess the patient's use of coping and stress management strategies.	Coping and stress management strategies can improve quality of life by reducing fatigue and helping the patient manage fatigue better.

Continued

ASSESSMENT OF FATIGUE	RATIONALE
Monitor for medication and treatment side effects known to be associated with fatigue.	Fatigue is a side effect associated with many medications and treatments.
Evaluate the effectiveness of measures used to address fatigue through ongoing assessment.	Evaluating the effectiveness of measures to address fatigue allows for evaluation of therapy effectiveness.

Table 35.1 Fatigue Visual Analog Scale

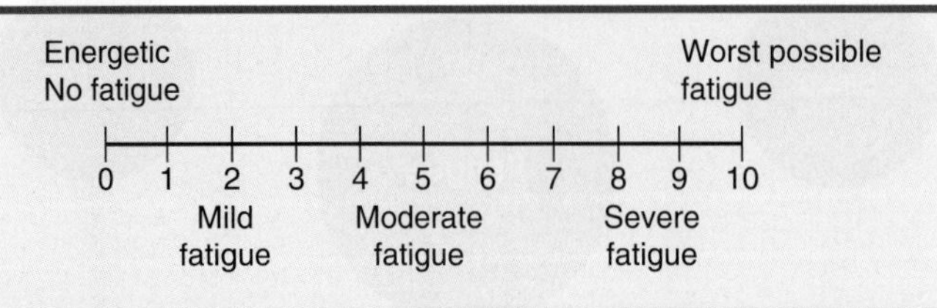

Table 35.2 Fatigue Assessment Scale (FAS)

The following 10 statements refer to how you usually feel. For each statement, you can choose one of five answer categories, varying from never to always: 1 = never, 2 = sometimes, 3 = regularly, 4 = often, 5 = always.

	Never	Sometimes	Regularly	Often	Always
1. I am bothered by fatigue	1	2	3	4	5
2. I get tired very quickly	1	2	3	4	5
3. I don't do much during the day	1	2	3	4	5
4. I have enough energy for everyday life	1	2	3	4	5
5. Physically, I feel exhausted	1	2	3	4	5
6. I have trouble starting things	1	2	3	4	5
7. I have problems thinking clearly	1	2	3	4	5
8. I have no desire to do anything	1	2	3	4	5
9. Mentally, I feel exhausted	1	2	3	4	5
10. When I am doing something, I can concentrate well	1	2	3	4	5

Total the responses. A total FAS score < 22 indicates no fatigue, a score ≥ 22 indicates fatigue.

From Michielsen HJ, De Vries J, Van Heck GL. Psychometric qualities of a brief self-rated fatigue measure: the fatigue assessment scale. *J Psychosom Res.* 2003;54:345.

Expected Outcomes

The patient will:

- report that fatigue has resolved or improved.
- implement strategies to compensate for fatigue.
- balance rest and activities based on patient priorities.
- maintain role performance and take part in desired activities of daily living.

INTERVENTIONS TO REDUCE FATIGUE	RATIONALE
Implement collaborative interventions aimed at treating underlying factors contributing to fatigue.	Fatigue may improve or resolve with treatment of an underlying contributing factor.
Notify the health care provider (HCP) if manifestations of fatigue persist or worsen.	Achieving an effective treatment plan often requires adjustments in therapy.
Encourage the patient to share their feelings about being fatigued.	The patient needs to know you consider the fatigue significant and understand that fatigue may profoundly disrupt a person's life.
Have the patient keep a fatigue diary or log for 1–2 weeks, noting level of fatigue, activities, and type of fatigue experienced.	An evaluation of a 1- or 2-week fatigue log or diary can assist in determining the exent of the fatigue.

INTERVENTIONS TO REDUCE FATIGUE	RATIONALE
Review with the patient their current commitments and schedule to help them prioritize activities and schedule rest periods.	The patient may need to adjust their schedule temporarily to be less busy.
Assist the patient with identifying support persons to assist with completing commitments.	Allowing others to assist with certain commitments can increase rest time for the patient.
MOBILITY: Help the patient develop an exercise plan, encouraging participation in moderate-intensity exercise.	Stretching, yoga, and moderate-intensity exercise can help relieve the effects of fatigue.
SLEEP: Encourage the patient to get adequate sleep, and implement measures to address impaired sleep if present.	An adequate amount of sleep helps to prevent and alleviate fatigue.
Encourage the patient to limit naps to early afternoon and less than 1 hour per day.	Oversleeping generally worsens fatigue.
Help the patient identify ways to conserve energy throughout the day, such as: • Organize work areas to keep frequently used items accessible. • Use adaptive devices. • Plan ahead to avoid rushing. • Have others perform activities that are taxing. • Stop working before becoming overly tired. • Work during the times when fatigue is the least.	Energy conservation activities play a key role in alleviating fatigue.
NUTRITION: Provide a nutritionally adequate diet, limiting caffeine.	Impaired nutrition increases the risk for fatigue because of inadequate energy sources.
Help the patient with activities of daily living, as needed.	Fatigue can interfere with the ability to complete activities of daily living.
FUNCTIONAL ABILITY: Help the patient develop ways to enhance participation in activities of daily living in the home, work, and socially.	Facilitating activities of daily living will help patients improve their functional ability.
STRESS AND COPING: Help the patient cope with fatigue by using positive coping and stress management strategies.	Improving the patient's ability to use stress management and coping strategies addresses many factors that contribute to fatigue.
SPIRITUALITY: Collaborate with the patient to select and implement spiritual support practices, such as meditation, yoga, mindful breathing, and tai chi.	Spiritual support practices help a patient improve health by focusing on mind and body connections.
Discuss prescribed medications known to be associated with fatigue with the HCP.	A change in the patient's medication regimen may lessen fatigue.
DEVELOPMENT: Implement measures to assist the patient in maintaining a positive self-image.	Persons with fatigue may have a negative self-image associated with stigma.
PAIN: Implement measures to address pain, if applicable.	Better pain control may lower the incidence of fatigue.
FUNCTIONAL ABILITY: Implement measures to address social isolation the patient may be experiencing.	Social isolation can negatively influence the quality of life.
Assist parents and caregivers in identifying support persons to assist with providing care.	Allowing others to assist with care can increase rest time for caregivers.
Encourage the parents to rest and sleep when the infant sleeps.	This increases the amount of time available for rest.
Pediatric	
Teach siblings about fatigue and what to do when their sibling is tired and does not want to play or is irritable.	Education can help siblings understand fatigue and how to support their sibling.
Discuss with school personnel the child's schedule and any changes or modifications needed.	Modifying the child's schedule can promote school attendance, completion of assignments, and general academic success.
Encourage the child to take part in play activities appropriate to age, developmental level, and abilities.	A child's normal role includes play activity.

COLLABORATION	RATIONALE
MOOD AND AFFECT: Treatment for coexisting Psychologic problems	Most people with depression report fatigue.
Cognitive behavior therapy	Cognitive behavior therapy helps reduce fatigue by helping the patient manage stressors that make fatigue worse.
Occupational therapy	Occupational therapy can recommend assistive devices and assist in modifying activities to help the patient function at their maximum ability.
CARE COORDINATION: Social work or case management	A social worker or case manager can help the patient and caregiver identify community resources to assist with fulfilling role responsibilities.

PATIENT AND CAREGIVER TEACHING

- Cause of fatigue, if known, and how long it will last
- Manifestations of fatigue
- Management of any underlying condition associated with fatigue
- Ways to manage fatigue
- Health-promoting behaviors, including nutrition, sleep
- Positive coping and stress management strategies
- Exercise plan with scheduled rest
- Energy-conserving strategies
- Relaxation techniques
- When to notify the HCP

DOCUMENTATION

Assessment

- Assessments performed
- Diagnostic and laboratory test results
- Manifestations of fatigue
- Screening test results

Interventions

- Discussions with other interprofessional team members
- Environmental modifications made
- Notification of the HCP about patient status
- Therapeutic interventions and the patient's response
- Teaching provided
- Referrals initiated

Evaluation

- Patient's status: improved, stable, declined
- Presence of manifestations of fatigue
- Response to teaching provided
- Response to therapeutic interventions

Allergy 36

Definition

Hypersensitivity induced by exposure to an allergen, resulting in harmful immune responses on subsequent exposures

Hypersensitivity reactions or exaggerated immune responses include allergic reactions and autoimmune reactions. Four types of hypersensitivity reactions exist (Table 36.1). Anaphylactic reactions are Type I reactions that occur suddenly after exposure to the offending allergen. Anaphylaxis is a rapid and severe response that can be systemic (generalized) or local (cutaneous).

Foods, drugs, pollens, dust, molds, bee venom, vaccines, or latex may all evoke hypersensitivity reactions. Allergic rhinitis, or hay fever, is the most common Type I reaction. Some allergens cause more than one type of hypersensitivity. Often, those who have a reaction to one type of allergen (e.g., pollen) will have a similar reaction to other antigens in the same or a similar class.

You play a key role in helping the patient make lifestyle adjustments so that there is minimal exposure to offending allergens. Teach the patient that even with drug therapy and immunotherapy, they will never be totally desensitized or completely symptom-free. Help the patient use preventive measures to control symptoms and reduce allergen exposure. If the allergen is a drug, have the patient avoid the drug. Encourage patients to make their allergies known to all health care providers and carry documentation stating their allergies.

Associated Clinical Problems

- Food Allergy: hypersensitive reaction that occurs with exposure to a specific food
- Latex Allergy: hypersensitive reaction to natural latex rubber products
- Risk for Latex Allergy: increased risk for a hypersensitive reaction to natural latex rubber products
- Risk for Anaphylaxis: increased risk for a life-threatening systemic or hypersensitivity reaction to an allergen
- Risk for Reaction to Contrast Media: increased risk for a reaction from receiving iodinated contrast media

Common Risk Factors

- Asthma
- Family history of allergies
- History of food and medication sensitivities
- Known allergies
- Previous reaction to related substances
- Unusual reactions to insect bites or stings

Latex Allergy

- Allergic rhinitis
- Atopic eczema
- Having certain food allergies
- History of multiple surgical procedures
- Long-term occupation exposure to latex products
- Spina bifida

Risk for Reaction to Contrast Media

- Dehydration
- Diabetes
- Heart failure
- Increased creatinine levels
- Kidney disease
- Medications: chemotherapy, metformin, nonsteroidal anti-inflammatory drugs (NSAIDs)
- Multiple myeloma
- Polycythemia
- Previous reaction to contrast media
- Sickle cell disease

Manifestations

- Diagnostic test results: positive results to skin tests, eosinophils in secretions
- Ears: diminished hearing; immobile or scarred tympanic membranes; recurrent ear infections
- Laboratory test results: positive results to blood tests, ↑ immunoglobulin E (IgE) levels, abnormal white blood cell (WBC) count
- Eyes: conjunctivitis, dark circles under the eyes, itchy eyes, watery eyes
- Nose: nasal voice, itchy nose, rhinitis; pale, boggy mucous membranes; sneezing; swollen nasal passages; recurrent nosebleeds; crease across the bridge of the nose ("allergic salute")
- Respiratory: cough, dyspnea, stridor, wheezing
- Skin: rashes, including urticaria, wheal and flare, papules, and vesicles; dryness, scaliness, scratches, itching
- Throat: continual throat clearing; red throat; swollen lips or tongue; palpable neck lymph nodes

Table 36.1 Types of Hypersensitivity Reactions

Type I: IgE Mediated	Type II: Cytotoxic	Type III: Immune Complex	Type IV: Delayed Hypersensitivity
Rate of Development			
Immediate	Minutes to hours	Hours to days	Several days
Examples			
Allergic rhinitis Anaphylaxis Asthma Atopic dermatitis	Goodpasture syndrome Graves disease Transfusion reaction	Acute glomerulonephritis Rheumatoid arthritis SLE	Contact dermatitis (e.g., poison ivy)

Food Allergy
- Abdominal cramps
- Diarrhea
- Food intolerances
- Vomiting

Latex Allergy
- Type I reaction: anaphylaxis
- Type IV reaction: dryness, redness, swelling, crusting of the skin
- Irritant reaction: redness, fissuring, cracking of the skin, blistering

Anaphylaxis
- Initial: itching, redness, diarrhea, vomiting, abdominal cramps, difficulty breathing
- Severe: laryngeal edema, vascular collapse, ↓ blood pressure (BP), shock, respiratory distress

Reaction to Contrast Media
- Mild reaction: hives, itching, rhinorrhea, nausea, vomiting, diaphoresis, coughing
- Moderate reaction: headache, facial edema, ↑ pulse, ↑ BP, palpitations, dyspnea
- Severe reaction: dysrhythmias, laryngeal edema, bronchospasm, pulmonary edema, seizures, syncope

Key Conceptual Relationships

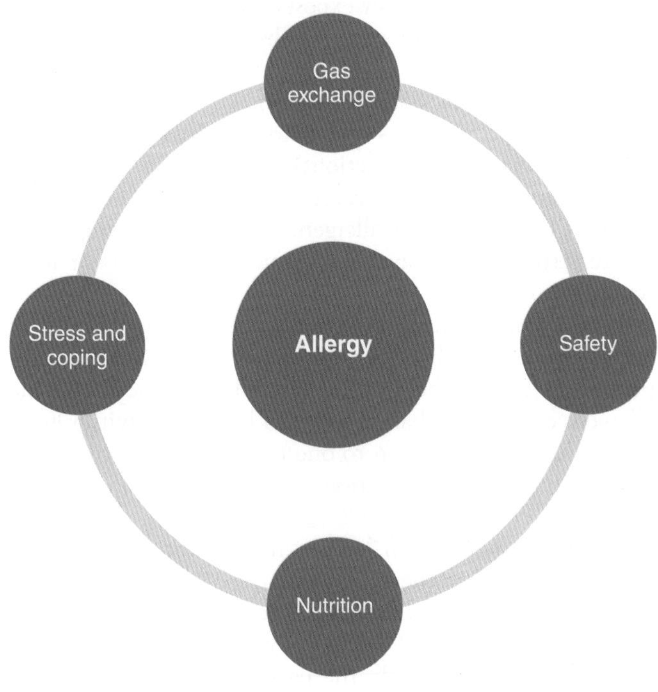

ASSESSMENT OF ALLERGY	RATIONALE
Identify patients who need emergency management for an allergic reaction so that they can be stabilized.	Identifying an acute allergic reaction allows for early intervention.
Assess for risk factors that may increase the risk of having allergies or an allergic reaction.	A thorough history helps identify factors that influence the presence of allergies.
Obtain information about family allergies and atopic diseases, such as asthma, eczema, and allergic rhinitis.	Family history, including information about atopic reactions in relatives, is important in identifying at-risk patients.

ASSESSMENT OF ALLERGY	RATIONALE
Obtain a detailed allergy history, including: • What the suspected allergen is • Any history of atopic diseases, such as asthma, eczema, or allergic rhinitis • Allergy symptoms • Age when symptoms first started • Speed of onset of symptoms after contact with the allergen • Duration of symptoms • Severity of reaction • Frequency of occurrence • Reproducibility of symptoms on repeated exposure • Details of any previous treatment, including the use of medications to treat allergies	A thorough history helps identify allergens and guides intervention.
If medication allergies are present, obtain additional medication history, including: • Generic and trade names of the suspected medication(s), including the strength and formulation • Reason for taking the medication • Number of doses taken or number of days on the medication before the reaction • Route of administration	All health care providers (HCPs) need to be aware of medication allergies so that offending medications can be avoided or pretreatment administered.
If a food allergy is suspected, obtain additional allergy history, including: • Any foods that are avoided and why • Who suspected a food allergy and why • Any response to eliminating and reintroducing foods	A thorough history helps identify food allergies and guides intervention.
Review social and environment factors, including exposure to pets, trees and plants, air pollutants, floor coverings, and types of cooling and heating systems.	Identifying potential allergens assists in guiding interventions that aim to reduce exposure.
Perform a complete physical assessment and monitor indicators of allergy on an ongoing basis:	
• Manifestations of allergies and allergic reactions	Identifying manifestations of allergies and allergic reactions allows for early intervention.
• WBC count with differential	The eosinophil count is high in Type I hypersensitivity reactions.
• IgE antibodies	Serum IgE levels are generally high in Type I hypersensitivity reactions, which serves as a diagnostic indicator of allergy.
• Sputum, nasal, and bronchial secretions tests	Eosinophils may be present in sputum, nasal, and bronchial secretions.
• Skin tests	Allergy skin testing is often an important step in diagnosing allergies.
Assist with performing skin and blood allergy testing.	Allergy testing is often an important step in diagnosing allergies.
STRESS AND COPING: Assess the effects of lifestyle and stress level on allergic symptoms.	Many allergic reactions, especially asthma and urticaria, may be worsened by fatigue and stress.
Evaluate the effectiveness of measures used to reduce allergic reactions through ongoing assessment.	Ongoing assessment allows for the evaluation of therapy effectiveness.
Pediatric	
Obtain details of the mother's diet if the child is breastfed.	A thorough history helps identify food allergies and guides intervention.

Expected Outcomes

The patient will:

- not experience an allergic reaction.
- be free from complications related to allergies.
- identify allergens.
- implement strategies to reduce exposure to allergens.
- describe measures to implement in the event of an allergic reaction.

INTERVENTIONS TO REDUCE ALLERGY	RATIONALE
GAS EXCHANGE: Initiate emergency measures to manage an acute system reaction or anaphylaxis: • Ensure patent airway. • Administer prescribed IV fluids. • Administer prescribed epinephrine. • Apply prescribed high-flow oxygen. • Position the patient flat, with their legs raised. If in respiratory distress, the patient may prefer to sit up, with their legs elevated. • Remove the trigger. • Administer prescribed inhaled β_2-agonist and nebulized epinephrine for lower and upper respiratory tract involvement.	An anaphylactic reaction is a life-threatening event that requires immediate medical and nursing interventions.
Administer prescribed immunotherapy.	Immunotherapy is the recommended treatment for the control of allergic symptoms when the allergen cannot be avoided or drug therapy is not effective.
Administer medications as prescribed, including:	
• Epinephrine	Parenteral epinephrine is the drug of choice to treat an anaphylactic reaction.
• Antihistamines	Antihistamines block the effects of histamine, reducing manifestations if a reaction occurs or with exposure to the antigen.
• Sympathomimetic/decongestants	Various agents offer symptomatic relief of allergy symptoms.
• Leukotriene receptor antagonists (LTRAs)	LTRAs block leukotriene, a major mediator of the allergic inflammatory process, reducing the symptoms of allergic rhinitis.
• Corticosteroids	Nasal corticosteroid sprays are effective in relieving the symptoms of allergic rhinitis.
• Mast cell stabilizers (cromolyn)	Mast cell–stabilizing agents inhibit the release of histamines, leukotrienes, and other agents from the mast cell after antigen–IgE interaction.
• Antipruritic drugs	Topically applied antipruritic drugs protect the skin and provide relief from itching.
SAFETY: Ensure that the patient's allergies are listed on all medical and dental records and place an alert band.	All HCPs need to be aware of the patient's allergies so that safety precautions may be implemented.
Encourage the patient to wear a medical alert bracelet listing the drug allergy.	The patient has the responsibility to make their allergies known to all HCPs.
Help the patient make lifestyle adjustments so that there is minimal exposure to offending allergens.	Effective treatment of allergies includes reducing exposure to the offending allergen.
Assist the patient with implementing environment control measures, such as sleeping in an air-conditioned room, damp dusting daily, and covering mattresses and pillows with hypoallergenic covers.	Effective treatment of allergies includes reducing exposure to the offending allergen.
Assist the patient with keeping a daily or weekly food or other type of diary with a description of any untoward reactions.	Diaries with a description of any untoward reactions are useful in determining relationships between ingested foods or environment exposure and allergic reactions.
STRESS AND COPING: Encourage the use of positive stress management and coping behaviors.	Many allergic reactions, especially asthma and urticaria, may be worsened by fatigue and emotional stress.
Notify the HCP if manifestations of allergies persist or worsen.	Achieving an effective treatment plan often requires adjustments in therapy.

INTERVENTIONS TO REDUCE LATEX ALLERGY	RATIONALE
Use latex avoidance protocols for those patients with a positive latex allergy test or a history of signs and symptoms related to latex exposure. • Post signs noting latex allergy. • Put a latex allergy alert band on the patient. • Eliminate all latex-containing products from the patient's environment. • Place latex-free products in the patient's room.	Use of nonlatex products eliminates exposure to latex and reduces the risk of a reaction.
Encourage patients to avoid foods associated with latex food syndrome: banana, avocado, chestnut, kiwi, tomato, water chestnut, guava, hazelnut, potato, peach, grape, and apricot.	Some foods with proteins similar to the proteins in rubber may cause an allergic reaction in people who are allergic to latex.
Assist the patient in identifying latex products in the home environment.	Identification and removal of latex products will reduce the risk of an allergic reaction.
Help the patient find and obtain alternatives to latex-containing products.	Finding latex-free products will promote adherence with latex avoidance.

INTERVENTIONS TO REDUCE THE RISK OF A REACTION TO CONTRAST MEDIA	RATIONALE
Depending on patient risk, notify the HCP regarding the administration of prophylaxis medications.	Prophylactic measures may be needed prior to the procedure to reduce the risk of a reaction.
Ensure that the patient is well hydrated before the procedure.	Hydration decreases the incidence of renal problems induced by contrast media.
Hold metformin and other oral hypoglycemic agents for 48 hours prior to the procedure.	Oral hypoglycemic agents are associated with the development of lactic acidosis after receiving contrast media.

COLLABORATION	RATIONALE
NUTRITION: Dietitian	Collaborating with a dietitian offers the patient further information and support for implementing an avoidance diet.
Support groups	The patient and caregiver may find tips for allergy avoidance and locating products, as well as support for managing allergies, from peers.
School counselor, school social worker, or school psychologist	School personnel can provide the services necessary to ensure a child with allergies, particularly to food, is in a safe environment at school.

PATIENT AND CAREGIVER TEACHING

- About allergies and the cause of the allergic reaction, if known
- Manifestations of allergies and allergic reactions
- Methods of allergy testing
- Ways to avoid or reduce exposure to allergens
- What to do if an allergic reaction occurs
- Safe use of medications
- How to use commercial kits containing automatic injectable epinephrine
- Importance of having a medical alert bracelet
- Need to inform providers about allergies
- When to notify the HCP or seek emergency care about a reaction

DOCUMENTATION

Assessment
- Assessments performed
- Diagnostic and laboratory test results
- Manifestations of allergy

Interventions
- Discussions with other interprofessional team members
- Medications given
- Notification of HCP about patient status
- Therapeutic interventions and the patient's response
- Teaching provided
- Referrals initiated

Evaluation
- Patient's status: improved, stable, declined
- Manifestations of allergy
- Response to teaching provided
- Response to therapeutic interventions

Impaired Immunity 37

Definition

Impaired ability of the body to resist disease

Immunity is the ability of the body to resist disease. An optimal immune response protects the body against invasion by pathogens and destroys mutated cells and dead or damaged cell substances. When the immune system does not work as it should, there is an increased risk for infection and other problems. Persons with a suppressed immune response are *immunocompromised*. The patient may have leukopenia, a decrease in the total white blood cell (WBC) count (granulocytes, monocytes, and lymphocytes) or granulocytopenia, a deficiency of granulocytes, which include neutrophils, eosinophils, and basophils. Neutrophils play a major role in the immune response. They are closely monitored in clinical practice as an indicator of a patient's risk for infection.

Immunosuppression is a result of many conditions and diseases. It can be an expected effect, a side effect, or an unintentional effect of certain drugs. The most common cause from treatment is the use of chemotherapy and immunosuppressive therapy. Patients who are immunosuppressed are at significant risk for infection. Impaired immunity blunts normal inflammatory responses, leading to diminished signs and symptoms of infection. With advancing age, there is a decline in the immune response. Older people are more susceptible to infections like pneumonia from pathogens that they were relatively immunocompetent against before. Their antibody response to immunizations, such as the flu vaccine, is lower.

Common Causes and Risk Factors

- Age
- Alcohol use disorder
- Being unimmunized
- Burns
- Cancer
- Chronic kidney disease
- Chronic obstructive pulmonary disease (COPD)
- Diabetes
- Exposure to pollutants
- High-risk sexual behavior
- Impaired immune function
- Intravenous (IV) drug use
- Malnutrition
- Medications: biologic response modifiers, chemotherapy, and corticosteroids
- Poor hand hygiene
- Pregnancy
- Radiation therapy
- Rheumatoid arthritis
- Systemic lupus erythematosus
- Trauma
- Unsanitary conditions; food and water contamination

Manifestations

- Dyspnea
- Fatigue
- Fever
- Headache
- Impaired wound healing
- Infection, including recurrent or unusual infections
- Lymphadenopathy
- Malaise
- Night sweats
- Pain, including dysuria, abdominal pain, sore throat
- ↑ Pulse
- ↑ Respiratory rate
- Sores in the mouth
- Vaginal discharge or itching
- Weight loss
- Diagnostic test results: positive culture results
- Laboratory test results: abnormal WBC count

Pediatric

- Impaired growth and development

Related Concepts and Clinical Problems

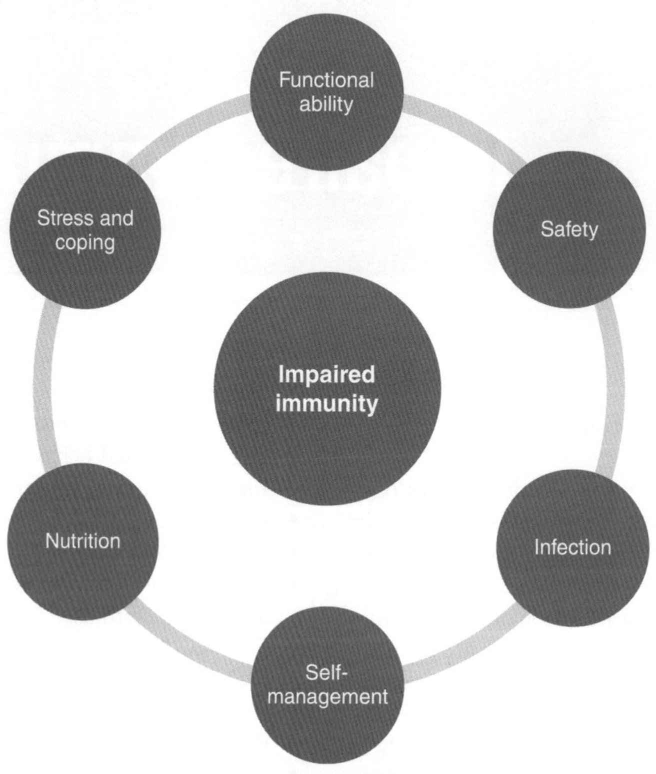

ASSESSMENT OF IMMUNE FUNCTION	RATIONALE
Assess for the potential cause of impaired immunity.	Identifying the cause of impaired immunity allows for early intervention.
Assess risk factors that influence the patient's immune response.	A thorough history can identify patients at risk for immune compromise.
Obtain a complete vaccination history.	The vaccination history helps to identify protective immune responses and risk of infection.
Evaluate the patient's underlying health status.	Underlying health status has a significant influence on the patient's immune system function.
Perform a complete physical assessment and monitor indicators of immune function on an ongoing basis:	
• Manifestations of impaired immunity	Identifying manifestations of impaired immunity allows for early intervention.
• Vital signs	Changes in vital signs are often present with an infection.
• WBC count with differential	Evaluation of the WBC count and differential can reveal leukopenia and neutropenia.
• Antinuclear antibody test (ANA)	An ANA test is standard in determining the presence of autoimmune disease.
• C-reactive protein (CRP) and erythrocyte sedimentation rate (ESR)	Inflammatory markers usually increase with the general inflammation that may accompany an altered immune response.
• Human immunodeficiency virus (HIV) testing	HIV attacks and impairs the body's natural defense system against infection.
• Immunoglobulin levels	People who do not produce sufficent antibodies are at higher risk for infection.

ASSESSMENT OF IMMUNE FUNCTION	RATIONALE
Calculate the absolute neutrophil count (ANC).	The ANC reflects the number of neutrophils available for combating bacterial infection, with lower-than-normal values associated with an increased risk of infection.
Obtain culture specimens (e.g., sputum, throat, blood, lesions, wounds, urine, feces), as ordered.	Cultures determine the type of pathogen present and guide treatment.
Assist with performing a bone marrow aspiration.	Bone marrow aspiration and biopsy are done to examine cell morphology and determine the cause of impaired immune system function.
INFECTION: Monitor for the signs and symptoms of infection on an ongoing basis.	Identifying an infection allows for early intervention.
NUTRITION: Obtain a diet history, including usual daily caloric intake, diet choices, and use of nutrition support.	Optimal nutrition supports the growth and activity of WBCs.
STRESS AND COPING: Assess the current and past use of stress management and coping strategies.	Stress makes the body more vulnerable to pathogens by depressing the immune system.
Evaluate the effectiveness of measures used to improve immune system function through ongoing assessment.	Ongoing assessment allows for evaluation of therapy effectiveness.
Pediatric	
DEVELOPMENT: Assess the child's growth and development level.	Immune system disorders or their treatment may affect growth, development, and the performance of age appropriate activities.

Expected Outcomes

The patient will:

- achieve optimal immune system function.
- be free from infection.
- adhere to the prescribed therapeutic regimen.

INTERVENTIONS TO PROMOTE IMMUNE FUNCTION	RATIONALE
Implement collaborative interventions addressed in treating the underlying cause of an immune problem.	Impaired immunity may improve with treatment of the underlying cause.
Notify the health care provider (HCP) if manifestations of impaired immune responses persist or worsen.	Achievement of an effective treatment plan often requires adjustments in therapy.
Implement strict hand hygiene by the patient and all who have contact with them.	Hand hygiene is an important infection prevention measure and should be done before, during, and after patient contact.
Determine the type and start any transmission-based precautions.	Precautions protect the patient from potential sources of pathogens and infection.
Place a surgical mask on patients when they leave their rooms.	Wearing a mask reduces the patient's exposure to environment contaminants and pathogens.
Use sterile technique when changing dressings or performing invasive procedures.	Using sterile technique protects the patient from pathogens and potential sources of infection.
Implement neutropenic precautions: • Place the patient in a private room. • Screen visitors and staff for signs of infection. • Prohibit the use of live plants or cut flowers. • Avoid fresh fruits and vegatables. • Avoid unpasteurized drinks. • Limit invasive procedures when possible.	Neutropenic precautions protect the patient from pathogens and potential sources of infection.

Continued

INTERVENTIONS TO PROMOTE IMMUNE FUNCTION	RATIONALE
Administer medications as prescribed:	
• Hematopoietic growth factors	Growth factors may prevent neutropenia or reduce its severity and duration.
• Immunoglobulin	IV immunoglobulin can be given as a replacement therapy for patients with specific deficiencies.
• **INFECTION:** Antimicrobials	The appropriate antimicrobial therapy will treat an underlying infection.
SELF MANAGEMENT: Administer vaccinations according to recommended schedules and patient needs.	Vaccinations that do not contain live organisms are given to prevent common infections, such as pneumococcus.
FUNCTIONAL ABILITY: Assist the patient with daily bathing.	Daily bathing protects the patient from potential sources of skin pathogens.
INFECTION: Have the patient brush their teeth with a soft toothbrush 2 to 4 times daily and floss once daily if it does not cause excess pain or bleeding.	Immunosuppression increases the risk of oral infections and periodontitis.
NUTRITION: Provide a nutritionally adequate diet, high in protein and vitamins and low in carbohydrates.	Optimal nutrition supports the growth and activity of WBCs.
SLEEP: Provide the patient with opportunities for adequate sleep.	Adequate rest provides the body with the energy needed for optimal immune system function.
STRESS AND COPING: Encourage the use of positive coping and stress management strategies.	Stress makes the body more vulnerable to pathogens by depressing the immune system.
FUNCTIONAL ABILITY: Help the patient prioritize activities and maintain some daily activity, such as walking, while avoiding crowds.	Continued participation in safe activities helps maintain physical and pulmonary function.
Implement measures to address any social isolation the patient experiences.	Social isolation that may be necessary because of isolation precautions can negatively influence the patient's quality of life.
Pediatric	
DEVELOPMENT: Institute measures to promote optimal growth and development.	Immune system disorders or their treatment may affect growth, development, and the performance of age-appropriate activities.

COLLABORATION	RATIONALE
NUTRITION: Dietitian	Collaborating with a dietitian offers the patient further information and support for implementing an optimal diet.
Support groups	The patient and caregiver may find tips from peers for living and coping with immune problems.
Dental care	Dentists perform periodic deep cleaning and recommend care to reduce the risk of oral infection.
Pediatric	
School counselor, school social worker, or school psychologist	Collaboration with school officials can help ensure the child receives an education equal to other students in a safe environment.

PATIENT AND CAREGIVER TEACHING

- Cause of impaired immunity, if known
- Factors that may be contributing to impaired immunity
- Role of immune system in maintaining health and preventing infection
- Manifestations of impaired immunity
- Diagnostic and laboratory tests used to monitor immune status
- Management of any underlying condition causing impaired immunity
- Hand hygiene techniques
- Measures being used to improve immune system function
- Measures to reduce the risk of exposure to pathogens
- Community and home transmission-based precautions
- Safe use of medications
- How to monitor temperature
- Signs and symptoms of infection
- Importance of proper nutrition
- Recommended health screenings and immunizations
- When to notify the HCP

DOCUMENTATION

Assessment

- Assessments performed
- Diagnostic and laboratory test results
- Manifestations of impaired immunity

Interventions

- Discussions with other interprofessional team members
- Medications given
- Notification of HCP about patient status
- Therapeutic interventions and the patient's response
- Teaching provided
- Referrals initiated
- Neutropenic precautions implemented

Evaluation

- Patient's status: improved, stable, declined
- Manifestations of impaired immunity
- Response to teaching provided
- Response to therapeutic interventions

Infection 38

Definition

Disease caused by the invasion of the body by pathogenic microorganisms

An infection occurs when a pathogen, or a microorganism that causes disease, invades the body, multiplies, and produces disease, usually causing harm to the host. The signs and symptoms of infection are a result of specific pathogen activity, which triggers inflammation and other immune responses. Infections are categorized as localized, disseminated, or systemic and as acute or chronic. A localized infection is limited to a small area. A disseminated infection has spread to areas of the body beyond the initial site of infection. Systemic infections have spread extensively throughout the body, often through the blood, and may be life-threatening.

Infections vary by severity, location, the patient's response to treatment, and the potential for harmful consequences. Infection, immunity, and inflammation are closely related. Having an infection means the immune system is already compromised, increasing the risk of a secondary infection. Infection stimulates an inflammatory response and affects temperature. You can assist the patient in managing any fatigue and pain. Monitor for problems with fluid and electrolyte balance. Helping the patient maintain adequate nutrition and rest is important to combating infection and supporting immune function. The experience of having a serious infection may be associated with anxiety and fear.

Many infectious diseases are more common in older adults. Infections may sometimes be difficult to diagnose in an older adult because they may not have the classic manifestations of infection. Instead, they may have lethargy, agitation, loss of appetite, incontinence, or changes in cognition. Fever may be absent, and coexisting conditions can mask manifestations further. Older adults also tend to have more complications from an infection.

Associated Clinical Problem

- Urinary tract infection (UTI): infection in the urinary system

Common Risk Factors

- Age
- Autoimmune disease
- Being unimmunized
- Being without housing
- Burns
- Cancer
- Chronic kidney disease
- Chronic obstructive pulmonary disease
- COVID-19
- Crowded or unsanitary living conditions
- Debilitation
- Diabetes
- High-risk sexual behavior
- Impaired immunity
- Impaired nutrition
- Intubation and mechanical ventilation
- Intravenous drug use
- Invasive lines
- Lack of preventive health care
- Liver disease
- Low socioeconomic status
- Medications: antimicrobials, biologic response modifiers, chemotherapy, corticosteroids
- Poor hand hygiene
- Radiation therapy
- Recent surgery
- Recent travel, particularly outside the United States or to an underdeveloped area
- Recurrent infections
- Transplant recipient
- Trauma

Pediatric

- Low birth weight
- Prematurity

Urinary Tract Infection

- Catheters, including indwelling catheters, external condom catheters, ureteral stents, nephrostomy tubes, intermittent catheterization
- Congenital defects with obstruction and urinary stasis
- Fistula
- Habitual delay of urination
- Incontinence
- Menopause
- Multiple sex partners
- Poor personal hygiene
- Obesity

- Obstruction from tumor, stricture, benign prostatic hypertrophy
- Pregnancy
- Sexually transmitted infection (STI)
- Shorter female urethra and colonization from normal vaginal flora
- Urinary retention
- Urinary tract instrumentation
- Urinary tract stones
- Use of spermicidal agents, diaphragms, bubble baths, feminine sprays

Manifestations

- Specific symptoms associated with the site of infection

Local

- Edema
- Exudate
- Loss of function
- Pain
- Redness
- Warmth

Systemic

- Anorexia
- Chills
- Diagnostic tests: positive culture results
- Fatigue
- Fever
- Increased pulse
- Increased respiratory rate
- Laboratory tests: ↑ white blood cell (WBC) count with a shift to the left
- Lymphadenopathy
- Malaise
- Nausea

Older Adult

- Cognitive changes
- Falling
- Incontinence

Pediatric

- Fussiness
- Irritability
- Poor feeding
- Sleepiness

Urinary Tract Infection

- Dysuria
- Flank pain
- Frequency
- Hematuria
- Hesitancy
- Nocturia
- Sediment in urine
- Suprapubic discomfort
- Urgency

Key Conceptual Relationships

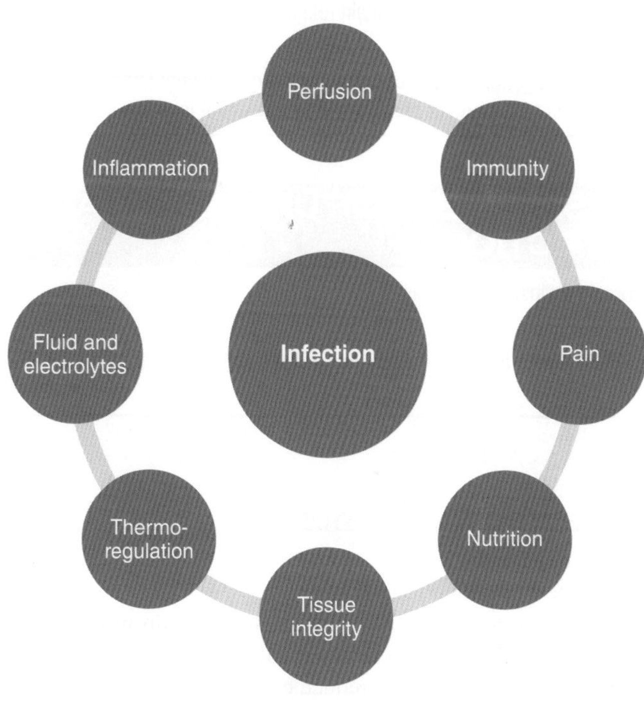

ASSESSMENT OF INFECTION	RATIONALE
Assess for the potential cause of the infection.	Identifying the cause of an infection assists in focusing interventions.
IMMUNITY: Assess risk factors that influence the patient's immune response.	A thorough history can identify patients at risk for immune compromise.
Obtain a complete vaccination history.	The vaccine history helps to identify protective immune responses and risk factors for infection.
Evaluate the patient's underlying health status.	Health status has a significant influence on the patient's risk for infection.
Perform a complete physical assessment and monitor indicators of infection on an ongoing basis:	
• Manifestations of infection	Identifying manifestations of infection allows for early treatment.

Continued

ASSESSMENT OF INFECTION	RATIONALE
• **INFLAMMATION:** Manifestations of inflammation	Infection stimulates an inflammatory response.
• **THERMOREGULATION:** Vital signs, including pulse oximetry	Fever, tachycardia, and tachypnea are common when infection is present.
• WBC count with differential	Elevated levels of B and T lymphocytes, neutrophils, and monocytes can indicate infection.
• Lactate levels	An increased lactate can result from impaired tissue oxygenation associated with infection.
Review the results of specific diagnostic tests related to the source of infection, such as chest radiograph, lumbar puncture, and computed tomography (CT) scanning.	Specific diagnostic tests are done to detect the source of infection.
Obtain culture specimens (e.g, sputum, throat, blood, lesions, wounds, urine, feces) as ordered.	Cultures determine the type of pathogen present and guide treatment.
NUTRITION: Obtain a diet history, including usual daily caloric intake, diet choices, and use of nutrition support.	Proper nutrition supports immune system function and reduces risk of infection.
FUNCTIONAL ABILITY: Assess the effects the infection is having on the patient and family and determine whether the infection is affecting the patient's ability to maintain relationships and perform activities of daily living.	Patients with a chronic or serious infection may have psychologic, financial, role-performance, and social problems.
Evaluate the effectiveness of measures used to combat infection through ongoing assessment of signs and symptoms of infection.	Ongoing assessment allows for evaluation of therapy effectiveness.

ASSESSMENT OF URINARY TRACT INFECTION	RATIONALE
Obtain a dipstick urinalysis.	A dipstick urinalysis can identify the presence of nitrites, WBCs, and leukocyte esterase, which can assist in identifying an infection.
FUNCTIONAL ABILITY: Assess the patient's ability to perform personal hygiene.	Appropriate personal hygiene can reduce the risk of developing a UTI.

Expected Outcomes

The patient will:

- be free from infection.
- be free from complications associated with an infection.
- adhere to the prescribed therapeutic regimen.
- implement measures to reduce exposure to potential infection.

INTERVENTIONS TO MANAGE INFECTION	RATIONALE
Implement collaborative interventions addressed at treating underlying risk factors associated with infection.	Treatment of underlying risk factors enhances the ability to combat infection.
Notify the health care provider (HCP) if manifestations of the infection persist or worsen.	Achieving an effective treatment plan often requires adjustments in therapy.
Implement strict hand hygiene by the patient and all who have contact with them.	Hand hygiene is an important preventive measure and should be done before, during, and after patient contact.
Determine and start any transmission-based precautions as needed.	Appropriate precautions protect the patient and others from potential sources of pathogens and infection.
Place a surgical mask on patients when they leave their rooms, if needed.	Wearing a mask reduces the patient's exposure to pathogens and reduces the risk of their transmitting infection.

INTERVENTIONS TO MANAGE INFECTION	RATIONALE
Administer medications as prescribed:	
• Antibiotics	The appropriate antibiotic therapy is necessary to treat a bacterial infection.
• **THERMOREGULATION:** Antipyretics	Antipyretics lower fever, which is a common physiologic response to inflammation.
• **PAIN:** Analgesics	Analgesics relieve pain caused by inflammation and infection.
• **INFLAMMATION:** Nonsteroidal antiinflammatory drugs (NSAIDs)	NSAIDs are important in managing pain, fever, and inflammation by suppressing the inflammatory response.
Administer antipyretics on a regular schedule.	Around-the-clock administration of antipyretics prevents acute swings in temperature, which can induce chills.
INFLAMMATION: Implement measures to reduce inflammation.	Infection stimulates an inflammatory response.
IMMUNITY: Implement measures to enhance immune system function.	A properly functioning immune system is necessary to combat infection.
NUTRITION: Provide a nutritionally adequate diet that is high in calories.	A high-calorie, nutritionally adequate diet provides the body with the necessary factors to promote healing.
Administer prescribed IV fluids.	A high fluid intake will replace fluid losses and assist in maintaining blood volume.
Encourage increased oral fluid intake.	A high fluid intake will replace fluid loss from perspiration and fever and decrease the pain associated with UTIs.
SLEEP: Provide the patient with opportunities for adequate sleep.	Adequate rest provides the body with the energy needed for optimal immune system function and resolution of infection.
FATIGUE: Help the patient prioritize activities and alternate rest and activity periods.	Limiting activities conserves energy and helps prevent fatigue.

INTERVENTIONS TO MANAGE A URINARY TRACT INFECTION	RATIONALE
Administer a prescribed urinary analgesic.	A urinary analgesic, such as oral phenazopyridine, may relieve the discomfort caused by severe dysuria.
Assist the patient with perineal hygiene, especially after using a bedpan or after a bowel movement; if fecal incontinence is present, in cleaning from front to back.	Proper perineal hygiene reduces risk of UTI from fecal and vaginal contaminants.
Encourage the patient to void every 3 to 4 hours.	Frequent voiding reduces urinary stasis, which increases risk of UTI.
Avoid unnecessary catheterization and remove indwelling catheters as soon as possible.	Avoiding unnecessary catheterization and early removal of indwelling catheters are the most effective means for reducing catheter-associated UTIs.
Encourage the patient to avoid caffeine, alcohol, citrus juices, chocolate, and highly spiced foods or beverages.	Caffeine, alcohol, citrus juices, chocolate, and highly spiced foods or beverages are potential bladder irritants.
Apply local heat to the suprapubic area or lower back by using a heating pad, taking a warm shower, or sitting in a tub of warm water filled above the waist.	Application of local heat to the suprapubic area or lower back may temporarily relieve the discomfort associated with a UTI.
Women's Health	
Avoid the use of harsh or scented soaps, perineal washes and sprays, and tight clothing.	The patient should avoid actions that disturb the balance of normal flora, which allows the overgrowth of bacteria that can cause UTIs.

COLLABORATION	RATIONALE
CARE COORDINATION: Social work	The social worker can explore resources that may be available to help the patient with an infection to obtain access to appropriate health care.
NUTRITION: Dietitian	Collaborating with a dietitian offers the patient further information and support for implementing the prescribed diet.
GAS EXCHANGE: Respiratory therapy	Respiratory therapists assess, plan, and implement interventions that address potential problems to promote optimal respiratory function.

 PATIENT AND CAREGIVER TEACHING

- Reason the patient developed the infection if known
- Manifestations of infection and signs of improvement
- Diagnostic and laboratory tests used to detect infection
- Measures used to manage the infection
- Hand hygiene techniques
- Safe use of medications, including side-effect management, and how they fit into the overall management plan
- How to monitor temperature
- Measures to reduce the risk of recurrent infection
- When to notify the HCP

DOCUMENTATION

Assessment

- Assessments performed
- Diagnostic and laboratory test results
- Manifestations of infection

Interventions

- Discussions with other interprofessional team members
- Medications given
- Notification of HCP about patient status
- Therapeutic interventions and the patient's response
- Teaching provided
- Referrals initiated
- Transmission-based precautions implemented

Evaluation

- Patient's status: improved, stable, declined
- Presence of manifestations of infection
- Response to teaching provided
- Response to therapeutic interventions

Risk for Infection 39

Definition

Increased risk for a disease caused by the invasion of the body by pathogenic microorganisms

We are constantly exposed to microorganisms. Although many do not pose a health threat, some cause human disease. These are known as *pathogens*. Pathogens are found in the form of bacteria, viruses, parasites, or fungi. Pathogens are routinely found on the skin; on the mucous membranes; in the linings of the respiratory, gastrointestinal, and urinary tracts; and in the mouth and eyes. Typically, a person's immune system can protect the body against pathogens, thus preventing the development of infection.

Many factors increase a person's susceptibility to developing an infection. Preventive actions aimed at decreasing infection risk by increasing the patient's defense mechanisms can be incorporated into the plan of care. Basic care includes recommended immunizations; adequate nutrition, rest, activity, and hydration; and personal hygiene. Older people are more susceptible to infections (e.g., pneumonia) from pathogens that they were relatively immunocompetent against at an earlier age. Their antibody response to immunizations (e.g., flu vaccine) is lower.

A person's beliefs influence infection prevention. For example, isolating a patient to prevent spread of infection is considered disrespectful and uncaring in some cultures. Some people believe that specific foods help the body to fight infection and retain balance. Even though specific vaccinations are recommended, personal beliefs influence whether or not a person chooses to be vaccinated.

Nurses play a key role in reducing the risk of infection by prioritizing infection control practices. Astute assessment and monitoring are part of preventing many infections. Nurses must be able to identify factors that place the patient at risk for infection and create a safe environment that addresses those risks. Provide education aimed at reducing infection risk to patients and caregivers. Ensure that patients and families understand the reason for infection control measures.

Associated Clinical Problems

- Risk for Cross-Infection: increased risk for the transmission of an infection from one person to another with different pathogens in the same environment
- Risk for Eye Infection: increased risk for an infection in the eye
- Risk for Oral Mucosa Infection: increased risk for an infection of the oral mucous membranes
- Risk for Surgical Site Infection: increased risk for an infection at the surgical site

Common Risk Factors

- Age
- Autoimmune disease
- Being without housing
- Burns
- Cancer
- Chronic kidney disease
- Chronic obstructive pulmonary disease (COPD)
- Crowded or unsanitary living conditions
- Debilitation
- Diabetes
- High-risk sexual behavior
- Impaired immune function
- Impaired nutrition
- Inadequate vaccination
- Indwelling urinary catheter
- Intubation and mechanical ventilation
- Invasive lines
- Intravenous (IV) drug use
- Lack of preventive health care
- Liver disease
- Low socioeconomic status
- Medications: antimicrobials, biologic response modifiers, chemotherapy, corticosteroids
- Occupation
- Poor hand hygiene
- Radiation therapy
- Recent surgery
- Recent travel, particularly outside the United States or to an underdeveloped area
- Recurrent infections
- Sickle cell anemia
- Transplant recipient
- Trauma (physical or emotional)

Pediatric
- Low birth weight
- Prematurity
- Prolonged rupture of membranes
- Maternal infection

Eye Infection
- Allergies
- Contact lens wear
- Eye surgery
- Inability to close eyes
- Ocular trauma

Pediatric
- Maternal sexually transmitted infection, including gonorrhea or chlamydia

Oral Mucosa Infection
- Alcohol use
- Decreased salivation
- Ineffective oral hygiene
- Mechanical factors, including braces and dentures
- Mouth breathing
- NPO status
- O_2 therapy
- Periodontal disease
- Tobacco use

Pediatric
- Cleft lip or palate

Surgical Site Infection
- Duration of the surgery
- Improper site preparation
- Length of preoperative hospital stay
- Number of types of pathogens in a wound
- Surgical technique
- Type of surgery

Key Conceptual Relationships

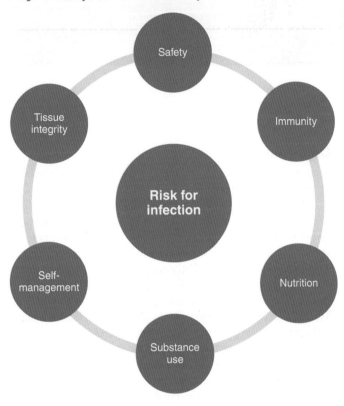

ASSESSMENT OF INFECTION RISK	RATIONALE
Assess risk factors that increase the patient's risk for infection.	A thorough history can identify patients at risk for infection.
IMMUNITY: Assess risk factors that influence the patient's immune response.	A thorough history can identify patients at risk for immune compromise.
Obtain a complete vaccination history.	The vaccine history helps to identify protective immune responses and risk factors for infection.
Evaluate the patient's underlying health status.	Health status has a significant influence on the patient's risk for infection.
Perform a complete physical assessment and monitor indicators of potential infection on an ongoing basis:	
• Manifestations of infection	Identifying an infection allows for early intervention.
• Vital signs	Changes in vital signs are an important indicator of infection.
• White blood cell (WBC) count with differential	Evaluation of the WBC count and differential can confirm an infection.
• Glucose and hemoglobin A1c	Hyperglycemia increases the risk of infection.
• Lactate levels	An increased lactate can result from impaired tissue oxygenation associated with infection.
Obtain culture specimens (e.g., sputum, throat, blood, lesions, wounds, urine, feces) as ordered.	Cultures determine whether a pathogen is present and guide treatment.

ASSESSMENT OF INFECTION RISK	RATIONALE
Review the results of specific diagnostic tests related to the potential source of infection, such as chest radiographs, lumbar punctures, and CT scans.	Specific diagnostic tests are done to detect the source of infection.
SUBSTANCE USE: Screen tobacco and/or other substance use problems.	Smoking and tobacco use cause oral irritation and increase the risk of general infection.
STRESS AND COPING: Assess the current and past use of stress management and coping strategies.	Stress makes the body more vulnerable to invasion by pathogens by depressing the immune system.
NUTRITION: Obtain a diet history, including usual daily caloric intake, diet choices, and use of nutrition support.	Proper nutrition supports immune system function and reduces the risk of infection.
Evaluate the effectiveness of measures used to reduce infection risk through ongoing assessment.	Identifying an infection allows for the early initiation of treatment.

Expected Outcomes

The patient will:

- be free from infection.
- adhere to the prescribed therapeutic regimen.
- identify infection risks and implement measures to reduce risk.
- report signs and symptoms of infection and follow screening procedures.

INTERVENTIONS TO REDUCE RISK OF INFECTION	RATIONALE
Implement collaborative interventions addressed at treating underlying risk factors for infection.	Treatment of underlying risk factors can reduce the risk of the patient developing an infection.
Notify the health care provider (HCP) if manifestations of infection are present.	Identifying an infection allows for early intervention.
Administer prescribed prophylactic antimicrobial medications.	Prophylactic antimicrobial medications can reduce the risk of the patient developing an infection.
SELF-MANAGEMENT: Administer needed vaccinations according to recommended schedules and patient needs.	Vaccinations are given to prevent common infections, such as pneumococcus.
Implement strict hand hygiene by the patient and all who have contact with them.	Hand hygiene is an important preventive measure and should be done before, during, and after patient contact.
Use sterile technique when performing invasive procedures.	Using sterile technique protects the patient from potential sources of pathogens and infection.
Maintain closed catheter systems, such as those used for hemodynamic monitoring, chest tubes, urinary catheters, and IV infusions, whenever possible.	Each time a system is opened, pathogens from the environment can enter the body, increasing risk for infection.
IMMUNITY: Implement neutropenic precautions, if needed.	Neutropenic precautions protect the patient from potential sources of pathogens and infection.
Ensure the patient is bathing daily.	Daily bathing protects the patient from potential sources of skin pathogens.
NUTRITION: Provide a nutritionally adequate diet.	Proper nutrition supports immune system function and reduces the risk of infection.
Maintain sufficient fluid intake, unless contraindicated.	Dehydration and dry mucous membranes increase risk of infection.
SLEEP: Provide the patient with opportunities for adequate sleep.	Adequate rest provides the body with the energy needed for optimal functioning of the immune system.
GLUCOSE REGULATION: Maintain glucose control for patients with diabetes.	Hyperglycemia increases risk of infection.
STRESS AND COPING: Encourage the use of positive coping and stress management strategies.	Stress makes the body more vulnerable to invasion by pathogens by depressing the immune system.

INTERVENTIONS TO REDUCE THE RISK OF EYE INFECTION	RATIONALE
Administer prescribed medications, such as eye drops, ointments, and artificial tears.	Prolonged dry eyes can cause an eye infection.
Encourage the patient to avoid eye irritants, including smoke, pollutants, hair spray, and air blowing in the eyes.	Eye irritation increases risk of an eye infection.

INTERVENTIONS TO REDUCE THE RISK OF ORAL MUCOSA INFECTION	RATIONALE
Have the patient avoid irritating food and fluids, such as highly spiced food or items with temperature extremes.	The intake of irritating foods and fluids increases risk of oral mucous membrane problems.
Provide oral care at least every 4 hours while the patient is awake.	Proper oral hygiene reduces risk of oral infections and periodontitis.
Provide frequent lip lubrication.	Keeping the lips moist helps prevent drying and cracking, which decreases infection risk.
SUBSTANCE USE: Promote smoking and tobacco cessation interventions.	Smoking and tobacco use cause oral irritation and increase risk of infection.

INTERVENTIONS TO REDUCE THE RISK OF SURGICAL SITE INFECTION	RATIONALE
TISSUE INTEGRITY: Provide wound care as ordered, using aseptic technique.	Using sterile technique protects the wound from potential sources of pathogens and infection.

COLLABORATION	RATIONALE
Dental care	Dentists perform periodic deep cleaning and recommend care to reduce risk of oral infection.
NUTRITION: Dietitian	Collaborating with a dietitian offers the patient further information and support for implementing the prescribed diet.
Pediatric	
School counselor, school social worker, or school psychologist	Collaboration with school officials can help ensure that the child receives an education equal to other students in a safe environment.

PATIENT AND CAREGIVER TEACHING

- Reason the patient is at risk for infection
- Management of conditions increasing infection risk
- Diagnostic and laboratory tests used to detect infection
- Hand hygiene
- Infection risks in everyday situations
- Measures to reduce the risk of exposure to pathogens
- Transmission-based precautions
- How to monitor temperature
- Signs and symptoms of infection
- Safe use of medications
- Recommended screenings and immunizations
- When to notify the HCP

 **DOCUMENTATION**

Assessment

- Assessments performed
- Diagnostic and laboratory test results
- Manifestations of infection

Interventions

- Discussions with other interprofessional team members
- Medications given
- Notification of the HCP about patient status
- Therapeutic interventions and the patient's response
- Teaching provided
- Referrals initiated
- Transmission-based precautions implemented

Evaluation

- Patient's status: occurrence of infection
- Presence of manifestations of infection
- Response to teaching provided
- Response to therapeutic interventions

Inflammation 40

Definition

Physiologic response to tissue injury or infection

Inflammation is the body's normal physiologic response to injury or illness. It occurs in all patients who have sustained any type of tissue trauma. Acute inflammation is the immediate response to tissue injury. It is short in duration. Inflammation that continues for weeks to years after the initial injury is termed chronic. The response to inflammation is the same regardless of the cause, and the manifestations are relatively consistent. The degree of inflammation depends on the severity and scope of the injury and the person's physiologic capacity. Risk factors include having an autoimmune disease and allergies, having a compromised immune system, exposure to pathogens with or without resultant infection, and being very young or old.

Many of the processes associated with inflammation also occur with infection. The pathologic processes may overlap, or one can trigger another. Inflammation is always present with infection but may occur in the absence of infection. Tissue integrity may be impaired. Pain, impaired mobility, and problems regulating temperature and fluid and electrolyte balance are common. Fatigue and stress are often present with acute inflammation or may be prolonged during chronic inflammation.

The nursing care of the patient with acute inflammation is directed at mediating the inflammatory process to promote tissue healing. Most treatment depends on the cause. Interventions for those with chronic inflammation are aimed at preventing or slowing tissue damage. Nurses play a key role in helping patients manage the symptoms that accompany inflammation, including pain, impaired mobility, and fatigue.

Common Causes

Acute

- Allergic reaction
- Anaphylaxis
- Appendicitis
- Bronchitis
- Burn injury
- Cholecystitis
- Electrical or chemical injury
- Foreign body injury
- Infections (viral, bacterial, parasitic, fungal)
- Insect bite or sting
- Joint strain or sprain
- Mechanical trauma (laceration, crush injury)
- Nephritis
- Radiation damage
- Septic shock
- Trauma

Chronic

- Asthma
- Cirrhosis
- Chronic obstructive pulmonary disease (COPD)
- Diverticulitis
- Fibromyalgia
- Inflammatory bowel disease
- Multiple sclerosis
- Myasthenia gravis
- Osteoarthritis
- Psoriasis
- Rheumatoid arthritis
- Systemic lupus erythematosus
- Tuberculosis

Manifestations

Local

- Edema
- Exudate
- Loss of function
- Pain
- Redness
- Warmth

Systemic

- Anorexia
- Enlarged lymph nodes
- Fatigue
- Fever
- Malaise
- Nausea
- Increased pulse
- Increased respiratory rate
- Laboratory tests: ↑ white blood cell (WBC) count with a shift to the left, ↑ inflammatory markers

Key Conceptual Relationships

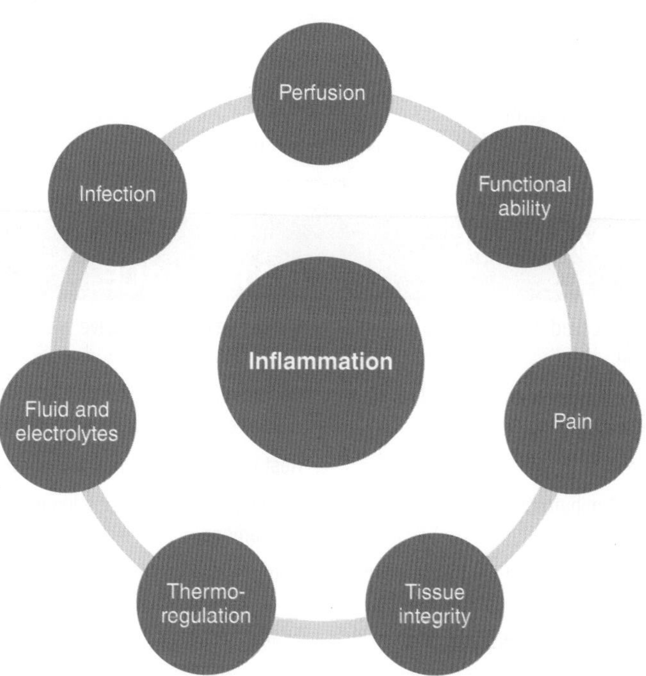

ASSESSMENT OF INFLAMMATION	RATIONALE
Assess for the potential cause of inflammation.	Identifying the cause of inflammation allows for early intervention.
Assess risk factors that may limit the patient's physiologic ability to respond to inflammation.	A decreased ability to respond to inflammation increases risk of an ineffective inflammatory response.
Determine the duration of the inflammatory process and the treatment measures that have already been initiated.	Knowing the disease trajectory guides treatment.
Perform a complete physical assessment and monitor indicators of inflammation on an ongoing basis:	
• Manifestations of inflammation	The manifestations of inflammation vary according to the cause and body area involved.
• Systemic symptoms associated with inflammation, such as anorexia, nausea, and fatigue	Systemic manifestations are related to increased levels of inflammatory markers.
• Vital signs	Changes in vital signs are often present with inflammation, especially when there is an infection.
• WBC count with differential	Because of the demand for neutrophils at the site of inflammation, the bone marrow releases more neutrophils, resulting in high WBC and neutrophil counts.
• C-reactive protein (CRP) and erythrocyte sedimentation rate (ESR)	Measures of inflammatory markers are usually increased with general inflammation.
FUNCTIONAL ABILITY: Assess for lifestyle effects of inflammation, such as the ability to interact with others, perform work and household duties, and engage in physical and social activities.	Chronic inflammation and resulting pain, fatigue, and limited mobility can affect the ability to participate in activities of daily living.
Evaluate the effectiveness of measures used to control inflammation through ongoing assessment.	Ongoing monitoring allows for evaluation of therapy effectiveness.

Expected Outcomes

The patient will:

- be free from complications of inflammation.
- be free from manifestations of inflammation.
- adhere to the prescribed therapeutic regimen.
- maintain role performance and take part in desired activities of daily living.

INTERVENTIONS TO MANAGE INFLAMMATION	RATIONALE
Implement collaborative interventions addressed at treating the underlying cause of the inflammation.	Inflammation may resolve with treatment of the underlying cause.
Implement protection, rest, ice, compression, and elevation (PRICE) measures within the first 24–48 hours after injury.	By minimizing swelling, the injured tissue and surrounding tissue are protected from additional damage.
• Protect and rest the injured area.	Rest helps the body use its nutrients for the healing process.
• Put ice on a sprain or strain for 20 minutes at a time every 2 or 3 hours.	Leaving ice in place for a longer period may cause additional tissue damage.
• Apply the compression wrap snugly but not so tight as to impede circulation.	Compression of the affected area helps to minimize swelling.
• Whenever possible, elevate the injured area above the level of the heart.	Elevation is useful in minimizing swelling.
Apply appropriate immobilization devices, such as splints or slings.	Stabilization limits movement of the injured area, helping to ease strain and tension in that area and thus decreasing pain.
Encourage the use of needed mobility aids, such as wheelchairs, walkers, or crutches.	Mobility aids minimize weight bearing to an injured extremity.
Apply heat after 24–48 hours for 20 minutes at a time every 2 or 3 hours.	Heat promotes healing by increasing circulation and removal of debris from the inflamed site.
PERFUSION: Implement venous thromboembolism (VTE) prophylaxis measures for the patient on bed rest.	VTE prophylaxis measures protect against thrombus formation.
TISSUE INTEGRITY: Keep edematous skin moisturized.	Moisturizers help create a protective layer over the skin, reducing the risk of injury and water loss.
Administer prescribed medications, including:	
• Corticosteroids	Corticosteroids reduce the swelling and pain that accompany inflammation by suppressing the immune system.
• Nonsteroidal antiinflammatory drugs (NSAIDs)	NSAIDs are important in the management of pain, fever, and inflammation by suppressing the inflammatory response.
• **PAIN:** Analgesics	Analgesics relieve pain caused by inflammation.
• **INFECTION:** Antimicrobials	Appropriate antimicrobial therapy treats an underlying infection that caused inflammation.
THERMOREGULATION: Implement measures to manage a fever.	Managing fever can increase the patient's comfort level.
NUTRITION: Provide a nutritionally adequate diet that is high in calories.	A high-calorie, nutritionally adequate diet provides the body with the necessary factors to promote healing.
FLUID AND ELECTROLYTES: Encourage increased oral fluid intake.	A high fluid intake will replace fluid loss from perspiration and fever.
Notify the health care provider (HCP) if manifestations of inflammation persist or worsen.	Achieving an effective treatment plan often requires adjustments in therapy.
STRESS AND COPING: Help the patient and caregivers cope with chronic inflammation by encouraging the use of positive coping behaviors.	Using positive coping behaviors will help the patient and caregiver manage the stress.
FATIGUE: Assist the patient with prioritizing activities and encourage them to alternate rest and activity periods.	Limiting activities conserves energy and helps prevent fatigue.
FUNCTIONAL ABILITY: Help the patient develop strategies to help them participate in activities of daily living in the home, at work, and socially.	Making activities of daily living easier will help patients cope with chronic inflammation and improve functional ability.

COLLABORATION	RATIONALE
CARE COORDINATION: Social work	The social worker can explore resources to help the patient obtain access to health care.
MOBILITY: Physical therapy	Physical therapists assess, plan, and implement interventions that address musculoskeletal problems.

PATIENT AND CAREGIVER TEACHING

- Cause of the inflammation, if known, and how long it may last
- Factors contributing to inflammation
- Manifestations of inflammation
- Management of conditions causing inflammation
- Measures being used to treat inflammation
- Safe use of medication
- Factors that increase inflammation and how to manage them
- Ways to prevent further injury
- When to notify the HCP

DOCUMENTATION

Assessment

- Assessments performed
- Diagnostic and laboratory test results
- Manifestations of inflammation

Interventions

- Discussions with other interprofessional team members
- Medications given
- Notification of the HCP about patient status
- Therapeutic interventions and the patient's response
- Teaching provided
- Referrals initiated
- VTE precautions implemented

Evaluation

- Patient's status: improved, stable, decline
- Presence of manifestations of inflammation
- Response to teaching provided
- Response to therapeutic interventions

Mobility

Activity Intolerance 41

Definition

Inadequate energy to complete daily activities or desired activities

The terms *activity intolerant* and *activity deconditioned* describe a lack or loss of physical fitness, such as may happen in patients with extended immobility or bed rest. The consequences of immobility include serious changes, such as decreased cardiac output, venous stasis, atelectasis, joint contracture, skin breakdown, constipation, urinary stasis, and infection.

Nurses have a role in helping patients improve their activity tolerance and prevent the negative effects of general immobility.

Associated Clinical Problem

- Risk for Activity Intolerance: increased risk for inadequate energy to complete daily or desired activities

Common Causes

- Anemia
- Cancer and cancer treatment
- Cardiopulmonary disease
- Chronic kidney disease
- General weakness
- Imbalance between oxygen supply/demand
- Impaired mobility or immobility
- Liver problems, such as hepatitis and cirrhosis
- Malnutrition
- Obesity
- Pain
- Prolonged bed rest
- Sedentary lifestyle

Manifestations

- Abnormal vital sign changes in response to activity
- Excessive decrease in oxygen saturation in response to activity
- Electrocardiogram (ECG) changes in response to activity
- Exertional discomfort or dyspnea
- Fatigue
- Impaired ability to perform activities of daily living (ADLs)
- Muscle weakness
- Diagnostic tests: stress testing may indicate myocardial ischemia in response to activity.

Key Conceptual Relationships

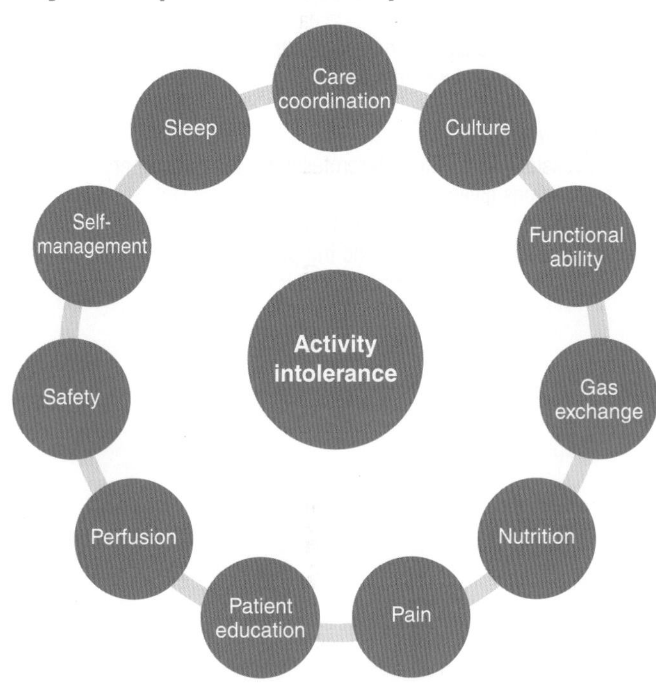

ASSESSMENT OF ACTIVITY TOLERANCE	RATIONALE
Assess for risk factors that may contribute to activity intolerance.	Identify factors that place the patient at risk for activity intolerance to allow for early intervention.
Assess for possible causes of activity intolerance.	Physical and psychologic factors, including medications and underlying health status, may affect energy level.
Perform a physical assessment and obtain diagnostic tests based on the patient's history, including:	
• **PAIN:** Comprehensive pain assessment	Experiencing pain negatively affects activity tolerance.
• Ability to progressively dangle, sit, and walk as allowed by condition	Assessment is needed to determine a safe level of activity and the need for assistance.
• Gait and musculoskeletal function	Physical mobility has a significant impact on the ability to perform role responsibilities independently.
• **GAS EXCHANGE:** Presence of dyspnea at rest or with exertion	Measures to address impaired respiratory function may be needed to enhance activity tolerance.
• **TISSUE PERFUSION:** Vital signs, comparing at rest with activity	Changes in heart rate, blood pressure, and respiratory rate characterize the presence of activity intolerance.
Assess readiness for activity after illness or surgery.	Physiologic stability is needed for upright posture.
SAFETY: Assess for fall risk.	Impaired mobility may increase the risk of falls.
FUNCTIONAL ABILITY: Assess the impact of activity intolerance on daily life, including the ability to perform work and household duties and engage in physical, mental, and social activities.	The severity and frequency of activity intolerance influence the patient's functional ability.
Evaluate the effectiveness of measures used to address activity tolerance through ongoing assessment.	Reviewing the effectiveness of interventions allows for evaluation and adjustment of therapy.

Expected Outcomes

The patient will:

- demonstrate increased tolerance for activity.
- participate in physical activity with heart rate, blood pressure, and breathing rate within normal exercise limits.
- implement strategies to enhance activity tolerance.
- take part in desired ADLs.

INTERVENTIONS FOR PROMOTING ACTIVITY TOLERANCE	RATIONALE
PERFUSION: Implement collaborative interventions aimed at treating factors contributing to activity intolerance.	Activity intolerance may improve or resolve with treatment of an underlying contributing factor.
Notify the health care provider (HCP) if manifestations of activity intolerance persist or worsen.	Achievement of an effective treatment plan often requires adjustments in therapy.
Encourage the person to share their feelings about experiencing activity intolerance.	The patient needs to know you consider the activity intolerance significant and you understand that it may profoundly disrupt a person's life.
Assist the patient in identifying personal strengths and abilities.	Identifying personal strengths will help the patient integrate those strengths into enhancing activity tolerance.
Set mutual goals to increase daily activity levels.	Encourage patient participation in planning activity.
SELF-MANAGEMENT: Provide encouragement and reinforcement for activity efforts.	A supportive relationship may improve the patient's motivation to continue activities.
Minimize cardiovascular deconditioning by positioning patient who is on bed rest in an upright position several times daily if possible.	Position changes help maintain orthostatic tolerance.
For the patient who is not yet able to ambulate, provide active, active assisted, or passive range of motion several times a day.	Range-of-motion exercises prevent contractures and stiffness while building strength to support eventual ambulation.

Continued

INTERVENTIONS FOR PROMOTING ACTIVITY TOLERANCE	RATIONALE
PERFUSION: While assisting with activity, observe for nausea, pallor, dizziness, confusion, and changes in vital signs.	Postural hypotension may occur after a period of bed rest or with hypovolemia.
Return the patient to the bed or chair if symptoms of hypotension do not resolve rapidly.	Returning the patient to the bed or chair can prevent possible fall and injury.
Monitor cardiovascular response to activity and stop activity for excessive tachycardia, bradycardia, dysrhythmias, or chest pain.	Activity may cause excessive myocardial oxygen consumption.
GAS EXCHANGE: Implement measures to address impaired respiratory function, if present.	Activity intolerance may be related to the presence of impaired respiratory function.
Set up portable oxygen or a long extension tubing for patients who need continuous oxygen when ambulating and ensure the patient can manage the tubing safely while ambulating.	Oxygen needs increase during exercise. However, managing the oxygen tubing may restrict motion.
Assist the patient with obtaining and learning to use any assistive devices, including canes and walkers.	Many assistive devices are available to assist the patient in accommodating for activity intolerance.
SAFETY: Encourage caregivers to use the right assistive devices and proper techniques to lift, move, transfer, and reposition the patient.	Using proper assistive devices reduces the risk of injury to the patient or caregivers.
Allow the patient who is fatigued extra time to carry out physical activities.	Allowing extra time can maintain patient independence and avoid frustration.
Encourage more frequent, short periods of activity rather than an extensive, exhausting effort.	Allow for cardiovascular recovery between activities.
SELF-MANAGEMENT: For those with extremely limited activity tolerance, help prioritize activities for the day.	Assistance with or modification of some activities may allow for completing other desired activities.
FUNCTIONAL ABILITY: Help the patient with ADLs, as needed.	Activity intolerance can interfere with the ability to complete ADLs.
SAFETY: Implement fall risk precautions if needed, including: • Wearing nonskid shoes • Maintaining clear paths • Having adequate lighting • Orienting the patient to the environment • Keeping the call light and personal possessions within reach • Keeping floors clean and dry • Having the patient call for assistance before getting out of bed	Fall precautions represent the best method of reducing the risk of injury.
NUTRITION: Provide a nutritionally adequate diet.	People with impaired nutritional status are at risk of activity intolerance as a result of inadequate energy sources.
PAIN: Implement measures to address pain, if applicable.	There is a strong association between activity intolerance and pain; reducing pain may improve activity tolerance.
CULTURE AND DEVELOPMENT: Institute measures to reduce any social isolation the patient may be experiencing.	Reduced activity tolerance may lead to social isolation. Social support may enhance motivation for activity.
SLEEP: Encourage the patient to get adequate sleep and implement measures to address impaired sleep, if present.	Activity intolerance may worsen after inadequate sleep.

COLLABORATION	RATIONALE
Physical therapy	Physical therapists assess, plan, and implement interventions that promote activity tolerance.
Occupational therapy	Occupational therapists can assist with devices and strategies to increase independence.
PERFUSION: Cardiac rehabilitation, pulmonary rehabilitation	Rehabilitation programs provide specialized support for patients with cardiac or pulmonary conditions in improving activity tolerance.
NUTRITION: Dietitian	Malnutrition causes significant morbidity as a result of the loss of lean body mass.
CARE COORDINATION: Social work or case management	A social worker or case manager can help the patient and caregiver identify community resources to assist with fulfilling role responsibilities and ADLs.
DEVELOPMENT: Child life specialist	A specialist can assist with support for play during restricted mobility or when the child has minimal energy.

PATIENT AND CAREGIVER TEACHING

- Progression of activity
- Cause of activity intolerance, if known
- Manifestations of activity intolerance
- Management of any underlying condition causing activity intolerance
- Measures to improve activity tolerance
- Measures to reduce the risk of complications
- Importance of taking medications as prescribed
- Anticipatory guidance regarding difficult situations
- Importance of proper nutrition, adequate sleep
- Role of physical therapy
- Safety modifications in the living environment
- Community and self-help resources available
- Safe use of adaptive devices
- When to notify the HCP

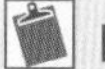

DOCUMENTATION

Assessment
- Assessment findings
- Tolerance for activity
- Diagnostic test results

Interventions
- Discussions with other members of the interprofessional team
- Environment modifications made
- Medications given
- Therapeutic interventions and the patient's response
- Referrals initiated
- Safety measures implemented, including fall precautions
- Support and assistive devices and personnel required for activity
- Notification of the HCP about diagnostic test results and assessment findings
- Teaching provided

Evaluation
- Patient's status: improved, stable, declined
- Diagnostic test results
- Patient's response to therapeutic interventions
- Presence of any manifestations of activity intolerance
- Patient's response to teaching

Musculoskeletal Problem 42

Definition

Impaired ability to move one or more extremities

The musculoskeletal system is composed of voluntary muscle and six types of connective tissue: bone, cartilage, ligaments, tendons, fascia, and bursae. The purpose of the musculoskeletal system is to protect body organs, provide support and stability for the body, store minerals, and allow coordinated movement. *Mobility* refers to purposeful physical movement. Large muscle movements, fine motor movements, and coordinated movements depend on the synchronized efforts of the musculoskeletal and nervous systems. Being mobile requires energy, muscle strength, skeletal stability, joint function, and neuromuscular coordination.

Mobility may affect the function of individual joints or groups of joints, such as when an older adult experiences limitation of joint movement and discomfort with joint movement. Many functional problems experienced by an older adult are related to musculoskeletal problems. Changes may affect the older adult's ability to complete self-care tasks and pursue other usual activities. Effects of musculoskeletal changes may range from mild discomfort and decreased ability to perform activities of daily living (ADLs) to severe, chronic pain and immobility.

At times, immobilization is intended as a therapeutic measure. For example, the temporary immobilization of a joint with a brace may be required for recovery after injury or surgery. Nurses have a role in helping patients manage immobilization devices and prevent the negative effects of general immobility. Patient and caregiver teaching are important nursing responsibilities when the patient has a musculoskeletal problem.

Associated Clinical Problems

- Bedridden: unable to move out of a reclining position or ambulate
- Decreased Muscle Tone: abnormally limp muscles with decreased resistance to passive movement
- Difficulty Balancing: impaired ability to maintain posture
- Disuse Syndrome: physical and psychosocial effects of inactivity that result in muscle weakness, restricted joint range of motion, reduced respiratory function, altered blood flow in the peripheral tissue, reduced bone density, and diminished mental function
- Hypertonicity: abnormally increased muscle tension
- Impaired Active Range of Motion: limited ability or strength to move a joint independently through its entire cycle of movement
- Impaired Balance: inadequate ability to maintain posture safely
- Impaired Bed Mobility: impaired ability to perform specific motions while in bed, such as turning side to side
- Impaired Mobility: limited ability to ambulate or otherwise reposition
- Impaired Sitting: impaired ability to be seated
- Impaired Standing: impaired ability to be in a fully upright position
- Impaired Transfer Ability: impaired ability to move to and from a bed, chair/wheelchair, and toilet
- Impaired Walking: impaired ability to ambulate upright with feet on the ground
- Impaired Wheelchair Mobility: difficulty managing a wheelchair around curbs, soft surfaces, and obstacles
- Limitation of Joint Movement: inability to demonstrate a full range of motion
- Muscle Weakness: inadequate strength of muscle movement
- Paralysis: inability to move one or more muscles
- Poor Muscle Tone: abnormally limp muscles with decreased resistance to passive movement
- Risk for Disuse Syndrome: increased risk for physical and psychosocial effects of inactivity
- Tremor: involuntary muscle quivering

Common Causes and Risk Factors

- Amputation
- Arthritic conditions, including gout, osteoarthritis, and rheumatoid arthritis
- Cerebral palsy
- Congenital disorders
- Deconditioning
- Degenerative neuromuscular conditions, including amyotrophic lateral sclerosis, Huntington disease, multiple sclerosis, muscular dystrophy, Parkinson disease
- Disuse atrophy
- Fibromyalgia
- Guillain–Barré syndrome
- Injury: fracture, joint dislocation, sprain, tendonitis
- Low back pain or herniated disk
- Malnutrition

- Metabolic bone disease, including osteomalacia, osteoporosis, Paget disease
- Myasthenia gravis
- Myositis
- Myotonia
- Obesity
- Orthopedic surgery
- Prolonged use of immobilization devices such as casts and braces
- Scoliosis
- Spinal cord injury
- Spinal stenosis
- Systemic lupus erythematosus

Manifestations

- Absence of full range of joint motion
- Altered gait
- Contractures
- Cramping
- Crepitation
- Inability to initiate muscle movement
- Joint swelling
- Muscle atrophy or weakness
- Muscle tremor
- Pain limiting movement
- Paresthesia
- Spastic movement
- Stiffness
- Uncoordinated movement
- Unstable posture
- Abnormal laboratory tests, including antinuclear antibodies (ANAs), sedimentation rate, anti-DNA antibody, and C-reactive protein
- Diagnostic tests: radiography and other imaging may reveal fractures and soft tissue damage

Key Conceptual Relationships

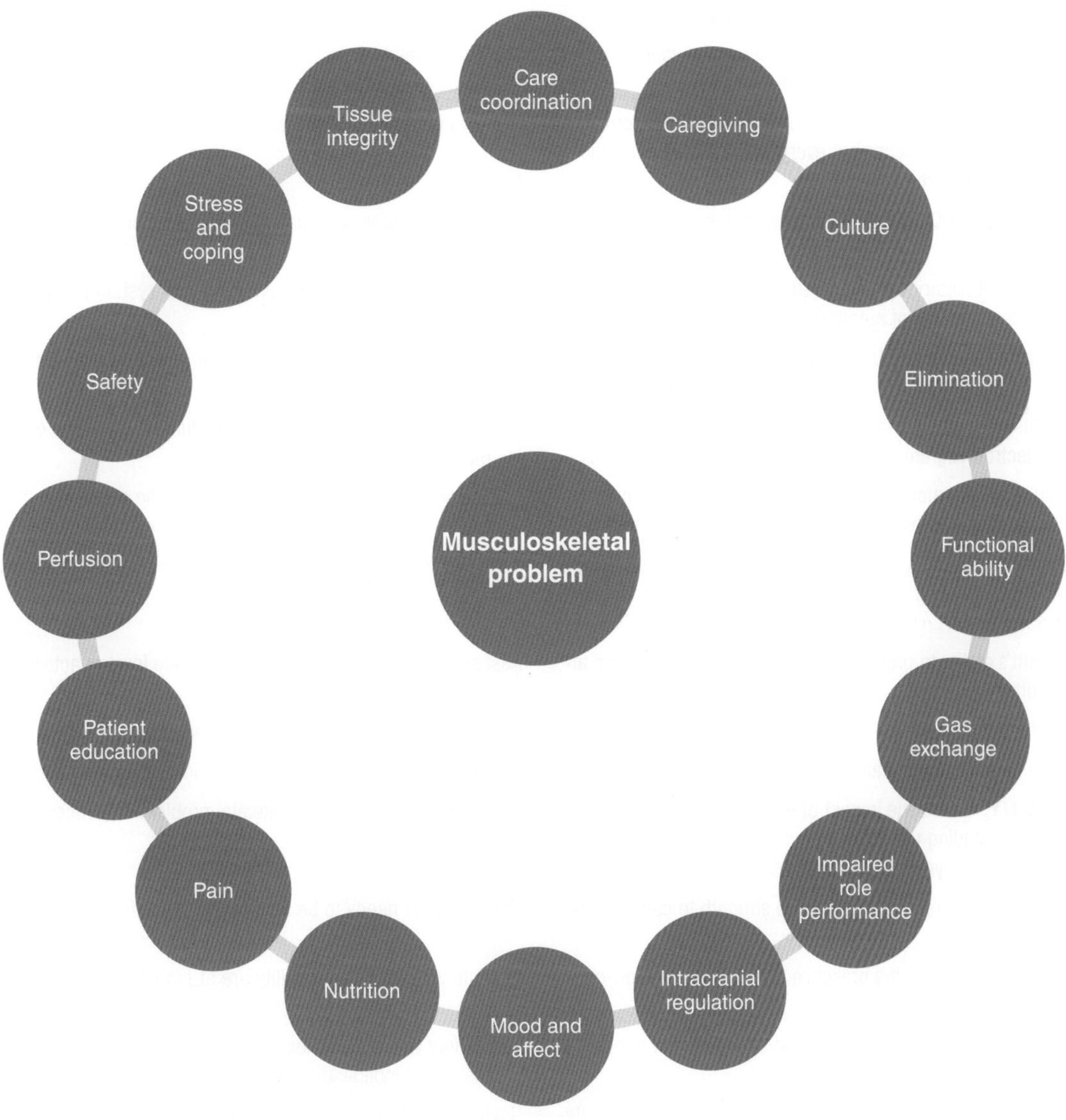

ASSESSMENT OF MUSCULOSKELETAL FUNCTION	RATIONALE
Assess for common causes and risk factors that may contribute to a musculoskeletal problem.	Identifying factors that place the patient at risk for a musculoskeletal problem allows for early intervention.
Record history of traumatic injuries, including: • Mechanism and circumstances of the injury, such as crush or stretch • Methods and duration of treatment • Current abilities and progress related to the injury • Any need for assistive devices and ongoing rehabilitation • Interference with ADLs	Trauma to the musculoskeletal system is a common reason for seeking care and can have a long-lasting impact on the patient's function.
Perform a physical assessment and obtain diagnostic tests based on the patient's history, including:	
• **PAIN:** Comprehensive pain assessment	Pain accompanies many musculoskeletal problems and may restrict movement.
• Gait and musculoskeletal function, including: • General posture and body build • Muscle size, symmetry, strength, and tone • Joint symmetry, contour, and range of motion • Limb length and other skeletal abnormalities	Assessment is needed to determine the presence and degree of a musculoskeletal problem.
• **PERFUSION:** Circulation, including pulse, sensation, color, capillary refill, and temperature, in an injured body part	Musculoskeletal trauma may cause nerve or vascular damage, with diminished perfusion causing further damage.
• **TISSUE INTEGRITY:** Skin integrity, using a standard tool, on admission and with reassessment every shift in acute care and every visit in home care	Identifying impaired tissue allows for rapid treatment.
• **INTRACRANIAL REGULATION:** Neurologic status	Changes in neurologic function often cause or accompany a musculoskeletal problem.
• **NUTRITION:** Diet history, including usual daily caloric intake, dietary choices, and use of nutrition support	Proper nutrition supports musculoskeletal system function and bone health.
• **ELIMINATION:** Bladder and bowel function	Incontinence may occur as a result of problems with ambulating to the toilet or with spinal cord injury.
Evaluate the results of diagnostic studies, including imaging studies, arthroscopy, electromyogram (EMG), bone scans, and myelogram.	Diagnostic tests are performed to evaluate for a cause of a musculoskeletal problem.
Evaluate the results of laboratory tests, such as ANAs, sedimentation rate, anti-DNA antibody, C-reactive protein, and rheumatoid factor.	Laboratory tests are useful in diagnosing the cause of a musculoskeletal problem.
Assess the patient's readiness for activity after illness or surgery using a standardized measure such as the Bedside Mobility Assessment Tool (BMAT 2.0); see Fig. 42.1.	Assessment is used to determine physiologic stability and avoid injury.
Evaluate the patient's ability to progressively dangle, sit, and walk as allowed by condition.	Assessment is needed to determine a safe level of activity and the need for assistance.
SAFETY: Assess for fall risk.	Impaired mobility may increase the risk for falls.
Assess the patient daily for appropriateness of activity and bed rest orders.	Prepare to mobilize the patient as soon as they are able.
FUNCTIONAL ABILITY: Assess the impact of the musculoskeletal problem on daily life, including the ability to perform work and household duties and engage in physical, mental, and social activities.	The severity of the musculoskeletal problem influences the patient's functional ability.
CAREGIVING: Assess the caregiver's ability and strength to safely assist with mobility.	The caregiver needs to be able to provide safe, effective care.
MOOD AND AFFECT: Screen for the presence of any coexisting psychologic problems.	Patients with impaired mobility are at high risk for depression.
STRESS AND COPING: Assess the patient's use of coping and stress management strategies.	The patient with a musculoskeletal problem may have difficulty coping with the loss of independence.
Evaluate the effectiveness of measures used to address a musculoskeletal problem through ongoing assessment.	Reviewing the effectiveness of measures to address a musculoskeletal problem allows for adjustment of care plans.

Test/assessment level	Description of test	Pass response	PASS =
Assessment level 1 Assessment of: • Sitting balance • Upper extremity and core strength • Ability to sit upright without getting tachycardic, diaphoretic and/or light-headed; i.e., sitting tolerance	**Sit and Shake:** From semi-reclined position or at EOB, ask patient to sit upright for up to 1 minute (if there is any concern regarding orthostatic hypotension or postural intolerance); then reach across midline and shake hands with caregiver – repeat with other hand. (Patient's feet may either be flat on floor or dangling.) **Safe mode**: Use sling and lift to assist to side of bed (e.g., sternal precautions, abdominal incision) or bed in chair position, then complete "Sit and Shake."	**Sit:** Able to follow commands and sit unsupported (i.e., unsupported by sling or bed surface) for up to 1 minute. **Shake:** Able to maintain seated balance while challenged by reaching across midline of trunk with one or both hands and shaking caregiver's hand.	**Pass** assessment level 1 "Sit and Shake" = **Proceed to assessment Level 2, "Stretch"** **Fail** = **Mobility level 1 patient** *As appropriate, follow critical care early/progressive mobility program protocol to advance through BMAT assessment levels.*
Assessment level 2 Assessment of: • Leg strength in preparation for weight bearing • Control and strength of leg muscles, including quadriceps and lower leg muscles • Foot drop	**Stretch:** While sitting upright unsupported, extend one leg and straighten knee (knee remains below hip level) and point toes/pump ankle between dorsiflexion/plantar flexion x 3 repetitions. (Patient's feet may either be flat on floor or dangling.) **Safe mode:** Continue to use sling and lift (mobile or overhead/ceiling), bed in fowler's or chair position to complete "Stretch."	**Stretch:** Able to extend leg and straighten knee = engage quadriceps; then able to pump ankle for 3 repetitions = AROM/move ankle between dorsiflexion/plantar flexion = engage calf muscles/skeletal muscle pump and assist with venous return/fluid shifts.	**Pass** assessment level 2 "Stretch" = **Proceed to assessment level 3, "Stand"** **Fail** = **Mobility level 2 patient**
Assessment level 3 Assessment of: • Ability to shift forward, raise buttocks and rise smoothly; balance and strength to rise • Standing tolerance for up to 1 minute, which allows for fluid shifts and other compensatory changes to occur • Static standing balance	**Stand:** With feet flat on floor about shoulder width apart, shift forward, raise buttocks/rise and stand upright for up to 1 minute (if there is any concern regarding orthostatic hypotension, postural intolerance or syncope). **Safe mode:** Use sit-to-stand lift and vest/sling, or ambulation vest/pants and lift. *Always default to using safe mode if concerned regarding orthostatic hypotension/syncopal event or other compensatory changes.*	**Stand:** Able to rise, maintain balance and upright standing position for up to 1 minute. *The majority of patients who exhibit orthostatic hypotension do so within the first minute of standing, which is the rationale for 1 minute.* Use walker, cane, crutches or prosthetic leg(s) as appropriate to assist.	**Pass** assessment level 3 "Stand" = **Proceed to assessment level 4, "step"** **Fail** = **Mobility level 3 patient**
Assessment level 4 Assessment of: • Pre-ambulation weight shift abilities • Further assessment of leg strength • Dynamic standing balance, which further allows for fluid shifts and other compensatory changes to occur • Cognitive ability to follow directions	**Step:** 1) March-or step-in-place taking small steps (not high-marching steps) x 3 repetitions; if able to pass then 2) Step forward with one foot, weight-bear/shift weight onto foot and return foot to starting position; repeat with other foot. **Safe mode:** Use ambulation vest/pants and lift; consider use of bed in chair position and egress from end-of-bed. *Always default to using safe mode if concerned regarding orthostatic hypotension/syncopal event, other compensatory changes or falls.*	**Step:** Able to perform both marching-in-place and forward step and return with one foot and then the other. Use walker, cane, crutches or prosthetic leg(s) as appropriate.	**Pass assessment level 4 "step"** = **Progress through discharge planning** Continue to complete BMAT per protocol; address medical issues and stability; use multidisciplinary approach: Work on discharge goals for best destination/placement; consider functional status, ongoing equipment needs and ADL's **Fail** = **Remain a mobility level 4 patient**

FIG. 42.1 *BMAT 2.0*. Based on Boynton T, Kumpar D, VanGilder C. The Bedside Mobility Assessment Tool 2.0. *American Nurse*. 2020;15.

Patient's BMAT mobility level	Assessment Level					
	1. Sit & Shake*	2. Stretch*	3. Stand*	4. Step*	Test options in safe mode *(See figure A, page one for description of basic test)*	Patient care and strengthening in safe mode SPHM Equipment to consider for patient care/strengthening NOTE: Consult with PT/OT per facility protocol
Mobility Level 1 = Fails/unable to "Sit and Shake" *As appropriate, follow critical care early/progressive mobility program protocol.*	**Fail**	NA	NA	NA	1) Perform with patient sitting upright in bed 2) Using lift and sling help patient sit at Edge of Bed (EOB) *As appropriate, follow critical care early/progressive mobility program protocol to advance through BMAT assessment levels.*	**Goals:** Avoid complications of immobility, engage and strengthen postural muscles and progress to level 2. 1) Edge of Bed (EOB) dangling with sling and lift: Work on sitting balance and reaching across midline; perform calf pump exercises 2) Bed in Fowler's or chair position: Sitting supported or unsupported to cross midline and shake hands; also perform calf pump exercises 3) Lift and repo sheet: For boosting and turning 4) Lift and multistraps: For turning and limb holding 5) Lift and sling: For bed to chair/commode transfer 6) Friction reducing device (FRD): For PROM/AROM exercises
Mobility level 2 = Passes "Sit and Shake;" Fails/unable to "Stretch"	Pass	**Fail**	NA	NA	1) Perform with patient sitting upright in chair position 2) While at EOB dangling and secured by sling and lift	**Goals:** Avoid complications of immobility, engage and strengthen postural and lower extremity muscles, assist with fluid shifts and progress to level 3. 1) FRD: Partial squats and leg AROM exercises – bed flat or tilt position 2) Lift and repo sheet: Boosting and turning 3) Lift and multistraps: Limb holding or turning 4) Lift and sling: Bed to chair/toilet transfer 5) In bed: Perform additional calf pump exercises
Mobility level 3 = Passes "Sit and Shake," and "Stretch;" Fails/unable to "Stand"	Pass	Pass	**Fail**	NA	1) Using sit-to-stand lift with vest: Evaluate patient's tolerance for standing upright and weight bearing; monitor patient's BP and HR; maintain balance for up to 1 minute. 2) Using standing/ambulation vest or pants and floor-based or ceiling lift: Starting with patient's feet flat on floor, instruct patient to rise and stand; monitor patient's BP, HR, standing balance and tolerance for up to 1 minute. As appropriate, after testing in safe mode, use walker, cane, crutches, prosthetic leg(s) to evaluate standing tolerance and to progress to "Step."	**Goals:** Strengthen muscles in upright position, assist fluid shifts, avoid falls and progress to level 4. 1) Sit-to-stand lift with vest/sling: Stand for 1–2 minutes; shift weight from one foot/leg to the other, 2–3 deep breaths 2) Squats using FRD with bed in tilt position 3) Lift and multistraps: Limb holding 4) Powered or non-powered sit-to-stand lift for bed to chair/toilet transfers (e.g., quick night-time transfer to and from toilet) 5) If using aid (walker, cane, crutches, prosthetic), after standing with sit-to-stand lift, work on standing with aid.
Mobility level 4 = Passes "Sit and Shake," "Stretch" and "Stand;" Fails/unable to "Step"	Pass	Pass	Pass	**Fail**	1) If a sit-to-stand lift with vest was used and patient passed "Stand:" evaluate first portion of "Step," march-in-place, while patient is still secure in vest attached to sit-to-stand lift. 2) Using ambulation vest or pants attached to lift: Evaluate "Step" by instructing patient to march-in-place. If able to perform march-in-place, instruct patient to advance step with one foot and return foot to starting position. If able to pass, repeat with other foot. Use walker, cane, crutches or prosthetic leg(s) as appropriate.	**Goals:** Improve standing tolerance and endurance with stepping and weight-shifts, balance and ambulation; avoid falls; consider mobility, functional status, and discharge goals. 1) Lift and ambulation vest/pants for standing, stepping-in-place, weight-shifting/balance activities, and walking 2) Set distance goals to improve endurance and confidence with lift and without lift after passing "Step." 3) If using aid (walker, cane, crutches, prosthetic) to pass "Step," assure that aid is always easily accessible and used for transfers in-room and during hallway ambulation.
Progress through Discharge planning = Passes all 4 assessments Review discharge goals; post-acute discharge planning	Pass	Pass	Pass	**Pass**	• Continue to complete BMAT per protocol; with any change in status adjust mobility level and goals as needed. • While improving/maintaining mobility, continue to address medical issues and stability as needed; evaluate other medical conditions/treatment plan prior to physician release. • Mobility goals may include: Independence with bed mobility and transfers; improve balance, standing tolerance, endurance with walking; independence with aid(s)-walker, cane, crutches, prosthetic(s).	**Multidisciplinary approach:** • Compare pre-admit status, including ability to perform ADLs, to discharge status; i.e., previous level of function (PLOF) compared to post-acute functional status; review rehabilitation goals–have they been met? • Review discharge goals and guide discharge recommendations; appropriate post-acute discharge destination and equipment needs.

FIG. 42.1 cont'd

Expected Outcomes

The patient will:

- return to the previous level of mobility or reach the maximum possible mobility.
- be free from or experience minimal complications of impaired mobility/immobility.
- use joint protection measures to improve activity tolerance.
- achieve independence in self-care and maintain optimal role function.

INTERVENTIONS FOR PROMOTING MUSCULOSKELETAL FUNCTION	RATIONALE
Implement collaborative interventions aimed at treating the underlying cause of the musculoskeletal problem.	Mobility problems may improve with treatment of the underlying musculoskeletal problem.
Provide proper joint protection: • Position the patient in good body alignment. • Apply splints, braces, or other immobilizers as prescribed. • Provide special positioning as needed, such as positioning patients with a partial or total hip replacement by a posterior approach that maintains leg abduction by placing an abductor splint/pillow between the legs.	Joint protection measures promote comfort and reduce the risk of further injury.

INTERVENTIONS FOR PROMOTING MUSCULOSKELETAL FUNCTION	RATIONALE
Use the safe mode strengthening action in the BMAT Bedside Mobility Assessment Tool (BMAT 2.0; see Fig. 42.1) to plan progressive activity. Provide active, active-assisted, or passive, range of motion as needed.	Safe progression of activity and exercises help prevent joint contracture and muscle stiffness.
Administer prescribed medications.	Medication therapy may be used to manage symptoms of musculoskeletal problems.
Notify the health care provider (HCP) if manifestations of the musculoskeletal problem persist or worsen.	Achievement of an effective treatment plan often requires adjustments in therapy.
Make needed environment modifications, such as providing chairs and toilet seats at raised height to accommodate the patient.	Environment modifications can facilitate optimal mobility.
PERFUSION: Implement measures to promote venous return in the affected extremities.	Enhancing venous return promotes fluid mobilization and adequate circulation, decreasing the risk of venous thromboembolism (VTE).
PAIN: Implement measures to manage pain, including treating pain before activity.	Pain restricts motion.
INTRACRANIAL REGULATION: Implement measures to address any neurologic problem the patient is experiencing.	Addressing changes in neurologic function may result in an improvement in a musculoskeletal problem.
STRESS AND COPING: Offer emotional support to the patient and family.	A lack of mobility may be frustrating and create a feeling of confinement.
Provide extra time to complete activities as needed.	Allowing extra time encourages independence.
Encourage the use of adaptive devices for mobility and ADLs.	The use of adaptive devices improves mobility and promotes independence.
Assist with implementing the plan of care developed by the occupational therapist.	The occupational therapist's plan of care is designed to promote performance of ADLs.
Assist with implementing the plan of care developed by the physical therapist.	The physical therapist's plan of care is designed to promote optimal mobility and physical function.
CARE COORDINATION: Assist the patient in obtaining any necessary adaptive devices and making any needed environment adaptations.	Adaptive devices and environment modifications can assist the patient in performing mobility to optimal ability.
SAFETY: Implement measures to reduce the risk of transfer injury: • Use lift devices and sufficient personnel to move or reposition the patient. • Use devices such as a trapeze, slide sheets, and mechanical lifts to move dependent or obese patients in bed. • Obtain special bariatric beds and lift devices for patients who are obese.	Precautions are needed to prevent the risk of transfer injury to the patient or physical injury to the staff.
TISSUE INTEGRITY: Implement measures to promote tissue integrity: • Reposition the patient frequently. • Keep linens clean, dry, and smooth. • Avoid dragging skin across linens when moving. • Provide a special mattress or bed. • Apply protectors over bony prominences, such as heels and elbows.	Patients with impaired mobility have an increased risk for impaired tissue integrity.
GAS EXCHANGE: Encourage the immobile patient to cough and deep breathe or use an incentive spirometer hourly when awake.	Diligent respiratory care can prevent atelectasis.
SAFETY: Implement fall risk precautions if needed, including: • Wearing nonskid shoes • Maintaining clear paths • Avoiding ambulating when the patient is sedated • Orienting the patient to the environment • Keeping the call light and personal possessions within reach • Keeping floors clean and dry • Having the patient call for assistance before getting out of bed • Keeping the bed in a low position	Fall precautions represent the best method of reducing the risk of injury in the patient at risk for falling as a result of musculoskeletal problems.
CLOTTING: Implement VTE prophylaxis as appropriate for the level of risk.	Implementing the VTE precaution bundle reduces the incidence of VTE.

Continued

INTERVENTIONS FOR PROMOTING MUSCULOSKELETAL FUNCTION	RATIONALE
NUTRITION: Implement measures to address body weight if the patient is overweight or obese.	Excess weight places additional stress on joints and restricts mobility.
Provide a nutritionally adequate diet.	Adequate nutrition is needed to build muscle mass and preserve strength.
FUNCTIONAL ABILITY: Help the patient with ADLs, as needed.	Impaired mobility often interferes with the ability to complete ADLs.
Help the patient develop strategies to help with participation in ADLs in the home, at work, and socially.	Making the performance of ADLs easier will help patients achieve maximal independence.
CULTURE: Institute measures to reduce any social isolation the patient may be experiencing.	Being immobile may lead to increased social isolation.
STRESS AND COPING: Encourage the use of positive coping and stress management strategies.	Coping and stress management strategies can improve quality of life by helping the patient better manage a musculoskeletal problem.
CAREGIVING: Implement measures to address caregiver role strain, if present.	Assessing the caregiver for signs of role strain is necessary to provide adequate support.

COLLABORATION	RATIONALE
Physical therapy	Physical therapists assess, plan, and implement interventions that promote musculoskeletal function.
Occupational therapy	Occupational therapy can recommend assistive devices and assist with skill development to help the patient achieve maximum independence.
NUTRITION: Dietitian	Malnutrition causes significant morbidity as a result of the loss of lean body mass.
Home safety evaluation	A home safety evaluation assesses a patient's home environment and provides suggestions for increasing safety.
CARE COORDINATION: Social work or case management	A social worker or case manager can help the patient and caregiver identify community resources to assist with support and obtaining durable medical equipment assistive devices.
Support groups	Support groups can play a major role in promoting the patient's adjustment to changes in function.
Disease or symptom management programs	Disease or symptom management programs help patients understand their treatment regimen and address the complex needs of those with chronic illness.
FUNCTIONAL ABILITY: Home health agency	A home health agency may be able to provide assistance with the patient's care and household maintenance.
MOOD AND AFFECT: Treatment for any coexisting psychological problems	Many persons with mobility problems report experiencing depression.

PATIENT AND CAREGIVER TEACHING

- Cause of a musculoskeletal problem, if known, and how long it may last
- Manifestations of a musculoskeletal problem
- Management of any underlying condition causing a musculoskeletal problem
- Measures being used to address the musculoskeletal problem or improve mobility
- Measures to reduce the risk of complications
- Safe use of mobility devices and therapeutic immobilizers
- Caregiver safety when assisting mobility
- Community and home precautions, if needed
- Importance of taking medications as prescribed
- How to perform range of motion and other exercises
- Anticipatory guidance regarding situations that may be problematic
- Importance of proper nutrition and sleep
- Modifications in the living environment to promote safety
- Available community and self-help resources
- Role of physical and occupational therapies
- Positive coping and stress management strategies
- Early recognition of problems and how to manage them
- Importance of long-term follow-up
- When to notify the HCP

DOCUMENTATION

Assessment

- Manifestations of musculoskeletal problem
- Extent of mobility and strength
- Comfort
- Diagnostic test results

Interventions

- Discussions with other members of the interprofessional team
- Environment modifications made
- Medications given
- Therapeutic interventions and the patient's response
- Referrals initiated
- Safety measures implemented, including fall precautions
- Teaching provided
- Progressive mobilization
- Use of mobility devices and therapeutic immobilizers
- Pain management
- Notification of the HCP about diagnostic test results and assessment findings

Evaluation

- Patient's status: improved, stable, declined
- Diagnostic test results
- Patient's response to therapeutic interventions
- Patient's response to teaching
- Progress in mobility

Pain 43

Definition

Unpleasant sensory and emotional experience associated with actual or potential tissue damage

Pain is a complex, multidimensional experience that can cause suffering and decrease quality of life. It is a major reason that people seek health care. We classify pain in many ways. Acute pain lasts for a short period and is associated with injury, surgery, illness, trauma, or painful medical procedures. Acute pain functions as a signal, warning the person of potential or actual tissue damage. It usually disappears when the underlying cause has resolved. Chronic pain does not have an adaptive role; it persists past the time when expected pain associated with tissue damage should subside. Chronic pain can be disabling and often is accompanied by anxiety and depression.

The pain experience affects all aspects of a person's life and is interrelated with many concepts. Culture and spirituality influence the expression of pain. Acute pain adversely affects mobility and sleep, leading to fatigue. Those with severe or chronic pain are more likely to describe their health as poor and have increased mortality. Different patient populations, including ethnic minorities, children, and adults with cognitive impairment, are at risk for inadequate pain management.

You are an important member of the interprofessional pain management team. Regularly screen all patients for pain. When pain is present, perform a thorough pain assessment, describing the patient's pain experience. You can provide quality patient care by identifying pain management goals with the patient and implementing pain management interventions, including teaching, advocacy, and support of the patient and caregiver.

Associated Clinical Problems

- Abdominal Pain: pain in the abdominal cavity
- Acute Pain: severe pain of a limited duration
- Arthritis Pain: pain associated with an inflammatory joint condition
- Chronic Pain: persistent pain that lasts for longer periods
- Fracture Pain: pain associated with a fracture
- Inadequate Pain Control: failure to achieve acceptable pain relief
- Labor Pain: pain associated with childbirth
- Phantom Pain: pain in a body part that is no longer present

Common Causes

- Acute ischemia
- Cancer
- Headache and migraines
- Infection
- Inflammation: cholecystitis, appendicitis, inflammatory bowel disease
- Labor and childbirth
- Low back pain
- Overuse injuries and strains
- Peripheral neuropathy and neuralgia
- Physical disability
- Surgery and diagnostic procedures
- Tissue trauma: lacerations, fractures, amputation, burns

Manifestations

- Affective responses: anxiety, fear, depression, irritability
- Expressive behavior: grimacing, moaning, crying, restlessness
- Family/caregiver reporting patient in pain
- Impaired sleep
- Not taking part in activities
- Physical responses: diaphoresis, ↑ heart rate, ↑ respiratory rate, changes in BP, pupil dilation, anorexia, nausea, muscle spasm, pallor
- Positioning to avoid pain
- Positive response to analgesia
- Presence of condition or procedure known to cause pain
- Protective behaviors: guarding, lack of movement, rubbing an area
- Reduced interactions with others
- Self-report of pain

Key Conceptual Relationships

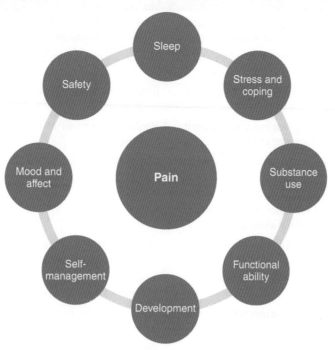

ASSESSMENT OF PAIN	RATIONALE
Determine the potential cause of pain.	Identifying the cause of pain allows for early intervention.
Note the patient's age, cognition, and ability to communicate.	Age, cognition, and ability to communicate affect the ability to report pain.
Perform a comprehensive pain assessment: • Onset • Location • Duration • Characteristics • Aggravating factors • Relieving factors • Treatments attempted • Severity	Assessment helps to determine the type and cause of pain and directs its treatment.
Use a formal pain scale appropriate for the patient's age, and cognition (Figure 43.1 and Table 43.1).	The consistent use of pain rating scales identifies the intensity of pain over time and evaluates the effectiveness of treatment.
Perform a complete physical assessment and monitor indicators of pain on an ongoing basis:	
• Manifestations of pain	Identifying pain allows for early intervention.
• Vital signs	Pain, particularly acute pain, is often accompanied by changes in heart rate, blood pressure, and respiratory rate.
• Physiologic and behavior responses, including grimacing, rubbing an area, groaning, and restlessness, especially in those unable to communicate effectively	Physiologic and behavior cues, such as crying, grimacing, moaning, groaning, or restlessness, are powerful indicators of the presence of discomfort.
Explore the patient's knowledge and beliefs about pain and expectations about pain management.	Patient beliefs, attitudes, and expectations influence responses to pain and pain treatment.
Assess for factors that decrease pain tolerance, such as fatigue.	Factors that decrease pain tolerance can interfere with the ability to achieve acceptable pain management.

Continued

ASSESSMENT OF PAIN	RATIONALE
Evaluate experiences with pain, including history of chronic pain, resulting disability, and the effectiveness of pain control measures, including analgesics.	Experience with pain influences the ways in which a person responds to the current experience of pain.
Assess the appropriateness of using patient-controlled anesthesia (PCA) therapy.	PCA therapy provides the patient with control in pain management.
Compare the amount of pain medication given with patient reports of pain.	If medication requests are frequent, medication dosage may need to be increased.
Determine the needed frequency of assessing pain and monitor patient satisfaction with pain management at specified intervals.	Nursing actions based on reassessment are key to providing optimal pain management.
CULTURE: Assess cultural factors influencing the pain response and how the patient views pain.	Culture influences responses to pain and pain treatment.
FUNCTIONAL ABILITY: Assess lifestyle effects of the pain, such as on the ability to sleep, enjoy life, interact with others, perform work and household duties, and engage in physical and social activities.	The pain experience affects all aspects of a person's life.
MOOD AND AFFECT: Assess mental status and screen for coexisting psychological problems.	Many patients with pain, particularly chronic pain, may have depression and other psychological problems.
SAFETY: Assess for adverse and risk factors for opioid-related harms and ways to mitigate patient risk.	Adverse effects, including respiratory depression, a decrease in cognition, or misuse, may require an adjustment in medication or dose.
SUBSTANCE USE: Obtain a history of the use of alcohol and other substances that could influence the use of analgesics.	Use of alcohol and other substances can alter effective doses of analgesics or lead to undertreatment.
Obtain blood and urine toxicology screens.	Diagnostic tests provide objective data about drug metabolites in the blood and urine.
STRESS AND COPING: Assess the current and past use of stress management and coping strategies.	A patient experiencing pain may rely on substance use or other negative behaviors as a means of coping with the stress.
Evaluate the effectiveness of the pain control measures used through ongoing assessment of the pain experience.	Achieving an effective treatment plan often requires adjustments in medications, dosage, or route to achieve maximal benefits while minimizing adverse effects.
Pediatric	
Determine the child's understanding of the cause of pain, if possible.	Pain assessment in children should not be based solely on behaviors.
Include the parent/caregiver rating of the child's pain.	Parents and nurses can rate a child's pain differently, with the parents' observation often being more accurate.
Assess the effect of pain on sleep and play.	A child who sleeps, plays, or both can be in pain; however, both can serve as distractions or show the adequacy of pain control.
Use the FLACC scale (Table 43.1) or other behavioral measure to assess pain in infants and young children.	Infants experience pain as measured by physiologic, behavior, metabolic, and hormonal responses.
Older Adult	
Be persistent in asking older adults about pain, conducting the assessment in an unhurried, supportive manner.	While many older adults believe that pain is a normal, unavoidable part of aging, pain in an older adult can result from multiple pathologic conditions.
Use the proper pain assessment tool, adapting as needed for older adults.	Older adults may not show objective signs of pain because of years of adaptation and increased pain tolerance.

Expected Outcomes

The patient will:

- report pain is alleviated or reduced to an acceptable level.
- have a reduction in pain behaviors.
- report an improved mood and coping.
- adhere to prescribed pharmacologic regimen.
- appropriately use pharmacologic and nonpharmacologic therapies to control pain.
- report adequate sleep.
- maintain role performance and take part in desired activities of daily living.
- recognize factors that increase pain and take preventive action.

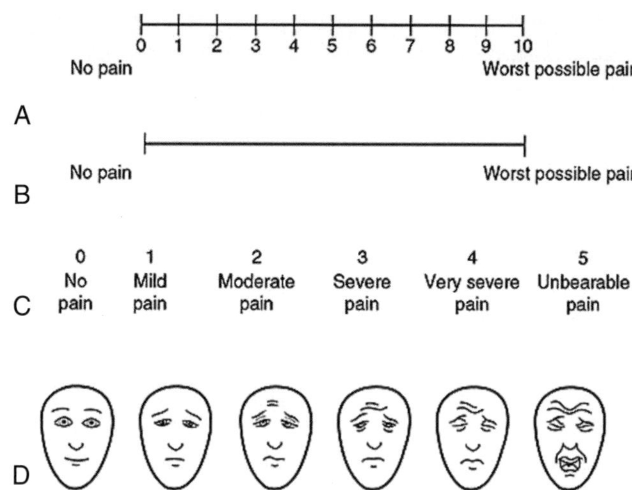

FIG. 43.1 Pain Intensity Scales. (A) 0 to 10 Numeric Scale. (B) Visual Analog Scale. (C) Descriptive Scale. (D) Faces Pain Scale. (Modified from Baird M: *Manual of Critical Care Nursing: Nursing Interventions and Collaborative Management*, ed 2. St. Louis: Elsevier; 2015. Source: Harding M, Kwong J, Roberts D, Hagler D, Reinisch C, eds. *Lewis's Medical-Surgical Nursing: Assessment and Management of Clinical Problems*, ed 12. St. Louis: Elsevier; 2022.)

Table 43.1 FLACC Scale

Behavior	0	1	2
Face	No particular expression or smile	Occasional grimace or frown, withdrawn, disinterested	Frequent to constant quivering chin, clenched jaw
Legs	Normal position or relaxed	Uneasy, restless, tense	Kicking or legs drawn up
Activity	Lying quietly, normal position, moves easily	Squirming, shifting, back and forth, tense	Arched, rigid or jerking
Cry	No cry (awake or asleep)	Moans or whimpers; occasional complaint	Crying steadily, screams, sobs, frequent complaints
Consolability	Content, relaxed	Reassured by touching, hugging, or being talked to, distractible	Difficult to console or comfort

Scoring:
0 = Relaxed and comfortable.
1–3 = Mild discomfort.
4–6 = Moderate pain.
7–10 = Severe discomfort/pain.

INTERVENTIONS TO MANAGE PAIN	RATIONALE
Mutually establish a pain management goal.	Mutually determining acceptable pain management goals gives the patient a sense of control.
Provide interprofessional care using a multimodal approach that integrates pharmacologic and nonpharmacologic measures to promote pain relief.	The expertise and perspectives of an interprofessional team can provide effective assessment and therapies for patients with pain.
Consider the patient's preferences, support of significant others, and expectations when selecting a pain relief strategy.	The patient's preferences, caregiver beliefs, and expectations influence responses to pain and pain treatment.
Provide the patient optimal pain relief with prescribed analgesics.	Pharmacologic therapy is the mainstay of effective pain management. Multimodal regimens achieve superior pain relief, enhance patient satisfaction, and decrease adverse medication effects.
Base the decision regarding range and medication selection orders on a thorough pain assessment.	Safe administration of range orders for analgesia should consider pain intensity, pain location, cause, characteristics of the pain, functional status, and previous response to analgesics.

Continued

INTERVENTIONS TO MANAGE PAIN	RATIONALE
Notify the health care provider (HCP) if the regimen is providing inadequate pain control.	An effective treatment plan often requires adjustments in medication, dosage, or route to achieve maximal benefits while minimizing adverse effects.
Notify the HCP about changes in pain or new reports of pain.	Changes in pain or new reports of pain may indicate a complication or new problem.
Medicate prior to an activity to increase participation while minimizing hazards with sedation.	Appropriate analgesic scheduling focuses on preventing or controlling pain.
Give pretreatment analgesia and/or nonpharmacologic strategies before painful procedures.	Appropriate analgesic scheduling focuses on preventing or controlling pain.
Encourage the patient to use adequate pain control measures before pain becomes severe.	Appropriate analgesic scheduling focuses on prevention or control of pain, rather than giving analgesics only after pain has become severe.
Implement measures to minimize pain in specific situations, such as splinting incisions with activity or applying splints or stabilization devices.	Stabilization helps to reduce strain and tension in an area, thus decreasing pain.
SUBSTANCE USE: Discuss with the patient and caregivers concerns about substance use.	Discussing concerns about addiction, tolerance, and physical dependence with patients and caregivers may ease concerns and promote adherence.
Collaborate with the patient, caregivers, and other health professionals to select and implement nonpharmacologic pain relief measures, including biofeedback, transcutaneous electrical nerve stimulation (TENS), hypnosis, relaxation, guided imagery, music therapy, activity therapy, acupressure, hot/cold application, and massage.	Nonpharmacologic pain relief measures can reduce the dose of analgesia needed to relieve pain, minimize the side effects of drug therapy, and increase the patient's sense of control.
Encourage the use of nonpharmacologic methods of pain relief before, after, and, if possible, during painful activities; before pain occurs or increases; and along with other pain relief measures.	Nonpharmacologic pain relief measures can reduce the dose of an analgesic needed to relieve pain and increase the patient's sense of control.
Encourage the patient with chronic pain to record pain intensity, medication use, response, and associated activities in a pain log or diary.	A pain log or diary can help determine the source of pain and therapies that promote effective pain management.
Support patients in using spiritual care practices.	Spiritual care helps relieve pain and improve health, well-being, and quality of life.
SAFETY: Implement measures to reduce or eliminate common side effects of drug therapy.	Appropriate management of side effects can increase the patient's comfort level.
Establish a therapeutic patient relationship: • Acknowledge the pain experience • Use active listening with therapeutic communication skills. • Provide a secure, relaxed atmosphere. • Convey acceptance of the patient's response to pain.	The development of a trusting nurse–patient relationship is a priority as the patient needs to feel confident that the reports of pain will be believed.
Encourage the patient to discuss the pain experience.	Acknowledging the patient's experience builds trust.
Control environment factors that influence the response to pain, such as room temperature, lighting, and noise.	Managing environment factors can increase the patient's comfort level.
Suggest distractions, including visitors, music, television and movies, gaming, and computer use.	Distraction shifts or moves attention away from discomfort and places focus elsewhere.
MOOD AND AFFECT: Implement measures to address problems that precipitate or increase the pain experience, such as depression.	Associated symptoms, such as anxiety, fatigue, fear, and depression, may worsen or be worsened by pain.
SLEEP: Promote adequate periods of rest and sleep and institute measures to address impaired sleep, if present.	Pain adversely affects mobility and sleep, leading to fatigue and worsening pain.
STRESS AND COPING: Help the patient and caregivers cope with the pain experience by using positive coping and stress management behaviors.	Providing more support increases the chance of achieving pain management goals.

INTERVENTIONS TO MANAGE PAIN	RATIONALE
FUNCTIONAL ABILITY: Help the patient develop strategies to help with taking part in activities of daily living in the home, at work, and socially.	Because the pain experience affects all aspects of life, making activities of daily living easier will help patients cope with pain and improve functional ability.
SAFETY: Provide a safe environment for the patient receiving opioid medications by initiating fall precautions.	Patients receiving opioid agents have an increased risk of falls.
Pediatric	
Use tactile and vocal stimuli, such as rocking and swaddling, to provide to comfort infants and young children.	Rocking, nonnutritive sucking, kangaroo care, and swaddling help reduce pain in infants and young children.
Encourage parent presence.	Most children feel more secure with their parents present, and most parents want to be present, including during painful procedures.
Collaborate with the patient and caregivers to select and implement nonpharmacologic pain relief measures, including puppetry, drawing, distraction, play therapy, storytelling, and massage.	Nonpharmacologic pain relief measures can reduce the dose of analgesia needed to relieve pain, minimizing the side effects of drug therapy and increasing the child's comfort.
DEVELOPMENT: Discuss with parents the potential for impaired development in the child with chronic pain and institute appropriate interventions.	Early identification allows for initiating the services and support needed by children with impaired development.
Older Adult	
SAFETY: Monitor older adults closely for respiratory depression and excess sedation when they receive opioid analgesics.	Older adults have a higher risk of respiratory depression with opioid use.
Titrate prescribed doses carefully and monitor for drug interactions.	The effects of analgesics are prolonged in older adults because of decreased drug metabolism and clearance.

INTERVENTIONS TO ADDRESS LABOR PAIN	RATIONALE
Determine the level of support provided by the labor partner(s), including the expectant father, significant others, and/or doula or coach.	The nurse supplements, supervises, and provides supportive care, depending on the support others provide.
Provide coaching on the use of breathing techniques.	Breathing techniques assist with pain managment during labor.
Consult the HCP about pain management if the pain is not controlled to an acceptable level.	Revisions to the pain management plan may be needed to prevent sleep deprivation, maternal exhaustion, and increased anxiety.
Encourage ambulation if possible.	Walking promotes more efficient contractions.
Encourage position changes every 20 to 30 minutes.	Position changes can prevent or correct malposition of the fetus, promote rotation and labor progress, and reduce lower back pain.

COLLABORATION	RATIONALE
Support groups	Support groups can provide the patient with support, validation, and education that increases the chance of achieving pain management goals.
Counseling	Counseling can help the patient develop better coping skills for managing pain.
MOOD AND AFFECT: Treatment for coexisting psychological problems, including depressed mood and emotional problems	Treating an underlying psychological problem will aid in achieving pain management goals.

PATIENT AND CAREGIVER TEACHING

- Cause of the pain, if known, and how long it may last
- Factors contributing to pain
- About pain and manifestations of pain
- Pain assessment methods and reason for frequent monitoring of pain
- Expectations about pain management
- Principles of pain management
- Safe use of medications for pain relief, including proper use and side effect management
- How to use patient-controlled analgesia
- Fears and risks of addiction
- Nonpharmacologic techniques to manage pain
- Anticipatory guidance about managing situations associated with pain
- Community and self-help resources available
- Positive coping and stress management strategies
- Relaxation techniques
- Importance of notifying HCP if pain is not relieved

DOCUMENTATION

Assessment

- Assessments performed
- Diagnostic and laboratory test results
- Manifestations of pain
- Screening test results

Interventions

- Discussions with other interprofessional team members
- Medications given
- Notification of HCP about patient status
- Therapeutic interventions and the patient's response
- Teaching provided
- Referrals initiated
- Safety measures implemented, including fall precautions

Evaluation

- Pain level
- Patient's status: improved, stable, declined
- Manifestations of pain
- Response to teaching provided
- Response to therapeutic interventions

Sensory Deficit 44

Definition

Impaired ability to hear, see, taste, smell, or correctly perceive touch

People receive external stimuli through the five senses: vision, hearing, taste, smell, and touch. Sensory perception involves how people receive that sensory input and, through various physiological processes, interpret the stimuli. Problems affecting sensory perception occur across the lifespan. They can be primary or secondary problems and can cause acute and chronic changes. There is a broad spectrum of presentation and age-related differences. Changes that occur during growth and development in early infancy affect visual acuity and hearing perception. Some sensory function declines as part of the normal aging process, with most people having noticeable changes in hearing and vision.

Functional senses support independence and participation in fulfilling activities. Thus a problem can have a significant negative impact on development, health, and well-being. Sensory deficits share many of the same consequences. These include a reduced overall quality of life and a higher risk for injury. Impaired vision and hearing contribute to development delay and learning disabilities in infants and children and a loss of functional ability in adults. Functional problems include difficulty establishing a career, impaired interpersonal relationships, social isolation, depression, and negative self-image. Many incur a financial burden through loss of income and the cost of treatment and assistive devices.

Specific sensory deficits are associated with particular problems. Poor vision can be devastating to activities of daily living and independence, also taking a toll on family members and caregivers. Since hearing is the basis for most social interaction and communication, having a hearing problem can lead to social isolation. Impaired smell and taste can affect nutrition. Tactile perception problems are associated with a high risk for injury.

Nurses can assess for problems with sensory function and implement measures to help patients function as fully as possible, enhancing their quality of life. Assisting the patient with finding ways to function safely within their environment reduces the risk of injury and promotes independence. Collaboration with interprofessional team members supports the patient with accessing and using necessary resources.

Associated Clinical Problems

- Hearing Problem: impaired ability to sense sound
- Smelling Problem: impaired ability to smell
- Tactile Perception Problem: impaired ability to perceive touch
- Taste Problem: impaired ability to taste
- Vision Problem: impaired ability to sense visual images

Common Causes

- Age
- Congenital conditions: Down syndrome, congenital malformations
- Family history
- Genetic conditions
- Lost, damaged, or lack of sensory aids
- Traumatic injury

Pediatric

- Low APGAR scores
- Prematurity

Hearing Problem

- Cerumen impaction
- Medications: Aminoglycosides, aspirin, chemotherapy, loop diuretics, nonsteroidal antiinflammatory drugs (NSAIDs)
- Noise exposure
- Recurrent infections

Smelling Problem

- Allergies
- COVID-19 infection
- Dementia
- Liver disease
- Medications: antihistamines, antibiotics, chemotherapy, decongestants, disease-modifying antirheumatic drugs (DMARDs), nasal sprays
- Nasal and sinus problems
- Neurodegenerative diseases: Parkinson disease, multiple sclerosis
- Smoking
- Upper respiratory infections

Tactile Perception Problem

- Alcohol use disorder
- Chemotherapy

- Diabetes
- Peripheral vascular disease
- Raynaud syndrome
- Spinal cord injury
- Stroke
- Third-degree burn

Taste Problem
- Chronic renal failure
- COVID-19 infections
- Endocrine problems: Cushing syndrome, diabetes, hypothyroidism
- Liver failure
- Medications: calcium channel blockers, chemotherapy, corticosteroids, DMARDs
- Neurologic problems: Bell palsy, multiple sclerosis, stroke
- Oral cancer, infections, inflammation
- Periodontal disease
- Smoking

Vision Problem
- Cataracts
- Diabetic retinopathy
- Foreign body in eye
- Glaucoma
- Infections
- Macular degeneration
- Ocular cancer
- Retinal detachment
- Stroke

Pediatric
- Retinoblastoma
- Retinopathy of prematurity

Manifestations

- Changes in role performance, lifestyle
- Depressed mood
- Self-report or validated report of a sensory deficit
- Social isolation

Pediatric
- Behavior problems
- Development delays

Hearing Problem
- Ear pain
- Tinnitus
- Vertigo
- Diagnostic testing: deficits present with audiometry, auditory brain stem response; abnormal tympanometry

Tactile Perception Problem
- Falling
- Impaired ability to perceive vibration, light touch
- Lack of coordination
- Lack of point discrimination
- Muscle weakness
- Numbness
- Pain
- Paresthesias
- Diagnostic testing: abnormal results of nerve biopsy, electromyography (EMG)

Taste Problem
- Malnutrition
- Weight loss
- Diagnostic testing: deficits present with identification testing

Vision Problem
- Eye pain
- Headache
- Diagnostic test results: abnormal visual acuity, peripheral vision; ↑ intraocular pressure; positive findings on ophthalmoscopy

Pediatric
- Eyes not moving in synchrony
- Lack of eye tracking

Key Conceptual Relationships

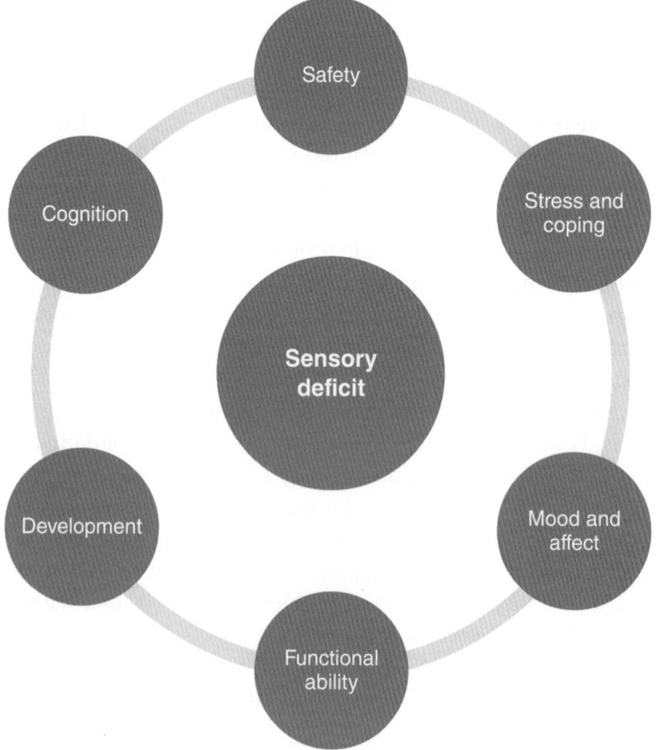

ASSESSMENT OF SENSORY PERCEPTION	RATIONALE
Assess risk factors for a sensory deficit.	Identifying factors that place patients at risk for a sensory deficit allows for early intervention.
Determine the potential cause of a sensory deficit.	Some sensory deficits may improve or resolve with treatment of the underlying cause.
Obtain a thorough history of the sensory deficit, including: • Onset, sudden or gradual • Duration • Symptoms experienced • Intensity or severity • Perceived consequences • Precipitating and aggravating factors • Treatment • Use of adaptive devices	A thorough history aids in determining the cause of a sensory deficit, helps identify contributing factors, and helps determine treatment.
Perform a physical assessment and monitor indicators of the sensory deficit on an ongoing basis:	
• **COGNITION:** Cognitive and mental status	Sensory deficits can cause changes in cognition and mental status.
• Hearing: ear examination, otoscopic examination, general ability to hear, Rinne and Weber tests, balance, cranial nerve function	Assessment helps determine the presence, degree, and cause of a hearing problem.
• Smell: nasal patency, visual inspection of nose	Assessment helps determine the presence and cause of a smelling problem.
• Tactile perception: gait; Romberg test; peripheral sensory stimuli testing, including monofilament tests	Assessment helps determine the presence and degree of a tactile perception problem.
• Taste: examine tongue and oral cavity, evaluate smell	Assessment helps determine the presence of a taste problem.
• Vision: eye examination, visual acuity, extraocular eye movements, ophthalmoscopic exam	Assessment helps determine the presence, degree, and cause of a vision problem.
Evaluate the results of diagnostic tests, including:	
• Hearing: audiometry, tympanometry, otoacoustic emissions, auditory brain stem response	Diagnostic testing helps determine the presence and degree of a hearing problem.
• Smell and taste: identification testing	Diagnostic testing can helps determine the presence and degree of a smelling or taste problem.
• Vision: measurement of visual acuity, peripheral vision, and intraocular pressure; ophthalmoscopy	Diagnostic testing helps determine the presence, degree, and cause of a vision problem.
• Tactile perception: nerve biopsy, EMG	Diagnostic testing helps determine the presence and degree of a tactile problem.
FUNCTIONAL ABILITY: Assess for lifestyle effects of having a sensory deficit, such as impaired ability to perform work and household duties and engage in physical and social activities.	A sensory deficit can adversely influence the ability to engage in role performance and desired activities.
STRESS AND COPING: Assess coping strategies used by patient and caregiver and how they are coping with a sensory deficit.	Quality of life for patients and caregivers is directly related to the coping strategies that they use.
Assess the patient's support system: • Who do they live with? • Are they employed? • Do they have friends and relatives accessible? • Have they used any community resources?	Support from others is an important aspect in self-managing a sensory deficit.
SELF-MANAGEMENT: Assess how the patient is managing coexisting health problems.	A sensory problem can be a barrier to the ability to engage in self-management of a health problem.
Evaluate the effectiveness of measures used to address a sensory deficit through ongoing assessment.	Ongoing monitoring allows for evaluation of therapy effectiveness.

Continued

ASSESSMENT OF SENSORY PERCEPTION	RATIONALE
Pediatric Obtain a prenatal history.	Identifying factors that place a child at risk for a sensory deficit allows for early intervention.
DEVELOPMENT: Perform age-appropriate sensory screenings.	Timely identification of a sensory deficit allows for early intervention.
Assess the child's level of physical and emotional development.	The effects of a sensory deficit and management depend on the child's age, development level, and health status.

Expected Outcomes

The patient will:

- report an improvement in or experience no further decline in sensory perception.
- implement strategies to compensate for sensory deficit.
- maintain role performance and take part in desired activities of daily living.
- implement health promotion behaviors to reduce the risk of sensory perception problems.
- remain free from injury.
- maintain contact with supportive resources.

INTERVENTIONS TO ADDRESS SENSORY DEFICITS	RATIONALE
Implement collaborative interventions addressed at treating underlying factors contributing to sensory deficit.	Certain sensory deficits may improve or resolve with treatment of contributing factors.
Notify the provider if a sensory deficit unexpectedly worsens.	Notifying the provider allows for early intervention.
Assist with implementing the plan of care developed by occupational therapy and other rehabilitation specialists.	Specialists' plans of care are designed to promote optimal performance of activities of daily living.
Encourage the patient to use recommended sensory aids.	Sensory aids support residual sensory function.
Assist the patient in identifying strengths and abilities.	Integrating personal strengths into the plan of care can enhance role performance.
Encourage the patient to identify and express their feelings about having a sensory deficit.	Expressing thoughts and feelings can improve psychological problems that often accompany having a sensory deficit.
Implement environment modifications, such as reducing background noise when communicating with a patient who has a hearing problem.	Environment modifications can assist with compensating for the sensory deficit.
SAFETY: Implement safety precautions.	Safety precautions decrease the higher risk for injury that accompanies many sensory deficits.
FUNCTIONAL ABILITY: Help the patient develop strategies to promote independent participation in activities of daily living.	Modifying activities of daily living will help patients be as independent as possible.
STRESS AND COPING: Help the patient and caregivers cope with the sensory deficit by using positive stress management and coping behaviors.	Quality of life for patients and caregivers is related to the stress management and coping strategies they use.
CARE COORDINATION: Assist the patient in obtaining necessary adaptive devices.	Adaptive devices can assist the patient in being as independent as possible.
COGNITION: Implement measures to address any change in cognition.	Sensory deficits can cause changes in cognition and mental status.
FUNCTIONAL ABILITY: Implement measures to address any social isolation the patient may be experiencing.	Social isolation can negatively influence quality of life in a person with a sensory deficit.

INTERVENTIONS TO ADDRESS SENSORY DEFICITS	RATIONALE
Pediatric	
DEVELOPMENT: Institute measures to promote the child's growth and development.	Age-appropriate activities are necessary for nurturing the child's growth and development.
FUNCTIONAL ABILITY: Encourage the child to take part in play activities appropriate to age, development level, and ability.	A child's normal role includes taking part in play activity.

INTERVENTIONS TO ADDRESS A HEARING PROBLEM	RATIONALE
SAFETY: Encourage the patient to use ear protection.	Using ear protection may help prevent further hearing loss.
Stop medications known to be associated with ototoxicity if a new hearing problem occurs and notify the health care provider (HCP).	Hearing loss may be reversible if ototoxic medications are stopped quickly.
Use strategies to promote effective communication. • Face the patient directly • Spotlight the face • Use gestures • Do not shout • Speak clearly, slowly, and with a normal tone • Do not overenunciate	Appropriate communication strategies contribute to the patient's well-being by reducing isolation.
Assist the patient with obtaining hearing aids or other assistive devices.	Assistive devices can help the patient in accommodating for diminished hearing.

INTERVENTIONS TO ADDRESS A SMELL PROBLEM	RATIONALE
Administer prescribed intranasal corticosteroid spray.	Intranasal corticosteroid spray can reduce inflammation in the nasal passages.

INTERVENTIONS TO ADDRESS A TACTILE PROBLEM	RATIONALE
TISSUE INTEGRITY: Provide appropriate foot care.	Appropriate skin and foot care can reduce the risk of injury.
Implement measures to reduce the risk of impaired skin integrity.	Safety measures decrease the risk of injury that accompanies having a tactile problem.
PAIN: Implement measures to address any pain the patient may be experiencing.	Pain often accompanies peripheral neuropathy, a common cause of a tactile problem.

INTERVENTIONS TO ADDRESS A TASTE PROBLEM	RATIONALE
Encourage the patient to make mealtime social.	Making mealtime pleasant may increase food intake.
Have the patient try a wide variety of foods and various spices and seasonings.	Experimenting with different foods may lead to the patient discovering foods that are more palatable.
SUBSTANCE USE: Promote tobacco cessation interventions.	Smoking, vaping, or chewing tobacco may cause or worsen taste problems.

INTERVENTIONS TO ADDRESS A VISION PROBLEM	RATIONALE
Administer prescribed medications, including:	
• β-Adrenergic eye drops	β-Adrenergic eye drops decrease production of aqueous humor.
• Prostaglandin analogs	Prostaglandin analogs decrease the outflow of aqueous humor between the uvea and sclera.
• Carbonic anhydrase inhibitors	Carbonic anhydrase inhibitors decrease the production of aqueous humor.
• Cholinergic agents	Cholinergic agents stimulate iris sphincter contraction, facilitating aqueous outflow.
• Adrenergic agonists	Adrenergic agonists decrease the production of aqueous humor.
Assist the patient with obtaining assistive devices or animal companions, including canes and guide dogs.	Assistive devices and companions help the patient in accommodating for diminished vision.
Encourage the use of adaptive strategies: • Appropriate lighting • Magnification • Technology aids, such as audio text, large print materials	Adaptive strategies assist the patient in accommodating for diminished vision.
Use appropriate communication strategies: • Announce your presence when entering a room. • Talk in a normal tone of voice. • Explain activity occurring in the room. • Announce when you are leaving so the patient is not talking to someone who is no longer there.	Appropriate communication strategies promote conversation with the person who has vision impairment.
Encourage the use of strategies to assist with activities of daily living: • Keep the environment organized and place all items in specific, consistent locations. • When walking, let the patient take your arm. • Provide descriptions of unfamiliar items. • Allow the patient to seat themselves. • Use items with bright, contrasting colors.	These measures facilitate independence for patients with vision problems.
Pediatric	
Administer prophylactic eye ointment to newborns.	Antibiotic eye ointment given to newborns reduces the chance of the infant acquiring an infection.

COLLABORATION	RATIONALE
Specialty medical care, including neurological, ophthalmology, otolaryngology, or audiology	Specialists can determine if a problem is present, the most likely cause, and provide treatment.
STRESS AND COPING: Counseling	Counseling and cognitive behavior therapy may be needed to assist in the patient managing problems from a sensory deficit.
Support groups	Support groups can play a major role in promoting adjustment to role changes and offering suggestions from peers for managing a sensory deficit.
Community-based support systems	Community agencies can provide various types of long-term support and assistance.
FUNCTIONAL ABILITY: Rehabilitation specialist, vocational rehabilitation	Specialty support services assist the patient in achieving maximum independence and well-being.
CARE COORDINATION: Social work	The social worker can explore resources that may be available to help the patient obtain access to health care and resources.
FUNCTIONAL ABILITY: Occupational therapy	Occupational therapists assess, plan, and implement interventions that promote a person's ability to fulfill role responsibilities.

COLLABORATION	RATIONALE
NUTRITION: Dietitian	The dietitian can provide the patient information and support for implementing the prescribed diet to address deficits in smell and taste.
School counselor, school social worker, or school psychologist	School personnel can provide the services necessary to ensure that a child with a sensory deficit is provided appropriate support at school.
MOOD AND AFFECT: Treatment for coexisting psychological problems, particularly depression	Treatment of underlying psychological problems is an important part of helping the patient cope with a sensory deficit.

 PATIENT AND CAREGIVER TEACHING

- Cause of a sensory deficit
- Normal age-related variations in sensory function
- Manifestations of a sensory deficit
- Management of underlying conditions associated with a sensory deficit
- Screening examinations and surveillance for hearing and vision problems
- Safe use of medications and how they fit into the management plan
- Measures to prevent further sensory decline
- Role of case management
- Role of occupational therapies
- Modifications in the living environment to promote safety
- Community and self-help resources available
- Sources of information and social support
- Positive coping and stress management strategies
- How to safely use adaptive devices
- Importance of long-term follow up
- When to notify the HCP

DOCUMENTATION

Assessment

- Assessments performed
- Diagnostic and laboratory test results
- Manifestations of a sensory deficit
- Screening test results

Interventions

- Discussions with other interprofessional team members
- Environmental modifications made
- Medications given
- Notification of HCP about patient status
- Therapeutic interventions and the patient's response
- Teaching provided
- Referrals initiated
- Safety measures implemented, including fall precautions

Evaluation

- Patient's status: improved, stable, declined
- Presence of manifestations of a sensory deficit
- Response to teaching provided
- Response to therapeutic interventions

Impaired Tissue Integrity 45

Definition

Damage, inflammation, or lesion of the skin or underlying structures

The skin's primary function is to protect the underlying body tissues. The skin acts as a barrier against invasion by bacteria and viruses and prevents excess water loss. The fat in the subcutaneous layer insulates the body and provides protection from trauma. Melanin is a substance in the skin that screens and absorbs ultraviolet radiation.

Tissue integrity is the state of structurally intact and physiologically functioning epithelial tissues, including the integument (skin, subcutaneous tissue) and mucous membranes. Disruptions to tissue integrity may result from illness, injury, or intentional trauma, such as a surgical incision. Tissue injuries and wounds heal by primary, secondary, or tertiary intention. *Primary intention healing* occurs when wound margins are well approximated, as in a sutured surgical incision or a simple laceration, and takes place more rapidly than the other types of healing. *Secondary intention healing* processes occur when wounds such as ulcerations have distant edges and granulation tissue gradually fills the gap to close the wound. *Tertiary intention healing* processes occur when a wound that must stay open because of infection or contamination can be sutured closed only much later, resulting in more scarring.

Nurses have an important role in protecting tissue integrity and supporting wound healing. Adequate nutrition and perfusion promote healing. Interventions aimed at promoting mobility and preventing infection reduce the risk of further injury. Skin and tissue damage is often visible to the individual and others. Addressing concerns about pain and self-image promotes patients' comfort.

Associated Clinical Problems

- Arterial Ulcer: open wound resulting from poor blood flow, usually on the foot
- Burn Wound: tissue damage caused by heat, ranging from superficial to full-thickness injury
- Diabetic Ulcer: wounds resulting from vascular complications of diabetes
- Dry Skin: ashy, cracked surface resulting from a lack of moisture
- Excoriation: loss of skin layers through scraping or abrasion
- Impaired Oral Mucous Membrane: disruption of the tissue of the lips or oral cavity
- Impaired Skin Integrity: loss of intact skin or mucous membrane barrier
- Lymphedema: localized swelling of the body caused by disruption to the lymph system, with an abnormal accumulation of lymph
- Malignant Wound: lesion resulting from cancerous cells infiltrating the skin and its supporting vessels, leading to tissue necrosis
- Perioperative Positioning Injury: localized damage to the skin and/or underlying soft tissue resulting from specific positioning during a lengthy surgery or procedure
- Positioning Injury: localized damage to the skin and/or underlying soft tissue resulting from positioning
- Pressure Injury: localized damage to the skin and/or underlying soft tissue, usually over a bony prominence or related to a medical or other device, from intense and/or prolonged pressure or pressure in combination with shear
- Surgical Wound: intentional incision through the skin or mucosa to reach underlying structures
- Traumatic Wound: avulsion, abrasion, or other opening in the skin from force
- Venous Ulcer: open wound resulting from high venous pressure, usually on the inner ankle

Common Causes

- Burns
- Cancer
- Diabetes
- Immune problems, including immune reaction, psoriasis, and dermatitis
- Impaired tissue perfusion
- Infection or infestation
- Inflammatory disorders, including acne
- Neuropathy
- Obesity
- Smoking
- Surgery
- Thermal or radiation injury
- Trauma

Manifestations

- Bleeding or bruising
- Exudate and drainage
- Fever
- Inflammation
- Loss of function
- Lymphedema
- Nerve damage
- Pain
- Pressure injury
- Primary lesions, including macules, papules, vesicles, plaques, wheals, and pustules
- Pruritis
- Secondary lesions, including fissures, ulcers, excoriations, scales, and scars
- Skin atrophy
- Traumatic wound
- Variations in pigmentation
- Diagnostic tests: positive wound culture may confirm infection
- Laboratory tests may show leukocytosis and hyperglycemia

Key Conceptual Relationships

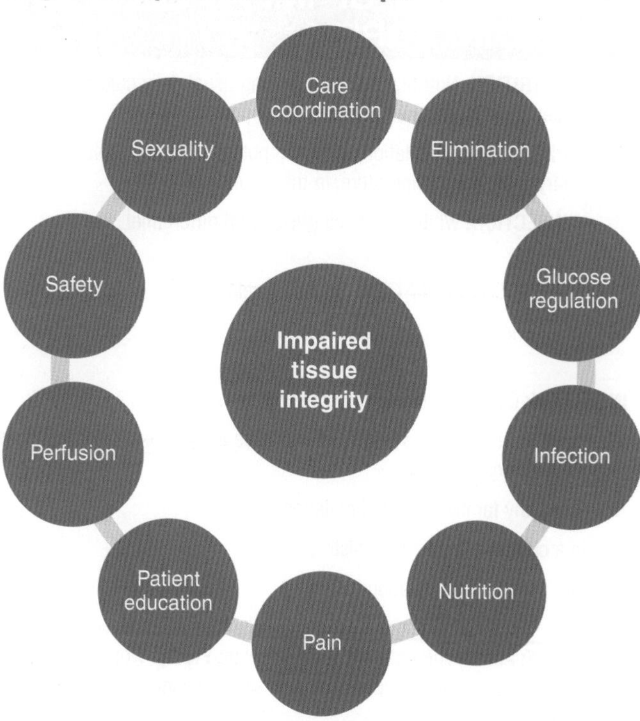

ASSESSMENT OF IMPAIRED TISSUE INTEGRITY	RATIONALE
Determine the cause of the wound.	The cause of the wound guides the selection of interventions.
Obtain a thorough history of the patient's skin problem, including: • Onset, sudden or gradual • Duration, recurrance • Any changes noted • Accompanying symptoms • Alleviating and aggravating factors • Treatments the patient has tried and response • Skin hygiene practices	A thorough history aids in evaluating the skin problem and helps direct treatment.
Evaluate the patient's underlying health status, noting factors that may delay wound healing.	Health status has a significant influence on the patient's wound healing.
Perform a complete physical assessment and monitor indicators of wound healing on an ongoing basis:	

• Thorough assessment of the wound on admission and with each dressing change, noting:
  • Location
  • Size (longest length, widest width), shape, undermining, and tunneling
  • Color of the wound and surrounding tissues
  • Type of tissue in the wound
  • Color, odor, and consistency of any drainage or exudate
  • Associated symptoms, including pain, bruising, and loss of function
  • Presence of drains in a surgical wound and tissue characteristics around the drains
	Redness of the surrounding tissue, foul odor, or purulent drainage may indicate wound infection. Early detection allows for prompt treatment.

• Compare affected and unaffected areas of the skin to detect differences.	Subtle changes in skin color such as blanching or erythema may be difficult to detect visually in persons with dark skin tones. Comparison to an unaffected skin area may help to identify changes.
• Vital signs	Elevations in pulse and temperature may occur with a wound infection.

Continued

ASSESSMENT OF IMPAIRED TISSUE INTEGRITY	RATIONALE
• **NUTRITION:** Nutrition status, including usual daily caloric intake, diet choices, and use of nutrition support	Proper nutrition supports wound healing.
• **PERFUSION:** Circulation, including pulse, sensation, color, capillary refill, and temperature, in the wound area	Inadequate perfusion is associated with poor wound healing.
• **INFECTION:** White blood cell (WBC) with differential	Evaluation of the WBC count and differential can confirm the presence of leukocytosis associated with infection.
• **GLUCOSE REGULATION:** Glucose levels	Hyperglycemia inhibits wound healing.
Assess for unrecognized tissue injuries.	Reduced blood flow to the tissues and diminished perception of pain makes skin more prone to injury.
INFECTION: Obtain wound culture specimens, as ordered.	Cultures determine whether a pathogen is present and guide treatment.
Inquire about the patient's history of exposure to irritants and ultraviolet (UV) radiation/sunlight.	Exposure to irritants may cause immediate skin disruptions or contribute to long-term damage.
Ask about any family history of melanoma.	Family history of melanoma increases the risk for the patient.
Obtain a complete medication history.	Some medications cause the skin to thin or be more sensitive to UV light.
Obtain a complete vaccination history.	Patients with wounds contaminated by foreign material may require a tetanus toxoid injection.
SEXUALITY: Assess the patient's feelings related to the wound, such as fear of disfigurement, depression, and sadness, and their impact on self-image.	These feelings can occur with skin problems that alter physical appearance.
Evaluate the effectiveness of measures used to enhance healing through ongoing assessment.	Wound healing may be difficult, and adjustments in therapy may be needed.
SUBSTANCE USE: Screen for the presence of tobacco and/or other substance use problems.	Smoking and tobacco use cause oral irritation and increase the risk of infection.
Use the mnemonic ABCDE to remember the early signs of melanoma during a skin assessment: • **A**symmetry: the shape of one half does not match that of the other half. • **B**order that is irregular: the edges are often ragged, notched, or blurred in outline. The pigment may spread into the surrounding skin. • **C**olor that is uneven: shades of black, brown, and tan may be present. Areas of white, gray, red, pink, or blue may be seen. • **D**iameter: there is a change in size, usually an increase. • **E**volving: the mole has changed during the past few weeks or months.	Early detection and treatment of melanoma improve outcomes.

ASSESSMENT OF A PRESSURE INJURY	RATIONALE
To do a pressure injury risk assessment, use a validated assessment tool such as the Braden Scale.	Using a consistent approach to risk assessment for pressure injuries supports planning for injury prevention, treatment, and monitoring outcomes.
Assess injury using staging categories based on those outlined by the National Pressure Ulcer Advisory Panel.	Standardized categories allow for effective documentation, communication, and treatment decisions.

Expected Outcomes

The patient will:

- avoid exposure to skin irritants.
- maintain integrity of skin and mucous membranes.
- demonstrate effective wound care.
- experience progress in wound healing.
- identify and report signs of wound infection.

INTERVENTIONS TO PROMOTE WOUND HEALING	RATIONALE
Implement collaborative interventions aimed at treating any underlying risk factor associated with the wound.	Treatment of underlying risk factors enhances wound healing.
Notify the health care provider (HCP) if the wound is not healing or worsens.	Achievement of an effective treatment plan often requires adjustments in therapy.
Provide appropriate wound care:	
• Cleanse wounds with normal saline or a nontoxic cleanser.	Nontoxic cleansers avoid damage to granulating tissue.
• Change dressing using sterile technique.	Sterile technique reduces the risk of wound infection
• Apply and reinforce a dressing appropriate for wound type and drainage.	Debridement or control of infection may require medications or specially impregnated wound dressings.
• **INFECTION:** Apply prescribed topical agents or therapeutic dressings, if needed.	Debridement or control of infection may require medications or specially impregnated wound dressings.
Assess and maintain function of special wound equipment or wound vacuum.	Therapies may be used to support the healing process.
Position the patient to avoid placing tension on the wound.	Pressure impedes the blood flow needed for healing.
Implement infection control procedures, including: • Strict handwashing. • Remind the patient not to touch the wound. • Keep the patient's environment as free as possible from contamination.	Infection control procedures help keep the wound free from further infection.
Administer prescribed antimicrobial therapy.	The patient may receive antimicrobials to prevent or manage a wound infection.
SEXUALITY: Assist the patient with managing any feelings of fear of disfigurement, scarring, and body image concerns.	The patient may be distressed at the thought or sight of an incision or wound because of fear of scarring or disfigurement.
Avoid inappropriate facial expressions that may make the patient feel ashamed of or concerned about the wound.	Avoid causing the patient emotional distress.
PAIN: Administer prescribed analgesics, timed to provide peak action during painful dressing changes or wound care.	The timing of analgesics can reduce the pain experience of major wound procedures.
Encourage nonpharmacologic methods of pain control, such as guided imagery and distraction.	Nonpharmacologic methods may decrease the needed dose or frequency of analgesic medications.
NUTRITION: Provide a nutritionally adequate diet, high in protein and vitamins.	Proper nutrition is needed to provide the nutrients necessary to support wound healing.
Implement measures to promote tissue integrity:	
• Use devices to reduce pressure (low-air-loss mattresses, foam mattresses, wheelchair cushions, padded commode seats, heel boots) as appropriate.	The use of devices reduces pressure on the skin and tissue to prevent injury.
• Reposition frequently on an individualized schedule based on risk factors, patient's overall condition, and type of mattress and support surface.	Pressure impedes the blood flow needed for healing.
• Keep bedding and other surfaces clean and dry.	Excess moisture leads to tissue maceration and accelerates injury.
• **ELIMINATION:** Prevent and manage incontinence as needed.	Excess moisture and caustic fluids contribute to tissue damage.
• Use devices (e.g., lift sheets, slide boards) and adequate help to avoid friction on the skin and shearing force when repositioning the patient.	Friction damages the skin.

Continued

INTERVENTIONS TO PROMOTE WOUND HEALING	RATIONALE
SAFETY: Implement measures to reduce the risk of positioning injury: • Use devices such as a trapeze, slide sheets, and mechanical lifts to move and position dependent or obese patients in bed. • Obtain special bariatric beds and lift devices for patients who are extremely obese. • Apply pressure-point padding over nerves, skin over bony prominences, earlobes, and eyes. • Maintain correct anatomic alignment, using devices as needed.	Precautions are needed to prevent the risk of positioning injury to the patient or physical injury to the staff.
PERFUSION: Implement venous thromboembolism (VTE) prophylaxis appropriate for the level of risk and measures to promote venous return in affected extremities.	Enhancing venous return and reducing the incidence of VTE promotes fluid mobilization and adequate circulation to promote wound healing.
IMMUNITY: Administer vaccinations as needed, according to recommended schedules and patient need.	Patients with wounds contaminated by foreign material may require a tetanus toxoid injection.
GLUCOSE REGULATION: Maintain glycemic control for patients with diabetes.	Hyperglycemia impairs wound healing and increases the risk of infection.

INTERVENTIONS TO MANAGE PRESSURE INJURIES	RATIONALE
Implement prevention measures for patients at risk for pressure injuries.	Preventing pressure injuries maintains quality of life.
Use devices to reduce pressure (low-air-loss mattresses, foam mattresses, wheelchair cushions, padded commode seats, heel boots) as appropriate.	Reduce pressure on skin and tissue to prevent injury.
MOBILITY: Reposition frequently on an individualized schedule based on risk factors, patient's overall condition, and type of mattress and support surface.	Pressure impedes the blood flow needed for healing.
Keep bedding and other surfaces clean and dry.	Excessive moisture leads to tissue maceration and accelerates injury.
Use devices (e.g., lift sheets, slide boards) and adequate help to avoid friction on skin and shearing force when repositioning the patient.	Friction damages skin.
ELIMINATION: Prevent and manage incontinence as needed.	Excessive moisture and caustic fluids contribute to tissue damage.
Assess and maintain the function of specialized wound equipment or wound vacuum.	Therapies may be used to promote the wound healing process.
Provide care of the wound incision site and pressure ulcer care, including prescribed topical agents or therapeutic dressings, if needed.	Debridement or control of infection may require medications or specially impregnated wound dressings
PAIN: Administer prescribed analgesics, timed to provide peak action during painful dressing changes and wound care.	This helps prevent the pain experienced during major wound procedures.
Encourage nonpharmacologic methods of pain control, such as guided imagery and distraction.	Nonpharmacologic methods may decrease the needed dose or frequency of analgesic medications.

COLLABORATION	RATIONALE
Wound, ostomy, and continence nurse (WOCN)	A WOCN can assess the patient and prescribe measures to promote optimal tissue integrity.
NUTRITION: Dietitian	The dietitian can recommend a diet with protein and other nutrients needed for wound healing.
CARE COORDINATION: Case management or social work	Resources may be available to help the patient obtain access to ongoing health care and secure needed supplies.

 PATIENT AND CAREGIVER TEACHING

- Process of wound healing and factors that affect wound healing
- How long it may take the wound to heal
- Management of underlying conditions influencing wound healing
- Skin hygiene practices
- Specific skin care and wound care regimens
- Obtaining, storing, and disposing of wound care supplies
- Prescribed topical and systemic medications, including proper administration and side effects
- Signs and symptoms of wound infection
- ABCDEF mnemonic for comprehensive monthly skin self-assessments
- Importance of proper nutrition and adequate rest
- How to protect the wound
- Measures to prevent wound recurrence, if appropriate
- Community and self-help resources available
- Where to find additional information
- When to notify the HCP or WOCN

DOCUMENTATION

Assessment

- Assessments performed
- Characteristics of lesions and wounds
- Laboratory results

Interventions

- Discussions with other members of the interprofessional team
- Environment modifications made
- Medications given
- Notification of HCP about patient status and assessment findings
- Therapeutic interventions and the patient's response
- Teaching provided
- Referrals initiated

Evaluation

- Patient's status: improved, stable, declined
- Characteristics of lesions and wounds
- Response to therapeutic interventions
- Response to teaching provided

Risk for Impaired Skin Integrity 46

Definition

At risk for loss of intact skin/tissue barrier

Being at risk for impaired skin integrity means the patient's skin is vulnerable to injury or unable to heal normally. Preventing pressure injuries is an important aspect of nursing care. A pressure injury is localized damage to the skin and/or underlying soft tissue. It usually occurs over a bony prominence or where tissue is in contact with a medical or other device. The injury occurs because of intense and/or prolonged pressure or pressure, in combination with shear. The most common sites for pressure injuries are the sacrum and the heels. Oxygen devices such as nasal cannulas may cause constant pressure above the ears, leading to tissue injury.

Preventing pressure injuries is challenging because the cause of pressure injuries varies by clinical setting. They are commonly seen in high-risk persons, such as older adults, those who are debilitated, or those who are chronically ill. Critical care patients are at high risk because of the use of medical devices, hemodynamic instability, and the use of vasoactive drugs. Foot ulcerations resulting from pressure or trauma are most likely to occur in persons with diabetes who have impaired circulation and neuropathy. The patient in surgery may be at risk for a perioperative positioning injury.

A primary nursing responsibility is identifying patients at risk for developing impaired skin integrity and implementing evidence-based injury prevention strategies for those at risk.

Associated Clinical Problems

- Risk for Diabetic Foot Ulcer: at risk for developing distal foot wounds as a result of vascular complications of diabetes
- Risk for Impaired Oral Mucous Membranes: at risk for disruption of the tissue of the lips or oral cavity
- Risk for Perioperative Positioning Injury: at risk for tissue damage as a result of specific positioning during a lengthy surgery or procedure
- Risk for Pressure Injury: at risk for injury as a result of prolonged pressure on tissue (Table 46.1)
- Risk for Stoma Complication: at risk for stoma injury as a result of positioning/weight of appliance, clothing, or other factors
- Risk for Thermal Injury: at risk of skin damage from excessive heat or cold

Common Risk Factors

- Critically ill
- Debilitation or chronic illness
- Diabetes
- Fluid imbalance
- History of prior pressure injury
- Immune problem, including immune reaction or posttransplantation
- Impaired circulation or mobility
- Impaired cognition
- Inadequate nutrition
- Medications: chemotherapy, corticosteroids, hypnotics, opioids, sedative-hypnotics
- Neurologic problems, including spinal cord injury and stroke
- Neuropathy
- Obesity
- Older adult

Risk for Impaired Oral Mucous Membranes

- Alcohol use
- Decreased salivation
- Ineffective oral hygiene
- Mechanical factors, including braces and dentures
- Mouth breathing
- Nothing by mouth (NPO) status
- Oxygen therapy
- Periodontal disease
- Tobacco use

Pediatric

- Cleft lip or palate

Risk for Pressure Injury

- Advanced age
- Anemia
- Contractures
- Devices in contact with the skin
- Elevated body temperature
- Friction
- Hip fracture
- Incontinence
- Low diastolic blood pressure (<60 mm Hg)
- Pain

Table 46.1 Manifestations of Pressure Injuries

Stage 1: Nonblanchable redness Intact skin with nonblanchable redness of a localized area, usually over a bony prominence. Darkly pigmented skin may not have blanching; its color may differ from the surrounding area.
Stage 2: Partial-thickness loss of dermis Presents as a shallow open ulcer with a red-pink wound bed, without slough. May also present as an intact or open/ruptured serum-filled or serosanguineous-filled blister, or a shiny or dry shallow ulcer without slough or bruising. Bruising indicates deep tissue injury.
Stage 3: Full-thickness skin loss Subcutaneous fat may be visible, with no exposure of bone, tendon, or muscle. Slough may be present but does not obscure the depth of tissue loss. May include undermining and tunneling. The depth varies by anatomic location.
Stage 4: Full-thickness tissue loss Exposed bone, tendon, or muscle. Slough or eschar may be present; often includes undermining and tunneling. Depth varies by anatomic location. Ulcers can extend into muscle and/or supporting structures. Exposed bone/muscle is visible or directly palpable.
Unstageable/Unclassified: Full-thickness skin or tissue loss (depth unknown) Occurs when the actual depth of ulcer is completely obscured by slough and/or eschar in wound bed. Until enough slough and/or eschar are removed to expose the base of wound, the true depth cannot be determined. Stage 3 or 4 injury.
Suspected Deep Tissue Injury (Depth Unknown): Purple or maroon localized area of discolored intact skin or blood-filled blister resulting from damage of underlying soft tissue from pressure and/or shear. The area may be preceded by tissue that is painful, firm, mushy, boggy, warmer, or cooler compared with adjacent tissue. Deep tissue injury may be hard to detect in those with dark skin tones. May include a thin blister over a dark wound bed and become covered by thin eschar. Evolution may be rapid, exposing additional layers of tissue, even with optimal treatment.

- Presence of excess moisture
- Prolonged surgery
- Shear
- Vascular disease

Risk for Thermal Injury
- Exposure to temperature extremes
- Radiation therapy
- Use of thermal devices

Key Conceptual Relationships

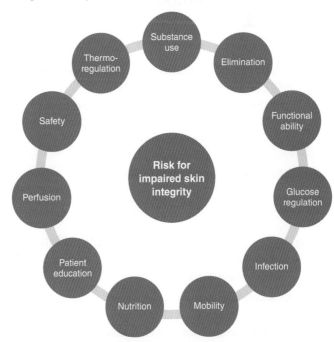

ASSESSMENT OF RISK FOR IMPAIRED SKIN INTEGRITY	RATIONALE
Assess for factors that increase the patient's risk for impaired skin integrity.	A thorough history can identify patients at risk for impaired skin integrity.
Evaluate the patient's underlying health status.	Health status has a significant influence on the patient's risk for infection.
Use a validated assessment tool, such as the Braden Scale (see Table 46.2), to do a pressure-injury risk assessment.	Using a consistent approach to risk assessment for pressure injuries supports planning for injury prevention, treatment, and monitoring outcomes.

Continued

ASSESSMENT OF RISK FOR IMPAIRED SKIN INTEGRITY	RATIONALE
Provide for patient privacy during any skin assessment or treatment by using a closed room or curtains and draping the patient modestly.	Ensuring privacy reflects respect for human dignity.
Assess skin and oral mucous membranes on admission, then as needed: • In acute care, reassess patients for pressure injuries at least every 24 hours. • In long-term care, reassess residents weekly for the first 4 weeks after admission and then at least monthly or quarterly. • In home care, reassess patients at every encounter.	Establishing a baseline supports planning for immediate care needs and provides a comparison for future assessments.
Perform a complete physical assessment and monitor for the development of wounds on an ongoing basis:	
• Inspect skin for color, integrity, scars, lesions, and signs of breakdown. • Inspect oral mucosa for moisture and intact surface. • Check facial and body hair for distribution, color, quantity, and hygiene. • Inspect nails for shape, contour, color, thickness, cleanliness, and dryness. • Palpate skin for temperature, texture, moisture, thickness, turgor, and mobility. • Assess skin near and in contact with medical devices such as oxygen tubing, casts, and braces.	A complete skin assessment helps to identify areas of concern and provides a baseline for comparison.
• Compare affected and unaffected areas of the skin to detect differences.	Subtle changes in skin color such as blanching or erythema may be difficult to detect visually in persons with dark skin tones. Comparison to an unaffected skin area may help to identify changes.
• **NUTRITION:** Nutrition status, including usual daily caloric intake, dietary choices, and use of nutrition support	Proper nutrition supports tissue integrity.
• **PERFUSION:** Circulation, including pulse, sensation, color, capillary refill, and temperature, in the wound area	Diminished perfusion is associated with an increased risk of impaired skin integrity.
• **MOBILITY:** Mobility and musculoskeletal function	Physical mobility problems and immobility have a significant impact on the risk of developing impaired skin integrity.
• **ELIMINATION:** Bowel and bladder function	Excessive moisture and caustic fluids associated with bowel and bladder incontinence increase the risk for tissue damage.
• **GLUCOSE REGULATION:** Glucose levels	Hyperglycemia is associated with impaired circulation and neuropathy, which increase the risk of impaired skin integrity.
Inquire about the patient's history of exposure to irritants and ultraviolet (UV) radiation/sunlight.	Exposure to irritants may cause immediate skin disruptions or contribute to long-term damage.
Obtain a complete medication history.	Some medications cause the skin to thin or be more sensitive to UV light.
Assess for unrecognized tissue injuries.	Reduced blood flow to the tissues and diminished perception of pain make the skin more prone to injury.
SUBSTANCE USE: Screen for the presence of tobacco and/or other substance use .	Smoking causes oral irritation, increasing the risk of impaired oral mucous membranes, and causes vasoconstriction, reducing tissue perfusion.
Evaluate the effectiveness of measures used to promote skin integrity through ongoing assessment.	Ongoing assessment allows for changes in the treatment plan.

Expected Outcomes

The patient will:

- avoid exposure to skin irritants.
- maintain integrity of skin and mucous membranes.
- recognize factors that may lead to impaired skin integrity and take preventative action.

Table 46.2 Braden Scale

Patients with a total score of 16 or less are considered at risk: 15 to 16 = low risk, 13 to 14 = moderate risk, 12 or less = high risk. Undertake and document risk assessment within 6 hours of admission or on the first home visit. Reassess if there is a change in the individual's condition and repeat regularly according to local protocol.

SENSORY PERCEPTION Ability to respond meaningfully to pressure-related discomfort	1. Completely limited: unresponsive (does not moan, flinch, or grasp) to painful stimuli as a result of diminished level of consciousness or sedation OR limited ability to feel pain over most of body surface.	2. Very limited: responds only to painful stimuli. Cannot communicate discomfort except by moaning or restlessness OR has a sensory impairment that limits the ability to feel pain or discomfort over ½ of the body.	3. Slightly limited: responds to verbal commands but cannot always communicate discomfort or need to be turned OR has some sensory impairment that limits the ability to feel pain or discomfort in 1 or 2 extremities.	4. No impairment: responds to verbal commands. Has no sensory deficit that would limit the ability to feel or voice pain or discomfort.
MOISTURE Degree to which skin is exposed to moisture	1. Constantly moist: skin is kept moist, almost constantly by perspiration, urine, etc. Dampness is detected every time patient is moved or turned.	2. Moist: skin is often but not always moist. Linens must be changed at least once a shift.	3. Occasionally moist: skin is occasionally moist, requiring an extra linen change approximately once a day.	4. Rarely moist: skin is usually dry; linens only require changing at routine intervals.
ACTIVITY Degree of physical activity	1. Bedfast: confined to bed.	2. Chairfast: ability to walk severely limited or nonexistent. Cannot bear own weight and/or must be assisted into chair or wheelchair.	3. Walks occasionally: walks occasionally during day but for very short distances, with or without assistance. Spends majority of each shift in bed or chair.	4. Walks frequently: walks outside the room at least twice a day and inside room at least once every 2 hours during waking hours.
MOBILITY Ability to change and control body position	1. Completely immobile: does not make even slight changes in body or extremity position without assistance.	2. Very limited: makes occasional slight changes in body or extremity position but unable to make frequent or significant changes independently.	3. Slightly limited: makes frequent though slight changes in body or extremity position independently.	4. No limitations: makes major and frequent changes in position without assistance.
NUTRITION Usual food intake pattern	1. Very poor: never eats complete meal. Rarely eats more than ⅓ of any food offered. Eats 2 servings or less of protein (meat or dairy products) per day. Takes fluids poorly. Does not take a liquid dietary supplement OR is nothing by mouth (NPO) and/or maintained on clear liquid or intravenous (IV) fluid for more than 5 days.	2. Probably inadequate: rarely eats a complete meal and generally eats only about ½ of any food offered. Protein intake includes only 3 servings of meat or dairy products per day. Occasionally will take dietary supplement OR receives less than optimum amount of liquid diet or tube feeding.	3. Adequate: eats over half of most meals. Eats a total of 4 servings of protein (meat, dairy products) each day. Occasionally will refuse a meal but will usually take a supplement if offered OR is on a tube feeding or total parenteral nutrition (TPN) regimen, which probably meets most nutritional needs.	4. Excellent: eats most of every meal. Never refuses a meal. Usually eats a total of 4 or more servings of meat and dairy products. Occasionally eats between meals. Does not require supplementation.
FRICTION AND SHEAR	1. Problem: requires moderate to maximum assistance in moving. Complete lifting without sliding against sheets is impossible. Frequently slides down in bed or chair, requiring frequent repositioning with maximum assistance. Spasticity, contractures, or agitation leads to almost constant friction.	2. Potential problem: moves feebly or requires minimum assistance. During a move, skin probably slides to some extent against sheets, chair, restraints, or other devices. Maintains relatively good position in chair or bed most of the time but occasionally slides down.	3. No apparent problem: moves in bed and in chair independently and has sufficient muscle strength to lift up completely during move. Maintains good position in bed or chair at all times.	

Source: Agency for Healthcare Research and Quality. Preventing Pressure Ulcers in Hospitals. www.ahrq.gov/patient-safety/settings/hospital/resource/pressureulcer/tool/pu7b.html.

INTERVENTIONS TO MAINTAIN SKIN INTEGRITY	RATIONALE
Implement collaborative interventions aimed at treating risk factors for impaired skin integrity.	Treatment of risk factors supports prevention of skin/tissue damage.
Notify health care provider (HCP) if a new wound develops.	The development of a wound requires prompt medical attention.
NUTRITION: Provide a nutritionally adequate diet, high in protein and vitamins.	Proper nutrition is needed to maintain tissue integrity.
Implement measures to promote tissue integrity:	
• Use devices to reduce pressure (low-air-loss mattresses, foam mattresses, wheelchair cushions, padded commode seats, heel boots) as appropriate.	The use of devices reduces pressure on the skin and tissues to prevent injury.
• Protect pressure points from medical devices such as oxygen tubing, feeding tubes, and casts.	Devices that remain in place over time can cause continuous pressure on the tissues.
• Reposition frequently on an individualized schedule based on risk factors, patient's overall condition, and type of mattress and support surface.	Pressure impedes the blood flow needed for healing.
• Keep bedding and other surfaces clean and dry.	Excess moisture leads to tissue maceration and accelerates injury.
• **ELIMINATION:** Prevent and manage incontinence as needed.	Excess moisture and caustic fluids contribute to tissue damage.
• Use devices (lift sheets, slide boards) to avoid friction on the skin and shearing force when repositioning the patient.	Friction damages the skin.
• Obtain adequate help and/or lifting devices to avoid dragging the patient's skin on the bedding surface.	Friction damages the skin.
SAFETY: Implement measures to reduce the risk of positioning injury: • Use devices such as a trapeze, slide sheets, and mechanical lifts to move and position in bed patients who are dependent or obese. • Obtain special bariatric beds and lift devices for patients who are extremely obese. • Apply pressure point padding over nerves, skin over bony prominences, earlobes, and eyes. • Maintain correct anatomic alignment, using devices as needed.	Precautions are needed to prevent the risk of a positioning injury to the patient or a physical injury to the staff.
Implement measures to assist the patient with mobility, encouraging ambulation and exercises to the extent of their ability.	Activity stimulates circulation and directly reduces the harmful effects of immobility.
PERFUSION: Implement venous thromboembolism (VTE) prophylaxis for the level of risk and measures to promote venous return in affected extremities.	Enhancing venous return and reducing the incidence of VTE promotes fluid mobilization and adequate circulation to maintain skin integrity.
GLUCOSE REGULATION: Maintain glycemic control for patients with diabetes.	Hyperglycemia impairs wound healing and increases the risk of infection.
FUNCTIONAL ABILITY: Assist with the patient with meeting needs related to nutrition, hydration, and personal hygiene.	Nutrition, hydration, and adequate personal hygiene reduce the risk of impaired skin integrity.
When removing tape or adhesive dressings, gently release the skin from the tape rather than pulling the tape away from the skin. Consider using an adhesive remover liquid rather than force to remove tape.	Removing adhesive dressings may lead to skin tears.

INTERVENTIONS TO REDUCE THE RISK FOR IMPAIRED ORAL MUCOUS MEMBRANES	RATIONALE
Have the patient avoid irritating food and fluids, such as highly spiced food or items with temperature extremes.	Irritating foods and fluids increase the risk of injury to the oral mucous membranes.
Provide oral care at least every 4 hours while the patient is awake.	Proper oral hygiene reduces the risk of impaired oral mucous membranes.
Provide frequent lip lubrication.	Keeping the lips moist helps prevent drying and cracking, which promotes skin integrity.
SUBSTANCE USE: Promote smoking and tobacco cessation interventions, as appropriate.	Smoking and tobacco use cause oral irritation and increase the risk of impaired oral mucous membranes.

INTERVENTIONS TO REDUCE THE RISK OF THERMAL INJURY	RATIONALE
Teach the patient to protect the skin from extreme temperatures and UV exposure.	Excess heat, cold, or UV exposure can cause acute and chronic tissue injury.
THERMOREGULATION: Implement measures to address alterations in temperature.	Maintaining normothermia reduces the risk of thermal injuries.
For patients receiving radiation therapy, reinforce specific skin care instructions.	Patients may need to avoid applying specific types of skin lotions or products during radiation therapy to minimize skin injury.
Monitor skin status when thermal interventions such as ice packs and heating pads are used. Provide frequent skin checks if thermal devices are needed for patients with impaired sensation, mobility, or consciousness.	Changes in sensation or inability to respond may lead to thermal injury if the patient is not closely monitored.

COLLABORATION	RATIONALE
Wound, ostomy, and continence nurse (WOCN)	A WOCN can assess the patient and prescribe measures to promote optimal tissue integrity.
NUTRITION: Dietitian	The dietitian can prescribe a diet with protein and other nutrients needed for optimal tissue health.
CARE COORDINATION: Case management or social work	Resources may be available to help the patient obtain access to ongoing health care.
MOBILITY: Physical therapy	Physical therapists assess, plan, and implement interventions that address problems associated with immobility.

PATIENT AND CAREGIVER TEACHING

- Causes of wounds and risks for developing a wound
- Management of conditions contributing to the increased risk of developing a wound
- Screening examinations and surveillance for skin integrity problems
- Skin hygiene practices
- Injury prevention from sun exposure and thermal injury
- Pressure injury prevention
- Early signs and symptoms of a skin integrity problem
- Proper nutrition
- Where to find additional information and support
- When to notify the HCP and seek care

DOCUMENTATION

Assessment

- Assessments performed
- Characteristics of lesions and wounds
- Laboratory results

Interventions

- Discussions with members of the interprofessional team
- Environmental modifications made
- Medications given
- Notification of the HCP about patient status and assessment findings
- Therapeutic interventions and the patient's response
- Teaching provided
- Referrals initiated

Evaluation

- Patient's status: improved, stable, declined
- Characteristics of lesions and wounds
- Response to therapeutic interventions
- Response to teaching provided

Anxiety 47

Definition

A subjectively distressing experience based on perception of psychological or physiologic threat.

Anxiety is a feeling of apprehension, uneasiness, or dread about the future and worry about the ability to predict or cope with those events. Anxiety can be episodic or chronic, mild or severe, adaptive or functionally impairing, and a symptom or a disorder. It is sometimes called the "fight-or-flight response" because it is the physiologic reaction that occurs in response to a perceived threat or impending danger. Although mild anxiety may be helpful in focusing attention, increasing amounts of anxiety tend to decrease problem-solving ability and other cognitive functions.

This concept focuses on anxiety as a normal experience in response to uncertainty. Anxiety is common in the context of uncertainty in health disruptions and medical procedures. However, a level of anxiety that interferes with daily life may represent an anxiety disorder, requiring additional resources and treatment. Anxiety affects many aspects of life, including relationships, role performance, and health. The person's ability to take part in activities of daily living and meet role expectations is an indicator of the severity. Depression or other emotional problems may interfere further with engaging in activities.

The nurse recognizes a range of anxiety, from mild anxiety to panic, and can intervene to help patients manage their anxiety (Table 47.1). Providing education about how to manage anxiety and helping the patient connect with community and self-help resources can help the patient cope with anxiety and promote quality of life.

Associated Clinical Problems

- Agitation: excessive, purposeless activity, usually associated with anxiety
- Death Anxiety: apprehension about the possibility or manner of death
- Fear: concern focused on a specific perceived threat

Common Risk Factors

Health Conditions

- Asthma
- Cancer
- Chronic infections
- Chronic obstructive pulmonary disease
- Declining health or terminal illness
- Degenerative neuromuscular disease
- Diabetes
- Drug or alcohol withdrawal
- Heart disease
- Irritable bowel syndrome
- Mood disorders, including depression
- Pheochromocytoma
- Substance use
- Thyroid disease
- Vestibular dysfunction

Situational

- Developmental or maturational crisis
- Impending death
- Major life change, such as a change in finances, environment, health, role, or status
- Presence or perception of stressors or threat
- Sensory impairment
- Separation from support system
- Situational crisis
- Traumatic incident
- Unfamiliar environment
- Value conflict
- Victim of violence

Pediatric

- Peer group problems
- School problems

Manifestations

- See Table 47.1
- Death anxiety
  - Fear of pain, dying process
  - Powerlessness
  - Sadness
  - Spiritual concerns, doubting beliefs
  - Worry about the impact of one's death on family
- Fear
  - Alarm
  - Apprehension
  - Increased tension
  - Panic
  - Self-report of fear
  - Terror

Table 47.1 Four Levels of Anxiety

Four Levels of Anxiety			
Mild Anxiety	**Moderate Anxiety**	**Severe Anxiety**	**Panic**
• Enhanced learning • Heightened awareness • Increase in senses, arousal • Increased motivation • Optimal functioning • Sleeplessness	• Decreased concentration • Decreased problem solving • Less alert, aware of surroundings • Narrowed perceptual field • Muscular tension • Increased heart rate, respiratory rate, and perspiration • Rapid speech	• Concentration progressively narrowed • Severely impaired cognition and attention • Changes in blood pressure (BP), palpitations • Headache, pupil dilation • Anorexia, nausea • Restlessness	• Complete lack of focus • Emotional and behavioral dysregulation • Marked functional impairment • Tendency to misperceive environment

Key Conceptual Relationships

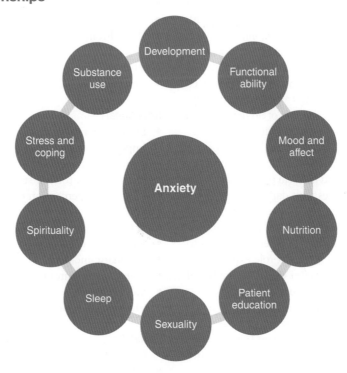

ASSESSMENT OF ANXIETY	RATIONALE
Assess for factors and health conditions that increase the risk for the patient experiencing anxiety.	Health conditions (e.g., hypoxia and hypoglycemia) may cause symptoms of anxiety.
Evaluate the patient's underlying health status.	Health status has a significant influence on mood.
Use a formal, patient-specific tool, such as the Beck Anxiety Inventory (Table 47.2) or the Posttraumatic Stress Disorder (PTSD) Checklist (Table 47.3), to detect the presence of anxiety.	Identifying the presence of anxiety allows for early intervention.
Assess the patient's perception of anxiety.	The patient's perception of the presence and level of anxiety may differ from other indicators of anxiety.
Perform a physical assessment and monitor indicators of anxiety on an ongoing basis:	
• Manifestations of anxiety	Identifying the presence of manifestations of anxiety allows for early intervention.

ASSESSMENT OF ANXIETY	RATIONALE
• Complete mental status examination, including appearance, attitude, mood and affect, speech, behavior, thought process and content, cognition, insight, and judgment.	Anxiety may affect cognition and other mental processes.
• Vital signs, comparing to baseline values	Anxiety may manifest in tachycardia and elevated BP, which will affect other health conditions.
STRESS AND COPING: Assess the current and past use of stress management and coping strategies.	A patient with anxiety may be relying on negative behaviors as a means of coping with stress.
MOOD AND AFFECT: Assess mental status and screen for coexisting depression or other problems.	Many patients with anxiety have coexisting depression or other psychological disorders.
Assess the patient's support system: • Who do they live with? • Are they employed? • Are friends and relatives accessible? • Have they used any community resources?	Interest and support from others are important aspects of managing anxiety.
FUNCTIONAL ABILITY: Perform a psychosocial assessment, evaluating for any lifestyle effects, such as problems with social interaction, ability to perform responsibilities, and ability to engage in physical activities.	Problems resulting from anxiety can affect all aspects of a person's life.
SUBSTANCE USE: Screen for the presence of alcohol, tobacco, and/or other substance use.	A patient with anxiety is at higher risk for substance use disorder.
SPIRITUALITY: Assess the patient's spiritual well-being.	There is a significant relationship between anxiety and spiritual well-being.
Evaluate the effectiveness of measures used to address anxiety through ongoing monitoring.	Monitoring the patient allows for evaluation of therapy effectiveness.
Pediatric	
Consider using a standardized anxiety scale, such as the Beck Anxiety Inventory for Youth.	Monitor changes in levels of anxiety.
Assess for separation anxiety.	Separation anxiety is identified by level of concern about being apart from a specific person.

Table 47.2 Beck Anxiety Inventory

The following is a list of common symptoms of anxiety. Please carefully read each item on the list. Indicate how much you have been bothered by that symptom during the past month, including today, by circling the number in the corresponding space in the column next to each symptom.

	Not at All	Mildly, But It Did Not Bother Me Much	Moderately—It Was Not Pleasant at Times	Severely—It Bothered Me a Lot
Numbness or tingling	0	1	2	3
Feeling hot	0	1	2	3
Wobbliness in legs	0	1	2	3
Unable to relax	0	1	2	3
Fear of worst happening	0	1	2	3
Dizzy or lightheaded	0	1	2	3
Heart pounding/racing	0	1	2	3
Unsteady	0	1	2	3
Terrified or afraid	0	1	2	3
Nervous	0	1	2	3
Feeling of choking	0	1	2	3
Hands trembling	0	1	2	3
Shaky/unsteady	0	1	2	3

Continued

Table 47.2 Beck Anxiety Inventory—cont'd

	Not at All	Mildly, but It Did Not Bother Me Much	Moderately—It Was Not Pleasant at Times	Severely—It Bothered Me a Lot
Fear of losing control	0	1	2	3
Difficulty in breathing	0	1	2	3
Fear of dying	0	1	2	3
Scared	0	1	2	3
Indigestion	0	1	2	3
Faint/lightheaded	0	1	2	3
Face flushed	0	1	2	3
Hot/cold sweats	0	1	2	3
Column Sum				

Scoring: Sum each column, then sum the column totals to achieve a grand score. The scores are classified as minimal anxiety (0–7), mild anxiety (8–15), moderate anxiety (16–25), and severe anxiety (30–63).
Source: Beck AT, Epstein N, Brown G, Steer RA. An inventory for measuring clinical anxiety: psychometric properties. *J Consult Clin Psychol.* 1988;56:893.

Table 47.3 Posttraumatic Stress Disorder (PTSD) Checklist

The following is a list of problems and complaints that people sometimes have in response to stressful life experiences. Please read each one carefully and circle the number that indicates how much you have been bothered by that problem in the last month.

No.	Response	Not at All	A Little Bit	Moderately	Quite a Bit	Extremely
1.	Repeated, disturbing memories, thoughts, or images of a stressful experience from the past?	1	2	3	4	5
2.	Repeated, disturbing dreams of a stressful experience from the past?	1	2	3	4	5
3.	Suddenly acting or feeling as if a stressful experience were happening again (as if you were reliving it)?	1	2	3	4	5
4.	Feeling very upset when something reminded you of a stressful experience from the past?	1	2	3	4	5
5.	Having physical reactions (e.g., heart pounding, trouble breathing, or sweating) when something reminded you of a stressful experience from the past?	1	2	3	4	5
6.	Avoid thinking about or talking about a stressful experience from the past or avoid having feelings related to it?	1	2	3	4	5
7.	Avoid activities or situations because they remind you of a stressful experience from the past?	1	2	3	4	5
8.	Trouble remembering important parts of a stressful experience from the past?	1	2	3	4	5
9.	Loss of interest in things that you used to enjoy?	1	2	3	4	5
10.	Feeling distant or cut off from other people?	1	2	3	4	5
11.	Feeling emotionally numb or being unable to have loving feelings for those close to you?	1	2	3	4	5
12.	Feeling as if your future will somehow be cut short?	1	2	3	4	5
13.	Trouble falling or staying asleep?	1	2	3	4	5
14.	Feeling irritable or having angry outbursts?	1	2	3	4	5
15.	Having difficulty concentrating?	1	2	3	4	5
16.	Being "super alert" or watchful/on guard?	1	2	3	4	5
17.	Feeling jumpy or easily startled?	1	2	3	4	5

Scoring: Sum the column totals to achieve a grand score. The scores are classified as 17–29, little to no severity; 28–29, some PTSD symptoms; 30–44, moderate to moderately high severity of PTSD symptoms; and 45–85, high severity of PTSD symptoms.
Source: Weathers F. Posttraumatic stress disorder checklist. In Reyes G, Elhai JD, Ford J (eds.): *Encyclopedia of Psychological Trauma.* Hoboken, NJ: Wiley; 2008.

Expected Outcomes

The patient will:

- identify when experiencing anxiety.
- identify and manage controllable sources of anxiety.
- manage anxiety response to a functional level.
- seek additional support as needed for anxiety disorder.

INTERVENTIONS TO MANAGE ANXIETY	RATIONALE
Implement collaborative interventions addressed at treating risk factors contributing to anxiety.	Treatment of risk factors can assist in improving the patient's mood.
Advocate for addressing health conditions, such as hypoxia or hypoglycemia, that may manifest through anxiety.	Anxiety may be a response to a physiologic state that can be treated.
Establish a therapeutic nurse–patient relationship: • Provide privacy and a calm, safe environment. • Use therapeutic touch, with the patient's consent. • Remain nonjudgmental. • Use active listening with therapeutic communication skills. • Respond honestly to patient questions and concerns.	A calm environment helps the patient feel safe and promotes trust between the patient and health care providers (HCPs).
Encourage the patient to talk about feelings and concerns.	Talking about feelings and concerns helps build rapport and decreases the patient's sense of isolation.
Help the patient identify triggers for anxiety.	Recognizing anxiety-producing situations prepares the patient to prevent or manage acute anxiety.
Assist the patient in obtaining information and developing appropriate problem-solving strategies in anxiety-provoking situations.	Developing problem-solving ability aids the patient in taking action to cope with difficulties, which can reduce anxiety.
STRESS AND COPING: Collaborate with the patient to select and implement complementary and spiritual support therapies, including relaxation, guided imagery, mindful breathing, yoga, and progressive muscle relaxation.	Complementary therapies can help reduce the manifestations of anxiety by promoting focus on mind and body connections.
Help the patient identify preferred diversionary activities while waiting for procedures or treatments.	Diversion may decrease anxiety temporarily.
Support family/caregivers of the patient who may also be anxious.	Family members may be able to provide significant support to the patient if they are able to manage their own anxieties.
Administer prescribed medications for ongoing anxiety, such as selective serotonin reuptake inhibitors (SSRIs), benzodiazepines, buspirone (Buspar), and tricyclic antidepressants.	Medications may be prescribed as part of the plan for managing chronic anxiety.
Assist the patient in identifying persons to whom they can express feelings openly.	Mood may be enhanced through sharing thoughts and feelings.
Assist the patient in reframing concerns as solvable problems.	Reframing may lessen or eliminate the source of anxiety.
FUNCTIONAL ABILITY: Help the patient develop strategies to increase participation in activities of daily living in the home, at work, and socially.	Anxiety may influence the ability to participate in activities of daily living.
MOOD AND AFFECT: Implement measures to assist the patient in managing any depression they may be experiencing.	Patients with anxiety often experience coexisting depression.
SLEEP: Provide the patient with opportunities for an environment conducive to adequate sleep.	A lack of adequate rest appears to be associated with increased anxiety.
NUTRITION: Encourage the patient to follow a nutritionally adequate diet.	It is believed that following a healthy, nutritionally sound diet lessens the incidence of anxiety.
Encourage participation in moderate-intensity exercise, such as walking, swimming, and bicycling.	Exercise raises levels of endorphins and may be helpful in the treatment of anxiety.
SEXUALITY: Implement measures to assist the patient in developing a positive self-image.	Patients with anxiety may have a negative self-image and low self-esteem.

Continued

INTERVENTIONS TO MANAGE ANXIETY	RATIONALE
SUBSTANCE USE: Implement measures to address substance use, if present.	A patient with anxiety is at higher risk for substance use disorder.
Pediatric	
Avoid showing medical equipment prior to use unless there is sufficient time for the child to play with and explore it safely, then process feelings.	The appearance of medical equipment can be frightening to a child.
Allow opportunities for the child to participate in play therapy, referring to a play therapy specialist as needed.	Play therapy provides insight into the child's coping and can help them cope with their emotions.

INTERVENTIONS TO MANAGE DEATH ANXIETY	RATIONALE
Encourage the patient to reflect upon what their life has meant and what makes them feel anxious about death.	Sharing encourages patients to acknowledge their anxiety and the value of their lives.
Assist the patient to reminisce and review their life in a positive manner.	Reminiscing encourages the patient to value their life by validating their accomplishments and self-worth.
SPIRITUALITY: Implement measures to address spiritual concerns.	There is a significant relationship between death anxiety and spiritual well-being.
Implement measures to assist the patient with managing grief.	Anticipatory grief is common among people who are facing the eventual death of a loved one or themselves.

INTERVENTIONS TO MANAGE SEPARATION ANXIETY	RATIONALE
Try gradual desensitization to the separation of concern.	A period of adjustment may be needed before separation anxiety resolves.
Provide access to objects that increase the sense of safety or transitional security objects, such as a blanket or favorite toy.	Having a security item provides a sense of safety in a new setting or situation.

COLLABORATION	RATIONALE
Child life specialist	A child life specialist can help the child manage anxiety related to health and health care through activities.
Behavioral counseling	Counseling may help patients manage moderate to severe anxiety or anxiety disorders.
Support groups and other mental health resources	Specialty mental health support services are available to assist the patient with managing the effects of anxiety.
MOOD AND AFFECT: Treatment for any coexisting psychological problems	Initiating treatment for depression or a coexisting psychological problem may assist with managing anxiety.
SPIRITUALITY: Pastoral care professional or preferred spiritual or religious leader	The patient with death anxiety may find comfort from their religious leaders, who provide support, perform spiritual counseling, and meet sacramental needs.

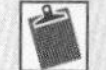 PATIENT AND CAREGIVER TEACHING

- Anxiety and its potential causes
- Recognizing the presence and extent of anxiety
- Managing sources of stress and perceived threat
- Promoting general wellness for strength to better cope with anxiety-producing situations
- Community and self-help resources, sources for information and social support
- Early recognition of problems and how to manage them
- Coping strategies and relaxation techniques
- Safe use of medications, including proper use and management of side effects, and how they fit into the overall management plan
- Importance of long-term follow-up
- When to notify the HCP and seek emergency assistance

DOCUMENTATION

Assessment

- Assessments performed
- Level of anxiety
- Manifestations of anxiety
- Screening test results

Interventions

- Discussions with other members of the interprofessional team
- Medications given
- Notification of the HCP about patient status
- Therapeutic interventions and the patient's response
- Teaching provided
- Referrals initiated

Evaluation

- Patient's status: improved, stable, declined
- Presence of any manifestations of anxiety
- Response to teaching provided
- Response to therapeutic interventions
- Plan for managing future situations

Impaired Cognition 48

Definition

An observable or measurable disturbance in thinking processes resulting from an abnormality in the brain or a factor interfering with normal brain function

Cognition is the mental action of acquiring knowledge and understanding through thought, experience, and the senses. Cognition refers to all the processes in human thought, including the reception, processing, storage, retrieval, and use of sensory input. Optimal brain function depends on the continuous perfusion of oxygenated and nutrient-rich blood. Decreased oxygen and glucose supply, as well as electrolyte and acid–base imbalances, significantly impair cognitive function. Cognitive changes from health conditions can be temporary or chronic. Depending on the cause, chronic states of impaired cognition can remain stable or decline over time.

Cognitive impairment can be devastating for the person and caregivers, particularly when the impairment is permanent, such as dementia. Ultimately, dementia adversely affects functional ability, role performance, and activities of daily living. Persons with dementia are at high risk for physical injury, impaired nutrition, and social isolation.

Delirium is a state of disturbed consciousness and altered cognition with a rapid onset over hours or a few days. It is common in older adults seen in emergency departments and is the most frequent complication of hospitalization for older adults. In a delirious state, the person experiences a reduced ability to focus, sustain, and shift attention. Memory, judgment, and orientation are impaired. Speech is rapid, rambling, and/or incoherent. Many conditions can lead to delirium, including dehydration, electrolyte imbalances, fever, hypoxia, sleep deprivation, adverse effects of medications, and illicit drug use. Delirium is often the first symptom of life-threatening problems such as pneumonia, urosepsis, or myocardial infarction. Delirium is usually reversible with prompt treatment. Nurses can make a difference by preventing conditions that lead to delirium, identifying the onset of delirium, and intervening for patient safety during states of impaired cognition.

Associated Clinical Problems

- Acute Confusion: disorientation regarding time, place, person, or situation occurring abruptly, over a short time interval
- Altered Thought Processes: disruption in mental activities such as conscious thought, orientation, problem solving, judgment, and comprehension
- Chronic Confusion: ongoing disorientation regarding time, place, person, or situation
- Confusion: mental state characterized by disorientation regarding time, place, person, or situation, causing a lack of orderly thought and an inability to choose or act decisively and perform the activities of daily living
- Delirium: state of disturbed consciousness and altered cognition with a rapid onset occurring over hours or days
- Diminished Judgment: inability to recognize the relationships of ideas and to form correct conclusions from data and experience
- Disorientation: state of mental confusion characterized by inadequate or incorrect perceptions of place, time, or identity
- Drowsy: sleepy or somnolent
- Impaired Abstract Thinking: inability to think flexibly or use concepts and generalizations
- Impaired Memory: inability to recall past experiences and prior learning
- Impaired Mental Alertness: diminished state of cognition with slowed, inactive thinking and decreased awareness of the environment
- Lack of Self-Awareness: diminished ability to explore and understand your own feelings, motivations, and behaviors
- Lethargy: state or quality of dullness, prolonged sleepiness, sluggishness, or serious drowsiness
- Limited Recall of Long-Past Events: diminished ability to remember experiences from years ago
- Limited Recall of Recent Events: diminished ability to remember experiences from recent hours
- Reduced Concentration: limited ability to focus on a mental task
- Restlessness: inability to rest or relax; unease or agitation
- Risk for Acute Confusion: increased risk for sudden short-term disorientation regarding time, place, person, or situation
- Risk for Confusion: increased risk for disorientation regarding time, place, person, or situation
- Risk for Delirium: increased risk for disturbed consciousness and altered cognition with a rapid onset
- Sedated: induced state of quiet, calmness, or sleep, by means of a medication
- Somnolence: condition of being sleepy or drowsy

Common Causes and Risk Factors

- Advanced age
- Cancer, chemotherapy
- Cardiovascular disease
- Chronic pulmonary disease
- Degenerative neurologic conditions, such as Parkinson disease, Huntington disease
- Dementia
- Depression
- Diabetes
- Environment exposures to lead or pesticides
- Hydrocephalus
- Intracranial tumor
- Immunologic disease, such as multiple sclerosis and systemic lupus erythematosus (SLE)
- Medication side effect
- Sensory deficit
- Stroke
- Substance use
- Traumatic brain injury

Delirium

- Electrolyte or fluid imbalance
- Hypoglycemia
- Hypoxia, anoxia
- Increased intracranial pressure
- Infection
- Intensive care unit stay
- Pain
- Sleep deprivation
- Substance use

Manifestations

- Agitation
- Altered cognitive functioning
- Altered personality or altered social functioning
- Decreased level of consciousness
- Deficits found through neuropsychometric testing
- Depression
- Diagnostic tests
- Diminished memory capacity
- Hallucinations
- Impaired judgment
- Inability to initiate purposeful behavior
- Lack of self-awareness
- Magnetic resonance imaging (MRI) and computed tomography (CT) imaging of brain lesions
- Misperception
- Personal care problem
- Reduced concentration
- Restlessness
- Wandering

Key Conceptual Relationships

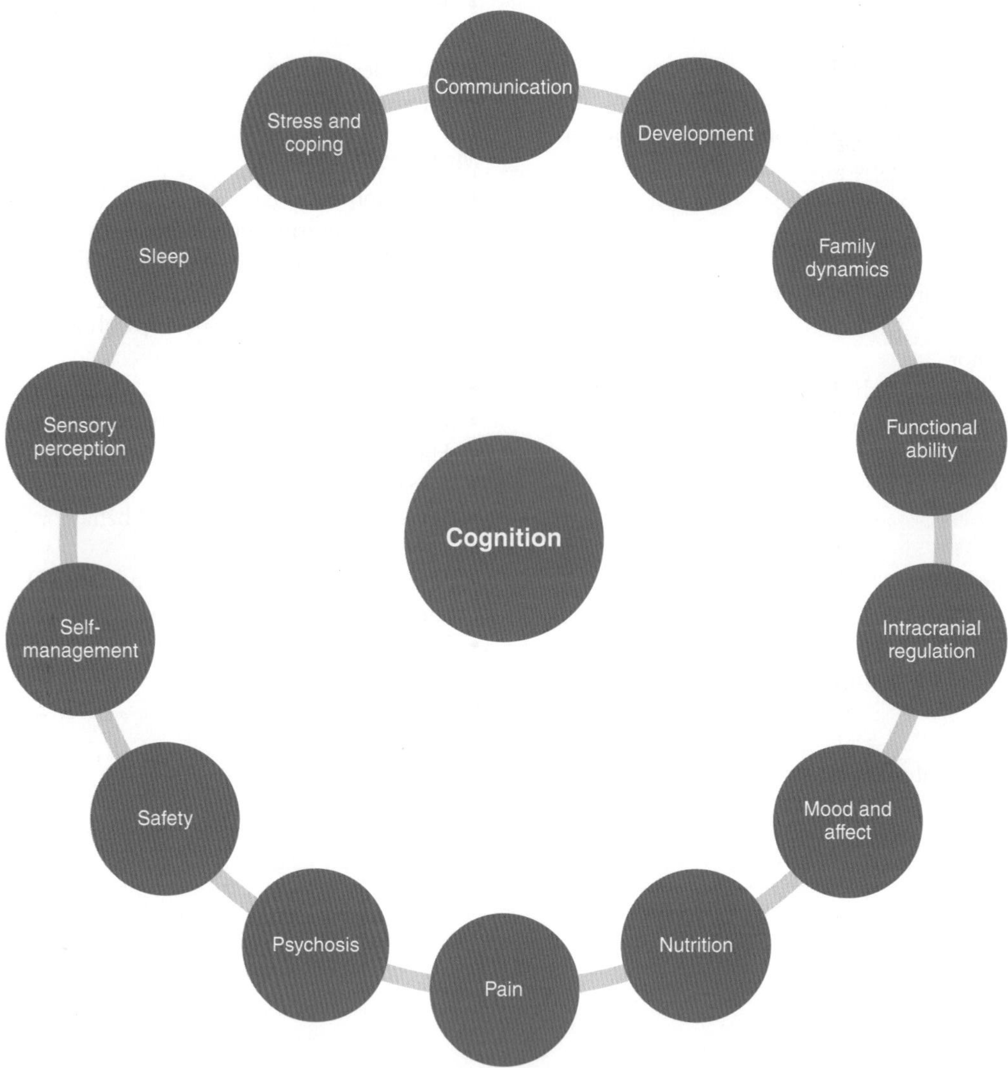

ASSESSMENT OF COGNITION	RATIONALE
Assess risk factors for impaired cognitive function, including intracranial disease, trauma, substance use, and chemical exposures.	Identifying factors or hazards that place the patient at risk for impaired cognition allows for early intervention.
Administer a brief screening tool for cognitive function, such as the Mini-Cog (Table 48.1).	Screening tools can guide the need for further evaluation and serve as a baseline for future comparison.
Obtain a thorough history of the patient's impaired cognition, including: • Onset, sudden or gradual • Frequency and severity of symptoms • Any fluctuation noted • Alleviating and aggravating factors	Abrupt changes may indicate physiologic causes of increased confusion that are acute and reversible.
Obtain a complete medication history, including prescribed and over-the-counter medications, herb and nutrition supplements, and recreational substances.	Impaired cognition can be associated with the use of medications and illicit substances.
Perform a physical assessment, focusing on underlying health status and potential causes of impaired cognition, and monitor indicators on an ongoing basis:	
• Identify manifestations of impaired cognitive function.	Identifying manifestations of impaired cognitive function allows for early intervention.

ASSESSMENT OF COGNITION	RATIONALE
• Assess level of consciousness, memory, logic and judgment, and any noticed change in behavior.	A thorough assessment can identify the current mental status and the presence of any deficits.
• Note any headaches, behavior changes, and seizures.	These manifestations are suggestive of a brain disorder.
• **COMMUNICATION:** Assess speech pattern and content, and difficulty in forming words or expressing ideas.	Identify the presence of any deficits.
• **MOOD AND AFFECT:** Screen for any coexisting psychological problems.	Many persons with dementia have coexisting psychological problems, particularly depression.
Review the results of diagnostic tests, including electrolyte panel, liver function tests, complete blood count, thyroid function tests, MRI, and CT scan.	Diagnostic tests may identify the most likely cause of impaired cognition.
SELF-MANAGEMENT: Determine the ability to meet self-care needs related to nutrition, elimination, hydration, and personal hygiene.	Unmet needs may lead to restlessness and health problems.
FUNCTIONAL ABILITY: Determine the patient's ability to perform basic and instrumental activities of daily living.	Impaired cognition affects functional status and the ability to fulfill roles and provide personal care.
If abnormalities are noted, perform an initial assessment, then ongoing monitoring with a standard cognitive assessment tool, such as the Mini-Mental State Examination (MMSE) (Table 48.2).	A standard assessment tool provides a baseline for future comparison and allows for changes to be tracked easily.
If abnormalities are noted, consult with health care team for specialized assessment.	Specific tools and processes may provide a more detailed assessment as a basis for care and treatment.
If the patient is unaware of changes, consult with family about the patient's cognitive function, including noting any problems with judgment, reduced interest in hobbies and activities, memory and behavior problems, problems managing finances, or consistent problems with thinking.	Family members and significant others can give important information in determining whether changes are acute or chronic and help establish the patient's baseline cognitive function.
Pediatric	
DEVELOPMENT: Assess for attainment and maintenance of development milestones and tasks.	Development progress is useful in assessing the mental status of the child.

Table 48.1 Mini-Cog

Administration

Tell the patient to listen carefully to and remember three unrelated words and then to repeat the words. *Example: apple, table, penny.* (This initial step is not scored.) The same three words may be repeated to the patient up to three tries to register all three words.

Tell the patient to draw the face of a clock, either on a blank sheet of paper or on a sheet with the clock circle already drawn on the page. After the patient puts the numbers on the clock face, ask them to draw the hands of the clock to read a specific time (11:10). The test is considered normal if all numbers are present in the correct sequence and position and the hands readably display the requested time.

Ask the patient to repeat the three previously stated words.

Scoring (Out of a Total of 5 Points)

Give 1 point for each word recalled without cues.

To score the clock drawing, give 2 points for a normal clock or 0 (zero) points for an abnormal clock drawing. A normal clock must include all numbers (1-12), each only once, in the correct order and direction (clockwise). There must also be two hands present, one pointing to the 11 and one pointing to the 2.

Interpretations

- Patients recalling none of the three words are classified as cognitively impaired (score = 0).
- Patients recalling all three words are classified as not cognitively impaired (score = 3).

Overall test:
0–2: Positive screen for dementia
3–5: Negative screen for dementia

Source: Borson S, Scanlan J, Brush M, et al. The Mini-Cog: a cognitive "vital signs" measure for dementia screening in multilingual elderly. *Int J Geriatr Psychiatry.* 2000;15:1021.

Table 48.2 Mini-Mental State Examination Sample Items

Orientation to Time
"What is the date?"
"What is the season?"
"What day of the week is it?"

Registration
"Listen carefully. I am going to say three words. You say them back after I stop. Ready? Here they are . . . HOUSE [pause], CAR [pause], LAKE [pause]. Now repeat those words back to me." (Repeat up to five times but score only the first trial.)

Naming
"What is this?" (Point to a pencil or pen.)

Reading
"Please read this and do what it says." (Show the examinee the words CLOSE YOUR EYES on the stimulus form.)"Please write a sentence."

ASSESSMENT OF DELIRIUM	RATIONALE
Administer a delirium rating scale, such as the Confusion Assessment Method (CAM) (Table 48.3), when confusion first appears, and use it for ongoing monitoring.	Standardizing the assessment allows for acute changes to be tracked easily.
Determine the potential cause of impaired cognition from delirium.	Treating the underlying cause usually contributes to the resolution of delirium.
Monitor neurologic status on an ongoing basis.	The patient's status will likely change over time.

Table 48.3 Confusion Assessment Method (CAM)

Delirium is diagnosed with the presence of features 1 and 2 and either 3 or 4.

Feature 1

Acute Onset and Fluctuating Course
Data usually obtained from a family member or nurse.
Shown by positive responses to the following questions:

- Is there evidence of an acute change in mental status from the patient's baseline?
- Did the (abnormal) behavior fluctuate during the day (i.e., tend to come and go or increase and decrease in severity)?

Feature 2

Inattention
Shown by positive response to the following question:

- Did the patient have problem focusing attention (e.g., being easily distractible or having problem keeping track of what was being said)?

Feature 3

Disorganized Thinking
Shown by a positive response to the following question:

- Was the patient's thinking disorganized or incoherent, such as rambling or irrelevant conversation, unclear or illogical flow of ideas, or unpredictable, switching from subject to subject?

Feature 4

Altered Level of Consciousness
Shown by any answer other than "alert" to the following question:

- Overall, how would you rate this patient's level of consciousness (alert [normal], vigilant [hyperalert], lethargic [drowsy, easily aroused], stupor [difficult to arouse], or coma [unarousable])?

Adapted from Inouye S, van Dyck C, Alessi C, et al. Clarifying confusion: the Confusion Assessment Method. *Ann Intern Med.* 1990;113:941.

Expected Outcomes

The patient will:

- maintain safety.
- (in cases of dementia) maintain functional ability for as long as possible.
- (in cases of delirium) demonstrate restoration of cognitive status to baseline.

INTERVENTIONS TO PROMOTE OPTIMAL COGNITION	RATIONALE
Introduce yourself when initiating contact, address the patient by name, and speak slowly.	This shows respect for the person in interactions.
Talk to the patient and often reorient to time, place, and person.	Reorienting as needed shows respect and regard.
Determine behavior expectations appropriate for the patient's cognitive status.	Setting goals based on current ability can help avoid frustration.
Provide a calendar with pertinent events.	Calendars serve as reminders and help maintain time orientation.
Provide and encourage the patient to use memory aids, including checklists, schedules, and reminder notices.	Reminders support memory of self-care tasks, medications, and appointments.
Present information in small, concrete portions, and reinforce and ask the patient to repeat important information.	Simple and clear information is easier to manage, and the repetition helps with recall.
Provide instructions in writing at the appropriate reading level.	Written instructions serve as reminders and resources over time.
Stimulate memory by repeating the patient's last expressed thought.	Reflecting information helps keep the patient on track with the topic.
Present changes in routine gradually, when possible.	Rapid change may be upsetting and increase cognitive impairment.
Place familiar objects and photographs in the patient's environment.	A stable environment may decrease anxiety and promote more independent actions.
Assign consistent health care team members.	Familiarity decreases anxiety, and familiar team members will be more attuned to subtle changes in cognition.
Schedule activities using the patient's usual patterns for sleep, medication use, elimination, food intake, and self-care in a consistent daily routine.	A consistent routine minimizes the patient's agitation and frustration.
Keep environment stimulation low, with adequate but nonglare lighting; quiet, soothing music; simple, familiar decor; and interaction in small groups. Remove or cover mirrors if the patient is frightened by them.	These measures help minimize the patient's agitation and frustration.
Use distraction, rather than confrontation, to manage agitated behavior.	Confrontation can increase agitation.
Provide cues such as current events, seasons, location, and seasonal and holiday decorations.	These cues provide assistance with orientation.
SAFETY: Maintain a safe, consistent physical environment.	Patients may have decreased judgment about safe actions.
FAMILY DYNAMICS: Encourage visitation by significant others, as appropriate, and include them in planning, providing, and evaluating care, to the extent desired.	Familiar persons may be comforting and help maintain orientation.
Limit decisions and numbers of options within daily decisions, such as asking whether a care activity could be done now or after lunch, rather than asking open-ended question about when it is preferred.	Decisions and numerous choices may frustrate the patient.
SLEEP: Allow for rest periods and undisturbed sleep.	Fatigue and interrupted sleep may increase chronic confusion and the risk of delirium.
Use television, radio, or music as part of a planned stimuli program based on the patient's preference but avoid arbitrary programming.	Familiar media may be comforting, while unfamiliar types of media may cause restlessness.
Encourage one-to-one and group activities based on the patient's cognitive abilities and interests.	Activities of interest may help engage the patient in interaction.
Encourage cognitive stimulation activities, such as reading, puzzles, and active participation in cultural or artistic activities.	Cognitive stimulation and creative tasks with social interaction promote the use of thinking and planning skills and the use of language.

Continued

INTERVENTIONS TO PROMOTE OPTIMAL COGNITION	RATIONALE
Administer prescribed medications, including:	
• Cholinesterase inhibitors, such as donepezil (Aricept) and the *N*-methyl-D-aspartate (NMDA) receptor antagonist memantine (Namenda)	Cholinesterase inhibitors may improve memory, awareness, and daily function for a period of time.
• Selective serotonin reuptake inhibitors (SSRIs), such as citalopram (Celexa) and fluoxetine (Prozac)	SSRIs are often used for the short-term treatment of depression, which is common with dementia.
• Antipsychotics, such as aripiprazole (Abilify) and haloperidol (Haldol), and benzodiazepines, such as lorazepam (Ativan)	Medications may reduce any associated behavioral problems, such as agitation, physical aggression, and disinhibition.
PAIN: Implement measures to treat pain as needed, without excess sedation.	Untreated pain may increase confusion and delirium.
SENSORY PERCEPTION: Encourage the patient's use of aids that increase sensory input, such as eyeglasses and hearing aids.	Accurate sensory input may improve cognition and communication.
FUNCTIONAL ABILITY: Assist the patient with meeting needs related to nutrition, elimination, hydration, and personal hygiene.	Unmet needs may lead to restlessness and further declines in health status.
INTRACRANIAL REGULATION: Implement measures to address increased intracranial pressure, if present.	Increased intracranial pressure is associated with changes in neurologic status and cognition.
NUTRITION: Implement measures to promote optimal nutrition.	The patient may not notice cues for hunger and thirst or be able to self-feed, leading to nutritional compromise.
STRESS AND COPING: Institute measures to provide caregiver support, if appropriate	Providing caregiving to a person with dementia can be highly stressful.

INTERVENTIONS TO MANAGE DELIRIUM	RATIONALE
If risk factors for delirium are identified, initiate specific interventions, such as oxygenation and glucose control.	Treatable factors may improve mental status in the presence of delirium.
Provide honest, reassuring, and simply stated information about what is happening and what can be expected to occur in the future in simple terms.	Simple, honest information may decrease anxiety and help build trust.
Psychosis: Acknowledge the patient's fears and feelings, but avoid validating misperceptions of reality.	Provide emotional support without reinforcing hallucinations or delusions.
Reduce environmental stimuli: • Maintain a well-lit environment that reduces sharp contrasts and shadows. • Remove excessive sensory stimuli (e.g., television or broadcast intercom announcements) when possible.	Eliminate stimuli that may support delusions.
Provide supervision and surveillance based on the assessed needs and safety risk of the patient.	Monitor for patient safety and implement therapeutic actions as needed.
If physical restraint is necessary, use the least restrictive measure that will support safety.	Minimize the use of restraints when possible to situations where endangerment exists.
If needed, administer prescribed medications for anxiety or agitation, limiting those with anticholinergic side effects.	Anticholinergics may worsen delirium.

COLLABORATION	RATIONALE
Stimulation program	Multiple modes of sensory stimulation may promote and protect cognitive capacity.
NUTRITION: Dietitian	Collaborating with a dietitian offers support for implementing a diet that promotes optimal nutrition.
Occupational therapy	Occupational therapists can recommend assistive devices and assist with skill maintenance to help the patient remain as independent as possible.
Legal assistance	Patients with early dementia should make plans in terms of advance directives, care options, financial concerns, and personal preferences for care.
SAFETY: Adult protective services	Adult protective services advocates for the well-being of older adults who may be in danger and have no one to assist them.
FUNCTIONAL ABILITY: Home health agency	A home health agency may be able to provide assistance with the patient's care and household maintenance.

PATIENT AND CAREGIVER TEACHING

- Cause of impaired cognition
- Management of underlying conditions causing impaired cognition
- Memory and orientation techniques and resources
- Measures being used to improve cognition
- Measures to reduce the risk of complications
- Taking medications as prescribed
- Modifying the living environment to promote safety
- Health promotion behaviors, including nutrition, sleep, and exercise
- Social support resources, community and self-help resources
- Sources of further information
- When to notify the health care provider (HCP)

DOCUMENTATION

Assessment

- Assessments of mental status and behavior
- Diagnostic and laboratory test results
- Manifestations of impaired cognition
- Screening test results
- Functional ability

Interventions

- Discussions with other members of the interprofessional team
- Environmental modifications made
- Medications given
- Notification of the HCP about diagnostic test results and assessment findings
- Therapeutic interventions and the patient's response
- Teaching provided
- Referrals initiated
- Safety measures implemented, including fall precautions
- Measures to address cognition:
    - Reorientation
    - Memory support methods
    - Diversional activities

Evaluation

- Status: improved, stable, declined
- Maintenance of safety
- Diagnostic test results
- Response to therapeutic interventions
- Continued manifestations of impaired cognition

Victim of Violence 49

Definition

Having been harmed or under threat of harm by another person

Violence, or physical action or words intended to hurt or cause harm, damage, or kill someone or something, is a public health crisis. It affects everyone, regardless of age, race, gender, or socioeconomic status. Interpersonal violence refers to violence between persons, Including child and elder abuse and neglect, intimate partner violence, and sexual abuse. Community violence is experienced outside the home (e.g., school, work, stores) from people who are not family members (e.g., strangers, classmates).

Action is needed to address the numerous emotional, social, and physical consequences of interpersonal violence. Besides injury, there is a risk for impaired growth and development in children. There is a risk for sexually transmitted diseases and pregnancy after sexual violence. Emotional consequences include depression, substance use, and suicidal ideation. Those who are victims of sexual violence have a high rate of posttraumatic stress disorder and guilt. Being a victim of mistreatment in childhood carries a higher chance of engaging in or demonstrating violent behavior as an adult.

All health care team members need to be vigilant for evidence of interpersonal violence with health care encounters. One of the few persons the victim may feel they can go to for help may be a health care provider (HCP). Nurses must routinely screen for violence and be able to intervene when there is a positive screen or when specific evidence suggests the patient has experienced violence. Offering support, assisting victims with getting the services they need, and helping them with referrals to community agencies are vital.

Associated Clinical Problems

- Rape-Trauma Syndrome: set of symptoms experienced by survivors of sexual assault
- Victim of Child Abuse: physical, emotional, or sexual abuse of a child
- Victim of Child Neglect: parental failure to meet a child's basic needs
- Victim of Elder Abuse: abuse of an older adult by the person's family/caregivers
- Victim of Elder Neglect: neglect of an older adult by the person's family/caregivers
- Victim of Intimate Partner Violence: victim of violence that occurs between people in a close relationship
- Victim of Sexual Assault: victim of any type of sexual activity in which one person does not agree to engage but is forced to comply

Vulnerability Factors

- Age
- Being disabled, having special needs
- Being female
- Chronic illness
- Community violence
- Family history of interpersonal violence
- History of arrests, incarcerations, interactions with law enforcement
- Impaired cognition
- Impaired development
- Impaired family function
- Lack of resources
- Poverty
- Social isolation
- Substance use

Risk for Child Abuse/Neglect

- Discord between parent and child temperament
- Having a teen parent
- Having a large number of siblings
- High level of parental stress
- Nonbiologic, transient caregivers in the home

Manifestations

- Aggression
- Decline from the prior level of functioning
- Denial
- Difficulty with forming intimate relationships
- Eating disorders
- Emotional problems
- Financial problems
- Impaired role performance for age
- Impaired sleep
- Impulse control problems
- Inability to trust
- Inappropriate sexual behavior
- Loneliness

- Malnutrition
- Mood problems, including depression, anxiety, avoidance, helplessness, guilt
- Negative self-image
- Physical injuries, injuries inconsistent with the history, and/or unusual injuries
- Poor hygiene
- Posttraumatic stress disorder
- Repeated and/or unexplained injuries
- Self-blame
- Social isolation
- Substance use
- Suicidal ideation
- Unmet medical needs
- Violent behavior

Pediatric
- Behavior problems
- Delinquency
- Failure to thrive
- Feeding problems
- Impaired growth and development
- School problems
- Sentinel injuries, such as intraoral injuries, bruising

Key Conceptual Relationships

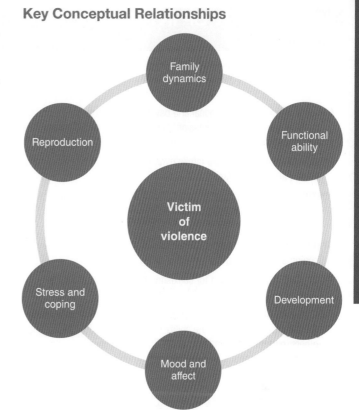

ASSESSMENT OF INTERPERSONAL VIOLENCE	RATIONALE
Assess the patient's immediate risk of danger, whether the perpetrator is present, their level of fear, and their self-appraisal of immediate and future safety needs.	A priority is to identify the risk or danger and initiate care that promotes patient safety.
Obtain a thorough history, assessing for factors that increase risk of being a victim of violence.	A thorough history that includes all risk factors is essential for the early identification of patients at risk of being a victim of violence.
Screen the patient at each encounter for interpersonal violence (Table 49.1).	Identifying victims of interpersonal violence through ongoing, confidential assessment promotes patient safety.
Obtain a history of the violence, including: • When it happened • Where it happened • Whether the perpetrator is known • Description of what happened • Whether there were others present • What the patient did after the injury • What others did (if present) • If multiple episodes, whether there is a pattern • Medical treatment obtained	The nature of the violence, the environment in which the violence occurred, the relationship between the perpetrator and the victim, and the context of the violence influence intervention and safety planning.
Perform a complete physical assessment or assist a specially trained person in performing the assessment, noting physical injuries.	A complete physical assessment is necessary to detect findings related to violence.
Assure the patient of their right to privacy and confidentiality, and refrain from asking about potential violence in the presence of the partner, family, or caregivers.	Providing information about the violence in the presnce of the perpetrator may put that victim in danger.

Continued

ASSESSMENT OF INTERPERSONAL VIOLENCE	RATIONALE
Complete evidence collection and obtain ordered specimens.	Documentation of visible injuries by written description, digital photographs, and/or body diagrams facilitates peer review and court testimony.
Assess to what degree emotional and psychologic responses are present, such as denial, anger, depression, posttraumatic stress disorder, fear, anxiety, and self-blame.	There are many emotional and psychological reactions that victims of interpersonal violence experience.
FAMILY DYNAMICS: Evaluate family dynamics and current level of functioning and observe family interactions.	Impaired family functioning is a risk factor for violence in the home.
CULTURE: Assess the role of culture and beliefs in the occurrence of interpersonal violence.	Culture factors that influence interpersonal violence include culture tolerance for violence, power dynamics related to gender, family structure, and stereotypical role views.
STRESS AND COPING: Assess for the use of stress management and coping strategies that the patient is using.	Patients experience stress in response to victimization.
MOOD AND AFFECT: Screen for coexisting psychological problems.	Identifying depression or other psychological problems and initiating treatment promotes positive patient outcomes.
FUNCTIONAL ABILITY: Perform a psychosocial assessment, evaluating the effects of violence on the ability to sleep, enjoy life, interact with others, perform work and household duties, and engage in physical and social activities.	Problems resulting from being a victim of interpersonal violence affect all aspects of a person's life.
Women's Health	
REPRODUCTION: Assess fetal well-being.	Violence may negatively affect fetal health and well-being.

ASSESSMENT FOR RISK FOR/VICTIM OF CHILD ABUSE/NEGLECT	RATIONALE
Ask the parent/caregiver to describe in detail the events surrounding all injuries, including information about the child's behavior before, during, and after the injury.	Consider the history in relation to the injurie. The parent/caregiver, if the perpetrator, may provide a history of events that is incomplete or inconsistent with the injuries seen.
FAMILY DYNAMICS: Assess the interactions and attachment level between the parent/caregiver and the child.	Negative parenting strategies and inappropriate discipline increase the risk of child abuse and neglect.
DEVELOPMENT: Assess the child's level of physical and emotional development.	Child maltreatment negatively affects development, with lasting cognitive and physical effects.

Table 49.1 Intimate Partner Violence Screening

1. Ask indirect questions:
   a. How does your partner treat you?
   b. Do you feel safe at home?
   c. Do you feel safe in your current relationship?
2. Ask direct questions:
   a. Have you been hit, kicked, punched, or otherwise hurt by someone within the past year? If so, by whom?
   b. Do you feel afraid of your partner?
   c. Has someone ever forced you to have sex when you did not want to?
   d. Is there a partner from a previous relationship who is making you feel unsafe now?
3. Ask about a history of partner violence:
   a. Have you ever had someone who hit you, hurt you, or threatened you?
   b. Have you ever had a partner who treated you badly?
   c. Has anyone forced you to have sexual activities that made you feel uncomfortable?

Expected Outcomes

The patient will:

- remain safe and free of harm.
- express their feelings.
- acknowledge and gain control over the effects of being a victim.
- identify and take part in counseling and supportive therapies.
- follow their personal safety plan, if needed.
- use strategies to address the psychological sequelae of being a victim.
- use appropriate resources.

INTERVENTIONS TO ADDRESS INTERPERSONAL VIOLENCE	RATIONALE
Provide appropriate collaborative care for injuries that are present.	An injured patient needs to be stabilized before further evaluation can proceed.
Provide the patient with adequate referrals or removal from the situation when interpersonal violence is present.	A priority intervention for a victim of violence is to initiate care that promotes patient safety.
Report the occurrence of interpersonal violence to legal authorities, following agency protocol and local and state laws.	It is a legal and ethical obligation to follow state laws for mandatory reporting.
Establish a therapeutic relationship with the patient: • Remain nonjudgmental. • Use active listening, with therapeutic communication skills. • Provide a secure, relaxed atmosphere.	The patient needs to talk about what happened and express their feelings and fears in a nonjudgmental atmosphere.
Assign a primary care nurse.	Maintaining the continuity of caregivers helps establish trust.
Encourage the patient to share feelings they may be experiencing, help them identify feelings of self-blame, and reassure them that their responses are normal and that they do/did not deserve to be victimized.	Acknowledging the situation and normal emotional responses, such as blaming themselves for what happened, helps the patient in dealing with the trauma associated with being a victim.
Assist the patient in developing a personal safety plan, including: • Where to go • Cash, credit cards, and debit cards • Personal documents, including court papers • Car keys • Medications • Items for childcare, such as formula and diapers • Clothing	The safety plan should include the resources needed if the patient needs to leave a situation suddenly.
Do not ask the patient why they stay in the relationship; focus instead on the perpetrator's behavior and protecting the patient.	Asking why they stay may increase a victim's sense of shame about abuse or be interpreted as blaming them for the situation.
Explore with the patient available support systems.	Adequate support mediates the effects of violence on the patient's physical and mental health.
STRESS AND COPING: Help the patient develop positive coping and stress management strategies.	Positive coping strategies help the patient respond to the stress associated with victimization and help promote the patient's sense of control.
CULTURE: Encourage the patient and family to establish their own goals and culturally considerate solutions for addressing violence.	Establishing their own goals and solutions promotes the patient and family's sense of control.
FAMILY DYNAMICS: Institute measures to promote optimal family function.	Promoting positive family interaction and communication will help the patient and family deal with the consequences of violence.
FUNCTIONAL ABILITY: Help the patient develop strategies to promote participation in activities of daily living in the home, work, and socially.	The effects of being a victim may influence the ability to take part in activities of daily living.
Establish a long-term follow-up process.	Long-term treatment is often necessary to address issues that accompany a history of being a victim of violence.
DEVELOPMENT: Implement measures to assist the patient in maintaining a positive self-image.	Persons who are victims of violence may experience a negative self-image.
Women's Health	
Address gynecologic needs, such as providing emergency contraception or treatment for sexually transmitted infections (STIs).	These measures reduce stress by decreasing the chance of unintended pregnancy and contracting an STI.

INTERVENTIONS TO ADDRESS RISK FOR/VICTIM OF CHILD ABUSE/NEGLECT	RATIONALE
Allow opportunities for the child to take part in play therapy, referring to a play therapy specialist if needed.	Play therapy provides insight into the child's coping and can help them cope with their emotions.
DEVELOPMENT: Institute measures to promote child growth and development.	Being a victim of interpersonal violence increases the risk of impaired growth and development.
FAMILY DYNAMICS: Institute measures to support positive parenting.	Using positive parenting strategies, effective communication strategies, and age-appropriate discipline reduces the risk of child abuse and neglect and reduces behavior problems in children who are victims.

INTERVENTIONS TO ADDRESS RISK FOR/VICTIM OF ELDER ABUSE/NEGLECT	RATIONALE
Assist the family who is planning to take care of an older family member at home to prepare for the stressors that will be involved.	Education and preparation can help the family prepare for the stress of caregiving.
Discuss with the family/caregiver the importance of accessing caregiver respite programs and support groups.	Respite may reduce caregivers' stress, which may in turn alleviate the potential for elder abuse.

COLLABORATION	RATIONALE
Psychological specialist for counseling	Counseling can help the patient overcome negative feelings that affect their relationships and quality of life.
Adult and/or child protective services	Protective services can help with placement while abuse is being investigated.
Support groups and other mental health resources for survivors, such as a rape crisis center	Specialty mental health support services are available to help the patient with managing the short- and long-term effects of being a victim of violence.
FAMILY DYNAMICS: Family-focused therapy	Promoting positive family interaction and communication will help the patient and family deal with the consequences of violence.
Emergency shelters and transition home services	Emergency shelters and transition homes offer a place to go for a patient in danger.
School counselor, school social worker, or school psychologist	School personnel can provide the services necessary to help ensure the child is in a safe environment at school.
MOOD AND AFFECT: Treatment for coexisting psychological problems, including depressed mood and emotional problems	Treatment of underlying psychological problems will help the victim cope.
Legal services	Legal services can help the patient with financial and legal matters, such as custody and support.

PATIENT AND CAREGIVER TEACHING

- Anticipatory guidance about expected feelings
- Measures being used to treat injuries and problems
- Need for any legal procedures
- Options for follow-up treatment
- Community and self-help resources available
- Positive coping and stress management strategies
- Early recognition of problems and how to manage them
- Importance of long-term follow-up
- When to notify the HCP and seek emergency assistance

DOCUMENTATION

Assessment

- Assessments performed
- Circumstances surrounding incidents
- Manifestations of being a victim of violence
- Screening test results

Interventions

- Discussions with other interprofessional team members
- Notification of the HCP about patient status
- Notification of the proper authorities
- Therapeutic interventions and the patient's response
- Teaching provided
- Referrals initiated
- Safety measures implemented

Evaluation

- Patient's status: improved, stable, declined
- Manifestations of being a victim of violence
- Response to teaching provided
- Response to therapeutic interventions

Violent Behavior 50

Definition

Physical or emotional force that causes injury to others or destruction of property

Being a perpetrator of violence is a complex phenomenon that has roots in many factors—biologic, social, culture, and economic. Poverty, being a victim of childhood violence, and substance use place a person at higher risk for being violent. There may be an organic brain or a psychiatric problem. Some perpetrators choose to be violent and may deny responsibility for the acts they commit. Those who are repeatedly violent often demonstrate other forms of destructive or antisocial behavior, often starting in childhood.

Nurses have an ethical responsibility to implement measures to reduce and prevent violence. These responsibilities include holding the person accountable and working with them to change their attitudes and behavior. To be effective in this role, nurses need to know when and how to respond when in their practice they encounter persons who are perpetrators of violence. Nurses will encounter perpetrators of violence in many settings. There may be patients who are aggressive or have risk-prone behaviors in acute psychiatric settings. Patients may come to the emergency department with hallucinations and delusions or under the influence of substances.

Associated Clinical Problems

- Abusive Behavior: mistreatment of another person
- Aggressive Behavior: forceful physical or verbal behavior that may or may not cause harm to others

Contributing Factors

- Access to guns and weapons
- Accumulated or chronic stress
- Acts on feelings of anger and hostility
- Antisocial behavior
- Desire for power or control
- Distrust of others
- Excess jealousy
- Family history of interpersonal violence
- Harmful masculinity ideals
- Impaired family function
- Low education level
- Negative self-image
- Organic brain disease
- Parenting during childhood
- Personal history of being abused, neglected, or bullied
- Personality disorder
- Poverty
- Presence of gangs or drugs in the environment
- Psychiatric illness
- Relationship problems
- Substance use
- Tendency to blame outside factors for what goes wrong
- Traumatic experiences
- Unemployment or unstable work history

Manifestations

- Aggression
- Anger
- Antisocial behavior
- Bullying
- Controlling behavior
- Destruction of property
- Divorce and separation from family
- Employment problems
- Impulsiveness
- Incarceration and legal problems
- Manipulative behavior
- Paranoia
- Perpetrating violence
- Risk-taking behavior
- Stalking
- Terrorizing
- Threats and threatening behavior

Key Conceptual Relationships

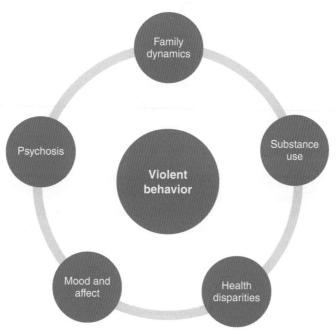

ASSESSMENT OF VIOLENT BEHAVIOR	RATIONALE
Assess for factors that influence the patient's capacity for violent behavior.	If the history identifies risk factors that increase the potential for violent behavior, specific interventions may reduce the patient's risk of committing violent behavior.
Assess for signs of aggression and imminent danger to others from the patient, including: • Access to guns or other weapons • Threats or plans to kill self or others • Rage for no apparent reason • Mumbling, staring, pacing, anxiety	If signs indicate escalating severity of violent behavior, action is needed to promote safety.
Perform a complete physical assessment, focusing on evaluating for organic disease and metabolic problems.	Many organic brain disorders and some metabolic problems, such as exposure to or ingestion of toxic chemicals, can lead to aggressive behavior.
SUBSTANCE USE: Screen the patient for substance use and evaluate the results of toxicology screening.	Substance use increases the risk of committing a violent act.
Assess the patient's verbal and nonverbal communication, noting signs of anger and agitation.	Communication can provide an assessment of the imminent risk of violence and allow for initiating measures to prevent behavior from escalating.
PSYCHOSIS: Assess mental status and screen for coexisting psychological problems.	Identifying depression or other coexisting problems and initiating treatment may assist with reducing violent behavior.
Obtain information about the patient from other sources, including family, friends, law enforcement, coworkers, and others who have had contact with the patient.	Collateral information is helpful in assessing the potential for violence.
FAMILY DYNAMICS: Obtain a social and family history and observe family and social interactions.	The family and social history can provide information as to potential exacerbating factors and predictors of violent behavior.
Evaluate the effectiveness of measures used to prevent or end violent behavior through ongoing assessment.	Ongoing monitoring allows for evaluation of therapy effectiveness.

Expected Outcomes

The patient will:

- admit to being a perpetrator of violence.
- be free from aggressive, abusive, or violent behavior.
- obtain and take part in treatment.
- identify factors contributing to their behavior.
- express empathy toward victim(s).
- appropriately express emotions.
- contact appropriate resources when necessary.
- refrain from substance use.

INTERVENTIONS TO END VIOLENT BEHAVIOR	RATIONALE
If there is a clear danger to a potential victim, follow agency protocol and procedure for duty to warn and notify the appropriate authorities.	There is an ethical and legal duty to warn when there is a clear and present danger to a specific victim or victims.
Start immediate deescalation measures at any signs of distress, including: • Acknowledge the situation. • Remove any triggers causing the behavior. • Redirect or distract the patient. • Set clear limits for the patient to follow. • Use nonthreatening body language. • Respond to expressed problems or concerns. • Have sufficient staff for a show of strength.	Instituting deescalation measures can help prevent agitation or angry behaviors from escalating into violence.
Contact the appropriate authorities if mental health treatment is needed.	Involuntary treatment should only occur as a last resort and be limited to persons who pose an imminent, serious risk of physical harm to themselves or others.
Observe the patient's behavior often while carrying out routine activities.	Close observation is necessary so intervention can occur quickly. Doing so while carrying out routine care avoids suspicion.
If the violent situation involves possible criminal behavior, contact law enforcement.	An aggressive, violent person may be behaving criminally, requiring intervention by law enforcement personnel.
Establish a therapeutic relationship with the patient: • Remain nonjudgmental. • Use active listening with therapeutic communication. • Speak in a calm, soft manner. • Be empathetic. • Maintain the patient's personal space.	Therapeutic communication is central to establishing a relationship with the patient and averting or defusing distress.
Administer prescribed medications to provide chemical restraint, such as benzodiazepines, typical and atypical antipsychotics, and ketamine.	Chemical restraints, involving the use of a drug to restrict the patient's movement or behavior, may be needed as a safety measure.
Place the patient in seclusion or physical restraints if ordered.	Seclusion and physical restraints may be needed to maintain the immediate physical safety of the patient and others.
Maintain a low level of environment stimuli: • Provide low lighting, low noise level. • Remove all dangerous objects.	Anxiety or agitation increases in a stimulating environment.
Develop a behavior contract with the patient, placing clear limits on what behavior will and will not be tolerated and outlining the consequences of being aggressive or violent.	Involving the patient in developing a behavior contract can help the patient address violent behavior and enhance adherence.
Allow the patient to express their feelings and concerns about their conduct and assist them in developing appropriate methods of expressing their feelings.	Listening to the patient's concerns may reveal their awareness of their feelings and help them develop appropriate means of expression.
Use motivational interviewing to initiate behavior change.	Helping patients identify why they might want to make a change and how they might do it is more effective than telling them they should.
Help the patient with identifying the negative consequences of their behavior and their responsibility to stop.	One of the first steps in behavior change is to identify the negative consequences of behavior and connect them to their conduct.

INTERVENTIONS TO END VIOLENT BEHAVIOR	RATIONALE
SUBSTANCE USE: Implement measures to address substance use.	Substance use cessation improves well-being and promotes positive outcomes.
FAMILY DYNAMICS: Institute measures to promote optimal family function.	Addressing dysfunctional family interaction and communication may help prevent further violence.
Establish a long-term follow-up process.	Long-term treatment is often necessary to address the issues that accompany a history of violent behavior.

COLLABORATION	RATIONALE
Psychological services that specialize in persons with a history of violent behavior, such as a batterer intervention program	Specialists offering specific psychological counseling techniques are part of effective treatment aimed at reducing violent behavior.
Peer support groups	Support groups provide mentorship and support.
PSYCHOSIS: Treatment for coexisting psychological problems	Initiating treatment for depression or another coexisting psychological problem may help with reducing violent behavior.
FAMILY DYNAMICS: Family-focused therapy	Therapy can address dysfunctional family interaction and help the family cope with the sequelae of a family member's actions.
HEALTH DISPARITIES: Social work or case management	Meeting needs for financial, food, shelter, and basic resources can reduce the incidence of abuse and neglect.

 PATIENT AND CAREGIVER TEACHING

- Nature of the behavior and the impact of that behavior on victims
- Need to stop the violent behavior
- Individual responsibility for their behavior
- Reason for interventions
- Treatment of coexisting problems, such as substance use
- Community and self-help resources
- Early recognition of problems and how to manage them
- Positive verbal and nonverbal communication skills
- Conflict resolution strategies
- Importance of regular, long-term follow-up
- When to notify the health care provider (HCP) and seek emergency assistance

 DOCUMENTATION

Assessment

- Assessments performed
- Manifestations of violent behavior

Interventions

- Discussions with other interprofessional team members
- Environment modifications made
- Medications given
- Notification of the HCP about patient status
- Notification of the proper authorities
- Therapeutic interventions and the patient's response
- Teaching provided
- Referrals initiated
- Safety measures implemented

Evaluation

- Patient's status: improved, stable, declined
- Presence of violent behavior
- Response to teaching provided
- Response to therapeutic interventions

Depressed Mood 51

Definition

Depressed mood lasting 2 weeks or longer and accompanied by a lack of pleasure or interest in most other activities

Mood refers to the way a person feels. *Affect* is the observable response or the way a person communicates those feelings. All people have normal, healthy changes in mood. Mood disorders represent a serious change in mood that interferes with a person's ability to function. Mood disorders include major depressive disorder, bipolar disorder, persistent depressive disorder, and seasonal affective disorder. The most serious consequence of having depression is suicide ideation. Around 25% of those with depression have suicide thoughts. Depression can cause physical illness, including cancer, heart disease, and diabetes.

Having depression affects many aspects of life, including relationships, role performance, and health. The person's ability to take part in activities of daily living and meet role expectations is an indicator of the severity. Some develop anxiety or other emotional problems that further interfere with engaging in activities. Others engage in substance use. Caregivers may feel helpless or inadequate because they cannot make the patient feel better.

Although depression in older adults is common, it is *not* a normal part of aging. It may be hard to recognize depression in an older adult. Sometimes, the signs of depression might be mistaken for other problems, such as dementia. An older adult's risk of depression tends to increase as their health deteriorates.

Nurses are in a key position to recognize the manifestations of depression and assist patients who need further assessment and treatment. The nurse's ability to respond if the patient is acutely distressed is important in maintaining patient safety. Providing education about how to manage depression and helping the patient connect with community and self-help resources can promote quality of life and participation in activities of daily living.

Associated Clinical Problems

- Lack of Initiative: lack of willingness to make decisions and take action
- Postpartum Depression: depression that occurs within the first year of having a child
- Sadness: feeling down because of grief, discouragement, or disappointment
- Self-Injurious Behavior: behavior with the intent of intentionally causing physical harm to oneself
- Self-Mutilation: intentionally injuring one's body
- Suicide Ideation: thinking about suicide or killing oneself
- Withdrawn Behavior: not wanting to communicate with other people

Common Risk Factors

- Adverse childhood events
- Being female
- Being LGBTQIA
- Family history
- Having a personality or psychiatric disorder
- Having a disabling or serious health condition
- Neuroticism
- Socially isolated
- Stressful life events, including death, divorce, monetary crisis, loss
- Substance use disorder
- Trauma
- Victim of interpersonal violence, including abuse and neglect

Postpartum Depression

- Ambivalence regarding pregnancy
- Being postpartum
- First pregnancy
- Lack of a partner
- Lack of a support network
- Risk for Suicide: increased risk for killing oneself

Manifestations

- Anger, hostility
- Anxiety
- Changes in eating pattern
- Despair
- Difficulty concentrating
- Failure to attend to self-care (appearance, hygiene)
- Fatigue
- Feelings of failure, worthlessness, hopelessness
- Flat affect
- General restlessness or agitation
- Guilt
- Impaired sleep
- Irritability

- Lack of initiative
- Loss of libido
- Memory changes
- Monotone speech
- Mood swings
- Negative self-image
- Not participating in usual activities
- Personality changes
- Powerlessness
- Sadness
- Self-injurious behaviors
- Sexual problems
- Suicide ideation

Pediatric
- Problems in school

Postpartum Depression
- Episodic tearfulness
- Hyperactivity
- Irrationality

Suicide Ideation
- Giving away possessions
- Planning for committing suicide
- Visiting or calling people to say goodbye

Key Conceptual Relationships

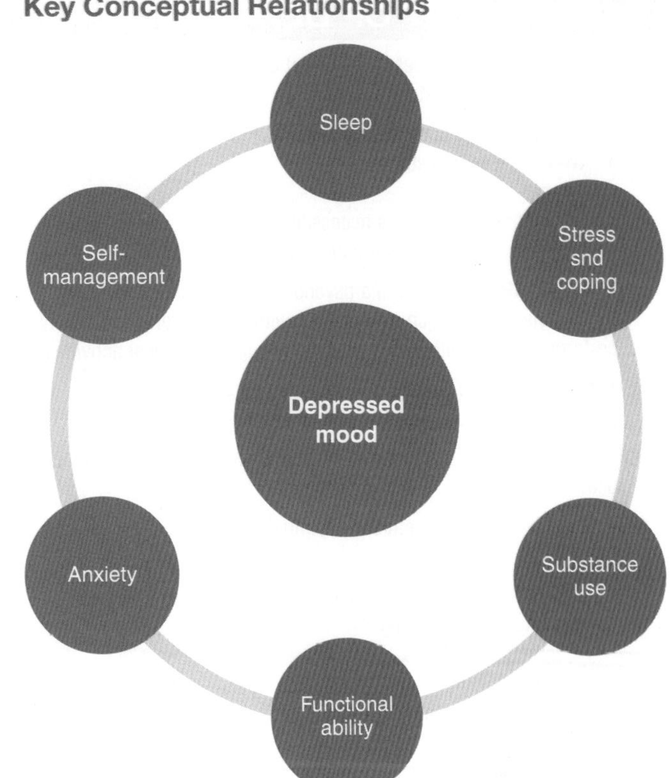

ASSESSMENT OF DEPRESSION	RATIONALE
Assess the patient through observation and directly question for suicide ideation (e.g., having a suicide plan).	Prompt referral to a mental health professional is needed if suicide ideation is present.
Assess for factors that increase risk for depression.	A thorough history can identify conditions or situations that place patients at risk for depression.
Evaluate the patient's underlying health status.	Underlying health status has a significant influence on mood.
Use a formal, patient-specific tool, such as the Patient Health Questionnaire (PHQ-9), to detect a depressed mood (Table 51.1).	Identifying a depressed mood allows for early intervention.
Perform a complete physical assessment and monitor for depression on an ongoing basis:	
• Manifestations of depression	Identifying depression allows for early intervention.
• Complete a mental status examination, including appearance, attitude, mood and affect, speech, behavior, thought process and content, cognition, insight, and judgment.	Depression is often accompanied by changes in mental status.
• Screen for coexisting anxiety or other problems.	Many patients with depression have coexisting anxiety or other psychological disorders.
Assess the patient regarding past or present experiences with self-injury, including: • Frequency of behaviors • Underlying motive or reason • What emotional response the patient receives	A thorough history can identify if the patient is participating in self-injurious behaviors and guide treatment.
Evaluate the results of diagnostic studies, such as a complete blood count (CBC), chemistry panel, thyroid panel, liver function tests, urinalysis, and toxicology screens.	Diagnostic test results can help determine whether there is a physiologic cause for depression.
CULTURE: Assess the role of culture in the patient's mood and affect.	Expression of mood is influenced by one's culture.

ASSESSMENT OF DEPRESSION	RATIONALE
STRESS AND COPING: Assess the current and past use of stress management and coping strategies.	A patient with a depressed mood may be relying on substance use or other negative behaviors as a means of coping with stress.
Assess the patient's support system: • Who do they live with? • Are they employed? • Are friends and relatives accessible? • Have they used any community resources?	Interest and support from others are important aspects of managing daily mood.
FUNCTIONAL ABILITY: Perform a psychosocial assessment, evaluating for lifestyle effects, such as problems with social interaction, ability to perform responsibilities, and ability to engage in physical activities.	Depression can affect all aspects of a person's life.
SELF-MANAGEMENT: Assess how well the patient is managing coexisting health problems.	Depression often exacerbates illnesses and can affect a person's motivation and capacity to engage in daily self-management.
SUBSTANCE USE: Screen for alcohol, tobacco, and/or other substance use.	A patient with depression is at higher risk for substance use disorder.
SPIRITUALITY: Assess the patient's spiritual well-being.	Those with higher levels of religious and spiritual involvement have lower rates of depression and suicide behavior.
Evaluate the effectiveness of measures used to address depression through ongoing monitoring.	Ongoing monitoring allows for evaluation of therapy effectiveness.
Older Adult Screen for depression with a tool specific to older adults.	Signs of depression among older adults can be different from those of younger adults.

Table 51.1 Patient Health Questionnaire-9

Over the last 2 weeks, how often have you been bothered by any of the following problems?

	Not at All	Several Days	More Than Half the Days	Nearly Every Day
1. Little interest or pleasure in doing things	0	1	2	3
2. Feeling down, depressed, or hopeless	0	1	2	3
3. Trouble falling or staying asleep, or sleeping too much	0	1	2	3
4. Feeling tired or having little energy	0	1	2	3
5. Poor appetite or overeating	0	1	2	3
6. Feeling bad about yourself or that you are a failure or have let yourself or your family down	0	1	2	3
7. Trouble concentrating on things, such as reading the newspaper or watching television	0	1	2	3
8. Moving or speaking so slowly that other people could have noticed, or the opposite—being so fidgety or restless that you have been moving around a lot more than usual	0	1	2	3
9. Thoughts that you would be better off dead or of hurting yourself in some way	0	1	2	3

To score, total each column, then add together. Total scores of 5, 10, 15, and 20 represent cutpoints for mild, moderate, moderately severe and severe depression, respectively.
PHQ-9. Retrieved from https://cde.drugabuse.gov/instrument/f226b1a0-897c-de2a-e040-bb89ad4338b9

Expected Outcomes

The patient will:

- report an improvement in mood.
- be free from self-harm.
- participate in role responsibilities and attend to self-care.
- adhere to prescribed therapeutic regimen, including engaging in counseling and medication use.
- use personal strategies to address depression.

- contact appropriate resources when necessary.
- refrain from substance use.

INTERVENTIONS TO ADDRESS DEPRESSION	RATIONALE
Initiate appropriate safety protocols and referrals if the patient is identified as being at risk for self-harm.	The risk of self-harm necessitates implementing\guidelines to keep the patient safe.
Implement measures to protect the patient from self-harm or suicide: • Removing sharp and glass objects from environment • Removing belts and strings from the environment • Providing constant one-to-one interaction if the risk for self-harm is high • Checking on the patient every 15 minutes	Providing a safe environment may prevent the patient from self-harming and suicide.
Implement collaborative interventions aimed at treating risk factors contributing to depression.	Treatment of causative or risk factors can assist in improving the patient's mood.
Establish a therapeutic nurse–patient relationship: • Use therapeutic touch, with the patient's consent. • Remain nonjudgmental. • Use active listening with therapeutic communication skills.	A nurse's words and actions that convey sincere acceptance and interest have a positive effect on the patient and help establish trust.
Encourage the patient to identify and express their feelings.	Mood may be enhanced through sharing thoughts and feelings.
Notify the health care provider (HCP) if manifestations of depression persist or worsen or if suicide ideation is present.	Achievement of an effective treatment plan often requires adjustments in therapy.
Administer prescribed medications:	
• Antidepressants	Antidepressants address neurotransmitter dysfunction that can partially cause depression.
• Mood stabilizers	Mood stabilizers are believed to assist with addressing neurotransmitter dysfunction.
STRESS AND COPING: Help the patient develop positive coping behaviors.	The use of positive coping skills equips the patient to manage mood problems.
Assist the patient in identifying persons to whom they can express feelings openly.	Mood may be enhanced through sharing thoughts and feelings.
Assist the patient in developing problem-solving strategies.	Developing problem-solving ability aids the patient in acting in their life and coping with difficulties, which can reduce depression.
Collaborate with the patient to select and implement complementary and spiritual support therapies, including relaxation, guided imagery, mindful breathing, acupressure, yoga, and massage.	Complementary therapies can help reduce the manifestations of depression and stress by focusing on mind and body connections.
ANXIETY: Implement measures to assist the patient in managing any anxiety they may be experiencing.	Patients with a depressed mood often experience coexisting anxiety.
STRESS AND COPING: Encourage the use of stress management strategies.	Stress from life issues may have a compounding effect on a person with a depressed mood.
DEVELOPMENT: Implement measures to assist the patient in maintaining a positive self-image.	Persons with depression may have a negative self-image and low self-esteem.
SUBSTANCE USE: Implement measures to address substance use.	A patient with depression is at higher risk for substance use disorder.
FUNCTIONAL ABILITY: Help the patient develop strategies to increase participation in activities of daily living in the home, at work, and socially.	Depression may influence the ability to participate in activities of daily living.
Assist the patient with performing personal care, if needed.	A certain level of personal hygiene is needed to ensure health and promote positive social interactions.
Encourage participation in moderate-intensity exercise, such as walking, swimming, and bicycling.	Exercise raises levels of endorphins and may be helpful in the treatment of depression.
CULTURE: Implement measures to promote positive social interaction.	Social interaction can decrease feelings of depression.
SLEEP: Provide the patient with opportunities for adequate sleep.	A lack of adequate rest has a negative effect on mood.

Continued

INTERVENTIONS TO ADDRESS DEPRESSION	RATIONALE
NUTRITION: Encourage the patient to follow a nutritionally adequate diet.	It is believed that following a healthy, nutritionally sound diet lessens the incidence of depression.
SPIRITUALITY: Implement measures to address spiritual concerns.	Enhancing spirituality may help some patients when incorporated into their overall treatment plan.

INTERVENTIONS TO REDUCE SELF-INJURIOUS BEHAVIORS	RATIONALE
Develop a safety plan with the patient.	A safety plan outlines behaviors that help the patient stay safe and healthy.
Assist the patient with reframing self-injurious behaviors as a habit that the patient can change.	Reframing promotes recognition of negative thought patterns and increases coping skills.
Help the patient identify positive behaviors they can use when they feel the urge to self-injure.	This helps the patient identify healthy, adaptive behaviors and promotes their sense of control.

COLLABORATION	RATIONALE
Psychological specialist for cognitive behavioral therapy (CBT) and counseling	CBT and counseling may be needed to effectively assist the patient in managing a depressed mood.
CARE COORDINATION: Social work or case management	The social worker can explore resources that may be available to help the patient obtain access to health care.
Support groups and other mental health resources	Specialty mental health support services are available to assist the patient with managing the effects of having depression.
FAMILY DYNAMICS: Family-focused therapy	Family-focused therapy provides long-term support for improving overall family functioning.
SPIRITUALITY: Pastoral care professional or preferred spiritual or religious leader	Those with higher levels of religious and spiritual involvement have lower rates of depression and suicide behavior.

PATIENT AND CAREGIVER TEACHING

- About depression and its potential causes
- Factors that may be contributing to depression
- Manifestations of depression
- Management of conditions contributing to depression
- Positive coping and stress management strategies
- Community and self-help resources
- Sources of information and social support
- Early recognition of problems and how to manage them
- Safe use of medications, including proper use and side effect management, and how they fit into the overall management plan
- Importance of health promotion behaviors, including nutrition and sleep
- Importance of long-term follow-up
- When to notify the HCP and seek emergency assistance

DOCUMENTATION

Assessment

- Assessments performed
- Diagnostic and laboratory test results
- Manifestations of a depressed mood
- Screening test results

Interventions

- Discussions with other interprofessional team members
- Environment modifications made
- Medications given
- Notification of the HCP about patient status
- Therapeutic interventions and the patient's response
- Teaching provided
- Referrals initiated
- Suicide precautions implemented

Evaluation

- Patient's status: improved, stable, declined
- Presence of manifestations of a depressed mood
- Response to teaching provided
- Response to therapeutic interventions

Emotional Problem 52

Definition

An emotional problem that is associated with significant impairment in quality of life, productivity, and interpersonal functioning

Emotional problem is a broad term that reflects a wide range of emotional states, including mood swings and euphoria. All people have normal variations in emotions. What distinguishes an emotional problem is that the person has difficulty regulating their emotions, which results in behaviors or feelings that impair quality of life and productivity.

Emotional problems are strongly linked to growth and development. An infant's expression of emotion is related to their degree of physical comfort and cues from adults. Most children learn to recognize and control their emotions in middle childhood. Thus traumatic experiences during childhood, including abuse, neglect, trauma, and adverse childrearing, are often associated with the development of emotional problems. Adolescents often have mood swings because of fluctuating hormone levels.

Although all people have impulses, most have learned how to control them by adulthood. People who are more impulsive often receive pleasure from acting on the impulse but may feel remorse or regret afterward. Compulsions are a way of avoiding or reducing certain emotions, especially anxiety. People may develop anxiety if they cannot act on an impulse or compulsion.

Having an emotional problem can affect many aspects of a person's life, including their relationships, role performance, and health. Decision-making ability is usually altered. Some persons may engage in substance use or other behaviors considered reckless or dangerous. The person may have difficulty regulating their emotions such that their actions can be harmful to themselves or other people, property, or animals.

Nurses are in a key position to identify a person with an emotional problem and assist patients who need treatment and support. Providing education about how to manage their emotions and helping the patient connect with community and self-help resources can promote quality of life and participation in activities of daily living.

Associated Clinical Problems

- Compulsive Behavior: performing an act persistently and repetitively without it leading to an actual reward or pleasure
- Euphoria: exaggerated feeling of well-being not justified by reality
- Impulsive: predisposition toward rapid, unplanned reactions without regard for the consequences
- Low Self-Control: inability to control one's impulses, emotions, or behaviors
- Mood Swing: periods of variation about how one feels, changing from a sense of well-being to depression

Common Causes and Risk Factors

- Bipolar disorder
- Dementia
- Family history
- Panic disorder
- Schizophrenia
- Substance use
- Traumatic brain injury

Euphoria and Mood Swings

- Central nervous system infections
- Hormone changes
- Medication: corticosteroids
- Multiple sclerosis
- Stress
- Stroke
- Thyroid problems

Impulsivity

- Autism spectrum disorders
- History of childhood trauma, abuse, neglect
- Pediatric autoimmune neuropsychiatric disorders associated with streptococcal infections (PANDAS)

Manifestations

- Anxiety
- Changes in self-image
- Depression
- Self-negating talk
- Social isolation
- Suicidal thoughts

Pediatric

- Problems in school

Compulsive Behavior
- Distress if unable to take part in the repetitive behavior
- Excess cleaning or handwashing
- Feeling pleasure while performing the behavior
- Ordering and arranging things in a very particular way

Euphoria
- Agitation
- Distractibility
- Elevated and expansive mood
- Excess movement
- Hypersexual impulses
- Inflated self-esteem
- Insomnia
- Irritability
- Racing thoughts

Impulsivity
- Anxiety or excitement while acting on the impulse, with relief or pleasure after
- Explosive anger or acts of violence
- Guilt
- Hair pulling
- High-risk sexual behaviors
- Impatient
- Inability to control impulses
- Lying
- Stealing

Low Self-Control
- Impulsive
- Insensitive to others

Mood Swings
- Absence of eye contact
- Difficulty in using facial expressions
- Embarrassment about not being able to express emotions
- Excess, uncontrollable, or involuntary crying or laughter
- Expression of emotions inconsistent with the triggering factor
- Uncontrollable bursts of exaggerated and unintended emotional expression

Key Conceptual Relationships

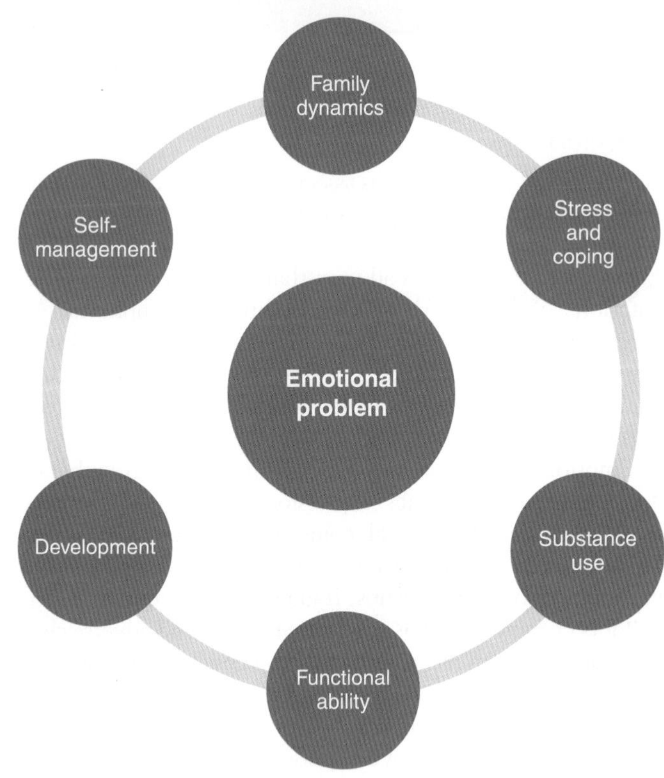

ASSESSMENT OF EMOTIONS	RATIONALE
Assess risk factors that influence having an emotional problem.	A thorough history can identify conditions or situations that place patients at risk for having an emotional problem.
Evaluate underlying health status.	Health status has a significant influence on emotional status and mood.
Perform a complete physical assessment and monitor indicators of an emotional problem on an ongoing basis:	
• Manifestations of an emotional problem	Identifying an emotional problem allows for early intervention.
• Mental status examination, including appearance, attitude, mood and affect, speech, behavior, thought process and content, cognition, insight, and judgment.	An emotional problem is often accompanied by a change in mental status.
Evaluate the results of diagnostic studies, such as a complete blood count, chemistry panel, thyroid panel, liver function tests, urinalysis, and toxicology screens.	Diagnostic test results can help determine whether there is a physiologic cause for an emotional problem.
STRESS AND COPING: Assess the current and past use of stress management and coping strategies.	A patient with an emotional problem may be relying on substance use or other negative behaviors as a means of coping with stress.

ASSESSMENT OF EMOTIONS	RATIONALE
Assess the patient's support system: • Who do they live with? • Are they employed? • Are friends and relatives accessible? • Have they used any community resources?	Interest and support from others are important aspects of managing an emotional problem.
FUNCTIONAL ABILITY: Perform a psychosocial assessment, evaluating for lifestyle effects, such as problems with social interaction, ability to perform responsibilities, and ability to engage in physical activities.	Issues resulting from an emotional problem can affect all aspects of life.
SELF-MANAGEMENT: Assess how well the patient is managing coexisting health problems.	Having an emotional problem can affect a person's motivation and capacity to engage in daily self-management.
SUBSTANCE USE: Screen for alcohol, tobacco, and/or other substance use.	A patient with an emotional problem is at higher risk for substance use disorder.
Evaluate the effectiveness of measures used to manage an emotional problem through ongoing monitoring.	Ongoing monitoring allows for evaluation of therapy effectiveness.

Expected Outcomes

The patient will:

- maintain self-control.
- report an improvement in manifestations.
- participate in role responsibilities.
- adhere to prescribed therapeutic regimen, including engaging in counseling and medication use.
- use appropriate resources when necessary.

INTERVENTIONS TO IMPROVE EMOTIONAL STATUS	RATIONALE
Implement collaborative interventions aimed at treating an underlying risk factor contributing to an emotional problem.	Treatment of underlying causative or risk factors can assist in improving emotional status.
Establish a therapeutic nurse–patient relationship: • Provide privacy and a safe environment. • Use therapeutic touch, with the patient's consent. • Remain nonjudgmental. • Be attentive and use active listening.	A nurse's words and actions that convey sincere acceptance and interest have a positive effect on the patient and help establish trust.
Notify the health care provider (HCP) if manifestations of an emotional problem persist or worsen.	Achievement of an effective treatment plan often requires adjustments in therapy.
Administer prescribed medications:	
• Antidepressants, especially selective serotonin reuptake inhibitors (SSRIs)	SSRIs may help reduce impulsive or compulsive behavior and other mood problems.
• Mood stabilizers, such as lithium and certain antiseizure agents	Mood stabilizers help regulate mood swings and may reduce impulsive and compulsive behaviors by regulating neurotransmitter levels in the brain.
• Atypical antipsychotics, such as aripiprazole (Abilify)	Antipsychotics may reduce manifestations of an emotional problem by regulating neurotransmitter levels in the brain.
Assist the patient in identifying persons to whom they can express feelings openly.	Mood may be enhanced through sharing thoughts and feelings.
Encourage the patient to keep a journal, noting emotions, stressors, medication use, and other potential factors that may influence emotions.	Journal analysis can help identify triggers of untoward emotional reactions.
Limit choices and reduce environment stimuli during periods of euphoria or elation.	Overstimulation can agitate an elated patient.
STRESS AND COPING: Help the patient develop positive coping behaviors.	Positive coping skills equip the patient to manage an emotional problem.

Continued

INTERVENTIONS TO IMPROVE EMOTIONAL STATUS	RATIONALE
Encourage moderate-intensity exercise, such as walking, swimming, and bicycling.	Exercise raises levels of endorphins and may be helpful in reducing mood fluctuations.
Assist the patient in developing problem-solving strategies.	Problem-solving abilities aid the patient in taking action in their life and coping with difficulties, which can reduce emotional problems.
Collaborate with the patient to select and implement complementary and spiritual support therapies, including relaxation, guided imagery, mindful breathing, acupressure, yoga, and massage.	Complementary therapies can help the patient manage an emotional problem and stress by focusing on mind and body connections.
DEVELOPMENT: Encourage the patient to express feelings about themselves and implement measures to enhance self-image.	Higher self-esteem may reduce mood swings and impulsivity.
NUTRITION: Encourage the patient to follow a nutritionally adequate diet, with reduced caffeine intake.	Caffeine is a stimulant and may trigger mood swings and impulsive or compulsive behaviors.
CULTURE: Implement measures to promote positive social interaction.	Social interaction can decrease feelings of isolation and loneliness.
SLEEP: Provide the patient with opportunities for adequate sleep.	A lack of adequate rest has a negative effect on mood and self-control.
STRESS AND COPING: Encourage the use of stress management strategies.	Stress from life issues may intensify an emotional problem and contribute to mood swings.
SUBSTANCE USE: Implement measures to address substance use.	Substance use compounds an emotional problem in many patients.

COLLABORATION	RATIONALE
Psychological specialist for cognitive behavioral therapy (CBT) and counseling	CBT and counseling may assist the patient in managing an emotional problem.
CARE COORDINATION: Social work or case management	The social worker can explore resources to help the patient obtain access to health care.
Support groups and other mental health resources	Specialty mental health support services are available to assist the patient with managing the effects of having an emotional problem.
FAMILY DYNAMICS: Family-focused therapy	Family therapy focuses on the cause of an emotional problem, symptoms, and treatments, resulting in improved patient outcomes.
SPIRITUALITY: Pastoral care with a professional or preferred spiritual or religious leader	Pastoral care can assist patients with their emotional, psychological, and spiritual coping.

PATIENT AND CAREGIVER TEACHING

- Factors contributing to the emotional problem
- Manifestations of the emotional problem
- Management of a condition contributing to the emotional problem
- Early recognition of problems and how to manage them
- Health promotion behaviors, including nutrition, sleep, and exercise
- Positive coping and stress management strategies
- Positive verbal and nonverbal communication skills
- Community and self-help resources available
- Sources of information and social support
- Safe use of medications, including side effect management, and how they fit into the overall management plan
- Importance of long-term follow-up
- When to notify the HCP and seek emergency assistance

 DOCUMENTATION

Assessment

- Assessments performed
- Manifestations of an emotional problem
- Screening test results

Interventions

- Discussions with other interprofessional team members
- Medications given
- Notification of the HCP about patient status
- Therapeutic interventions and the patient's response
- Teaching provided
- Referrals initiated
- Safety measures implemented

Evaluation

- Patient's status: improved, stable, declined
- Presence of manifestations of an emotional problem
- Response to teaching provided
- Response to therapeutic interventions

Impaired Psychological Status 53

Definition

State in which there is a loss of contact with reality

Psychosis is a state in which there is a loss of contact with reality. Perception, thoughts, mood, affect, and behavior are altered in a patient experiencing a psychotic episode. The person may have delusions and hallucinations that interfere with activities of daily living.

Psychoses are categorized as primary or secondary. *Primary psychosis* is usually chronic and stems from a psychiatric condition, such as schizophrenia. Persons with primary psychosis are more likely to have multiple episodes and greater disability. *Secondary psychosis* often arises from a medical condition. Psychosis can occur with dementia and delirium, be a sign of another medical condition, or be a result of substance use. Those with a secondary cause have a greater chance of recovering from a psychotic episode.

Psychosis has a variety of symptoms. There are two categories: positive and negative symptoms. Positive symptoms are changes in thoughts and feelings that "add to" or distort normal function. These include hallucinations and delusions. With negative symptoms, there is a loss of experience or something is "taken away." Examples include the inability to respond to people emotionally and the lack of speech.

Because reality is distorted, those with psychosis have considerable problems with social and role functions. They may struggle with maintaining employment and housing and attending to their basic needs. Caregivers may feel helpless or inadequate because they cannot make the patient feel better. Depression and anxiety are common. Suicide is a common cause of death. Nurses are in a key position to provide psychosocial care that helps the person improve their interpersonal and social function.

Associated Clinical Problems

- Delusions: fixed beliefs or thoughts that are false or not real
- Hallucinations: sensory perception experiences that occur without an external stimulus
- Suspicion: feeling that someone or something cannot be trusted

Common Risk Factors

- Acute substance intoxication
- Adverse child-rearing
- Carbon monoxide poisoning
- Child abuse
- Chromosomal conditions, including Klinefelter syndrome, fragile X syndrome
- Central nervous system infections, including encephalitis, meningitis, Lyme disease
- Delirium
- Dementia
- Endocrine problems
- Epilepsy
- Exposure to heavy metals, including arsenic, mercury
- Family history
- Head injury
- History of psychotic episode(s)
- Medications: anticholinergics, antiseizure agents, corticosteroids, sedative-hypnotics
- Neurodegenerative disorders, such as multiple sclerosis
- Perinatal trauma
- Personality disorder
- Psychiatric illness
- Schizophrenia
- Stroke
- Substance use

Manifestations

- Abnormal motor behavior
- Affect inappropriate to the situation
- Agitation
- Anhedonia
- Boundary problems
- Broadcasting
- Catatonia
- Delirium
- Delusions
- Disorganized speech
- Disorganized thinking
- Failure to attend to self-care
- Flat affect
- Fluctuating mental status
- Hallucinations
- Illusions
- Lack of speech (alogia)
- Lack of or not engaging in social interaction
- Not taking part in usual activities
- Thought insertion
- Suicidal ideation
- Suspicion
- Withdrawal

Key Conceptual Relationships

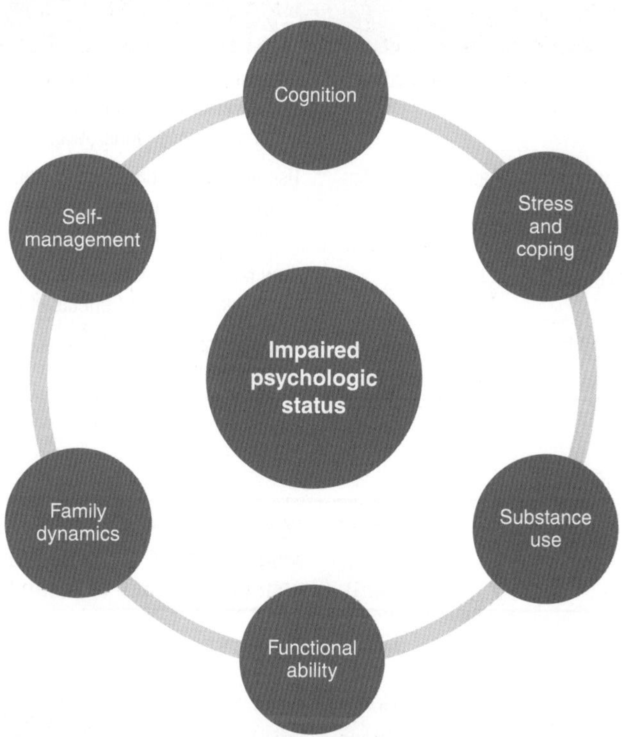

ASSESSMENT OF PSYCHOLOGICAL STATUS	RATIONALE
Assess risk factors contributing to impaired psychological status.	Treatment of secondary causes of psychoses may result in resolution of impaired psychological status.
Assess the patient through observation and direct questioning for suicidal ideation.	Prompt referral to a mental health professional is needed if suicidal ideation is present.
Evaluate the patient's underlying health status.	Underlying health status has a significant influence on psychological status.
Use a valid, reliable tool, such as the Brief Psychiatric Rating Scale (Table 53.1) or the Positive and Negative Syndrome Scale, to detect impaired psychological status.	Identifying impaired psychological status allows for early intervention.
Perform a complete physical assessment and monitor indicators of psychological status on an ongoing basis:	
• Manifestations of a depressed mood	Identifying a depressed mood allows for early intervention.
• Complete a mental status examination, including appearance; attitude, mood, and affect; speech; behavior; thought process and content; cognition; insight; judgment.	Impaired psychological status is often characterized by observable changes.
Evaluate the results of diagnostic studies, such as a complete blood count (CBC), chemistry panel, thyroid panel, liver function tests, urinalysis, and toxicology screens.	Diagnostic test results can help distinguish between a primary or secondary cause of psychosis.
STRESS AND COPING: Assess the current and past use of stress management and coping strategies.	A patient with an impaired psychological status may be relying on substance use or other negative behaviors as a means of coping.
Assess the patient's support system: • Who they live with • Employment status • Accessible friends and relatives • Use of community resources	Interest and support from others are important aspects of care management.
FUNCTIONAL ABILITY: Perform a psychosocial assessment, evaluating for lifestyle effects, such as problems with social interaction, ability to perform responsibilities, and ability to engage in physical activities.	Problems resulting from an impaired psychological status can affect all aspects of a person's life and inhibit their functioning within society.

ASSESSMENT OF PSYCHOLOGICAL STATUS	RATIONALE
SUBSTANCE USE: Screen for alcohol, tobacco, and/or other substance use.	A patient with a psychological problem is at higher risk for substance use disorder; psychotic symptoms may be a response to intoxication or substance withdrawal.
SAFETY: Screen patients receiving antipsychotic medication therapy for adverse effects.	Use of antipsychotics agents can cause extrapyramidal symptoms, metabolic syndrome, neuroleptic malignant syndrome, and liver and immune system problems.
FAMILY DYNAMICS: Evaluate family dynamics, current level of functioning, and family interactions.	How family members act toward and react to the patient may contribute to symptoms and effects of management.
Evaluate the effectiveness of measures used to address psychological status through ongoing monitoring.	Ongoing monitoring allows for evaluation of therapy effectiveness.

Table 53.1 Brief Psychiatric Rating Scale

	Not Present (1 point)	Very Mild (2 points)	Mild (3 points)	Moderate (4 points)	Moderately Severe (5 points)	Severe (6 points)	Extremely Severe (7 points)
SOMATIC CONCERN—preoccupation with physical health, fear of physical illness, hypochondriasis	☐	☐	☐	☐	☐	☐	☐
ANXIETY—worry, fear, overconcern for present or future, uneasiness	☐	☐	☐	☐	☐	☐	☐
EMOTIONAL WITHDRAWAL—lack of spontaneous interaction, isolation deficiency in relating to others	☐	☐	☐	☐	☐	☐	☐
CONCEPTUAL DISORGANIZATION—thought processes confused, disconnected, disorganized, disrupted	☐	☐	☐	☐	☐	☐	☐
GUILT FEELINGS—self-blame, shame, remorse for past behavior	☐	☐	☐	☐	☐	☐	☐
TENSION—physical and motor manifestations of nervousness, overactivation	☐	☐	☐	☐	☐	☐	☐
MANNERISMS AND POSTURING—peculiar, bizarre, unnatural motor behavior (not including tic)	☐	☐	☐	☐	☐	☐	☐
GRANDIOSITY—exaggerated self-opinion, arrogance, conviction of unusual power or abilities	☐	☐	☐	☐	☐	☐	☐
DEPRESSIVE MOOD—sorrow, sadness, despondency, pessimism	☐	☐	☐	☐	☐	☐	☐
HOSTILITY—animosity, contempt, belligerence, disdain for others	☐	☐	☐	☐	☐	☐	☐
SUSPICIOUSNESS—mistrust, belief that others harbor malicious or discriminatory intent	☐	☐	☐	☐	☐	☐	☐
HALLUCINATORY BEHAVIOR—perceptions without normal stimulus correspondence	☐	☐	☐	☐	☐	☐	☐
MOTOR RETARDATION—slowed or weakened movements or speech, reduced body tone	☐	☐	☐	☐	☐	☐	☐
UNCOOPERATIVENESS—resistance, guardedness, rejection of authority	☐	☐	☐	☐	☐	☐	☐
UNUSUAL THOUGHT CONTENT—unusual, odd, strange, bizarre thought content	☐	☐	☐	☐	☐	☐	☐
BLUNTED AFFECT—reduced emotional tone, reduction in formal intensity of feelings, flatness	☐	☐	☐	☐	☐	☐	☐
EXCITEMENT—emotional tone, agitation, increased reactivity	☐	☐	☐	☐	☐	☐	☐
DISORIENTATION—confusion or lack of proper association for person, place, or time	☐	☐	☐	☐	☐	☐	☐

Scoring: Sum the total score for the 18 items. Monitor serial results as a measure of response to treatment.
From Mendez M. *The Mental Status Examination Handbook*. Elsevier; 2022.

Expected Outcomes

The patient will:

- identify when experiencing symptoms.
- be free from self-harm.
- have reduced or no symptoms, including delusions and hallucinations.
- take part in role responsibilities and attend to self-care.
- adhere to prescribed therapeutic regimen, including engaging in counseling and medication use.
- implement measures to address medication side effects.
- contact proper emergency resources when necessary.
- maintain continuing contact with the appropriate community resources.
- refrain from substance use.

INTERVENTIONS TO IMPROVE PSYCHOLOGICAL STATUS	RATIONALE
Initiate safety protocols and referrals if the patient is at risk for self-harm.	The risk of self-harm from delusions or hallucinations requires measures to keep the patient safe.
Implement measures to protect the patient from self-harm or suicide: • Remove sharp and glass objects from the environment. • Remove belts and strings from the environment. • Provide constant 1-to-1 interaction if the risk for self-harm is high. • Check on the patient every 15 minutes.	These measures help maintain a safe environment to prevent the patient from self-harming and suicide.
Implement collaborative interventions aimed at treating factors contributing to impaired status.	Treatment of secondary causes of psychoses may result in resolution of impaired psychological status.
Notify the health care provider (HCP) if manifestations of a psychological problem persist or worsen.	Achieving an effective treatment plan often requires adjustments in therapy.
Notify the HCP if adverse medication effects occur.	The presence of some adverse effects, including extrapyramidal symptoms and liver problems, may require an adjustment in medication or dose.
Establish a therapeutic nurse–patient relationship: • Provide privacy and a safe environment. • Remain nonjudgmental. • Use active listening with therapeutic communication skills.	Words and actions that convey sincere acceptance and interest have a positive effect on the patient and help establish trust.
Assign a primary care nurse.	This establishes trust and boundaries so that changes can be immediately processed.
Reduce environment stimuli: • Maintain a well-lit environment that reduces sharp contrasts and shadows. • Remove excessive sensory stimuli (e.g., television or broadcast intercom announcements) when possible.	Excessive environment stimuli may precipitate or support delusions and hallucinations.
Administer prescribed medications:	
• First-generation antipsychotic agents, such as haloperidol (Haldol)	First-generation agents reduce the transmission of dopamine at key dopaminergic pathways in the brain, reducing positive symptoms.
• Second-generation antipsychotic agents, such as risperidone (Risperdal) and quetiapine (Seroquel)	Second-generation agents have fewer extrapyramidal side effects and are effective in reducing positive and negative symptoms.
• Anticholinergics, such as benztropine (Cogentin), bromocriptine	Anticholinergics are an adjunct therapy used to treat extrapyramidal side effects from antipsychotic agents.
• Benzodiazepines, such as alprazolam (Xanax)	Benzodiazepines provide tranquilization or sedation for the patient who has agitated or violent behavior.
SELF-MANAGEMENT: Provide the patient with resources to promote adherence to medication therapy and assist with managing side effects.	Education and discussion of side effects may assist the patient with expectations of treatment and limit the resistance to continued compliance.
COGNITION: Implement reality orientation measures.	Cognitive impairments and disturbances with reality are common manifestations of a psychotic episode.

INTERVENTIONS TO IMPROVE PSYCHOLOGICAL STATUS	RATIONALE
FUNCTIONAL ABILITY: Help the patient develop strategies to increase participation in activities of daily living.	These strategies address apathy and lack of interest in participating in activities of daily living that accompany psychosis.
Encourage participation in moderate-intensity exercise, such as walking, swimming, and bicycling.	Psychotic symptoms and the sedating effects of antipsychotic agents can lead to decreased activity.
NUTRITION: Implement measures to reduce weight gain.	Psychotic symptoms and the sedating effects of antipsychotic agents can lead to weight gain.
SUBSTANCE USE: Implement measures to address substance use.	A patient with a psychological problem is at higher risk for substance use disorder.
STRESS AND COPING: Help the patient develop positive coping behaviors.	Positive coping skills equip the patient to manage psychological problems.
Assist the patient in identifying persons to whom they can express feelings openly.	Mood may be enhanced through sharing thoughts and feelings.
Assist the patient in developing appropriate problem-solving strategies.	Developing problem-solving ability aids the patient in acting in coping with challenges.
Encourage the use of stress management strategies.	Stress from life issues may have a compounding effect on a person with a depressed mood.
FUNCTIONAL ABILITY: Implement measures to promote positive social interaction.	Positive social interaction can decrease feelings of social isolation.
Assist the patient with performing personal care, if needed.	A certain level of personal hygiene is needed to ensure health and promote positive social interactions.

COLLABORATION	RATIONALE
Psychological specialist for cognitive behavior therapy, cognitive enhancement therapy	Cognitive behavior therapy, cognitive enhancement therapy, and other therapies are part of the comprehensive treatment of psychosis.
CARE COORDINATION: Social work or case management	The social worker can explore resources to help the patient obtain access to health care.
Support groups and other mental health resources	Specialty mental health support services are available to assist the patient with managing the effects of having a psychological condition.
FAMILY DYNAMICS: Family-focused therapy	Family therapy focuses on the cause of psychosis, symptoms, and treatments, resulting in improved patient outcomes.
FUNCTIONAL ABILITY: Social skills training	Assisting the patient in developing social skills will help them maintain relationships with others.
Vocational rehabilitation	Specialty support services can assist the patient in achieving maximum independent functioning and well-being.

PATIENT AND CAREGIVER TEACHING

- Factors that contribute to impaired psychological status
- Management of a condition contributing to impaired psychological status
- Effects of psychosis on the family and option of family therapy
- Social services and community support for the patient and family
- Early recognition of episodes and how to manage them
- Safe use of medications, including proper use and side effect management, and how they fit into the overall management plan
- Community and self-help resources
- Positive coping and stress management strategies
- Relaxation techniques
- Anticipatory guidance about situations and stressors that may increase the risk of an episode
- Health promotion behaviors, including nutrition, sleep, exercise
- Importance of long-term follow-up
- Crisis line contact information
- When to notify the HCP or seek emergency services

 **DOCUMENTATION**

Assessment

- Assessments performed
- Diagnostic and laboratory test results
- Manifestations of impaired psychological status
- Screening test results

Interventions

- Discussions with other interprofessional team members
- Environment modifications made
- Medications given
- Notification of the HCP about patient status
- Notification of the proper authorities
- Therapeutic interventions and the patient's response
- Teaching provided
- Referrals initiated
- Safety measures implemented

Evaluation

- Patient's status: improved, stable, declined
- Manifestations of impaired psychological status
- Response to teaching provided
- Response to therapeutic interventions

Caregiver Role Strain 54

Definition

Distress in providing health-related care for a family member or significant other

Caregivers are family members or significant others who give or assist with direct patient care; provide emotional, social, spiritual, and possibly financial support for the patient; and manage and coordinate health care services. Approximately one in four adults in the United States provides daily care to someone. Caregiving involves providing psychological, or development needs beyond routine childcare and parenting.

The most common caregivers are spouses, adult children, parents, grandparents, and life partners. The most common family caregivers are older adult females. Other examples include but are not limited to those who care for spouses or parents with Alzheimer disease, grandparents who care for a grandchild with a development disorder, parents who care for an adult child with a spinal cord injury, and life partners who care for loved ones with a chronic illness.

It is important for nurses to be aware of the role caregivers play in health care delivery, the impact of this role on caregivers' lives, and supportive interventions needed to care for caregivers. How caregivers deal with caregiving depends on their perception of the experience and their coping abilities. What is stressful for one person may not be stressful for another. Important factors that influence how caregivers perceive and react to the challenges of caregiving include their level of knowledge; their feelings of anticipatory loss and grief; and the availability of material, practical, and spiritual resources needed for self-care. Nurses are an important source of support for family caregivers.

Associated Clinical Problems

- Compassion Fatigue: negative emotions and/or lack of empathy as a result of chronic exposure to difficult situations or extended caregiving
- Conflicting Caregiver Attitude: caregiver's attitude conflicts with the patient's preferences and/or the treatment plan
- Difficulty with Caretaking Responsibilities: sense of burden and effort in managing the care of a family member
- Risk for Caregiver Role Strain: increased risk for stress in performing the role of family caregiver

Common Causes and Risk Factors

- Change in living conditions to accommodate family member
- Change in roles and relationships within family unit
- Difficulty providing care
- Family conflict regarding caregiving decisions
- Financial strain resulting from patient's or caregiver's inability to work
- Having underlying health problems
- Inability to meet personal self-care needs, such as socialization, sleep, eating, exercise, and rest
- Inadequate information or skills related to caregiving tasks, such as bathing, drug administration, and wound care
- Lack of respite or relief from caregiving responsibilities
- Need to juggle day-to-day activities, decisions, and caregiving
- Other people's lack of understanding of the time and energy needed for caregiving
- Providing and coordinating complex health care

Manifestations

- Anger
- Anxiety
- Depression
- Denial
- Exhaustion
- Frustration
- Health problems
- Impaired sleep
- Irritability
- Lack of concentration
- Resentment
- Social withdrawal
- Stressed

Related Concepts and Clinical Problems

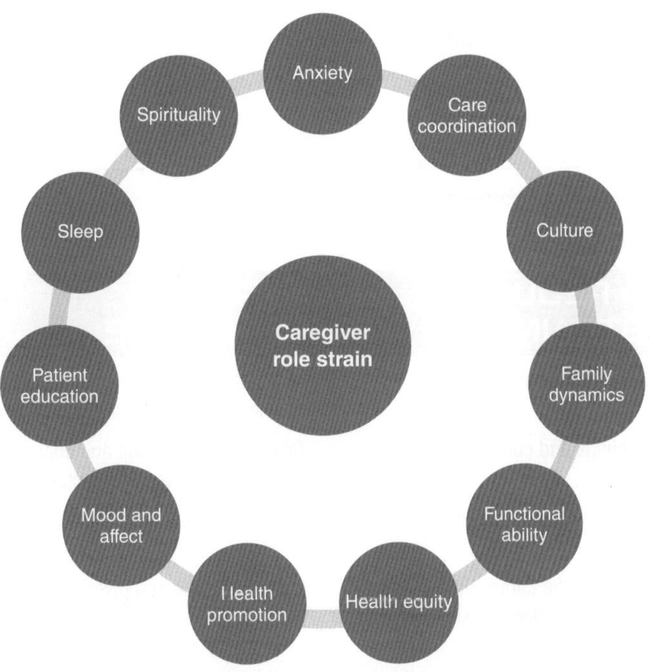

ASSESSMENT OF CAREGIVER ROLE STRAIN	RATIONALE
CULTURE: Identify all the caregivers involved with a patient's care.	The designated family spokesperson may be someone other than the direct caregiver(s).
Have the caregiver describe their typical day.	Establish a sense of the caregiver's role responsibilities.
Evaluate the patient and caregiver's relationship prior to the initiation of caregiving.	A history of tense or troubled relationships increases risk for role strain.
Ask the caregiver about their experience of the role and what helps them cope.	Focus on strengths and using positive coping strategies.
Evaluate the caregiver's underlying health status.	Health status has a significant influence on the ability to provide care.
HEALTH PROMOTION: Assess the caregiver's self-health management, including nutrition, sleep habits, exercise participation, and meeting personal health needs.	Maintaining physical health is important in being able to manage the physical and emotional work of caregiving.
CULTURE: Assess the caregiver's social interactions outside the caregiving relationship and the quality of available social support.	Maintaining social relationships helps to avoid isolation.
Assess the caregiver's current use of resources for information, caregiving support, and practical assistance.	Determining what resources have been useful is a foundation for teaching about other options.
Determine the caregiver's knowledge of and access to respite resources and services.	Having periods of relief to maintain personal health and relaxation may help lessen role strain.
PATIENT EDUCATION: Assess the caregiver's development and mental status and readiness to learn.	Determine the caregiver's readiness for new information related to providing care.
FAMILY DYNAMICS: Evaluate family dynamics, current level of functioning, and family interactions.	The strain of caregiving can exacerbate underlying tension among family members, such as sibling rivalry.
STRESS AND COPING: Assess and periodically monitor for indicators of caregiver role strain and stress.	Ongoing monitoring is needed to identify changes in stress level that may require additional intervention.

Expected Outcomes

The caregiver will:

- maintain their own physical and emotional health.
- be free from caregiver role strain.
- appropriately use support.

The patient will:

- receive safe care.
- maintain a positive relationship with the caregiver.

INTERVENTIONS TO REDUCE CAREGIVER ROLE STRAIN	RATIONALE
Acknowledge the ongoing contributions of the caregiver.	Acknowledgment demonstrates respect for the caregiver as a person and their contribution to the care of the patient.
Encourage the caregiver to talk about feelings and concerns about caregiving.	Talking about feelings and concerns helps build rapport and decrease the caregiver's sense of isolation.
Work with the caregiver to develop a routine that supports caregiving and maintaining a personal schedule.	Having a routine with personal time for the caregiver lessens role strain.
HEALTH PROMOTION: Encourage and support the caregiver in planning to maintain personal physical health with nutrition, physical activity, and adequate sleep.	Maintaining the caregiver's physical health is important in being able to manage the physical and emotional work of caregiving.
FUNCTIONAL ABILITY: Encourage the caregiver to maintain meaningful relationships outside of the home (friends, churches, hobbies, sports).	Relationships outside the home help the caregiver avoid social isolation and receive social support to manage stress.
PATIENT EDUCATION: Provide clear information about how to care for the patient at a level appropriate for the caregiver.	Information about how to provide care can make caregiving effective and ease stress.
Help the caregiver connect with local resources for help with practical issues, such as transportation and meals.	Community resources may be available to assist the caregiver.
CARE COORDINATION: Provide for consistent follow-up caregiver assistance through phone calls and/or home health or community nurse care.	Access to health professionals is an important source of information and support.
Encourage the caregiver's use of positive coping and stress management strategies.	Positive coping and stress management promote the caregiver's sense of control and ease stress levels.
Identify family options for respite care and explain local options for professional respite care.	Families may be able to share care responsibilities and/or may need assistance.
Recommend that the caregiver accept the help of others and suggest specific ways that others can contribute, such as: • Providing a meal • Doing an errand • Providing respite while the caregiver takes time for personal needs, exercise, and relaxation • Taking care of household cleaning and tasks	It may be difficult for the caregiver to ask for or accept help in the role.
FAMILY DYNAMICS: Institute measures to promote optimal family function and refer the patient and family to family-focused therapy, as appropriate.	Promoting positive family interaction and communication will help the family cope with the patient's illness and caregiving.
MOOD AND AFFECT: Implement measures to assist the caregiver in managing any depression, anxiety, or other psychological problem.	Caregiver role strain is associated with depression, anxiety, and other psychological problems.
SLEEP: Institute measures to address impaired sleep, if present.	Impaired sleep is a manifestation of caregiver role strain and increases the overall stress level.

COLLABORATION	RATIONALE
STRESS AND COPING: Support group	Groups provide emotional support and are an important source of practical insider information.
CARE COORDINATION: Social work or case management	Social workers and case managers can explore resources to help the patient and caregiver.
FUNCTIONAL ABILITY: Home health agency	A home health agency may provide assistance with the patient's care and household maintenance.
SPIRITUALITY: Pastoral care professional or the caregiver's preferred spiritual or religious leader or faith community	The caregiver may receive comfort and support from their religious leaders and faith community as they provide support, perform spiritual counseling, and offer practical assistance.
SAFETY: Adult protective services	Adult protective services advocates for the well-being of older adults who may be in danger or have no one to assist them.

PATIENT AND CAREGIVER TEACHING

- Factors that contribute to role strain
- Manifestations of role strain
- Importance of self-care, including nutrition, sleep, and exercise
- Benefits of sharing responsibilities with others
- Community and self-help resources
- Sources of information and social support
- Positive coping and stress management strategies
- Communication with health professionals
- Anticipatory guidance regarding problem situations

DOCUMENTATION

Assessment

- Perception of caregiving
- Caregiver health status
- Current coping strategies
- Manifestations of role strain

Interventions

- Measures initiated to promote self-care
- Teaching provided about resources
- Discussions with other members of the interprofessional team
- Referrals initiated

Evaluation

- Use of coping strategies
- Ongoing health status
- Unmet needs of patient and/or caregiver
- Manifestations of role strain
- Response to teaching provided

Difficulty Coping 55

Definition

Inadequate personal ability to manage problems, stress, or responsibilities

Stress is a response to perceived (real or imagined) demands or threats to one's well-being. Responses to the same stressor vary greatly. What one person perceives as stressful may not seem stressful to someone else. Stress can be physiologic, emotional, or psychological.

The stress response involves increases in cardiac output (resulting from the increased heart rate and increased stroke volume), blood glucose levels, oxygen consumption, and metabolic rate. Dilation of skeletal muscle blood vessels increases blood supply to the large muscles and supports quick movement. Increased cerebral blood flow increases mental alertness. For example, in stressful situations such as blood loss, increased extracellular fluid and the shunting of blood away from the gastrointestinal system help to maintain adequate circulation to vital organs. However, if stress is excessive or prolonged, these same physiologic responses can lead to harm. When a person sustains chronic, unrelieved stress, the body's defenses can no longer keep up with the demands. Chronic stress is a major factor in causing and worsening health conditions.

Coping is an effort to manage stressors. Coping strategies are positive or negative behaviors and actions to help deal with stress. Positive coping includes activities such as exercise and spending time with friends and family. Healthy coping helps you handle your stressors so that they do not overwhelm you. Negative coping may include substance use and denial. The consequences of poor coping can be physical, psychosocial, or both. Poor coping may lead to a decline in physical health status, depression and anxiety, a reduction in functional ability, and a change in social or financial status. Family and social relationships may suffer.

High levels of stress are common among patients, caregivers, and health care team members. How people deal with their stress is critical to their well-being. In addition to current stresses, many people have experienced adverse childhood events or other traumatic situations. Trauma-informed care involves empathetic, supportive recognition surrounding the significance and special needs of individuals who have previously experienced trauma. Nurses play a key role in helping persons recognize stress and implementing measures to enhance the ability to manage stressful events.

Associated Clinical Problems

- Denial: unconscious defense mechanism in which emotional conflict and anxiety are avoided by refusal to acknowledge those thoughts, feelings, desires, impulses, or facts that are consciously intolerable
- Denial About Illness Severity: avoiding acknowledgment about the seriousness of a health issue
- Difficulty Coping With Pain: inadequate ability to manage the experience of pain
- Difficulty Coping With Postpartum Changes: inadequate ability to manage physical and emotional changes from childbirth
- Impaired Acceptance of Health Status: inability to reconcile a significant change in health
- Impaired Adjustment: inability to make changes in response to stressful new circumstances
- Ineffective Community Coping: inability to manage community stressors using positive strategies
- Ineffective Family Coping: inability to manage family stressors using positive strategies
- Risk for Ineffective Family Coping: increased risk for inability to manage family stressors using positive strategies
- Ineffective Individual Coping: inability to manage personal stressors using positive strategies.
- Lack of Resilience: difficulty in weathering periods of stress and change successfully throughout life
- Posttrauma Response: pertaining to any emotional, mental, or physiologic consequences after a major illness, injury, or experience
- Risk for Posttrauma Syndrome: increased risk for emotional, mental, or physiologic consequences after a major illness, injury, or experience
- Risk for Difficulty Coping: increased risk for inability to manage stressors using positive coping strategies
- Stress Overload: inability to cope with perceived (real or imagined) demands or threats to one's mental, emotional, or spiritual well-being
- Moral Distress: response to situations where there is a moral problem, but those who have a responsibility to do something cannot act in a way that preserves their integrity

- Parental Stress: parent's or guardian's response to the demands or threats of raising a child
- Relocation Stress: difficulty coping with perceived threat in movement from one environment to another
- Risk for Relocation Stress: increased risk of inability to cope with movement from one environment to another

Common Causes and Risk Factors

- Cultural belief conflicts
- Disability
- Disruption in family routine
- Family configuration changes, including birth, divorce, death, and marriage
- Family member with disability, chronic illness, or poor health
- Impaired role performance
- Inadequate resources or social support
- Having a terminal or serious illness
- Lack of motivation
- Military combat
- Natural or human-made disasters
- Neurobiologic imbalances
- New, unpredictable situation
- Overwhelming life circumstances
- Pathologic fatigue
- Prolonged grief reaction
- Significant incident involving a family member, such as crime or jail
- Victim of interpersonal violence
- Witnessing horrific events

Common Health Disorders with a Stress Component

- Anxiety
- Depression
- Dyspepsia
- Eating disorders
- Fatigue
- Fibromyalgia
- Headaches
- Hypertension
- Insomnia
- Irritable bowel syndrome
- Low back pain
- Menstrual irregularities
- Peptic ulcer disease
- Sexual dysfunction

Manifestations

- Difficulty concentrating
- Inability to communicate effectively
- Inability to meet needs and role expectations
- Increased occurrence of illness
- Negative self-image
- Self-report of inability to cope or manage stress
- Sleep problems
- Substance use
- Withdrawal

Physical Manifestation of Acute Stress

- Decreased digestion and peristalsis
- Decreased secretions
- Excessive perspiration
- Increased glucose
- Increased heart rate
- Increased respiration rate
- Increased systolic blood pressure (BP)
- Muscle tension
- Peripheral vasoconstriction

Pediatric

- School problems

Denial

- Does not admit the influence of stressors on life
- Minimizes or dismisses symptoms
- Nonadherence

Risk for Ineffective Family Coping

- Abandonment or neglect
- Inability to meet family members' needs
- Negative family interactions

Risk for Relocation Stress

- Expresses concern over move
- Increased dependency
- Need for excessive reassurance
- Unwillingness to move

Key Conceptual Relationships

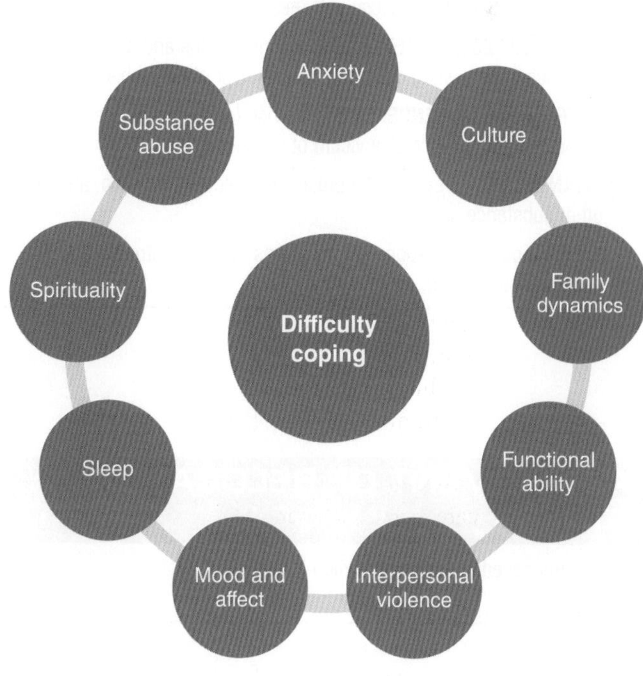

ASSESSMENT OF STRESS AND COPING	RATIONALE
Assess risk factors for stress.	Identifying factors that place the patient at risk for stress allows for early intervention.
Encourage the patient to identify sources of stress.	Verbalizing sources of stress may support coping and problem solving.
Assess underlying health status and determine any physiologic sources of stress.	Disease processes may contribute to overall stress.
Use a formal, patient-specific stress assessment scale, such as the Holmes Social Readjustment Rating Scale (Table 55.1), to identify sources of stress.	An assessment tool can help identify the level and sources of stress.
Perform a complete physical assessment and monitor indicators of the stress response on an ongoing basis.	Identifying the presence of the stress response allows for early intervention.
Ask about current and previously used methods of coping with difficult situations.	The health care team can build a plan of care on the patient's previous strengths and positive coping strategies.
Have the patient complete a formal tool assessing coping strategies, such as the Ways of Coping Scale or the Brief COPE (Table 55.2).	Scales can be used to identify strategies used for coping with or responding to stressors.
FAMILY DYNAMICS: Assess the patient's social resources and support system: • Who lives with them? • Are friends and relatives accessible? • Have they used any community resources?	Social support and other resources may be useful in coping with stressors.
Develop an ecomap for the patient.	An ecomap, a diagram that shows the social and personal relationships of a person with their environment, may help identify stresses and resources.
FAMILY DYNAMICS: Evaluate family dynamics, current level of function, and family interactions.	How family members act and react to the patient's stress affects how the patient copes.
CULTURE: Assess the person's perception of cultural conflicts that may increase stress.	Differences in views regarding gender roles, family relationships, spirituality, and other factors may present a cultural conflict that increases stress.
FUNCTIONAL ABILITY: Perform a psychosocial assessment, evaluating the effects of stress on daily life, including the ability to sleep, enjoy life, interact with others, perform work and household duties, and engage in physical and social activities.	Difficulty coping with stress can affect all aspects of a person's life.
MOOD AND AFFECT, ANXIETY: Assess mental status and screen for the presence of coexisting depression, anxiety, or other problems.	Patients with stress may have coexisting depression, anxiety, or other psychological disorders.
INTERPERSONAL VIOLENCE: Assess the risk for the patient being a perpetrator of violence or a victim of violence.	Violence may be present as an ineffective method of coping with stress.
SUBSTANCE USE: Screen for the presence of alcohol, tobacco, and/or other substance use.	A patient under stress is at higher risk for substance use disorder.
Evaluate the patient's response to measures to reduce stress through ongoing assessment.	Ongoing assessment allows for evaluation of therapy effectiveness.

ASSESSMENT OF RELOCATION STRESS	RATIONALE
Assess the speed at which relocation is occurring.	Relocation stress is often increased when the relocation is rushed or must occur quickly.

Table 55.1 Social Readjustment Rating Scale

Event	Event Value	Event	Event Value
1. Death of a spouse	100	22. Change in responsibilities at work	29
2. Divorce	73	23. Son or daughter leaving home	29
3. Marital separation	65	24. Trouble with in-laws	29
4. Jail term	63	25. Outstanding personal achievement	28
5. Death of a close family member	63	26. Spouse begins or stops work	26
6. Personal injury or illness	53	27. Begin or end school	26
7. Marriage	50	28. Change in living conditions	25
8. Fired at work	47	29. Revision of personal habits	24
9. Marital reconciliation	45	30. Trouble with boss	23
10. Retirement	45	31. Change in work hours or conditions	20
11. Change in health of family member	44	32. Change in residence	20
12. Pregnancy	40	33. Change in schools	20
13. Sex difficulties	39	34. Change in recreation	19
14. Gain of a new family member	39	35. Change in church activities	19
15. Business readjustment	39	36. Change in social activities	19
16. Change in financial state	38	37. Change in sleeping habits	16
17. Death of a close friend	37	38. Change in number of family get-togethers	15
18. Change to different line of work	36	39. Vacation	13
19. Change in number of arguments	35	40. Christmas	12
20. Mortgage or loan over $10,000	31	41. Minor violations of the law	11
21. Foreclosure of mortgage or loan	30	Total Points	

Directions for completion: Add up the point values for each of the events that you have experienced during the past 12 months.

Below 150 points:

The amount of stress you are experiencing as a result of changes in your life is normal and manageable. There is only a 1 in 3 chance that you might develop a serious illness over the next 2 years based on stress alone. Consider practicing a daily relaxation technique to reduce your chance of illness even more.

150–300 points:

The amount of stress you are experiencing as a result of changes in your life is moderate. Based on stress alone, you have a 50/50 chance of developing a serious illness over the next 2 years. You can reduce these odds by practicing stress management and relaxation techniques on a daily basis.

Over 300 points:

The amount of stress you are experiencing as a result of changes in your life is high. Based on stress alone, your chances of developing a serious illness during the next 2 years approaches 90%, unless you are already practicing good coping skills and regular relaxation techniques. You can reduce the chance of illness by practicing coping strategies and relaxation techniques daily.

Source: Holmes TH, Rahe RH. The social readjustment rating scale. *J Psychosom Res.* 1967;11:213.

Table 55.2 Brief COPE

These items deal with ways you've been coping with the stress in your life since you found out you were going to need to have this operation. There are many ways to try to deal with problems. These items ask what you've been doing to cope with this one. Obviously, different people deal with things in different ways, but I'm interested in how you've tried to deal with it. Each item says something about a particular way of coping. I want to know to what extent you've been doing what the item says—how much or how frequently. Don't answer based on whether it seems to be working or not—just whether you're doing it. Use these response choices. Try to rate each item separately in your mind from the others. Make your answers as true for you as you can.

1 = I haven't been doing this at all
2 = I've been doing this a little bit
3 = I've been doing this a medium amount
4 = I've been doing this a lot

Continued

Table 55.2 Brief COPE—cont'd

1. ______ I've been turning to work or other activities to take my mind off things.
2. ______ I've been concentrating my efforts on doing something about the situation I'm in.
3. ______ I've been saying to myself, "This isn't real."
4. ______ I've been using alcohol or other drugs to make myself feel better.
5. ______ I've been getting emotional support from others.
6. ______ I've been giving up trying to deal with it.
7. ______ I've been taking action to try to make the situation better.
8. ______ I've been refusing to believe that it has happened.
9. ______ I've been saying things to let my unpleasant feelings escape.
10. ______ I've been getting help and advice from other people.
11. ______ I've been using alcohol or other drugs to help me get through it.
12. ______ I've been trying to see it in a different light, to make it seem more positive.
13. ______ I've been criticizing myself.
14. ______ I've been trying to come up with a strategy about what to do.
15. ______ I've been getting comfort and understanding from someone.
16. ______ I've been giving up the attempt to cope.
17. ______ I've been looking for something good in what is happening.
18. ______ I've been making jokes about it.
19. ______ I've been doing something to think about it less, such as going to movies, watching TV, reading, daydreaming, sleeping, or shopping.
20. ______ I've been accepting the reality of the fact that it has happened.
21. ______ I've been expressing my negative feelings.
22. ______ I've been trying to find comfort in my religion or spiritual beliefs.
23. ______ I've been trying to get advice or help from other people about what to do.
24. ______ I've been learning to live with it.
25. ______ I've been thinking hard about what steps to take.
26. ______ I've been blaming myself for things that happened.
27. ______ I've been praying or meditating.
28. ______ I've been making fun of the situation.

Scales are computed as follows (with no reversals of coding):
Self-distraction, items 1 and 19
Active coping, items 2 and 7
Denial, items 3 and 8
Substance use, items 4 and 11
Use of emotional support, items 5 and 15
Use of instrumental support, items 10 and 23
Behavioral disengagement, items 6 and 16
Venting, items 9 and 21
Positive reframing, items 12 and 17
Planning, items 14 and 25
Humor, items 18 and 28
Acceptance, items 20 and 24
Religion, items 22 and 27
Self-blame, items 13 and 26
From Carver CS. You want to measure coping but your protocol's too long: consider the Brief COPE. *Int J Behavior Med.* 1997;4:92.

Expected Outcomes

The patient will:

- demonstrate positive adaptive coping strategies.
- report decreased levels of stress.
- recognize factors that may lead to increased stress and take preventive action.
- participate in effective problem solving.
- implement health promotion behaviors.

INTERVENTIONS TO PROMOTE COPING	RATIONALE
Implement collaborative interventions aimed at treating any risk factor contributing to stress.	Treatment of causative or risk factors can assist in reducing the patient's stress level.
Assist the patient in setting their own manageable short- and long-term goals and identifying resources and culturally considerate strategies to help meet goals.	Establishing their own goals and strategies respects the patient's cultural norms and values and changes the focus from stress to problem solving.
INTERPERSONAL VIOLENCE: Provide the patient with adequate referrals or options for removal from the situation when interpersonal violence or the risk is present.	Planning for safety helps to manage stresses and may prevent additional stressful or dangerous situations.
Establish a therapeutic nurse–patient relationship: • Promote a calm, predictable environment. • Remain nonjudgmental. • Use active listening with therapeutic communication skills. • Be empathetic. • Avoid false reassurances.	A therapeutic environment demonstrates respect and establishes rapport, which may help alleviate stress and provide methods of support.
Encourage verbalization of positive coping strategies used successfully in the past.	Focus the patient on integrating strengths into the stress management plan.
Communicate clearly with simple words and allow the patient time to respond.	In acute stress, comprehension may be decreased.
Encourage postponement of important decisions during times of high stress unless decisions are time sensitive.	Ideally, the patient should avoid making major decisions during times of difficulty coping.
Encourage the patient to talk about their needs, feelings, and concerns.	Talking about feelings and concerns helps build rapport and decrease the patient's stress.
Help the patient identify triggers for stress.	Helping the patient recognize stress-producing situations helps them to better prevent or manage stress.
Assist the patient to recognize and refute negative thoughts and transform them into positive thoughts or solvable problems.	Reframing may enhance the ability to cope.
In an acute situation, coach the patient to do relaxation breathing or imagery.	Relaxation breathing and imagery are effective and simple to do almost anywhere.
Emphasize the use of problem-focused coping strategies when it is possible to change or control a problem, such as setting priorities, collecting information, and seeking advice.	Problem-focused coping strategies allow a person to look at a challenge objectively, act to address the problem, and thereby reduce the stress.
Collaborate with the patient to select and implement complementary and spiritual relaxation strategies, including biofeedback, imagery, massage, meditation, muscle relaxation, music, Qigong, relaxing breathing, tai chi, and yoga.	Complementary therapies help reduce the manifestations of stress by focusing on mind and body connections.
Encourage the use of emotion-focused coping strategies when a situation is unchangeable or uncontrollable, such as discussing feelings with a friend or taking a warm, relaxing bath.	Managing stress through emotion-focused coping may decrease stress levels.
Assist the patient in developing appropriate problem-solving strategies in known stress-provoking situations.	Developing problem-solving ability aids the patient in taking action in their life and coping with difficulties, which can reduce stress.
FUNCTIONAL ABILITY: Allow extra time for the patient to manage activities of daily living.	Stress may slow thinking and physical responses.
CULTURE: Help the patient to identify available sources of social support.	Social support and other resources may be useful in coping with stressors.
Administer prescribed medications for stress, such as selective serotonin reuptake inhibitors (SSRIs), benzodiazepines, buspirone (Buspar), and tricyclic antidepressants.	Medications may be prescribed as part of the plan for managing stress.
SAFETY, MOOD, AND AFFECT: Determine the risk of the patient inflicting self-harm and refer for immediate assistance if at risk.	Stressful situations may increase the risk for suicide.
MOOD AND AFFECT, ANXIETY: Implement measures to assist the patient in managing any depression or anxiety they may be experiencing.	Patients experiencing stress may have coexisting depression or anxiety.

Continued

INTERVENTIONS TO PROMOTE COPING	RATIONALE
Reinforce and teach aspects of care management with the patient and caregiver, such as medication and treatments.	Provide information to support problem-focused coping strategies.
Encourage the patient to maintain a daily routine.	Stability reduces stress and allows the patient to incorporate stress-reducing strategies more easily.
SLEEP: Provide the patient with opportunities for adequate sleep.	A lack of adequate rest is associated with increased stress.
NUTRITION: Encourage the patient to follow a nutritionally adequate diet.	A nutritionally sound diet supports overall health.
Assist the patient with developing a regular physical activity plan, considering capabilities, daily routine, and personal preferences.	Exercise raises levels of endorphins and may be helpful in reducing stress.
SUBSTANCE USE: Implement measures to address substance use.	A patient under stress is at higher risk for substance use disorder.
SPIRITUALITY: Implement measures to address any spiritual concerns.	There is a significant relationship between stress and spiritual well-being.
Pediatric	
Avoid showing medical equipment prior to use unless there is enough time for the child to safely play with and explore it, then process feelings.	The appearance of medical equipment can be frightening to a child, causing stress.
Provide opportunities for the child to participate in play therapy, referring to a play therapy specialist as needed.	Play therapy provides insight into the child's coping and can help them cope with their emotions.

INTERVENTIONS TO PROMOTE EFFECTIVE FAMILY COPING	RATIONALE
FAMILY DYNAMICS: Encourage problem solving and communication among family members by: • Clarifying what they want and need from each other • Having them verbalize and share their feelings with each other • Having them appraise their current situation • Discussing their concerns and problems • Reviewing each family member's role expectations • Assisting them with developing solutions	Open communication among family members helps the family to identify and find ways to cope with stress.
Implement measures to address caregiver role strain, if present.	Supporting the caregiver may allow that person to support the patient more fully.

INTERVENTIONS TO MANAGE RISK FOR/RELOCATION STRESS	RATIONALE
Maintain as much consistency as possible in daily care, including caregivers, routines, and environment.	Consistency provides the patient with security, which promotes adjustment and reduces stress.
Help the patient plan to maintain desired relationships with others after the move, such as video, letters, phone calls, texts, and visits.	Being unable to maintain desired contact with family and friends increases relocation stress until a support system is established in the new location.

COLLABORATION	RATIONALE
Counseling	Counseling can help patients modify their attitudes and behaviors and promote positive coping and stress management skills.
Support groups	Peers with similar circumstances can play a major role in assisting the patient with coping with stressors and the effects of stress.

COLLABORATION	RATIONALE
SPIRITUALITY: Pastoral care professional or their preferred spiritual or religious leader	The patient who is experiencing stress may find comfort from their religious leaders who provide support, perform spiritual counseling, and meet sacramental needs.
MOOD AND AFFECT: Treatment for any coexisting psychological problems, including depressed mood and emotional problems	Treatment of underlying psychological problems will assist with managing stress.
DEVELOPMENT: Child life specialist	A child life specialist can help the child manage health and health care–related stress through activities.

PATIENT AND CAREGIVER TEACHING

- Common causes of stress
- Recognition of stress and stress response
- Emotion-focused and problem-focused coping strategies
- Relaxation techniques
- Lifestyle changes to influence stress level
- Anticipatory guidance regarding situations that may increase stress
- Health promotion behaviors, including nutrition, sleep, and exercise
- Community and self-help resources
- Sources of information and social support
- When to notify the health care provider

DOCUMENTATION

Assessment

- Stress level
- Manifestations of stress
- Screening test results

Interventions

- Coaching in strategy use
- Discussions with other members of the interprofessional team
- Therapeutic interventions and the patient's response
- Teaching provided
- Referrals initiated

Evaluation

- Patient's status: improved, stable, declined
- Stress level
- Evidence of coping
- Use of healthy/unhealthy strategies for coping
- Response to teaching provided

Grief 56

Definition

A pattern of physical and emotional responses to bereavement, separation, or loss

Grief is a normal reaction to a loss, such as the death of a loved one or the loss of what might have been, such as an imagined future. Grief may be experienced during life transitions and in response to other changes, such as a decline in health altering a family member's role. Grief involves both psychological and physiologic responses. It is a powerful and intense experience that affects all aspects of a person's life.

There are five stages in the Kübler-Ross model of grief: denial, anger, bargaining, depression, and acceptance. Not every person experiences all the stages of grieving, and the stages are not always progressive. It is common to reach a stage and then go backward. For example, a person may have reached the stage of bargaining and then revert to the denial or anger stage.

Another model of grief is the grief wheel. After the loss, a person feels shock, with numbness, denial, and an inability to think clearly. Next is the protest stage, with anger, guilt, sadness, fear, and searching. Then comes the disorganization stage, with despair, apathy, anxiety, and confusion. The next stage is reorganization, in which a person gradually returns to normal functioning but feels different. The final stage is the new normal. Trying to go back to the "old" normal, which is not there anymore, causes anxiety and stress. The challenge is to accept the new normal.

The manner in which a person grieves depends on such factors as the type of loss, the relationship with the person who has died (e.g., spouse, parent), physical and emotional coping resources, concurrent life stresses, cultural beliefs, and personality. Additional factors that affect the grief response include mental and physical health, economic resources, religious influences or spiritual beliefs, family relationships, social support, and time spent preparing for the death. Issues that occurred before the death, such as family conflict or marital problems, may affect the grief response. Nurses have a role in helping persons manage grief during illness, death and dying, and other transitions that bring a sense of loss.

Associated Clinical Problems

- Anticipatory Grief: feelings of grief that develop before, rather than after, a loss
- Complicated Grief: prolonged and intense mourning after a death, loss, or separation
- Disenfranchised Grief: relationship to the deceased person or loss is not socially sanctioned and cannot be shared openly
- Dysfunctional Grieving: failure to follow a course of normal grieving to resolution, including becoming overwhelmed and using maladaptive coping
- Risk for Dysfunctional Grieving: increased risk for failure to follow a course of normal grieving to resolution, including becoming overwhelmed and using maladaptive coping

Common Causes

- Death of a significant person
- Loss of health, role, lifestyle, or independence
- Negative change in perceived life trajectory
- Response to a change

Anticipatory Grief

- Potential loss of a significant person, job, or health

Dysfunctional Grieving/Risk for Dysfunctional Grieving

- Lack of social support
- Multiple losses
- Perinatal loss
- Psychological problems
- Socioeconomic difficulty, such as loss of income or insurance

Manifestations

- Anger
- Anxiety
- Changes in appetite
- Depression
- Despair
- Fear
- Guilt
- Helplessness
- Illness
- Inability to make decisions or concentrate
- Physical problems
- Sadness
- Sleeping problems

Pediatric
- Developmental regression

Anticipatory Grieving
- Death anxiety
- Denial of impending loss
- Expressing distress regarding potential loss

Key Conceptual Relationships

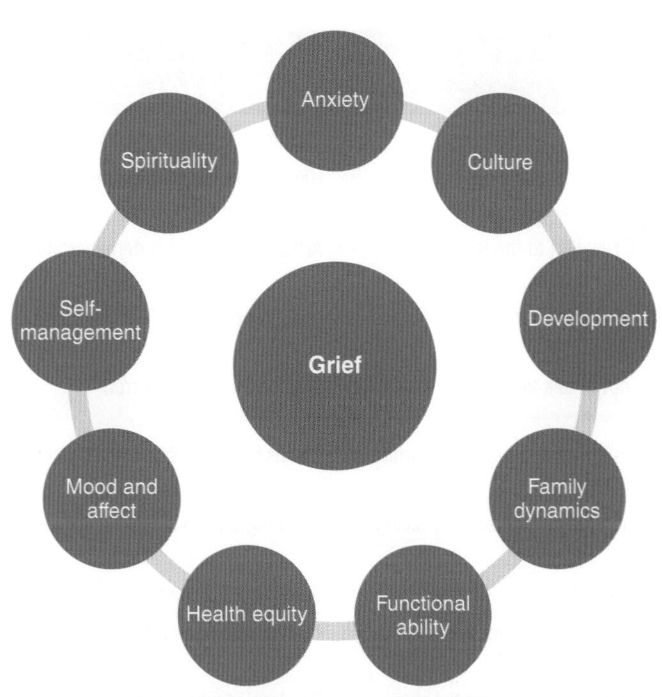

ASSESSMENT OF GRIEF	RATIONALE
Assess how the person is manifesting grief and how it is affecting their life and health.	Knowing how the person is managing grief allows the nurse to develop an effective plan to help the person cope with their loss.
Assess for the presence of factors that may hinder grieving.	Being aware of factors that may complicate grief allows the nurse to develop an effective plan to help the person cope with their loss.
Determine the significance and meaning of the loss to the person.	The significance of the loss is highly individual.
Assess for and identify positive coping strategies used in the past.	Coping strategies used successfully represent the person's strengths and can assist with the current stresses.
Assess for complicated or dysfunctional grief involving maladaptive coping strategies.	Extended grief may require additional support.
FAMILY DYNAMICS: Evaluate family dynamics, the current level of functioning, and family interactions.	The loss of a loved one changes the family system and creates the need for family members to reorganize.
SPIRITUALITY: Assess the influence of spiritual and religious beliefs on grief.	Spiritual beliefs and practices greatly influence a person's reaction to loss and the meaning attributed to loss.
CULTURE: Assess the influence of culture and social practices on grief.	Each culture has rituals that influence the expression of grief.
MOOD AND AFFECT AND ANXIETY: Screen for the presence of any psychological problems, including depression and anxiety.	The presence of depression, anxiety, or other psychological disorders can complicate grief.
FUNCTIONAL ABILITY: Evaluate the lifestyle effects of grief, including the ability to sleep, enjoy life, interact with others, perform work and household duties, and engage in physical and social activities.	A prolonged delay in return to normal activities may indicate complicated or dysfunctional grieving.
Pediatric	
Assess the child's development level and degree of understanding.	The child's development level affects how they understand loss and how the loss of a significant other affects them.

Expected Outcomes

The patient will:

- discuss the meaning of the loss.
- articulate support needs.
- identify ways to support others in the loss.
- use positive coping strategies.
- progress through the stages of grief.

INTERVENTIONS FOR RESOLVING GRIEF	RATIONALE
Use presence and therapeutic communication.	Therapeutic communication shows respect for human dignity.
Assign a primary nurse.	Having a primary nurse facilitates the development of a trusting relationship.
Assist in identifying the nature of the loss, reaction to the loss, and feelings about the loss.	Articulating the loss demonstrates respect.
Listen to the person's story and encourage them to verbalize memories related to past and current losses.	Prior losses may affect current grief.
If the patient is silent, respect the choice not to talk and remain available as needed.	Silence may be preferred.
Establish a caring, calm environment that allows the patient and family to express feelings such as anger, fear, and guilt.	Discussion of feelings helps work toward the resolution of grief.
Accept and support the patient's progression through personal grieving stages.	The progression of grief is individual.
Share information about grief stages, as needed.	Stages are commonly experienced and eventually progress.
Recognize that family members may have been caregivers and institute measures to support role changes.	Loss of role is an additional type of loss.
FAMILY DYNAMICS: Support family function by encouraging them to share their feelings.	The loss of a loved one changes the family system and creates the need for family members to reorganize.
CULTURE: Provide support or assistance in completing cultural and social activities and traditions related to loss or bereavement.	Cultural traditions and rituals may give comfort.
SPIRITUALITY: Provide support or assistance in completing religious and spiritual rituals related to loss or bereavement.	Participating in religious and spiritual rituals may give comfort.
Identify sources of community support for ongoing grief resolution.	Groups and individuals in the community may have special insight into the type of loss and provide ongoing support.
CAREGIVING: Identify sources of support and possible care needs of the surviving family.	A surviving spouse or partner may have depended on the deceased partner for care.
SELF-MANAGEMENT: Encourage the person to follow a nutritious diet with regular eating habits, get adequate rest, and participate in physical activity.	These measures help the patient to stay healthy and physically feel better.
MOOD AND AFFECT, ANXIETY: Institute measures to address any psychological problems, including depression and anxiety.	The presence of depression, anxiety, or other psychological disorders complicates grief.
Pediatric	
Encourage the expression of feelings in ways comfortable and developmentally appropriate to the child, such as writing, drawing, or playing.	Children have different levels of understanding about loss and may grieve differently.
Answer children's questions associated with the loss.	Provide honest communication at the development level of the child.
For a school-aged child, encourage continued participation in school, social, and extracurricular activities.	Participation in usual activities helps movement through the grief process.

INTERVENTIONS FOR LOSS OF AN EXPECTED CHILD	RATIONALE
Recognize that parents who have a miscarriage grieve and experience sorrow because of the loss of the child.	Recognition validates that the loss is real.
Provide emotional support during the labor and delivery process when a stillbirth is expected.	The care the nurse provides greatly influences the parents' perception of loss and how they respond to it.
Obtain mementos of the child, including footprints, handprints, pictures, caps, gowns, and blankets, as appropriate, for the family to keep.	The mementos that were in contact with the child are limited and may be precious to the family.
CULTURE: Affirm the value of the individuals beyond the parent role.	Recognize that the parental role may play an important role in cultural expectations.
SPIRITUALITY: Assist the family in obtaining spiritual care as desired, such as baptism or blessings.	This respects the family's spiritual beliefs and promotes grieving.

COLLABORATION	RATIONALE
Counseling	Additional support may be needed to resolve grief, particularly complicated or dysfunctional grief, and support coping.
Support group for grieving persons	Groups and persons in the community may have special insight into the type of loss and provide ongoing support.
SPIRITUALITY: Pastoral care professional or their preferred spiritual or religious leader	Many derive spiritual comfort from their religious leaders, who can provide support, perform spiritual counseling, and meet sacramental needs.
HEALTH EQUITY: Social worker or case management	Social workers and case managers may assist with financial concerns, including insurance and medical bills.
Child life specialist	A child life specialist can help the child manage grief through activities.
School counselor or school psychologist	These persons can provide support services for the grieving child at school.

PATIENT AND CAREGIVER TEACHING

- Stages of grief and what to expect
- Community and self-help resources
- Sources of information and social support
- Positive coping and stress management strategies
- Factors that predispose the patient to complicated grief
- Anticipatory guidance regarding situations that may aggravate grief
- Health promotion behaviors, including nutrition, sleep, exercise
- When to notify the health care provider and seek further assistance

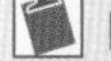

DOCUMENTATION

Assessment

- Response to grief

Interventions

- Therapeutic communications
- Assistance with spiritual and cultural care preferences
- Discussions with other members of the interprofessional team
- Teaching provided
- Referrals initiated

Evaluation

- Progress toward resolution of grief
- Response to teaching
- Response to therapeutic interventions

Substance Use 57

Definition

Dependence on a substance that leads to detrimental effects on physical or mental health or the welfare of others

Substance use disorder (SUD) involves several types of substances, ranging from those widely used and accepted like tobacco and alcohol to illegal drugs like heroin and cocaine. SUD results from continued, frequent substance use. Consequences occur over time as SUD progresses. Although each substance is its own disorder (i.e., alcohol use disorder, tobacco use disorder, opioid use disorder), the same overarching criteria are used for diagnostic purposes.

SUD does not exist in isolation. There are many interrelated concepts, depending on the patient's situation. When stress, coping, and family dynamics are ineffective, the persons within these systems are at risk for SUD. Problems at work, school, or home often result. Many patients with SUDs receive acute care for problems associated with substance use. Every drug associated with SUD harms some tissue or organ. SUD causes specific health problems, such as liver damage related to alcohol use, or problems resulting from injuries, such as falls.

You are likely to encounter patients with a substance-induced disorder. Your ability to be able to respond to a patient who is acutely intoxicated or in withdrawal is important in maintaining patient safety. The health care setting offers an opportunity for screening and providing teaching about substance use. You have a responsibility to motivate patients to change their behavior and refer them to programs that offer treatment. A nonjudgmental environment that provides education and access to community resources can assist the patient with cessation and positive coping.

Associated Clinical Problems

- Alcohol Dependence: dependence on alcohol that has detrimental effects on physical or mental health or the welfare of others
- Drug Dependence: dependence on a drug that has detrimental effects on physical or mental health or the welfare of others
- Neonatal Abstinence Syndrome: conditions that occur in the postpartum period as a result of the abrupt discontinuation of drugs that the baby was exposed to in utero
- Tobacco User: person who is dependent on the drug nicotine because of using tobacco products
- Withdrawal Symptoms: physical and mental response after cessation or severe reduction in intake of a regularly used substance

Common Risk Factors

- Aggressive behavior
- Drug availability
- Family or personal history of substance use
- Having a disability
- Homelessness
- Mood disorder
- Poor tolerance for pain
- Poverty
- Severe psychological distress
- Stress
- Tobacco user
- Using a highly addictive drug

Pediatric

- Lack of parental supervision
- Experiencing stressful events
- Having parents who are not college educated
- Lacking college/career plans
- Low self-esteem
- Overweight
- Peer pressure

Older Adult

- Decrease in finances
- Loss of social support
- Recent and multiple losses

Withdrawal Symptoms

- Cessation of substance use
- Coexisting psychological condition
- History of substance use

Neonatal Abstinence Syndrome

- Perinatal drug exposure

Manifestations

- Physiologic
  - Fatigue
  - Headaches

    - Mood changes
    - Seizure disorder
    - Sexual problems, erectile dysfunction
    - Sleep problems: insomnia, drowsiness
    - Slurred speech
    - Standard doses of sedatives do not have a therapeutic effect
    - Tremors
    - Unkempt appearance; appears older than age
    - Watery or reddened eyes
    - Weight loss
    - Withdrawal symptoms occur without the substance
- Behavior
    - Absenteeism, tardiness
    - Citations for driving while intoxicated or impaired
    - Defensive or evasive answers to questions about SUD and its importance in the person's life
    - Difficulty fulfilling work obligations or keeping a job
    - Financial problems, including those related to spending for substances
    - Increasing isolation; estranged from friends or family
    - Leisure activities that involve alcohol and/or other drugs
    - Marital conflict, separation, or divorce
    - Trauma from falls, auto accidents, fights, or burns
- Diagnostic tests: Positive toxicology screen

Pediatric

- Being secretive about where they go with friends
- Drastic changes in behavior and in relationships with family and friends
- Exaggerated efforts to prevent family members from entering their room
- Missing school, a sudden disinterest in school activities or work, or a decline in grades
- Sudden requests for money without a reasonable explanation; missing items or money in the home

Women's Health

- Not receiving prenatal care
- Victim of domestic violence

Withdrawal Symptoms

- Anxiety
- Cravings
- Increased pulse
- Irritability
- Nausea
- Palpitations
- Sleep problems
- Sweating
- Tremors

Manifestations Associated With Common, Specific Substances

- Alcohol: hyperactivity, ↑ BP
- Cannabis: muscle cramping
- Opioids: fever, muscle aches, nausea and vomiting, pupil dilation, runny nose, watery eyes
- Sedatives/hypnotics: fever, hallucinations, orthostatic hypotension, seizures
- Stimulants: delirium, fever, ↑ BP, psychosis, pupil dilation, seizures, suicidal ideation
- Tobacco: attention deficits, depression, ↑ appetite

Neonatal Abstinence Syndrome

- Diarrhea
- Difficulty feeding
- Failure to thrive
- Fever
- Increased respiratory rate
- Irritability and high-pitched crying
- Nasal stuffiness
- Seizures
- Sleeplessness
- Sneezing
- Sweating
- Vomiting

Key Conceptual Relationships

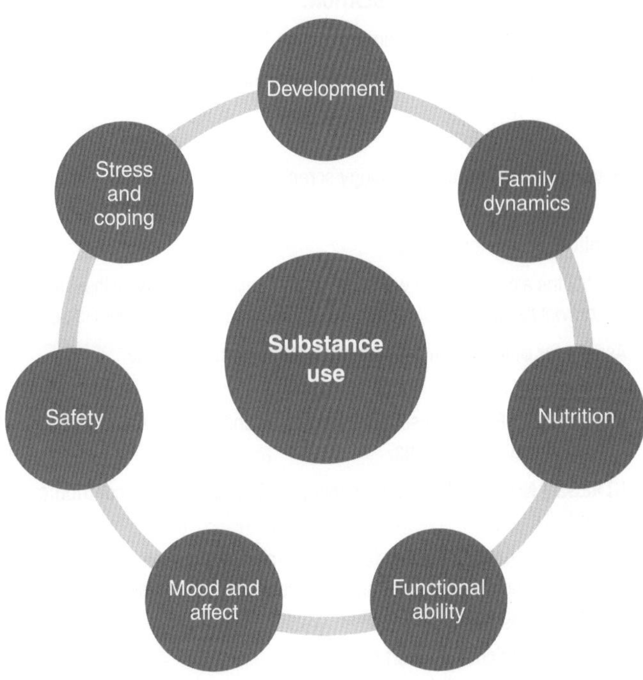

HEALTH AND ILLNESS CONCEPTS

ASSESSMENT OF SUBSTANCE USE	RATIONALE
Identify patients in need of emergency management for withdrawal or toxicity so that they can be stabilized.	Because withdrawal and severe intoxication both have potentially life-threatening side effects, rapid identification is imperative to early treatment.
Use screening tests to detect alcohol, tobacco, and/or other substance use problems, such as the T-ACE, CAGE, or brief universal screening questions (Box 57.1).	Screening is a simple, effective way to identify patients who need further assessment for SUD.
If a patient has a positive screen, follow up with a detailed assessment to identify specific problems. Use a formal, patient-specific tool to identify specific problems, such as the Alcohol Use Disorders Identification Test (AUDIT) (Table 57.1) or the Drug Abuse Screening Test (DAST-10) (https://cde.drugabuse.gov/instrument/e9053390-ee9c-9140-e040-bb89ad433d69).	The consistent use of SUD scales helps identify SUD.
If the patient admits to substance use, obtain a general history of alcohol and drug use first, and then identify daily patterns of consumption; obtain information on routes, dose, and duration of use; history of drug treatment; and incidence of previous withdrawals.	The purposes of a substance use assessment are to determine whether SUD exists and if present, the severity, so that appropriate treatment can be implemented.
Determine when the patient last used the substance.	Knowing the time of last use helps predict the onset of withdrawal and helps anticipate drug interactions.
Determine the patient's willingness and motivation to make an attempt to quit.	The patient must be motivated and willing to quit to regain and maintain abstinence.
Collect information about the substance use habits of peers and household members.	If a person's family and peers use substances, peer pressure may influence the patient to use substances, thus hindering recovery.
Obtain a complete medication history and determine the actual amount of medication the patient takes.	SUD can involve the inappropriate use and misuse of prescription drugs.
Perform a complete physical assessment, noting physical and behavioral manifestations of SUD.	Identifying manifestations of SUD allows for early intervention.
• **INTRACRANIAL REGULATION:** Neurologic status	Substance use places the patient at risk for changes in cognition and seizures.
• **PSYCHOSIS:** Psychological status	Withdrawal may be associated with changes in mentation and psychosis.
• **GAS EXCHANGE:** Vital signs, including pulse oximetry	Because of the frequency of respiratory distress, assessment of airway and breathing patterns is a top priority in a patient with acute toxicity resulting from substances.
Obtain blood and urine toxicology screens.	Diagnostic tests provide objective data about drug and alcohol metabolites in the blood and urine.
Monitor serum electrolytes.	Electrolyte imbalances can develop with the ingestion of various substances.
Identify the alcohol withdrawal stage by determining the Clinical Institute Withdrawal Assessment of Alcohol Scale, Revised (CIWA-Ar) score (Table 57.2).	Identifying alcohol withdrawal allows for appropriate treatment and monitoring.
Assess for other health problems related to substance use.	Drugs associated with SUD harm the body and cause specific health problems, such as lung cancer related to smoking.
MOOD AND AFFECT: Assess mental status and screen for coexisting psychological problems.	Many patients use substances to obtain relief from depression, anxiety, or other psychological disorders.
STRESS AND COPING: Assess coping strategies that may contribute to SUD.	A patient with SUD may have relied on substance use or other negative coping behaviors to deal with stress.
FAMILY DYNAMICS: Assess family dynamics and current level of functioning and observe family interactions. Determine the extent of enabling behaviors.	How family members act and react to the patient's SUD affects the course of SUD and how the patient views themselves.
Assess the patient's support system: • Who do they live with? • Are they employed? • Are friends and relatives accessible? • Have they used any community resources?	Interest and support from others are important aspects in achieving abstinence from substances.
Assess the role that substance use plays in the patient's life.	It is important to understand the role substance use has in the person's life and its meaning to their unique life experience.
FUNCTIONAL ABILITY: Perform a psychosocial assessment, evaluating for lifestyle effects of SUD, such as on the ability to sleep, enjoy life, interact with others, perform work and household duties, and engage in physical and social activities.	Problems associated with SUD affect all aspects of a person's life.

ASSESSMENT OF SUBSTANCE USE	RATIONALE
Evaluate the patient's response to measures to address substance use through ongoing assessment.	Identifying continued substance use allows for the evaluation of therapy effectiveness.
Women's Health	
Periodically screen pregnant patients for substance use by interviewing the woman privately.	Identifying the newborn at risk for conditions associated with maternal SUD and withdrawal is important for initiating care.
Perform a complete physical assessment of the woman and fetus presenting with complications related to SUD.	A complete physical assessment provides specific care.
Older Adult	
Screen for substance use with a screening tool specific to older adults.	Patterns of substance use among older adults are generally different from those of younger adults.
MOOD AND AFFECT: Assess for a depressed mood.	Overall emotional well-being influences substance use in older adults.

ASSESSMENT OF NEONATAL ABSTINENCE SYNDROME	RATIONALE
Assess the newborn's status using a standardized assessment tool, such as the Modified Finnegan Neonatal Abstinence Scale (https://www.mdcalc.com/modified-finnegan-neonatal-abstinence-score-nas).	Identifying manifestations of neonatal abstinence syndrome and their severity allows for appropriate treatment and monitoring.

Box 57.1 Universal Screening Questions

- How often in the past year have you had 5 (men) or 4 (women) or more drinks in a day?
- How many times in the past year have you used an illegal drug or prescription medication for nonmedical reasons?
- In the past year, how many days have you smoked cigarettes or used tobacco products?
- In the past year, have you ever drunk or used drugs more than you meant to?
- Have you felt you wanted or needed to cut down on your drinking or drug use in the past year?
- Do you sometimes drink beer, wine, or other alcoholic beverages? If so, how many does a week do you usually drink and how many drinks do you have?

Table 57.1 Alcohol Use Disorders Identification Test (AUDIT)

Please answer each question by checking 1 circle in the second column.		Score
How often do you have a drink containing alcohol?	• Never	(0)
	• Monthly or less	(1)
	• 2–4 times per month	(2)
	• 2–4 times per week	(3)
	• 4+ times per week	(4)
How many drinks containing alcohol do you have on a typical day when you are drinking?	• 1 or 2	(0)
	• 3 or 4	(1)
	• 5 or 6	(2)
	• 7–9	(3)
	• 10 or more	(4)
How often do you have 6 or more drinks on 1 occasion?	• Never	(0)
	• Less than monthly	(1)
	• Monthly	(2)
	• Weekly	(3)
	• Daily or almost daily	(4)

Continued

Table 57.1 Alcohol Use Disorders Identification Test (AUDIT)—cont'd

Please answer each question by checking 1 circle in the second column.		Score
How often during the last year have you found that you were not able to stop drinking once you had started?	• Never	(0)
	• Less than monthly	(1)
	• Monthly	(2)
	• Weekly	(3)
	• Daily or almost daily	(4)
How often in the last year have you failed to do what was normally expected of you because you were drinking?	• Never	(0)
	• Less than monthly	(1)
	• Monthly	(2)
	• Weekly	(3)
	• Daily or almost daily	(4)
How often during the last year have you needed a first drink in the morning to get yourself going after a heavy drinking session?	• Never	(0)
	• Less than monthly	(1)
	• Monthly	(2)
	• Weekly	(3)
	• Daily or almost daily	(4)
How often during the last year have you had a feeling of guilt or remorse about drinking?	• Never	(0)
	• Less than monthly	(1)
	• Monthly	(2)
	• Weekly	(3)
	• Daily or almost daily	(4)
How often during the last year have you been unable to remember what happened the night before because you had been drinking?	• Never	(0)
	• Less than monthly	(1)
	• Monthly	(2)
	• Weekly	(3)
	• Daily or almost daily	(4)
Have you or someone else been injured as a result of your drinking?	• No	(0)
	• Yes, but not in the last year	(2)
	• Yes, during the last year	(4)
Has a relative, friend, or other health worker been concerned about your drinking or suggested that you cut down?	• No	(0)
	• Yes, but not in the last year	(2)
	• Yes, during the last year	(4)

Scoring for AUDIT: Questions 1–8 are scored 0, 1, 2, 3, or 4. Questions 9 and 10 are scored 0, 2, or 4 only. The minimum score (nondrinkers) is 0, and the maximum possible score is 40. A score of 9 or more indicates hazardous or harmful alcohol consumption.
Source: Babor TF, Higgins-Biddle JC, Saunders JB, Monteiro M. *The Alcohol Use Disorders Identification Test,* ed 2. Geneva, Switzerland: WHO Press; 2001.

Table 57.2 Clinical Institute Withdrawal Assessment of Alcohol Scale, Revised (CIWA-Ar) CIWA-Ar Categories, With the Range of Scores in Each Category, Are as Follows

Category	Range
Agitation	0–7
Anxiety	0–7
Auditory disturbances	0–7
Headache	0–7
Clouding of sensorium	0–4
Paroxysmal sweats	0–7
Tactile disturbances	0–7
Tremor	0–7
Visual disturbances	0–7

Table 57.2 Clinical Institute Withdrawal Assessment of Alcohol Scale, Revised (CIWA-Ar) CIWA-Ar Categories, With the Range of Scores in Each Category, Are as Follows—cont'd

Patient:________________ **Date:**________________ **Time:**________________ (24 hour clock, midnight = 00:00)

Pulse or heart rate, taken for one minute:________________ **Blood pressure:**________

NAUSEA AND VOMITING – Ask "Do you feel sick to your stomach? Have you vomited?" Observation.
0 no nausea and no vomiting
1 mild nausea with no vomiting
2
3
4 intermittent nausea with dry heaves
5
6
7 constant nausea, frequent dry heaves and vomiting

TREMOR – Arms extended and fingers spread apart. Observation.
0 no tremor
1 not visible, but can be felt fingertip to fingertip
2
3
4 moderate, with patient's arms extended
5
6
7 severe, even with arms not extended

PAROXYSMAL SWEATS – Observation.
0 no sweat visible
1 barely perceptible sweating, palms moist
2
3
4 beads of sweat obvious on forehead
5
6
7 drenching sweats

ANXIETY – Ask "Do you feel nervous?" Observation.
0 no anxiety, at ease
1 mild anxious
2
3
4 moderately anxious, or guarded, so anxiety is inferred
5
6
7 equivalent to acute panic states as seen in severe delirium or acute schizophrenic reactions

AGITATION – Observation.
0 normal activity
1 somewhat more than normal activity
2
3
4 moderately fidgety and restless
5
6
7 paces back and forth during most of the interview, or constantly thrashes about

TACTILE DISTURBANCES – Ask "Have you any itching, pins and needles sensations, any burning, any numbness, or do you feel bugs crawling on or under your skin?" Observation.
0 none
1 very mild itching, pins and needles, burning or numbness
2 mild itching, pins and needles, burning or numbness
3 moderate itching, pins and needles, burning or numbness
4 moderately severe hallucinations
5 severe hallucinations
6 extremely severe hallucinations
7 continuous hallucinations

AUDITORY DISTURBANCES – Ask "Are you more aware of sounds around you? Are they harsh? Do they frighten you? Are you hearing anything that is disturbing to you? Are you hearing things you know are not there?" Observation.
0 not present
1 very mild harshness or ability to frighten
2 mild harshness or ability to frighten
3 moderate harshness or ability to frighten
4 moderately severe hallucinations
5 severe hallucinations
6 extremely severe hallucinations
7 continuous hallucinations

VISUAL DISTURBANCES – Ask "Does the light appear to be too bright? Is its color different? Does it hurt your eyes? Are you seeing anything that is disturbing to you? Are you seeing things you know are not there?" Observation.
0 not present
1 very mild sensitivity
2 mild sensitivity
3 moderate sensitivity
4 moderately severe hallucinations
5 severe hallucinations
6 extremely severe hallucinations
7 continuous hallucinations

HEADACHE, FULLNESS IN HEAD – Ask "Does your head feel different? Does it feel like there is a band around your head?" Do not rate for dizziness or lightheadedness. Otherwise, rate severity.
0 not present
1 very mild
2 mild
3 moderate
4 moderately severe
5 severe
6 very severe
7 extremely severe

ORIENTATION AND CLOUDING OF SENSORIUM – Ask "What day is this? Where are you? Who am I?"
0 oriented and can do serial additions
1 cannot do serial additions or is uncertain about date
2 disoriented for date by no more than 2 calendar days
3 disoriented for date by more than 2 calendar days
4 disoriented for place/or person

Total **CIWA-Ar** Score______
Rater's Initials______
Maximum Possible Score 67

The ***CIWA-Ar*** *is not* copyrighted and may be reproduced freely. This assessment for monitoring withdrawal symptoms requires approximately 5 minutes to administer. The maximum score is 67 (see instrument). Patients scoring less than 10 do not usually need additional medication for withdrawal.

Source: University of Maryland School of Medicine. CIWA-Ar. http://umem.org/files/uploads/1104212257_CIWA-Ar.pdf.

Expected Outcomes

The patient will:

- admit to SUD.
- achieve and maintain abstinence.
- be free from complications resulting from withdrawal syndrome.
- adhere to a prescribed therapeutic regimen, including engaging in behavior counseling and group therapy.
- have an improved quality of life, sense of well-being, and mental health.
- be productive in the family, work, and society.
- verbalize acceptance of responsibility for behavior.
- identify coping mechanisms to use in response to cravings and urges to use substances.
- maintain ongoing contact with the appropriate community resources.

INTERVENTIONS TO ADDRESS SUBSTANCE USE	RATIONALE
Institute resuscitation protocols according to agency policy when the patient is experiencing acute toxicity.	The goal of emergency management is to prevent life-threatening complications that occur because of substance use.
GAS EXCHANGE: Administer O_2 therapy and provide appropriate respiratory support.	Many agents affect the respiratory system, and measures are needed to prevent and correct hypoxia.
Establish a therapeutic relationship with the patient: • Remain nonjudgmental. • Be genuine and honest. • Use active listening with therapeutic communication skills. • Provide a secure, relaxed atmosphere. • Avoid blaming.	The development of a trusting nurse–patient relationship is a priority for the patient with SUD because patients often hide, deny, or minimize substance use.
Assign a primary care nurse.	This establishes trust and boundaries so that changes can be immediately processed.
Use motivational interviewing to initiate behavior change.	Helping patients identify why they would want to make a change and how they might do it is more effective than telling them they should.
Assist the patient in recognizing that SUD exists by discussing, in a caring manner, the impact of SUD on their life.	A key step in cessation is assisting patients in seeing relationships between SUD and their personal lives.
Develop achievable goals and cessation plan with the patient.	Goal achievement enhances self-esteem and promotes a positive expectation of future goals, which motivates the patient to change behavior.
Discuss with the patient the potential problem in relating to family and friends who continue to use substances.	Prepare the patient for the obstacles that occur in relation to family and friends who still use substances.
STRESS AND COPING: Help the patient develop positive coping behaviors.	Positive coping strategies provide an alternative way to manage stress without the use of substances.
Encourage the use of stress management strategies.	Positive stress management techniques promote the patient's sense of control by providing a concrete plan for responding to stressful situations before they occur.
Administer prescribed medications for the treatment of SUD, such as nicotine replacement therapy or methadone.	Medications can help reestablish normal brain function and decrease cravings.
SPIRITUALITY: Assist the patient in self-examination of spirituality and implement measures to address the patient's spiritual state.	Surrendering to faith in a power greater than oneself has been found to be effective in abstinence efforts for many persons.
Assist patients in developing practical ways to resist cravings after abstinence, such as talking to someone, getting busy with a task, or leaving an invoking situation.	Using cognitive and behavioral activities to manage cravings helps maintain abstinence.
Collaborate with the patient to select and implement complementary therapies, including relaxation, guided imagery, distraction, acupressure, yoga, and massage.	Complementary therapies can reduce cravings and anxiety, increasing the likelihood of maintaining abstinence.

INTERVENTIONS TO ADDRESS SUBSTANCE USE	RATIONALE
Work with the patient to identify behaviors that contribute to SUD and life problems (e.g., family problems, job-related problems, legal difficulties).	When patients take responsibility for behavior, they are more prepared to take responsibility for learning effective behaviors.
FUNCTIONAL ABILITY: Help the patient develop strategies to help with participation in activities of daily living in the home, at work, and socially.	Because SUD affects all aspects of life, making coping with activities of daily living easier will help patients improve functional ability.
Provide reinforcement for positive actions.	The patient with SUD often needs to learn to accept self as an individual with positive attributes to maintain abstinence.
FAMILY DYNAMICS: Institute measures to promote optimal family function and refer the patient and family to family-focused therapy, as appropriate.	Promoting positive family interaction and communication will help the patient and family deal with the substance use.
NUTRITION: Implement measures to achieve and maintain optimal nutrition.	Malnutrition is prevalent among persons with substance use disorder.
Women's Health	
Maintain a nonjudgmental attitude and make clear the primary interest is the newborn's welfare, not punishing the woman.	A nonjudgmental, supportive approach based on medical concern is most effective.

INTERVENTIONS TO ASSIST THE TOBACCO USER	RATIONALE
Encourage participation in moderate-intensity exercise, such as walking, swimming, and bicycling.	Exercise is associated with a short-term reduction in the desire to smoke and tobacco-related withdrawal symptoms.
Help the patient recognize cues associated with smoking or vaping, such as being with others who smoke or drink alcohol.	Avoiding cues associated with smoking or vaping will help the patient maintain abstinence.
Women's Health	
DEVELOPMENT: Explore with the woman and family the risk for injury to the fetus and woman when the pregnant woman smokes, is exposed to secondhand smoke, or engages in substance use.	Provides safety information regarding fetal well-being.

INTERVENTIONS TO MANAGE WITHDRAWAL	RATIONALE
Institute resuscitation protocols according to agency policy when the patient is experiencing withdrawal.	The goal of emergency management is to prevent life-threatening complications that occur because of substance withdrawal.
Administer prescribed medications.	Medication therapy can decrease manifestations of withdrawal syndrome.
FLUID AND ELECTROLYTES: Administer prescribed intravenous fluid therapy.	Careful fluid replacement corrects dehydration and promotes renal clearance of substances.
THERMOREGULATION: Institute measures to manage fever.	Reducing fever will increase patient comfort and lower metabolic demands.
SAFETY: Provide a safe environment for the patient with neuromuscular manifestations by instituting fall and seizure precautions.	Withdrawal may be accompanied by changes in cognition and the potential for seizures.
COGNITION: Provide a quiet, nonstimulating, well-lit environment.	Sensory stimuli can increase delirium.
PSYCHOSIS: Implement measures to address hallucinations and reorient the patient.	Withdrawal may be associated with changes in mentation that necessitate reality orientation.
Allow the family members to participate in patient care as possible.	Family participation may decrease anxiety and help with reality orientation.

Continued

INTERVENTIONS TO MANAGE WITHDRAWAL	RATIONALE
Implement measures to protect the patient from self-harm by: • removing sharp and glass objects from environment. • removing belts and strings from the environment. • providing a 1-to-1 constant interaction if risk for self-harm is high. • checking on the patient every 15 minutes.	These measures may prevent the patient from self-harming.
Notify the health care provider (HCP) if withdrawal symptoms persist or worsen.	Achievement of an effective treatment plan often requires adjustments in therapy.

INTERVENTIONS TO ADDRESS NEONATAL ABSTINENCE SYNDROME	RATIONALE
REPRODUCTION: Implement measures to address risks that may be present during the perinatal period.	Providing nursing care that addresses the increased risks to the mother and newborn associated with SUD is essential for optimal maternal and newborn outcomes.
Administer prescribed medications for withdrawal.	Medication therapy can decrease manifestations of withdrawal and promote the comfort and well-being of the newborn.
Implement comforting techniques and environment modifications: • Quiet area with low lights • Providing a quiet environment • Swaddling or "kangaroo" care • Pacifier use • Gentle handling	These measures can decrease manifestations of neonatal abstinence syndrome and reduce or eliminate the need for medication.
Encourage the mother to breastfeed the newborn.	Breastfeeding appears to reduce the severity of neonatal abstinence syndrome.
If able, encourage mother and newborn rooming-in.	Maternal rooming-in appears to reduce the severity of neonatal abstinence syndrome.
Follow reporting requirements and notify appropriate agencies when newborns have signs and symptoms of substance use disorder.	Allows for appropriate support and follow-up for the mother and newborn.
Arrange for long-term pediatric care to begin immediately after hospital discharge.	The newborn affected by neonatal abstinence syndrome will be discharged from the hospital with residual signs that may last for months.

COLLABORATION	RATIONALE
Residential treatment	Residential treatment typically focuses on detoxification, providing initial intensive counseling, and preparing the patient for treatment in a community-based setting.
Behavior counseling	Counseling helps patients modify their attitudes and behaviors related to SUD, promote healthy life skills, and persist with treatment and abstinence.
Group therapy, such as Alcoholics Anonymous	Group therapy helps patients modify their attitudes and behaviors related to SUD through peer feedback.
FAMILY DYNAMICS: Family-centered treatment	This provides long-term support by addressing enabling influences on SUD patterns and improving overall family functioning.
Social services, vocational rehabilitation, workshops, or other resources, as appropriate	Patients recovering from SUD might have a myriad of needs that must be addressed to maintain abstinence.
MOOD AND AFFECT: Treatment for coexisting psychological problems, including depressed mood and emotional problems	Treatment of underlying problems is important to achieve and maintain abstinence.

 PATIENT AND CAREGIVER TEACHING

- Impact of substance use and the benefits of cessation
- Characteristics of SUD
- Risks associated with SUD
- Effects of SUD on the family and enabling behaviors
- Expectations associated with cessation plan
- Manifestations to expect during withdrawal
- Measures being used to treat withdrawal
- Lifestyle changes to maintain abstinence
- Ways to manage cravings
- Community and self-help resources
- Coping and stress management strategies
- Importance of long-term follow-up
- Role of case management
- Signs of relapse
- When to notify the HCP

DOCUMENTATION

Assessment

- Assessments performed
- Diagnostic and laboratory test results
- Manifestations of a substance use problem
- Manifestations of withdrawal
- Screening test results

Interventions

- Discussions with other interprofessional team members
- Environmental modifications made
- Medications given
- Notification of the HCP about patient status
- Therapeutic interventions and the patient's response
- Teaching provided
- Referrals initiated
- Safety measures implemented

Evaluation

- Patient's status: improved, stable, declined
- Presence of manifestations of substance use
- Response to teaching provided
- Response to therapeutic interventions

Continuity of Care Problem 58

Definition

Inadequate coordination across aspects of health care, including a lack of consistency in being able to see the same provider, poor communication and transfer of information across providers and settings, and a lack of follow-up or monitoring

All patients likely would prefer efficiently coordinated health care; it is especially important for those with multiple and complex chronic conditions. *Care coordination* is a set of activities purposefully organized to deliver the necessary services and information for optimal health and care across settings and time. The patient is the central member of the care coordination team.

Five key attributes of care coordination are an interorganizational and interprofessional team that includes the patient, communication and information exchange, a proactive plan of care with goals, a targeted set of purposeful activities, and outcomes and proactive follow-up. A lack of care coordination results in fragmented care, hospital readmissions, extended illness, and additional complications.

Nurses are responsible for providing care coordination in many settings. Priority populations for care coordination are those who are most at risk or frail. This may include a focus on serving children with special health care needs, the frail elderly population, those in crisis situations or experiencing catastrophic events, and persons at the end of life. Those in the second tier of risk and need for care coordination are those with complex situations, including people with cognitive impairments, multifaceted medical or mental health conditions, disabilities, low incomes, or unstable health insurance coverage.

Associated Clinical Problems

- Lack of Trust in Health Care Provider (HCP): inability or unwillingness to take the risk that a particular provider will ensure a good health outcome
- Risk of Dissatisfaction with Health Care: increased risk for finding the health care experience inadequate or unsatisfying
- Unfamiliar with Process for Obtaining Community Resources: lack of knowledge about available resources
- Unrealistic Expectation About Treatment: having much lesser or greater hopes for a particular therapy than is warranted based on the current evidence

Common Risk Factors

- Behavior and psychological problems
- Children with special needs
- Functional deficits
- History of nonadherence
- Hospitalization related to cancer, stroke, diabetes, chronic obstructive pulmonary disease (COPD), and heart failure
- Lack of a support system
- Low health literacy
- Multiple chronic conditions
- Older age
- Polypharmacy
- Preterm infants
- Recent hospitalization
- Receiving palliative care and end-of-life care

Manifestations

- Difficulty with arranging follow-up care
- Decreased patient confidence in self-managing care
- Decreased patient satisfaction
- Increased emergency department visits or hospital readmissions
- Ineffective communication among providers and with the patient
- Medication discrepancies

Key Conceptual Relationships

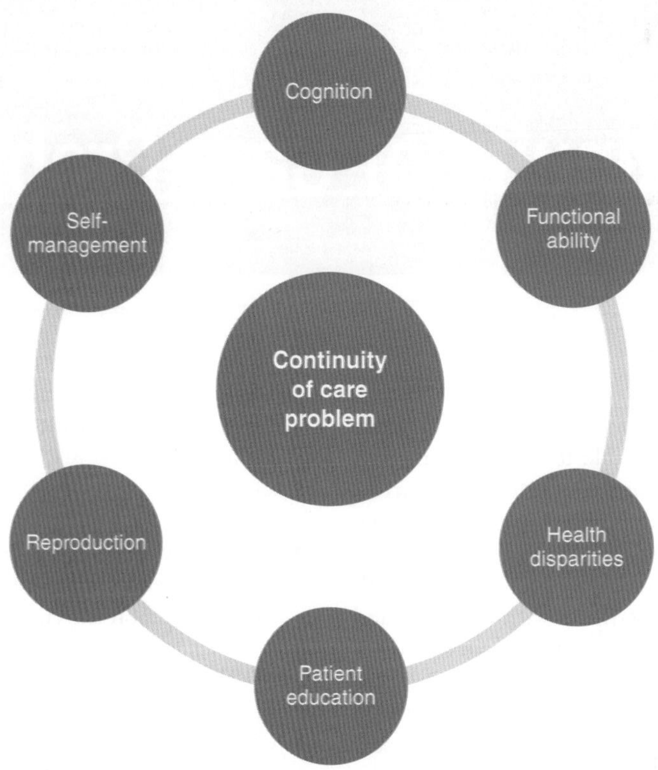

ASSESSMENT OF CONTINUITY OF CARE	RATIONALE
Perform a complete physical assessment and determine the patient's care needs:	
• **FUNCTIONAL ABILITY:** Functional assessment of the patient's ability to perform activities of daily living and carry out recommended therapy	This establishes a baseline to determine the patient's need for support.
• **COGNITION:** Cognition and ability to manage information	Managing information about a complex health situation can be challenging.
• Determine the patient's sources of informal and family support and living arrangements.	Assessment will help identify current resources and any environment challenges.
• **PATIENT EDUCATION:** Assess the patient's understanding of their health status, conditions, and care needs.	Knowing the patient's understanding of their health status establishes a baseline for teaching.
Elicit information from the patient and/or caregiver regarding any concerns they have at each encounter.	Addressing the concerns of the patient and/or caregiver assists the health care team in prioritizing care.
Assess the patient's goals for discharge and continued care.	Identify any gaps between the patient's goals and their current status.
HEALTH EQUITY: Assess the patient's socioeconomic status, including education, income, and employment status.	Patients with socioeconomic risk factors are more likely to experience problems with care coordination.
Determine what resources the patient requires to be able to carry out the prescribed therapy, considering access to care, financial and health insurance resources, and mobility.	Identify any gaps that exist between expected and actual self-care.
Review the patient's eligibility for resources, such as insurance, Medicare, or veteran status, and previous use of services.	Resource use and availability will vary by patient.
Determine whether there is any conflict between the patient's wishes and those of the health care team.	A contributing factor to discontinuity of care is when the patient or patient's decision maker and the health care team do not agree on goals or strategies.

ASSESSMENT OF CONTINUITY OF CARE	RATIONALE
Evaluate the quality of the patient's care coordination on an ongoing basis.	Periodic review of the patient's care coordination will allow for any needed adjustments.
Pediatric	
Assess the premature infant for needs associated with problems of breathing, feeding, temperature regulation, the heart, the brain, blood, and immunity.	Premature infants have complex needs that require coordinated long-term care.
Assess the situation of the child with special needs who may require collaboration among multiple care systems and providers, including medical, social, behavior, and education professionals.	Children with special needs often require multiple services for long-term support.
Women's Health	
REPRODUCTION: During a high-risk pregnancy, assess for support needs in the areas of patient education, nutrition, and social work.	High-risk pregnancy requires collaboration among multiple providers for an optimal birth outcome.

Expected Outcomes

The patient will:

- experience coordinated health care with a collaborative health team.
- adhere to the prescribed therapeutic regimen.
- maintain ongoing contact with appropriate community resources.

INTERVENTIONS TO ENHANCE CARE COORDINATION	RATIONALE
Ensure team members are aware of the goals of patient care.	All members of the health care team knowing the goals of care helps coordinate aims for care.
Arrange a health team conference for the patient and caregivers, as needed, to discuss goals, treatment options, and planning for complex health situations.	Conferences with health team members allow for discussions so that team members can collaborate toward shared goals.
Encourage patients to have the support person of their choice present with them at HCP visits.	Support persons can listen and take notes, helping the patient with information recall.
Offer patients information, resources, and opportunities to ask questions about prescribed therapies.	Information forms a basis for effective decisions about their care.
Help patients and caregivers make and keep a list of all current HCPs and services and their contact information, and encourage patients to take a copy of this information to appointments.	Having organized information promotes optimal communication.
Encourage the patient to keep a listing of scheduled appointments and diagnostic testing in one place, such as on a paper or online calendar.	Keeping track of complex scheduling promotes adherence.
Encourage the patient to keep a running list of questions and concerns in a health journal or online document to discuss with providers at the next scheduled visits.	Help the patient remember important questions to ask during appointments.
SELF-MANAGEMENT: Implement measures including medical record keeping and systems for monitoring health progress.	These measures promote the patient's self-health management.
Help the patient organize health instructions in one location, such as a drawer or file.	Keep information readily available for reference.
Assist patient to arrange a family conference, as needed, to discuss complex caregiving.	Family members who are caregivers can collaborate toward shared goals.
Encourage the patient to use health portal resources, when available.	Access to laboratory results, visit summaries, and other health information will help the patient and caregiver coordinate care.

Continued

INTERVENTIONS TO ENHANCE CARE COORDINATION	RATIONALE
Ensure discharge care is arranged while the patient is still hospitalized, including making appointments, following up for laboratory or test results, and securing equipment and services.	Ensure that the patient's care needs are met after the transition from the hospital.
Pediatric Help the patient and/or caregiver identify pertinent information, medications, and equipment to share with other caregivers, such as teachers and the school nurse.	This is important for maintaining care continuity while the child is attending school.

COLLABORATION	RATIONALE
Patient advocate or health navigator	Navigators provide specialized support for complex case coordination.
Disease or symptom management programs	Disease or symptom management programs help patients understand their treatment regimen and address complex needs with chronic illness.
HEALTH DISPARITIES: Social services or case management	Support may be needed to obtain financial, transportation, or other resources.
School nurse, counselor, and school social worker	Ensure the needs of the child are being met in the school environment.

PATIENT AND CAREGIVER TEACHING

- Coordinated care services
- Follow-up visits and long-term care
- Managing and tracking health data
- Keeping track of questions for providers
- Treatment plans
- Safe use of medications
- Scheduling timely posthospital follow-up
- Community and self-help resources
- Sources of information and social support
- When to notify the HCPs and which ones to notify for particular issues

DOCUMENTATION

Assessment

- Functional status
- Needs for support

Interventions

- Discussions with other members of the interprofessional team
- Teaching provided
- Referrals initiated

Evaluation

- Experience of care
- Health status
- Response to teaching provided

Impaired Communication 59

Definition

Impediment or blockage to exchanging thoughts, messages, or information

Communication is an exchange of ideas between people, a process of interaction in which symbols are used to create, exchange, and interpret messages. The messages may be transmitted through spoken or written language as well as through nonverbal means such as gestures, facial expressions, or body movements. Communication is important in building human relationships.

Health problems can result in communication difficulties. A person having difficulty finding words, speaking appropriately, or articulating speech may have aphasia. The problem may be sensory aphasia, in which language is not understood, or motor aphasia, in which words cannot be formed or expressed. Aphasia may be complete or partial, affecting specific language functions. Other persons may have weakness of the muscles involved in speech.

Communication is used in the context of health to seek assistance, collaborate, reassure, and teach. Miscommunication can be dangerous, even deadly, in health care settings, while effective communication promotes safe and high-quality health care. Even patients and health team members who are able to speak clearly and receive messages can be constrained by the lack of a common language. Nurses have a role in promoting effective communication and advocating for patients when barriers prevent patients from communicating effectively.

Associated Clinical Problems

- Communication Barrier: obstacle to exchanging thoughts, messages, or information
- Dysphasia: language function is disordered or absent because of an injury to certain areas of the cerebral cortex
- Expressive Dysphasia: impaired ability to form or express words
- Impaired Verbal Communication: impaired ability to exchange thoughts, messages, or information using language

Common Causes and Risk Factors

- Altered perception
- Altered vision, speech, or hearing
- Anatomic defects
- Autism
- Central nervous system problem
- Cultural differences
- Development delay
- Environment barriers
- Facial trauma, surgery
- Lack of common language
- Laryngeal cancer
- Musculoskeletal problems affecting processes of speech
- Presence of medical equipment, such as endotracheal tube
- Psychological problems, such as schizophrenia or bipolar disorder

Manifestations

- Absence of eye contact
- Absence of verbalization
- Difficulty comprehending communication
- Difficulty expressing thoughts verbally, including aphasia, dysphasia, apraxia, dyslexia
- Difficulty forming words or sentences
- Difficulty in the use of facial or body expressions
- Difficulty producing speech
- Slurring
- Stuttering
- Use of language unknown to health team members
- Diagnostic tests
  - Vision acuity test showing impaired vision
  - Audiometry showing hearing impairment
  - Speech evaluation showing impaired speech

Key Conceptual Relationships

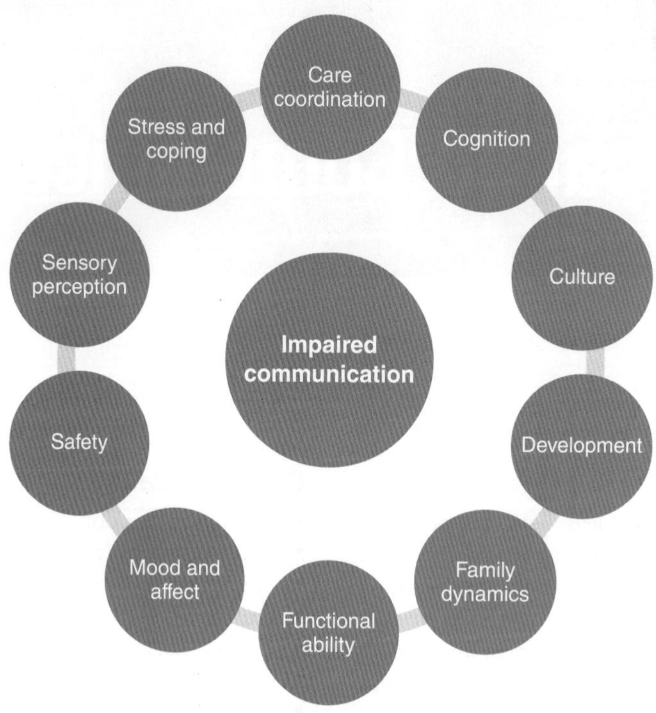

ASSESSMENT OF COMMUNICATION	RATIONALE
Assess for the potential cause of the patient's impaired communication.	Identifying factors that place the patient at risk for impaired communication allows for early intervention.
Perform a physical assessment, noting any factors that may influence communication:	
• Speech-language comprehension	Assessment is done to determine baseline function and detect the presence of any problems.
• **COGNITION:** Cognitive and mental status	Impairments in cognition and mental status can negatively influence communication.
• **SENSORY PERCEPTION:** Presence of sensory deficits and the patient's use of corrective measures, such as the use of glasses and/or hearing aids	Sensory deficits can be a major barrier to perceiving communication.
Obtain a formal speech pathology evaluation as appropriate.	A formal speech and language evaluation will determine whether any problems are present and outline the patient's strengths and weaknesses in communication.
Determine the patient's primary language and literacy level.	This allows the health care team to provide communication in appropriate language and context for the person.
CULTURE: Assess patient's preferences for communication, such as the use of silence, amount of personal space, and use of eye contact.	Cross-cultural differences in communication influence individual preferences for eye contact, silence, and personal space.
FAMILY DYNAMICS: Evaluate family dynamics, current level of functioning, and family interactions.	Having a family member with impaired communication affects how family members interact with each other.
FUNCTIONAL ABILITY: Perform a psychosocial assessment, evaluating for any lifestyle effects of having impaired communication, such as the ability to enjoy life, interact with others, perform work and role duties, and engage in social activities.	Problems resulting from having a communication problem can affect multiple aspects of a person's life.
MOOD AND AFFECT: Assess for the presence of any coexisting psychological problems, particularly depression.	Being unable to communicate effectively can lead to depression and other psychological problems.

ASSESSMENT OF COMMUNICATION	RATIONALE
STRESS AND COPING: Assess coping strategies used by patient and caregiver, and determine how they are coping with the presence of the communication impairment.	Quality of life for patients and caregivers is partly related to the coping strategies that they use.
Evaluate the patient's response to measures to enhance communication through ongoing assessment.	Ongoing assessment allows for adjustment of interventions as needed.
Pediatric	
DEVELOPMENT: Assess the child's development level, including level of speech and language comprehension.	The effects of impaired communication and management depend on the child's age and development level.

Expected Outcomes

The patient will:

- use effective communication techniques.
- be able to communicate needs.
- demonstrate congruent verbal and nonverbal behavior.
- demonstrate understanding of received communication.

INTERVENTIONS TO PROMOTE COMMUNICATION	RATIONALE
Get the patient's attention before speaking and show respect. Speak in a clear voice, using simple language. If the patient appears comfortable with eye contact, maintain eye contact at the patient's level.	Therapeutic communication techniques support effective communication.
Listen actively and validate verbal and nonverbal communication.	Validation ensures accurate receipt of intended communication.
Use caring, comfort-related touch, such as holding the patient's hand, if that is acceptable to the patient.	Some patients may find touch comforting; others may prefer not to be touched.
Use communication tools and technology, such as pen and paper, picture boards, flashcards, or typing on a computer or mobile phone, with patients who are nonverbal and/or endotracheally intubated.	Providing alternative communication methods allows nonverbal patients to express needs and concerns.
Continue to explain information and provide conversation for the nonverbal patient.	Show respect for the patient by acknowledging their presence.
Allow extra time to communicate with patients who have expressive or receptive communication challenges.	Allowing extra time can help reduce the patient's level of frustration.
Use comfortable silence to allow for reflection time or for the patient to organize thoughts.	Avoid filling up all space with talking.
Use techniques of paraphrasing, clarifying, exploring, and reflecting.	These techniques ensure accurate and therapeutic communication.
Use specific techniques with patients who have minimal strength or ability to respond: • Use close-ended questions that are easy to answer. • Avoid limiting communication in other situations by using open-ended questions.	The patient's frustration may be decreased with simplified responses.
Assign staff consistently.	When communication is difficult, staff who have experience with the patient's forms of communication my decrease patient frustration.
CULTURE: For patients and caregivers who speak a language different from the health care provider (HCP), use an approved interpreter or interpreter phone service.	Professional translation allows for the most effective communication. Asking family members to translate may impose an unfair burden on them and may lead to inaccurate communication of technical information.

Continued

INTERVENTIONS TO PROMOTE COMMUNICATION	RATIONALE
When working with an interpreter: • Speak slowly. • Maintain eye contact with the patient. • Talk to the patient, not the interpreter. • Use simple language with as few medical terms as possible. • Speak one or two sentences at a time to allow for easier interpretation. • Avoid raising your voice during the interaction. • Obtain feedback to be certain the patient understands. • Plan on taking twice as long to complete the interaction.	Communicating via an interpreter requires extra effort for effective messaging.
SENSORY PERCEPTION: If the patient has uncorrected hearing loss, reduce background noise, make eye contact before beginning to speak, and speak clearly, without overenunciating.	Eliminate competing sounds. Avoid distorting the voice, which makes lip reading more difficult.
FAMILY DYNAMICS: Include a family member/caregiver who can provide information about health history and patient preferences if the patient is unable to communicate verbally or if the patient's articulation is difficult to understand.	A family member who communicates effectively with the patient may decrease the patient's stress in communication.
For the patient who is unable to communicate effectively: • Speak to the patient respectfully and often, even if there is no apparent response. • Encourage family members to speak calmly and interact with the patient.	Family members may need reassurance to interact if the patient is unconscious or confused.
SAFETY: Ensure that nonverbal patients have a method to obtain help, such as a call bell that is in reach.	Providing a method to call for help addresses safety and allows the patient to express other needs.
Teach about health issues or provide conversation on the patient's preferred topics, such as travel, hobbies, or family, during the process of care and when waiting for procedures.	Talking about topics of interest to the patient demonstrates respect for patient preferences and interests while providing social interaction.
SENSORY PERCEPTION: Encourage patients with sensory aids, such as glasses or hearing aids, to use them.	Aids may be forgotten or intentionally ignored.
COGNITION: Implement measures to address impaired cognition, if present.	Addressing impaired cognition may have a positive effect on communication difficulties related to disorientation.
FUNCTIONAL ABILITY: Help the patient develop strategies for communication during activities of daily living (ADLs).	Making ADLs easier to perform will help patients be as independent as possible.
STRESS AND COPING: Help the patient and caregivers cope with the presence of a communication problem by using positive stress management and coping behaviors.	Quality of life for patients and caregivers is related to the stress management and coping strategies they use.
Pediatric	
Observe behavior cues in preverbal children and collaborate with parents or caregivers to interpret the cues.	Family caregivers may recognize the child's behavior patterns and be able to interpret differences in cries and other behaviors.
DEVELOPMENT: Assist the parent/caregiver of a child with referrals for specialized assessment and intervention for language and related development delays.	Early intervention supports language development.

COLLABORATION	RATIONALE
Speech therapy	Experts in speech and hearing may be needed to support the patient's communication.
Audiologist	Experts in speech and hearing may be needed to support the patient's communication.
STRESS AND COPING: Counseling	Counseling can assist the patient in managing problems from having impaired communication.

COLLABORATION	RATIONALE
Support groups	Groups of patients who are experiencing the same problem can assist in rehabilitation and decrease social isolation.
MOOD AND AFFECT: Treatment for any coexisting psychological problems, particularly depression	Being unable to communicate effectively can lead to depression and other psychological problems.
CARE COORDINATION: Social work or case management	A social worker or case manager can help the patient and caregiver identify helpful community resources.

PATIENT AND CAREGIVER TEACHING

- Cause of the communication problem and how long it may last
- Management of conditions contributing to the communication problem
- Role of speech therapy
- Using alternate forms of communication
- Congruence of verbal and nonverbal communication
- Community and self-help resources
- Sources of information and social support
- Maintaining role performance and taking part in desired ADLs
- When to notify the HCP

DOCUMENTATION

Assessment

- Assessments performed
- Diagnostic and laboratory test results
- Manifestations of impaired communication
- Method and content of communication

Interventions

- Discussions with other members of the interprofessional team
- Environmental modifications made
- Therapeutic interventions and the patient's response
- Teaching provided
- Referrals initiated
- Use of alternate forms of communication

Evaluation

- Patient's status: improved, stable, declined
- Ability of patient to send and receive messages effectively
- Response to teaching provided

Socioeconomic Difficulty 60

Definition

Challenges to health based on income, education, financial security, and perceptions of social status and social class

Health equity is an outcome achieved when all persons have the opportunity to attain their health potential and no one is disadvantaged. *Health disparities* are differences in the incidence, prevalence, mortality rate, and burden of diseases that exist among specific populations because of social, economic, or environment disadvantages. Health disparities affect population groups based on gender, age, ethnicity, socioeconomic status, education, geography, sexual orientation, disability, or special health care needs.

Limited access to high-quality, accessible, and affordable health care services clearly is associated with an increased incidence of illness and complications and a reduced lifespan. People with chronic health problems, such as diabetes, may have difficulty obtaining health care insurance. These issues must be considered in the broader context of social justice. The health care system and health care providers (HCPs) may also contribute to the problem of health disparities.

Discrimination and bias based on a patient's race, ethnicity, gender, age, body size, sexual orientation, or ability to pay may result in less aggressive or negative treatment practices. Discrimination can result in the delay of a proper diagnosis because of assumptions made about the patient. Factors such as bias and prejudice can affect health care–seeking behaviors. Sometimes, discrimination is difficult to identify, especially when it occurs at the institution level. Because the overt discriminatory behaviors of an HCP may not be immediately evident to the patient or the HCP, they may be difficult to confront. Even well-intentioned providers who try to eliminate bias in their care can demonstrate their prior beliefs or prejudices through nonverbal communication.

Nurses can support access to care and health equity through their actions. Advocacy includes providing adequate follow-up care for all patients, especially those who are experiencing health care disparities. When disparities are observed, consider the possibility that the person has experienced discrimination and/or abuse. Professional nurses are legally and ethically responsible to be patient advocates.

Associated Clinical Problems

- Difficulty Obtaining Medication: financial or logistic obstacles to acquiring prescribed drugs
- Employment Problem: inability to find or maintain consistent employment
- Financial Problem: lack of funds to support a healthy lifestyle
- Housing Problem: inadequate or unstable place of residence
- Lack of Access to Transportation: inadequate availability of travel for health care and wellness activities

Common Causes and Risk Factors

- Age
- Biased clinical decision-making
- Disability status
- Education
- Ethnicity and race
- Food insecurity
- Gender
- HCP's attitude
- High health care costs
- Income status
- Occupation
- Lack of health care services
- Lack of transportation to services or HCPs
- Mistrust
- Provider–patient communication problems
- Sexual orientation
- Unemployment
- Unstable housing

Manifestations

- Variable health outcomes for groups with social, economic, or environment disadvantages

Key Conceptual Relationships

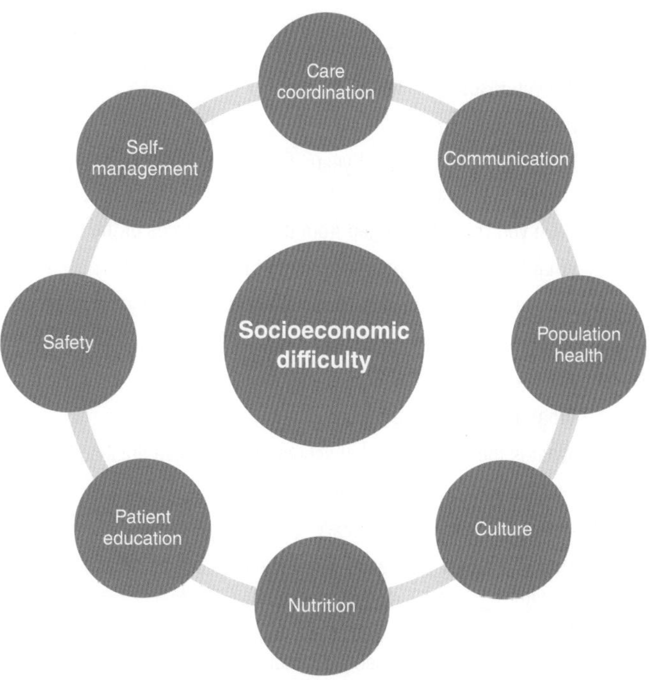

ASSESSMENT OF SOCIOECEONOMIC DIFFICULTY	RATIONALE
Assess for socioeconomic issues in the health history.	Awareness of disproportionate health risks can help identify those in need of resources.
CULTURE: Explore patient beliefs, values, meaning of illness, preferences, and needs.	Understand the patient's viewpoint so you can respect those beliefs in planning care.
Administer formal social determinants of health screening tools, such as the Protocol for Responding to and Assessing Patient's Assets, Risks, and Experiences (PRAPARE) (Table 60.1).	A formal screening tool can help determine patient needs.
SELF-MANAGEMENT: Assess the influence of socioeconomic status on the patient's current level of adherence to any prescribed therapeutic regimen.	Identify whether there is a gap between expected and actual self-care as a result of socioeconomic problems.
Develop an ecomap for the patient.	An ecomap is a diagram that shows the social and personal relationships of a person with their environment.
NUTRITION: Assess for food insecurity.	Persons or families with limited financial resources may have food insecurity. Less expensive, "filling" foods are more energy dense (high fat) and lack nutritional value, increasing the risk for obesity.
PATIENT EDUCATION: Assess health literacy level, including the ability to: • read and understand information. • understand instructions. • weigh risks and benefits. • make decisions.	This allows you to provide health information about resources at an understandable level.
Determine the patient's degree of awareness of available community and other resources that can assist with addressing problems.	Identify gaps in the patient's knowledge regarding available resources.
Review the patient's eligibility for various resources, such as insurance, food assistance, and unemployment, and previous use of services.	Resource use and availability will vary by patient.
Evaluate the patient's socioeconomic status on an ongoing basis.	A periodic review of the patient's socioeconomic status will allow for adjustments to be made as their circumstances change.

Table 60.1 PRAPARE (Protocol for Responding to and Assessing Patient's Assets, Risks, and Experiences)

Category	Question	Text
Personal Characteristics	1	Are you Hispanic or Latino?
	2	Which race(s) are you?
	3	At any point in the past 2 years, has seasonal or migrant farm work been your or your family's main source of income?
	4	Have you been discharged from the armed forces of the United States?
	5	What language are you most comfortable speaking?
Family and Home	6	How many family members, including yourself, do you currently live with?
	7	What is your housing situation today?
	8	Are you worried about losing your housing?
	9	What address do you live at?
Money and Resources	10	What is the highest level of school that you have finished?
	11	What is your current work situation?
	12	What is your main insurance?
	13	During the past year, what was the total combined income for you and your family members you live with?
	14	In the past year, have you or any family members you live with been unable to get any of the following when it was really needed? (food, clothing, utilities, child care, phone, medicine, any health care)
	15	Has lack of transportation kept you from medical appointments, meetings, work, or from getting things needed for daily living?
Social and Emotional Health	16	How often do you see or talk to people that you care about and feel close to?
	17	Stress is when someone feels tense, nervous, anxious, or can't sleep at night because their mind is troubled. How stressed are you?

Adapted from National Association of Community Health Centers. PRAPARE. https://prapare.org/.

Expected Outcomes

The patient will:

- attain a high-quality, longer life, free from preventable disease, disability, injury, and premature death.
- achieve health equity.
- experience social and physical environments that promote good health.
- experience quality of life, healthy development, and healthy behaviors across all life stages.

INTERVENTIONS FOR PROMOTING HEALTH EQUITY	RATIONALE
Establish a therapeutic relationship with the patient: • Build rapport and trust. • Find common ground. • Maintain eye contact, if comfortable for the patient. • Show genuine interest.	This helps to establish a positive relationship.
Maintain awareness of personal biases or assumptions and treat people with respect.	Even well-intentioned providers who try to eliminate bias in their care can demonstrate their prior beliefs or prejudices through nonverbal communication.
CULTURE: Choose health interventions adapted to the language and culture of the person to facilitate communication and decision making.	Language adaptation and cultural meanings of information should be considered in providing patient-centered care.
COMMUNICATION: Offer language assistance and tailored print and multimedia materials to those who have limited English proficiency and/or other communication needs.	Language assistance can give patients ready and timely access to all health care and related services.
PATIENT EDUCATION: Provide information attuned to the patient's level of health literacy.	The degree to which individuals can obtain, process, and understand basic health information to make decisions affects health outcomes.

INTERVENTIONS FOR PROMOTING HEALTH EQUITY	RATIONALE
Encourage patients to have the support person of their choice present with them at HCP visits.	Support persons may reduce the presence of bias that health care professionals may have but not be aware of.
Become knowledgeable about health disparities and discrimination affecting minority groups and other populations in your local health care settings.	Awareness of common issues may present opportunities for systematic change.
SELF-MANAGEMENT: Assist the patient in determining the resources needed to be able to follow any prescribed therapeutic regimen.	Help close any gaps that exist between expected and actual self-care.
Assist the patient and caregivers in navigating the health care system for sources of low-cost or free wellness care and access to health insurance.	Affordable health care services increase access to care.
Aim to schedule health services that are convenient and attentive to the patient's work commitments and transportation availability.	Developing a schedule that considers transportation and other factors promotes accessibility and helps meet the patient's needs.
Encourage the use of mail order or delivery services for medications and durable equipment.	Having medications and durable equipment delivered by mail order or delivery service can combat transportation problems.
PATIENT EDUCATION: Consider socioeconomic factors when preparing to teach the patient about health topics.	Knowing the patient's background and present or past occupation may assist in determining the vocabulary and examples to use during teaching.
Review the patient's complete medication list and discuss potential lower-cost alternatives with the HCP.	Patients want HCPs to consider their ability to pay when prescribing medications.

COLLABORATION	RATIONALE
CARE COORDINATION: Social work or case management	Social workers and case managers can help the patient obtain access to health care and other resources.
Pharmacists	Pharmacists can help identify medication resources available to the patient.

PATIENT AND CAREGIVER TEACHING

- Available resources
- How to access resources
- Communication with health providers
- Sources of information and social support
- Where to find additional information

DOCUMENTATION

Assessment

- Assessments performed
- Manifestations of socioeconomic difficulty
- Screening test results

Interventions

- Discussions with other members of the interprofessional team
- Therapeutic interventions and the patient's response
- Teaching provided
- Referrals initiated

Evaluation

- Access to health care and other resources
- Response to teaching provided

Risk for Disease 61

Definition

A characteristic, condition, or behavior that increases the likelihood of developing a disease or being injured

Health promotion is the process of supporting people to increase their control over and improve their health. The World Health Organization defines *health* as "a state of complete physical, mental, and social well-being and not merely the absence of disease and infirmity." Health promotion includes interventions for a person, family, community, population, and environment. Nurses have a role in promoting health and preventing disease throughout the lifespan.

Health promotion activities take place through three levels of prevention. *Primary prevention* refers to strategies for optimizing health and disease prevention. Nurses play a key role in providing health education focused on nutrition, exercise, immunizations, safe living and work environments, hygiene and sanitation, protection from environment hazards, avoidance of harmful substances, protection from accidents, and effective stress management. The goal of *secondary prevention* is to identify those in an early stage of a disease so that prompt treatment can be initiated. Early treatment provides an opportunity to cure disease, limit disability, or delay the consequences of advanced disease. Secondary prevention measures typically involve screening tests. *Tertiary prevention* involves minimizing the effects of disease and disability through collaborative disease management. The aim is to optimize the management of a condition and minimize complications so that the person can achieve the highest level of health possible.

Good nutrition, physical activity, and a healthy body weight are essential for overall health and well-being. A healthful diet, regular physical activity, and maintaining a healthy weight decrease a person's risk of developing or worsening serious health conditions. Key health promotion points include the following:

- Many people do not eat a healthy diet and are not physically active, which has led to a dramatic increase in obesity and related conditions such as heart disease, stroke, and type 2 diabetes.
- Poor oral health, particularly periodontal (gum) disease, has been linked to diabetes, heart disease, and stroke. Poor oral health in pregnant women is associated with premature births and low birth weight.
- Tobacco use is the most preventable cause of disease, disability, and death in the United States. Smoking and vaping also affect those who are exposed to secondhand smoke.
- Infant risk for sudden infant death syndrome (SIDS) can be dramatically decreased with simple interventions.
- Untreated sexually transmitted infections (STIs) can lead to serious long-term health consequences, including reproductive health problems, infertility, fetal and perinatal health problems, cancer, and transmission of infections.

Associated Clinical Problems

- Health Seeking Behavior Alteration: lack of interest in actions that promote wellness
- High-Risk Sexual Behavior: engaging in actions that increase the probability of sexually transmitted disease, injury, or unwanted pregnancy
- Impaired Exercise Behavior: inadequate and/or irregular physical activity
- Risk for Exposure to Secondhand Smoke: increased risk for disease from inhaling tobacco or marijuana smoke present in the physical environment
- Risk for Sudden Infant Death Syndrome: infant at increased risk for unexpected death
- Risk-Prone Health Behaviors: actions that increase the likelihood of injury or illness
- Sedentary Lifestyle: chronic inactivity

Common Risk Factors

- Age
- Exposure to air pollution
- Exposure to risks in the workplace
- Dangerous social settings
- Diabetes
- Gender
- Genetics
- High cholesterol levels
- Hypertension
- Lack of immunization for communicable diseases
- Lack of interest and/or motivation for health behaviors
- Lack of resources
- Limited access to clean water and sanitation
- Low socioeconomic status
- Nutrition choices

- Overweight or obesity
- Physical inactivity
- Poor personal hygiene
- Substance use, including tobacco and alcohol
- Time in the sun without protection
- Unsafe home environment
- Unprotected sex

Manifestations

- Expressed interest in improving health
- Presence of risk factors
- Presence of health condition

Key Conceptual Relationships

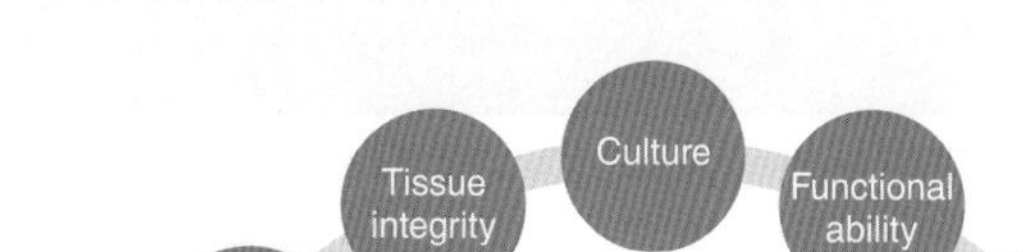

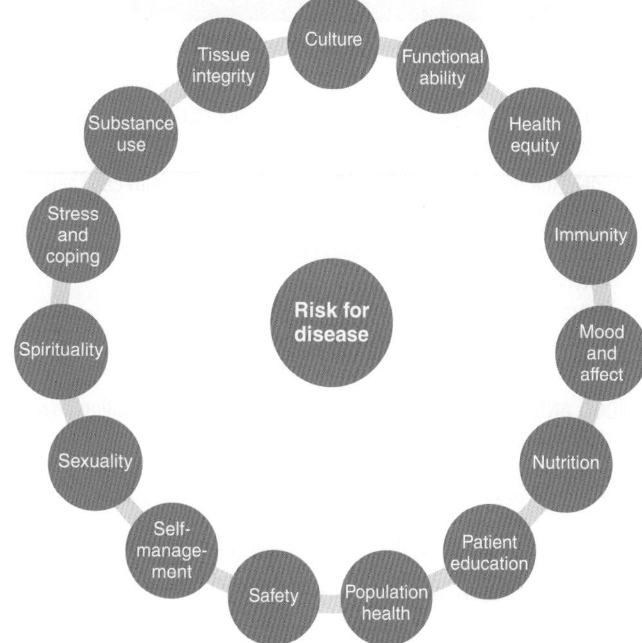

ASSESSMENT OF RISK FOR DISEASE	RATIONALE
Assess personal definition of health, facilitators and barriers to health, and motivation to change health behaviors.	Unique perceptions of health and illness affect choices and behaviors.
Perform a complete patient-centered health risk assessment appropriate to the patient's age, addressing: • Diet • Exercise behaviors • Hygiene behaviors • Immunization history • Self-examinations and screening behaviors • Sexual behaviors • Sleep habits • Substance use • Sun protection behaviors • Weight	Health risk assessments are designed to evaluate the risk for disease or disability and identify health-promoting behaviors.
Perform a complete physical assessment and evaluate underlying health status.	Health status has a significant influence on risk for disease.
Obtain appropriate biometric measures: • Height, weight, body mass index (BMI), waist circumference • Blood pressure • High-density lipoprotein/low-density lipoprotein, total cholesterol, triglycerides • Glucose, hemoglobin A1c levels	Biometric health measures reflect health status.
Assess the patient's and community's strengths and health concerns.	The health care team can base the plan of care on the patient's strengths.
CULTURE: Evaluate the influence of cultural perspectives on the patient's health management.	Cultural beliefs and practices may affect choices for health actions.

Continued

ASSESSMENT OF RISK FOR DISEASE	RATIONALE
PATIENT EDUCATION: Assess the patient's level of health literacy.	Knowing the patient's health literacy level allows you to present information in an understandable way.
HEALTH EQUITY: Assess the patient's socioeconomic risk factors, including education level, income, employment, and living conditions.	Socioeconomic factors contribute to a person's state of health.
Evaluate the person's access to resources, including health care and health insurance.	Inability to obtain supplies, lack of insurance or transportation, or other resources may prevent self-care behaviors.
CULTURE: Assess the patient's support system and availability of caregivers: • Who lives with them? • Are friends and relatives accessible? • What community resources have they used? • Has anyone served or is able to serve as a caregiver?	Interest and support from others are important aspects of managing health.
MOOD AND AFFECT: Screen for depression and other coexisting psychological problems at each encounter.	Depression is a common condition in many age groups that may affect the motivation to adopt healthy behaviors.
SAFETY: Screen for the presence of safety and fall risks.	Identifying specific risk factors for injury allows for the development of a customized injury prevention plan.
Evaluate the patient's health promotion needs on an ongoing basis.	A periodic review of the patient's health promotion needs allows for adjustments.
Pediatric Screen for health problems relevant to the adolescent and/or suggested by the patient history, such as anemia, hearing and vision problems, oral health problems, abnormal sexual maturation, abnormal physical growth, body image problems, eating disorders, poor nutrition, poor self-concept, low self-esteem, difficult relationships, abuse, and learning problems.	Many health behaviors begin in adolescence; risk behaviors have immediate and long-term effects on health and quality of life.

Expected Outcomes

The patient will:

- state awareness of their individual risk for disease.
- incorporate healthy lifestyle behaviors.
- identify potential health risks and participate in screenings.
- describe the benefits of following health promotion behaviors.

INTERVENTIONS TO DECREASE RISK FOR DISEASE	RATIONALE
Reinforce confidence in making behavior changes and taking actions to reduce the risk of disease.	Building confidence in decision making promotes self-efficacy.
Acknowledge the patient's and caregiver's expertise in managing chronic conditions.	Acknowledging self-management successes promotes self-efficacy and trust.
Encourage setting realistic and attainable goals, such as adding one or two additional vegetable servings daily.	Goal achievement enhances self-efficacy, promotes positive expectations, and supports behavior change.
Use motivational interviewing to help the patient identify unhealthy behaviors and choose healthier options.	Helping patients identify why they want to make a health change and how they might do it is more effective than telling them they should.
Provide positive reinforcement for achieving health goals.	Positive reinforcement promotes the patient's confidence in continuing healthy behaviors.
SELF-MANAGEMENT: Assist the patient in identifying ways to incorporate healthy behaviors in daily activities.	The patient may find it easier to add or adopt new behaviors that fit with existing routines and habits.
Encourage all patients to seek regular wellness care and screenings.	Risks and health concerns identified during wellness care and screening allow for early intervention.

INTERVENTIONS TO DECREASE RISK FOR DISEASE	RATIONALE
IMMUNITY: Encourage and administer vaccinations according to recommended schedules and patient need.	Vaccinations are given to decrease the risk of acquiring an infection.
Assist the patient with developing a regular physical activity plan, considering capabilities, daily routine, and personal preferences.	Regular physical activity is critical to improving health at every age.
NUTRITION: Implement measures to assist the patient in implementing the appropriate diet to achieve or maintain a healthy body weight.	The appropriate diet is a critical part of achieving an optimal weight.
Foster communication between the patient and caregiver and the health care team. Encourage patients to keep a list of health-related questions and concerns to ask at the next encounter.	Patients may forget to ask important questions during the appointment.
Encourage the patient to use health portal resources when available.	Access to laboratory results, visit summaries, and other health information may help the patient understand the current condition and treatment plan.
FUNCTIONAL ABILITY: Encourage the patient to maintain a culturally acceptable level of personal hygiene and grooming.	Some personal hygiene is needed to ensure health and promote positive social interactions.
STRESS AND COPING: Collaborate with the patient to select and implement mindfulness, meditation, and other positive strategies.	Introducing additional coping strategies will assist the patient with managing stress and changes in health status.
CULTURE: Implement measures to develop and promote positive social interaction.	Positive social interaction fosters physical and emotional health.
SPIRITUALITY: Encourage spirituality as a source of support for healthy behaviors and coping with the change.	Religious or spiritual beliefs may support the patient's health goals.
TISSUE INTEGRITY: Encourage the use of sun protection and avoidance of extended sun exposure.	Cumulative sun exposure over the lifetime increases the risk for skin cancer.
COMMUNITY HEALTH: Assist persons and community groups with developing resources for promoting healthy behaviors.	Supportive resources may be available through government and nongovernment sources.
HEALTH EQUITY: Assist the patient and caregivers in navigating the health care system for sources of low-cost or free wellness care and access to health insurance.	Affordable health care services increase access to care.
Pediatric	
SAFETY: Provide the parent/caregiver tips on injury prevention strategies tailored to the patient/child's specific development stage and curiosity level.	Anticipatory guidance helps to prevent common injuries.
Provide guidance to the parent/caregiver of an infant regarding: • Appropriate infant nutrition and habits, including recommendation of breastfeeding, if feasible. • Establishing bedtime rituals that reduce or eliminate disturbances in the sleep–wake cycle	Anticipatory guidance helps to prevent and manage development issues.
Assist youth in role playing to develop decision-making and assertiveness skills.	Being assertive and able to make decisions reduces stress and enhances health.
Encourage participation in school, extracurricular, and community volunteer activities.	Increased student engagement enhances mental and physical well-being.
Assist parents in establishing norms for parental monitoring of friends and activities.	Youth with clear, consistent limits and parental monitoring are less likely to engage in persistent risky behavior.
Assist the school-aged child and their parent/caregiver regarding: • Family involvement in the child's school and other activities • Learning personal hygiene skills (e.g., toileting, washing hands, brushing teeth) • Developing friendships	Anticipatory guidance helps to prevent and manage developmental issues.
Build a trusting relationship with the adolescent and parent/caregiver: • Encourage adolescents to be actively involved in decisions regarding their own health care. • Discuss normal development milestones and associated behaviors. • Facilitate a sense of responsibility for self and others. • Facilitate the development of sexual identity.	Anticipatory guidance helps to prevent and manage development issues.

INTERVENTIONS TO DISCOURAGE HIGH-RISK SEXUAL BEHAVIOR	RATIONALE
SEXUALITY: Encourage the patient to follow safe sex practices. Provide information on safe sex and avoidance of STIs.	Following safe sex practices can decrease the risk of acquiring an STI.
SEXUALITY: Assist the patient with understanding options, selecting contraception, and instructions for use, if desired.	Contraception decreases the risk of an unplanned pregnancy.

INTERVENTIONS TO DECREASE RISK FOR EXPOSURE TO SECONDHAND SMOKE	RATIONALE
Discuss the importance of tobacco avoidance with the patient and family.	Set the expectation to never start smoking or vaping.
SUBSTANCE USE: Review ways to provide a smoke-free environment for the patient and others.	Secondhand smoke can affect the health of others, particularly family members with reactive airway problems.

INTERVENTIONS TO DECREASE RISK FOR SIDS	RATIONALE
Encourage parents and caregivers to: • Place the infant on their back every time they sleep; avoid putting them to sleep on the stomach or sides. • Use a firm, noninclined sleep surface, such as a firm crib mattress covered by a fitted sheet. • Room-share without bed-sharing. • Keep soft objects and loose bedding out of the crib. • Avoid smoke exposure. • Breastfeed if possible. • Offer a pacifier at nap time and bedtime. • Do not hang a pacifier around the infant's neck. • Avoid overheating by placing not more than one layer on the infant than an adult would wear to be comfortable in that environment. • Immunize the infant according to recommendations from the American Academy of Pediatrics. • Do not use commercial devices marketed to reduce the risk of SIDS (e.g., wedges, positioners, special mattresses). • Car seats, strollers, swings, infant carriers, and infant slings are not recommended for routine sleep in the hospital or at home. • Do not rely on home cardiorespiratory monitors as a way to reduce the risk of SIDS. • Supervised awake "tummy time" counteracts the effects of regular back sleeping on muscle development or flattening of the head.	These measures are believed to be effective in reducing the risk of SIDS.

COLLABORATION	RATIONALE
HEALTH EQUITY: Social services or case management	Support may be needed to obtain financial, transportation, or other resources.
SUBSTANCE USE: Tobacco cessation support and resources	Tobacco cessation is challenging, so additional support is helpful in promoting cessation and continued abstinence.
STRESS AND COPING: Support groups	Interacting with others who face similar challenges may provide practical information and a sense of support.
Wellness programs	Many wellness programs focus on weight management, smoking cessation, screening, diabetes management, and other behaviors to promote health.
Counseling	Counseling can empower patients to make healthy and informed choices about their lifestyle.
Dental care	Maintaining oral health and good dentition promotes overall health.
MOOD AND AFFECT: Treatment for any coexisting psychological problems, including depressed mood and emotional problems	Depression is a common condition in many age groups that may affect the motivation to adopt healthy behaviors.
SEXUALITY: Recommend providers with experience in lesbian, gay, transgender, queer (questioning), intersex, agender (LGBTQIA) issues, as appropriate.	Experienced providers provide evidence-based screening and care.

PATIENT AND CAREGIVER TEACHING

- Wellness care
- Recommended screenings specific to the patient's age and risk status
- Risks, benefits, contraindications, and side effects of scheduled immunizations
- Anticipatory guidance for developmental issues
- Lifestyle changes to promote health
- Management of current health conditions and prevention of complications
- Where to find additional information
- Importance of long-term follow-up and communication with the health care team
- When to notify the health care provider

DOCUMENTATION

Assessment

- Health risk
- Current management of health behaviors
- Manifestations of any health condition

Interventions

- Discussions with other members of the interprofessional team
- Teaching provided
- Referrals made

Evaluation

- Patient's response to therapeutic interventions
- Progress toward health goals
- Response to teaching provided
- Presence of continued manifestations of a health condition

Dying Process 62

Definition

Progress toward the end of life

Death and the process of dying are highly individualized. *End-of-life (EOL) care* is the term used for health services related to death and dying. EOL care focuses on the physical and psychosocial needs of the patient and family. The goals for EOL care are to provide comfort and supportive care during the dying process, improve the quality of the patient's remaining life, help ensure a dignified death, and provide emotional support to the family.

Palliative care focuses on reducing the severity of disease symptoms. According to the World Health Organization, the overall goals of palliative care are to prevent and relieve suffering and improve the quality of life for patients with serious life-limiting illnesses. Patients may receive palliative care services in settings including the home, long-term and acute care, mental health facilities, rehabilitation centers, and prisons.

Palliative care often includes hospice care near the end of life. Hospice is not a place but a concept of care that provides compassion, concern, and support for persons in the last phases of a terminal disease. The main goals of hospice care are to assist the patient to live fully, as comfortably as possible, and to die pain-free and with dignity. Hospice programs emphasize symptom management, advance care planning, spiritual care, and family support. Hospice care is provided when a person has 6 months or fewer to live and that person or their health care proxy decides to forgo potentially curative treatments. It is important that the person be referred to hospice as early as possible to facilitate palliation of the physical, emotional, and spiritual distresses common at the end of life.

The palliative care team is an interprofessional collaboration involving the patient, nurses, family physicians, social workers, pharmacists, chaplains, and other health care professionals. Communication among the team members is important to provide optimal care.

Associated Clinical Problem

Fear of Death: dread about the end of life and/or the process of dying

Common Causes

- Cancer
- Chronic obstructive pulmonary disease
- Dementia
- End-stage kidney disease
- Heart failure
- Life-limiting illness
- Trauma

Manifestations

Behavioral

- Altered decision making
- Anxiety about unfinished business
- Decreased socialization
- Fear of loneliness
- Fear of meaninglessness of one's life
- Fear of pain
- Helplessness
- Life review
- Peacefulness
- Restlessness
- Saying goodbyes
- Unusual communication
- Visionlike experiences
- Withdrawal

Physiologic

- Blurred vision
- Cheyne–Stokes respirations and tachypnea
- Cold, clammy skin
- Cyanosis of nose, nail beds, and knees
- Decreased perception of pain and touch
- Difficulty maintaining body posture and alignment
- Difficulty speaking
- Gradual decrease in urine output
- Gradual loss of ability to move
- Grunting, gurgling, or noisy and congested breathing
- Hypotension
- Incontinence of urine and stool
- Increased heart rate; later, a slow, weak, and irregular pulse
- Loss of facial muscle tone
- Loss of gag reflex
- Mottling on hands, feet, arms, and legs
- Slowing or cessation of gastrointestinal function
- Swallowing becoming more difficult
- Waxlike skin

Key Conceptual Relationships

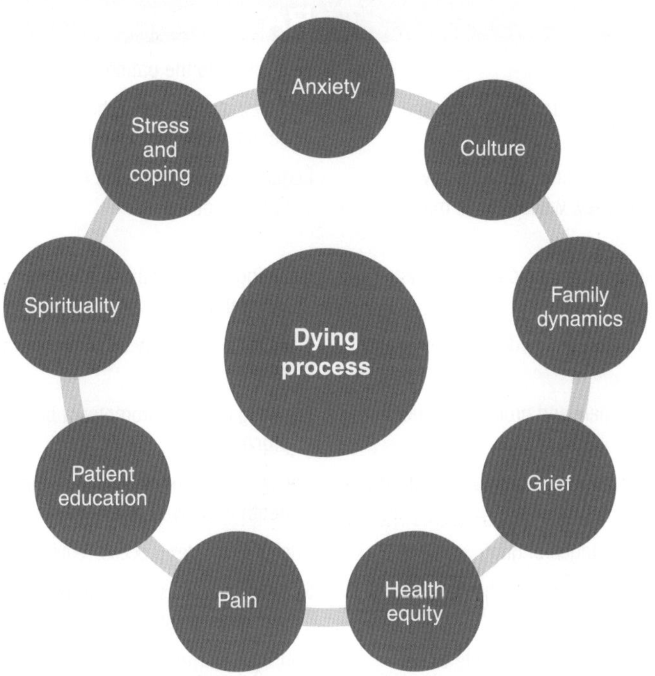

ASSESSMENT OF THE DYING PROCESS	RATIONALE
Knowing where patient and family understanding of prognosis and level of anticipatory grief.	Knowing where the patient and family are in the grief process allows the care team to develop an individualized plan of care.
Encourage the patient and family to share feelings about death and determine their wishes for EOL care.	Assess values and preferences.
Perform a physical assessment and monitor the deterioration of physical and mental capabilities as needed.	Changes in the level of care may be needed as the patient deteriorates.
PAIN: Assess the patient's level of pain and discomfort.	Identify the need for interventions to alleviate pain.
Assess prior experiences with grief and loss.	Past grief experiences often resurface and affect the meaning of the current experience.
CULTURE: Assess cultural expectations related to the dying process.	Beliefs may support specific practices related to dying, death, and loss.
SPIRITUALITY: Assess the role of spirituality in the dying process.	Beliefs may support specific practices related to dying, death, and loss.
ANXIETY: Assess the patient for anxiety and fear of death or dying.	Identify needs for support.
Determine whether decisions exist about organ donation, advance directives, living wills, and extreme measures of care.	Legal documents provide a means for the patient to state their care wishes before they are no longer able to do so.
STRESS AND COPING: Assess for caregiver role strain.	Daily care of the person with a terminal illness can be overwhelming for family caregivers.

Expected Outcomes

The patient will:

- make decisions about EOL care preferences.
- experience a peaceful death.

INTERVENTIONS TO SUPPORT THE DYING PROCESS	RATIONALE
Assist the patient in identifying care priorities.	This respects the patient's values and preferences.
Communicate your willingness to discuss death and dying with the patient and family.	Your being open about the topic demonstrates readiness to discuss details when the patient and family are ready.
Encourage the patient to complete legal documents, such as advance directives and health care power of attorney, while able to make decisions.	Legal documents provide for continuity of care after the patient is unable to make decisions.
CULTURE: Respect the patient's and family's specific care requests.	Including specific care requests promotes patient autonomy and respects cultural beliefs.
Include the family in care decisions and activities, as desired by the patient and family.	The desire for family involvement may vary and could provide emotional comfort.
PAIN: Institute measures to treat pain routinely and proactively, monitoring for breakthrough pain.	Ensuring comfort promotes a better quality of life during the dying process.
Implement measures to assist the patient with managing anticipatory grief, if appropriate.	Anticipatory grief is common among people who are facing the eventual death of a loved one or their own death.
Support the patient and family through the stages of grief.	Grief is a complex process, requiring different interventions during each phase.
SPIRITUALITY: Facilitate obtaining spiritual support for the patient and family.	Spiritual practices and spiritual advisors may provide comfort related to the meaning of life and death.
Offer preferred foods and beverages while the patient is able to eat.	Sharing favorite meals may provide comfort to the patient and family, even if not much is ingested by the patient.
Encourage the patient and family to verbalize their feelings of sadness, loss, and forgiveness and to touch, hug, and cry, if desired.	The patient and family may be experiencing intense feelings that are difficult to express.
Include family members in providing basic comfort care as the patient and family wish.	The family may find caregiving either comforting or overwhelming.
Facilitate discussion of funeral arrangements in advance or after death, as the patient and family prefer.	Discussion of after-death arrangements may be either comforting or upsetting.
STRESS AND COPING: Implement measures to reduce caregiver role strain and provide respite options.	Respite care and other measures can reduce exhaustion and illness for family caregivers.
When the patient appears unresponsive, converse with them and remind the family to speak as though the patient is alert, using a soft voice and gentle touch.	The patient near death may seem withdrawn from the physical environment and may maintain the ability to hear but be unable to respond.
Encourage the family to talk with and reassure the dying person.	Sharing feelings and talking provide comfort for the patient and family.
Provide support to the family as EOL nears:	
• Facilitate the family's efforts to remain at the bedside.	Visiting should be open, within the patient's wishes.
• Explain common physical changes at the EOL to family members and notify them when death is impending.	The physical manifestations associated with dying may be upsetting.
• Provide information and emotional support to the family if the patient experiences restlessness or delirium.	Common manifestations at the EOL may be upsetting to the family.
• Provide for patient and family privacy as desired.	Dying is an intimate process.
Implement comfort measures as EOL nears: • Keep the oral cavity moist. • Keep linens and clothing dry and clean. • Position the patient comfortably, often with the head of the bed elevated. • Clean secretions from the eyes and nose. • Keep lights at a low level. • Apply artificial tears as needed.	These interventions promote the patient's and family's comfort.
After the patient's death:	
• Provide respectful postmortem care.	This respects the dignity of the patient and family.
• Encourage the family to participate in after-death care if desired.	Participating in care may provide comfort for the family.
• Provide resources for follow-up grief and loss care to the family.	Grief is a continuing challenge after a loss.

COLLABORATION	RATIONALE
Hospice care, if desired	Hospice services may be helpful to the patient and family in achieving a peaceful death.
SPIRITUALITY: Pastoral care professionals or their preferred spiritual or religious leader	Many derive spiritual comfort from their religious leaders, who support patients, perform spiritual counseling, and meet sacramental needs.
HEALTH EQUITY: An attorney or financial representative	These persons can draft legal documents, such as wills and advance directives, and offer guidance on financial arrangements.

PATIENT AND CAREGIVER TEACHING

- About the dying process
- Common physical changes at the EOL
- Specific physiologic care needs
- Medications for comfort
- Managing pain proactively
- Grief process
- Caregiver respite
- Legal issues related to death and dying
- Resources for follow-up grief and loss care

DOCUMENTATION

Assessment

- Time of death
- Assessments performed
- Patient and family coping
- Learning needs

Interventions

- Teaching provided
- Medications given
- Notification of the health care provider about patient status
- Direct care provided
- Pain management interventions delivered

Evaluation

- Patient preferences honored
- Pain minimized
- Progress in grief work

Deficient Knowledge 63

Definition

Lacking information on a specific topic

Learning is the process through which a person acquires knowledge, skills, or attitudes. However, learning may not result in any observable change. A patient who understands instructions and is fully informed may choose not to change a behavior.

Nurses teach patients using various methods, such as direct instruction, coaching, counseling, and behavior modification. Teaching may be formal, such as giving a planned presentation to a group of patients and their caregivers, or informal, such as teaching a patient about medications before giving them. Although learning may occur without teaching, a teacher helps to organize information and skills to make learning more efficient. In patient teaching, the teaching–learning process involves the patient, the patient's caregiver(s), and the health professionals.

The types of learning that a patient will need to manage health are reflected in three domains: cognitive, psychomotor, and affective. Learning about the cause of a disease or the actions of a medication is cognitive learning, and methods such as lecture, discussion, and written material are appropriate. *Psychomotor learning* means acquiring physical skills, such as giving an insulin injection. Such learning requires handling equipment and practicing physical skills. *Affective learning* involves changing values to incorporate new beliefs about health and health management and requires making a personal investment in the change. Knowing what to do (cognitive) and how to do it (psychomotor) is not enough for behavior change. The patient must value the behavior (affective) enough to make it part of everyday life.

The teaching process and the nursing process involve the development of a plan that includes assessment, goal setting, implementation, and evaluation. The teaching process, like the nursing process, may not always flow in linear order, but the steps serve as checkpoints. The role of the nurse in patient education is to assess patient needs, motivation, and ability; assist the patient in forming goals; plan educational interventions to achieve goals; and evaluate patient learning outcomes. Formal patient education courses or classes are useful to address needs common to a group of patients. Formal courses are often taught using a plan with standard content. In contrast, informal teaching often occurs in one-on-one sessions with the patient and/or family. An informal approach represents most of the patient education done by nurses. Patient education takes place during patient encounters when a medication, diet, or treatment is explained or questions are answered about the patient's concerns. "Teach-back" is a commonly used strategy to ensure comprehension: after the nurse presents information or demonstrates a skill to the patient, the patient is asked to teach that information back to the nurse. Patients may also complete education activities through self-directed learning using written material or media on health topics, diseases, treatments, or skills.

When a patient is diagnosed with a complex health condition, consider referring the patient to a nurse educator specialist. For example, some organizations have diabetes educators who provide additional support for patients learning about the many aspects of diabetes self-management. Wound and ostomy care nurses may provide specific instructions to patients about care of a new stoma. Nurses in cardiac rehabilitation provide patient education to support healthy lifestyle changes after a cardiac event.

Associated Clinical Problem

- Behavior Change Process: effortful phases starting from having no interest ib or attention for a particular health issue to eventually incorporating a specific health behavior into daily life

Common Topics for Patient Education

- Breastfeeding
- Child development
- Community services
- Contraception
- Diagnostic testing
- Diet plan
- Disease process
- Exercise
- Fall prevention
- Fetal development
- Fluid volume management
- Infant care
- Infant feeding
- Labor and delivery
- Medication regimen
- Oral hygiene
- Pain management
- Parenting

- Patient-controlled analgesia
- Peritoneal dialysis
- Physical therapy
- Pregnancy
- Safety precautions
- Safe sexual behaviors
- Symptom management
- Therapeutic regimen
- Travel health

Common Causes

- Changes in health or perception of health
- Limited recall of information

Manifestations

- Assessed lack of knowledge or misinformation about a new disease, medication, treatment, or care regimen
- Inability to perform skills needed for health management
- Nonadherence
- Poor self-management of health condition
- Verbalized lack of knowledge or need for learning

Key Conceptual Relationships

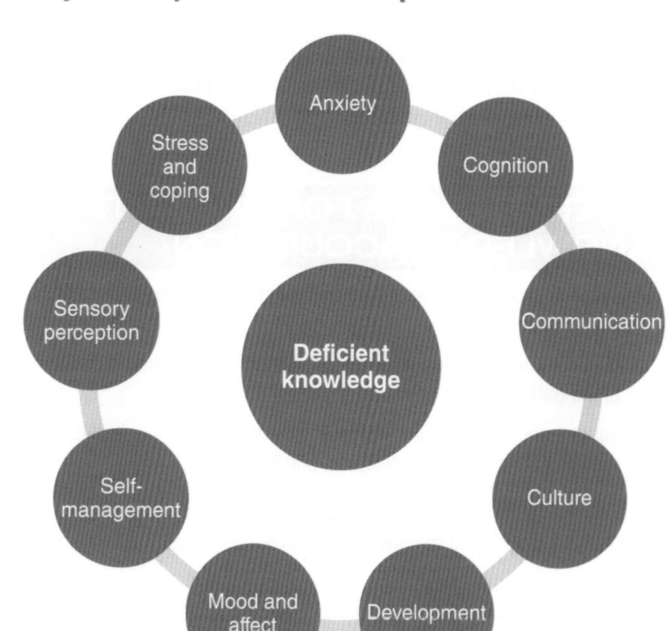

ASSESSMENT OF KNOWLEDGE	RATIONALE
Determine what the patient needs to know to achieve optimal function and self-manage their health.	Patients need specific knowledge to self-manage their own conditions optimally.
Assess the patient's physiologic status.	Pain, hunger, bladder pressure, fatigue, sedation, and other physical issues may prevent concentration on learning.
Assess the patient's readiness to learn.	Time may be needed to address emotional aspects of new health conditions.
Identify the patient's preferred methods of learning.	Patients have different learning styles, so tailoring the delivery method enhances engagement.
Assess current knowledge, beliefs, skills, and previous experiences related to the specific topic.	Building the teaching plan on current knowledge and prior experiences enhances knowledge acquisition.
COGNITION: Assess the patient's ability to comprehend the information.	The ability to understand may vary during illness or by cognitive level.
Assess the patient's education level and determine whether they have specialized education or training.	Specialized knowledge can serve as examples or analogies.
CULTURE: Identify health beliefs and cultural practices that may affect instructional content.	Respecting individual beliefs promotes a therapeutic relationship.
Determine the primary language the patient uses and assess their literacy level.	The health care team can provide communication in the appropriate language and context for the person.
MOOD AND AFFECT: Assess mental status and screen for the presence of any coexisting psychological problems.	Psychological factors have a major influence on the patient's ability to learn.
Pediatric	
DEVELOPMENT: Assess the child's level of physical and emotional development.	Education delivery depends on the child's age, development level, and health status.

Expected Outcomes

The patient will:

- describe the purpose of treatments and medications.
- explain how to take medications and complete therapies.
- demonstrate health-related skills safely.
- identify resources for additional information.

INTERVENTIONS FOR PROMOTING KNOWLEDGE ACQUISITION	RATIONALE
Respect the expertise of the patient and family in managing previous health issues.	Respecting patient and caregiver expertise encourages self-efficacy.
CAREGIVING: Include family/caregivers in teaching with the permission of the patient.	Family/caregivers may need information to assist the patient and can help reinforce information.
Set mutual and SMART goals with the patient: SMART = **s**pecific, **m**easurable, **a**chievable, **r**elevant, and **t**ime-based.	Clear goals promote mutual understanding.
Develop a teaching plan specific to the patient's needs:	
• Adjust teaching to the patient's level of knowledge.	Building the teaching plan on the patient's current knowledge level promotes knowledge acquisition.
• Organize information into small chunks of related topics.	Chunking improves retention.
• Tailor the content to the patient's cognitive, psychomotor, and affective abilities and development level.	Abilities for understanding, enacting, and physical skills may vary with individuals and with development.
• **DEVELOPMENT, COGNITION:** Provide information in a logical sequence, starting with simple information or by addressing the patient's questions.	Build on simple information or information that is of the highest priority to the patient.
• **SELF-MANAGEMENT:** Prioritize information critical to the patient for self-management of their health.	Endless information is available on health topics, but time and attention are limited, so patients need specific knowledge to self-manage their own conditions optimally.
Incorporate techniques of motivational interviewing, including: • Listening rather than telling • Expressing empathy through reflective listening • Not criticizing the patient • Respecting that change is up to the patient • Avoiding argument and direct confrontation • Helping the patient recognize the "gap" between where they are and where they hope to be	Respect the patient as an adult learner and autonomous decision maker.
Seek teachable moments, such as during medication administration, to provide or reinforce information.	Adults prefer immediately applicable information.
Establish optimal conditions for delivering the teaching:	
• Ensure an environment that provides privacy and is quiet enough for clear communication.	A noisy and active health care setting may make it difficult to focus.
• Teach when the patient is rested, not in pain, and not hungry.	Pain, hunger, bladder pressure, fatigue, sedation, and other physical issues may prevent concentration on learning.
• Ensure that basic needs are taken care of before and immediately after teaching sessions.	Taking care of needs prevents distractions during the teaching session.
• **SENSORY PERCEPTION:** Ensure the patient's use of perceptual aids, such as glasses and hearing aids.	Addressing sensory deficits promotes comprehension.
• Tailor the length of the session to the patient.	Ideally, a teaching session should be no longer than 15 to 20 minutes.
Promote effective communication:	
• Use simple language and explain health terminology.	Health terminology can be unfamiliar and confusing.
• Provide the patient with ample opportunity to ask questions.	Allowing time for questions encourages the patient's understanding.
• **COMMUNICATION:** Speak in a clear voice, use simple communication, maintain eye contact at the patient's level, get the patient's attention before speaking, and show respect.	Therapeutic communication techniques support effective teaching.

INTERVENTIONS FOR PROMOTING KNOWLEDGE ACQUISITION	RATIONALE
For patients and caregivers who speak a language different from that of the health care provider, use an approved interpreter or interpreter phone service.	Professional translation allows for the most effective communication when teaching.
Provide information through multiple forms of media, such as discussion, video, printed instructions, and demonstration.	Combining verbal and other methods improves information retention.
Encourage active engagement and participation by the patient and family.	Active participation improves retention.
Reinforce information and provide practice opportunities with feedback.	Repetition improves retention.
Provide the patient with reminders or memory aids.	Memory aids assist in recall over time.
STRESS AND COPING: Provide emotional support when the health condition requires changes.	Providing emotional support promotes rapport and acknowledges challenges.
Consider recommending support groups specific to the condition or situation.	Other persons who share the condition may provide practical ideas for daily management and social support for motivation.
Refer the patient to sources of additional information.	Patients may desire additional information after becoming comfortable with basic information or may use information as a way of coping.
Pediatric	
Provide the child with simple information about their condition and update the level of information as they develop.	The information provided to the child may need to be at a different level than that provided to parents/caregivers.
Incorporate play and active participation in teaching sessions.	Play is an effective way for children to learn and manage new information.

DOCUMENTATION

Assessment

- Readiness for learning
- Factors that may affect learning

Interventions

- Educational topics delivered
- Methods used
- Referrals initiated
- Materials given

Evaluation

- Progress in learning
- Demonstration of skills
- Ability to manage self-care
- Patient's response to the teaching

HEALTH CARE ENVIRONMENT

Health Literacy Problem 64

Definition

Limited ability to obtain and understand basic health information needed to make appropriate health decisions

Literacy is the ability to use printed and written information to function in society. *Health literacy* is the degree to which a person can obtain and understand basic health information needed to make appropriate health decisions. Almost 90% of U.S. adults have limited health literacy skills. Improving health literacy can advance community health. Persons with low levels of health literacy have trouble understanding and acting on health information, placing them at greater risk for hospital readmissions. Even those with high levels of health literacy may have a hard time understanding complex health information while they are sick or stressed.

Health illiteracy results in poor patient outcomes, not following treatment plans, limited self-management skills, and increased health disparities. It is challenging to assess health literacy because patients may be embarrassed to admit that they are having trouble understanding health information. Health professionals often overestimate the health literacy of patients. It is important for nurses to routinely assess a patient's health literacy level and provide information that the patient can understand.

Common Causes and Risk Factors

- Different spoken/written language than that of health staff
- Impaired cognition
- Impaired development
- Low education level
- Low reading level
- Low socioeconomic status
- Nodding or agreeing while unable to restate information
- Older adults
- Poor communication skills
- Sensory deficits
- Unfamiliarity with health-specific terminology

Manifestations

- Assessed lack of knowledge or misinformation
- Inability to navigate the health care system
- Inability to perform skills needed for health management
- Nodding or agreeing while unable to restate information
- Poor management of health condition

Key Conceptual Relationships

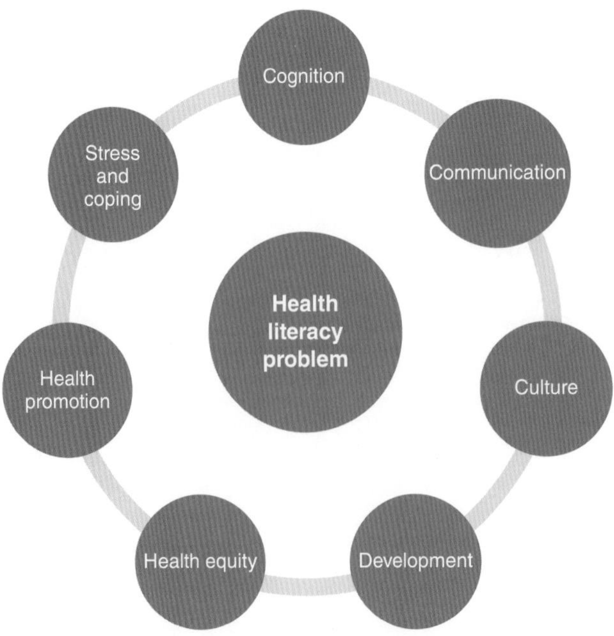

ASSESSMENT OF HEALTH LITERACY	RATIONALE
Determine the primary language the patient uses.	The health care team can provide communication in the appropriate language and context for the person.
Ask, "How often do you need to have someone help you when you read instructions, pamphlets, or other written material from your doctor or pharmacy?" Or use other standardized screening tools for health literacy, such as the Rapid Estimate of Adult Literacy in Medicine–Short Form (Table 64.1).	The Single-Item Literacy Screener (SILS) uses one question to identify adults who need help with reading, so it is quick to use in a clinical setting.
Observe for cues that may signal the presence of a literacy problem, such as: • Not completing forms • Deferring to others for information • Avoiding reading or writing in front of providers • Mispronouncing complex, multiple-syllable words • Written materials containing multiple spelling errors • Limited vocabulary	People with a literacy problem may not recognize or readily admit their reading difficulty.
Identify the patient's preferred method of learning.	Patients have different learning preferences, so tailoring the delivery method enhances engagement.
Assess the patient's education level.	Education level influences health literacy.
DEVELOPMENT: Assess the patient's development level.	Education needs to be tailored to the patient's development level.
Assess the patient's ability to restate health information that has been provided.	Assessing the patient's ability to restate information helps determine comprehension.
COGNITION: Assess the patient's ability to comprehend the information.	The ability to understand may vary during illness or by cognitive level.

Table 64.1 Rapid Estimate of Adult Literacy in Medicine–Short Form (REALM-SF)

How to Administer the REALM-SF

State: "Providers often use words patients do not understand. We are going to look at words providers often use with their patients to improve communication. Here is a list of medical words. Starting at the top of the list, please read each word aloud to me. If you do not recognize a word, you can say "pass" and move on to the next word." Then give the person the word list. If they take more than 5 seconds on a word, say "pass" and point to the next word. Hold the score sheet so that the patient cannot see it.

Behavior
Exercise
Menopause
Rectal
Antibiotics
Anemia
Jaundice
Total Score: ______

Scores and Grade Equivalents for the REALM-SF

Score	Grade Range
0	3rd grade and below; will not be able to read most low-literacy materials; will need repeated oral instructions and materials composed mainly of illustrations or audio- or videotapes
1–3	4th to 6th grade; will need low-literacy materials; may not be able to read prescription labels
4–6	7th to 8th grade; will struggle with most patient education materials; will not be offended by low-literacy materials
7	High school; will be able to read most patient education materials

Courtesy Terry B. Davis.

Expected Outcomes

The patient will:

- describe the purpose of treatments and medications.
- explain how to take medications and complete therapies.
- demonstrate health-related skills safely.
- identify resources for additional information.
- request translation services as needed.

INTERVENTIONS TO SUPPORT HEALTH LITERACY	RATIONALE
Create an environment in which the patient with a literacy problem can seek help or share their difficulties without feeling embarrassed.	This promotes trust and shows respect for the patient.
Offer verbal and written information in the patient's preferred language.	Comprehension is enhanced by using the language spoken by the patient.
COMMUNICATION: For patients and caregivers who speak a language other than that of the health care provider, use an approved interpreter or interpreter phone service.	Professional translation allows for the most effective communication when teaching.
If using interpretation services, plan ahead for prioritizing information and make eye contact with the patient while speaking.	Keep the focus on patient needs.
Include family/caregivers in teaching, with the permission of the patient.	Family/caregivers may need information to assist the patient and can help reinforce information.
Implement health literacy universal precautions using simple communications about health information.	When literacy screening is not feasible, assume that all patients may have difficulty understanding important health information and accessing health services.
Provide information in a logical sequence, in the order that the patient would follow, or start with addressing the patient's questions.	Build on simple information or information that is of the highest priority to the patient.
Plan frequent repetition and follow-up sessions.	Repetition reinforces learning.
Use teach-back to have the patient explain information and demonstrate skills.	Teach-back evaluates the effectiveness of teaching and learning.
Use various multimedia methods and technology to present and reinforce information as appropriate.	Visual methods may not require spoken language.
Give the patient a short, clear summary of written content, providing the main information.	Prioritize the most important information in a concise form for easier retention.
Help the patient and caregivers locate appropriate postdischarge groups and resources.	Cultural groups may provide social support and resources.
CULTURE: When available, use educational interventions that are culturally tailored to the health literacy needs of the patient.	Evidence supports some health education interventions specific to cultural groups.
HEALTH PROMOTION: Incorporate health promotion education that reflects the unique cultural interests and values of diverse groups.	Evidence suggests some health education interventions are more effective with certain cultural groups.

PATIENT AND CAREGIVER TEACHING

- Requesting and accessing interpretation services
- Community resources
- Sources of additional information

DOCUMENTATION

Assessment

- General literacy
- Health literacy

Interventions

- Adaptation of teaching
- Referrals initiated

Evaluation

- Progress in understanding health information
- Ability to manage self-care

Inadequate Community Resources 65

Definition

Deficiency in environment support for health

Population health focuses on improving the health status and health outcomes across a group of people, with the intention of improving health equity. A focus on the health of a specific geographic population is termed *community health*. The social environment and the physical environment affect health outcomes for individuals and populations.

Differences in local resources can have profound effects on the health and quality of life of community members. Many health disparities are associated with inadequate community resources, such as a lack of clean water or access to healthy foods. Government agencies, public health organizations, health care providers, and others can advocate to allocate resources in ways that promote health. Nurses can evaluate and influence factors, such as adequate food, safe housing, and accessible health facilities, that support the basic needs of the community.

Associated Clinical Problems

- Insufficient Health Services: limited access to primary, secondary, and tertiary health care
- High Crime Rate: frequent illegal activity and/or violence
- Insufficient Food Supply: inadequate options for purchasing healthy or fresh food
- Insufficient Water Supply: limited access to clean water
- Sanitation Problem: accumulation of garbage and/or sewage

Common Causes and Risk Factors

- Aging infrastructure
- Lack of affordable housing
- Lack of awareness
- Lack of community funding
- Lack of transportation
- Political decisions
- Poverty

High Crime Rate

- Easy access to guns and other weapons
- High unemployment rates
- Criminal activity and drugs in the environment

Manifestations

- Environment hazard reports
- Geographic or population-specific higher rates of illness
- Higher-than-expected crime rates
- Higher-than-expected mortality rates
- Lack of adequate sanitation
- Poor water quality
- Socioeconomic indicators, such as rates of reduced-cost/free school lunches provided
- Unusual illnesses

Key Conceptual Relationships

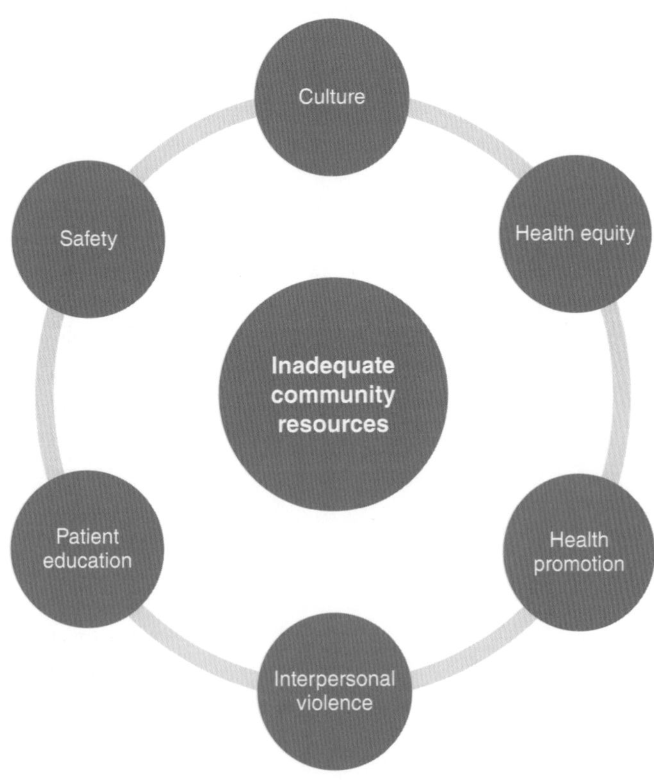

ASSESSMENT OF COMMUNITY RESOURCES	RATIONALE
Collaborate with community leaders to conduct a needs assessment that incorporates the perspectives of community members.	Involvement shows respect for the perspectives of community members.
Assess motivation and readiness for change in early discussions with the community.	Determining community members' initial engagement helps in planning next steps.
CULTURE: Identify the cultural health beliefs and practices of community members.	Incorporate and respect the cultural beliefs of community members to determine meaningful interventions.
Identify health concerns, strengths, and priorities with community partners.	Community partners are often gatekeepers who have knowledge of needs and priorities.
Define the objectives of advocacy and coalition building in the specific community to be assisted.	Collaboratively identify goals based on assessed needs.
Monitor indicators of inadequate community resources through ongoing data collection, analysis, and interpretation.	Data analysis is necessary for the purpose of planning, implementing, and evaluating public health interventions.
Assess food choices and the ability to access food, including: • Stores present in the area and ability of persons to access them • Types of foods in stores • Availability of locally sourced foods • Presence of food distribution resources for low-income persons, such as food banks and food pantries • Cost of food compared with other areas • Availability of specific food services, such as church meals and Meals on Wheels • Special Supplemental Nutrition Program for Women, Infants, and Children (WIC)	Food choices, resources, and access affect decisions related to food purchases and consumption.
Assess the ability to access water, including: • Sources of water for drinking, cooking, and hygienic care • Availability of water when needed • Presence of any contaminants in the water • Amount of water used per capita per day • Ability of persons to pay for water • Age of the infrastructure	Safe water is a fundamental human need.
Assess the availability of sanitation services, including: • Type of sewage and garbage disposal • Percent of households without indoor plumbing or with substandard plumbing • Ability of persons to pay for sanitation services • Age of the infrastructure	Adequate sanitation is necessary to reduce the spread of disease.
Assess resources for safe physical activity and exercise, such as sidewalks and parks.	Safe exercise options help support increasing physical activity.
Assess for available transportation, affordable housing, schools, and health care.	Infrastructure supports access to resources and enhances quality of life.
INTERPERSONAL VIOLENCE: Evaluate the rate of crime in the area, including: • Types of crimes committed • Number of crimes committed per capita • Number of persons who feel they have been victimized • When and where crimes occur	Gauging the extent of the crime problem means discovering how much crime there is, where and when it occurs most often, and who is most likely to be victimized.

Expected Outcomes

The community will:

- have access to adequate clean water and food supplies.
- avoid exposure to toxins.
- have access to a physically safe environment.

INTERVENTIONS FOR ACQUIRING COMMUNITY RESOURCES	RATIONALE
HEALTH EQUITY: Assist community members to navigate the health care system, including access to low-cost or free care; to solve billing issues; and to understand patient rights.	Community residents may need advocates to understand health care services and accessibility.
Initiate discussions in the community, directly or through social media, about the lack of community resources, such as food insecurity and lack of clean water, and their effects.	Discussing community resources enhances awareness of problems.
SAFETY: Determine whether groups of persons share the risk of any water- or sanitation-related environment injury and notify appropriate authorities of any concerns.	Groups of persons exposed to the same contaminants share similar health risks.
HEALTH PROMOTION: Provide community outreach programs to populations at risk.	Outreach programs provide information about the nature of community concerns and assist with resolving concerns.
Obtain consultation and support for community advocacy efforts to build coalitions and enhance conditions.	Seeking resources is often necessary to support building a coalition.
PATIENT EDUCATION: Participate in community information campaigns.	Informational campaigns increase awareness of community concerns.
Help mobilize community resources that will assist in achieving goals.	Resources may be available and unused.
Provide health care information and education to the public and legislators.	Education increases awareness of the health implications of policies and funding decisions.
Attend and speak at public forums about the positive effect of proposed health care services, projects, and legislation.	Be an advocate for legislation that supports community health.
Encourage participation by all segments of the community in a unified effort.	Inclusive activities strengthen the social network of the community.
Find legislative sponsors to propose health-related legislation.	Be an advocate for legislation that supports community health.
Strengthen contacts among individuals and groups to discuss common and competing interests.	Facilitating connections promotes collaborative work on health issues.
Develop strategies for managing conflict.	Facilitating positive interactions may strengthen the community network.
Evaluate the effectiveness of coalition building and community initiatives.	Identify the strengths of the process that may support future projects related to health.
Speak and write about successes in improving community health.	Successes support motivation and provide recommendations for future efforts.

DOCUMENTATION

Assessment
- Status of community resources
- Community needs and concerns

Interventions
- Advocacy
- Member involvement
- Facilitation
- Coalition building
- Policies and legislation

Evaluation
- Progress toward community goals

Health Care–Associated Complication 66

Definition

A detrimental patient condition that occurs during the process of receiving health care

Patient safety is a critical component of quality care. Unfortunately, there is always some risk associated with receiving health care. Health care–associated complications include a wide variety of problems. Human errors cause or contribute to some complications. Errors include incidents such as a wrong-site surgery or transfer injury from the improper use of a lift. The perioperative patient may sustain a burn or chemical injury during surgery. We consider these types of complications preventable. Other complications are not preventable, even with optimal care. Examples include delayed surgical recovery in a critically ill patient with multiple comorbidities or the unexpected occurrence of an adverse drug effect.

Reducing the risk of harm from complications requires the attention of all team members involved in the patient's care. Although it is not possible to eliminate all risk, nurses' astute assessment and monitoring are part of preventing many complications. Health care environments are complex, and a number of factors contribute to the potential for problems. There must be open communication about the patient's plan of care and discussion about potential areas of risk. The nurse can assess for factors that influence the occurrence of health care–associated complications and be a part of implementing prevention plans.

Associated Clinical Problems

- Adverse Drug Interaction: undesired, unintentional effect of a medication that occurs with usual use
- Delayed Surgical Recovery: slowed or delayed recovery from a surgical procedure
- Medication Side Effect: experiencing a secondary effect of drug therapy
- Risk for Perioperative Injury: risk for injury during surgery or a procedure
- Risk for Urinary Tract Injury: risk for urinary tract injury from urinary catheterization
- Transfer Injury: injury incurred when the patient is transferred or repositioned

Common Causes and Risk Factors

- Age
- History of a health care–associated complication
- Impaired cognition
- Obesity
- Severely compromised health status

Delayed Surgical Recovery

- Infection
- Prolonged, complex surgery
- Surgical complications

Medication Risk

- Kidney disease
- Liver disease
- Malnutrition
- Medication: antibiotics, anticoagulants, chemotherapy, diuretics, hypoglycemics, nonsteroidal antiinflammatory drugs (NSAIDs)
- Polypharmacy

Transfer Injury

- Improper use of equipment
- Lack of assistance and proper equipment

Risk for Urinary Tract Injury

- Improper catheter handling
- Long-term catheter use
- Multiple catheterizations
- Urethral size
- Urinary tract abnormalities
- Urinary tract catheterization
- Urinary tract trauma

Manifestations

- Anxiety and distress
- Need for more interventions
- Prolonged recovery

Delayed Surgical Recovery
- Impaired mobility
- Perception of more time needed to recover
- Unexpected pain

Medication Risk
- Acute kidney injury
- Delirium
- Falls
- Gastrointestinal bleeding
- Intracranial hemorrhage
- Kidney problems
- Liver problems
- Orthostatic hypotension

Risk for Perioperative Injury
- Burns
- Eye injury
- Fall from operating room table
- Infection acquired in operating suite
- Inhalation injuries
- Pressure injury
- Retained foreign objects
- Wrong-site or wrong-procedure surgery

Transfer Injury
- Falls
- Fractures
- Head injury

Risk for Urinary Tract Injury
- Fistula
- Hematuria
- Skin erosion
- Stone formation
- Urethral strictures, trauma

Key Conceptual Relationships

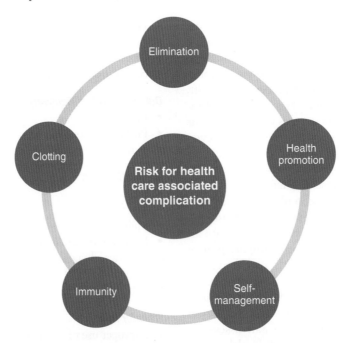

ASSESSMENT FOR A HEALTH CARE–ASSOCIATED COMPLICATION	RATIONALE
Identify patients in need of emergency management so that they can be stabilized.	Identifying an emergency allows for early intervention, improving patient outcomes.
Perform a risk assessment, focusing on factors that place the patient at risk for a health care–associated complication.	Patients at risk for complications need a prevention plan in addition to their therapeutic plan of care.
Evaluate the patient's underlying health status.	Health status has a significant influence on the development of complications.
Perform a physical assessment and obtain diagnostic tests based on the patient's risk assessment and health status.	The physical assessment and diagnostic tests are used to evaluate the risk or presence of a health care–associated complication so that appropriate treatment can be initiated.

ASSESSMENT FOR A HEALTH CARE-ASSOCIATED COMPLICATION	RATIONALE
Determine whether new assessment findings are possible medication effects or signs of another complication.	The potential for medication effects should be part of every differential diagnosis, especially in older adult patients and those who develop new symptoms after starting or adjusting the dose of a medication.
IMMUNITY: Obtain an allergy history.	A thorough history helps identify allergies and guides preventative actions.
Obtain a complete, accurate medication record.	An accurate medication record can identify high-risk drugs, discrepancies in medication use, potentially interactive drugs, and the use of relevant nonprescribed drugs and herb therapies, which contribute to medication risk.
Perform a safety assessment at the beginning of each procedure.	Identified risks can be addressed with a prevention plan prior to the start of the procedure.
Perform an assessment before attempting to reposition or transfer a patient, including: • Ability to assist and cooperate with instructions • Special precautions needed • Height and weight • Need for support or padding • Special medical considerations • Assistance needed (people, equipment) • Environment	Assessing the situation prior to performing patient transfer allows the nurse to plan the safest way to perform the procedure.
ELIMINATION: Assess for the continued need for urinary catheterization.	Using a catheter for the shortest time possible reduces the risk of complications.
SELF-MANAGEMENT: Assess the patient's ability to self-manage their health care regimen, including managing medications.	The risk for complications, especially medication related, is higher if the patient has difficulty managing their self-care regimen.
Evaluate the effectiveness of measures used to prevent a health care–associated complication through ongoing assessment.	Evaluating the effectiveness of measures to prevent health care–associated complications allows for evaluation of therapy effectiveness.
Women's Health Determine whether a woman is pregnant or breastfeeding.	The teratogenic effects of certain medications present a profound risk to the fetus or infant.

Expected Outcomes

The patient will:

- be free from health care–associated complications.
- describe measures to avoid health care–associated complications.

INTERVENTIONS TO ADDRESS A HEALTH CARE-ASSOCIATED COMPLICATION	RATIONALE
Implement collaborative interventions if the patient is experiencing an acute health care–associated complication.	The goal of immediate management is to prevent life-threatening complications that may occur because of the complication.
Implement collaborative interventions aimed at treating factors contributing to the risk for a health care–associated complication.	The risk of a complication may be reduced with a prevention plan addressing a contributing factors.
Notify the health care provider (HCP) if manifestations of a health care–associated complication persist or worsen.	Achieving an effective treatment plan often requires adjustments in therapy.
Provide ongoing information and reassurance to the patient who experiences a health care–associated complication.	Providing the patient with information about the complication enhances communication and patient understanding.

Continued

INTERVENTIONS TO ADDRESS A HEALTH CARE–ASSOCIATED COMPLICATION	RATIONALE
IMMUNITY: Institute measures to reduce exposure to allergens.	Measures to limit exposure to known allergens reduce the risk of complications.
SELF-MANAGEMENT: Implement measures to enhance the patient's ability to self-manage their health care regimen, especially medication therapy.	The risk for health care-related complications is higher if the patient has difficulty managing their health care regimen, including medication therapy.

INTERVENTIONS TO PROMOTE SURGICAL RECOVERY	RATIONALE
Implement measures to address postoperative symptoms, including pain and nausea.	Controlling symptoms such as pain and nausea can reduce postoperative recovery time.
Implement measures to enhance recovery after surgery, including: • Optimize nutrition. • Maintain fluid balance. • Maintain normothermia. • Promote early mobilization. • **CLOTTING:** Provide venous thromboembolism prophylaxis. • Manage pain. • Maintain normoglycemia. • Encourage pulmonary toilet.	Pathways for enhanced recovery after surgery support optimal patient outcomes and a reduced risk of complications.

INTERVENTIONS TO REDUCE MEDICATION RISK	RATIONALE
Discuss with the HCP if the patient is receiving known interacting medications or if you suspect an adverse effect.	HCP may consider making dose changes or changing or discontinuing the offending medication.
Notify the pharmacy and ensure the adverse effect is documented in the medication system.	Collaboration with pharmacists can minimize medication risk by increasing communication about the patient's treatment.
If the patient is experiencing undesirable side effects, encourage them to report those effects to the health care team.	Reporting undesirable side effects allows for the medications to be adjusted or measures instituted to address the side effects.

INTERVENTIONS TO REDUCE RISK FOR PERIOPERATIVE INJURY	RATIONALE
Perform the universal protocol at the beginning of each procedure: • Complete the preprocedural verification process. • Identify the operative site, involving the patient whenever possible. • Perform a "time-out," with briefing.	The risk of injury is reduced by involving the entire surgical team in the universal protocol and encouraging every team member to point out possible risks.
Follow routine perioperative checklists appropriate to the patient's surgery.	Checklist use can improve patient safety and the management of operating room incidents that occur.
Provide protective shielding.	Protective shielding reduces the risk of injury from nonionizing radiation.
TISSUE INTEGRITY: Pad areas at risk for pressure injury, such as heels and bony prominences.	Extended positioning on bony prominences and special positioning during surgical procedures increase risk for pressure injury.
Implement universal precautions and perform decontamination procedures between patients.	Precautions decrease the transmission of infection.
Assist with ensuring proper grounding and use of electrical equipment.	These measures reduce the risk of injury and harm from electrosurgical devices.
Follow agency counting procedures, and document surgical counts and actions taken if count discrepancies occur.	Measures must be taken to avoid unintended retention of a foreign object because it is a preventable, sentinel event.

INTERVENTIONS TO REDUCE TRANSFER INJURY	RATIONALE
Use the proper assistive devices and lifting techniques to lift, move, transfer, and reposition the patient.	The use of proper assistive devices reduces the risk of injury associated with patient handling.
Make environment adjustments prior to transfers, such as removing obstacles (furniture, intravenous line equipment, catheters) and adjusting seating/bed surface heights.	Environment adjustments can make the transfer easier and safer for the patient and the nurse.

INTERVENTIONS TO REDUCE RISK FOR URINARY TRACT INJURY	RATIONALE
Use the appropriate technique to insert the catheter.	Proper technique during catheter insertion minimizes the risk of trauma.
ELIMINATION: Institute measures to properly maintain the catheter: • Keep the catheter properly anchored. • Empty the bag before it is full. • Keep the bag below the level of the bladder. • Keep the tubing from kinking or becoming obstructed. • Remove an indwelling catheter as soon as possible.	Proper catheter protocol is essential to reduce the risk of trauma-related complications.
Ensure proper hygienic care: • Turn patient every 2 hours to cleanse area and change linens. • Use quilted pad under patient. • Use skin barrier creams. • Perform perianal care using only soap and water.	Proper hygienic care reduces the risk of injury and infection.

PATIENT AND CAREGIVER TEACHING

- Cause of the health care–associated complication
- Factors that may be contributing to a health care–associated complication
- Diagnostic and laboratory tests used to detect a health care–associated complication
- Management of a condition associated with the health care–associated complication
- Potential health care–associated complications
- Measures being taken to prevent health care–associated complications
- When to notify the HCP

DOCUMENTATION

Assessment

- Assessments performed
- Diagnostic and laboratory test results
- Manifestations of health care–associated complication
- Safety screening test results

Interventions

- Discussions with other members of the interprofessional team
- Environment modifications made
- Medications given
- Notification of the HCP about patient status
- Therapeutic interventions and the patient's response
- Teaching provided
- Referrals initiated
- Safety measures and checklists implemented

Evaluation

- Patient's status: occurrence of a health care–associated complication
- Manifestations of a health care–associated complication
- Response to teaching provided
- Response to therapeutic interventions

Risk of Environment Injury 67

Definition

Risk for adverse health associated with exposure to environment contaminants

There are many ways the environment contributes to a person's risk for injury. Exposure to pesticides, chemicals, waste, radiation, and pollution at work, in the home, and in the community can cause adverse health effects. The exact nature of the injury depends on the causative agent. Exposure to sources of ionizing radiation is one cause of injury. Radon gas, air travel, and living at a higher altitude are natural exposures. The most common human-made source of radiation is medical devices, including x-ray machines. Lead from contaminated dust and paint or corroded lead water pipes are common causes of lead poisoning.

Nurses have an important role in identifying those at risk for an environment-related injury. The nurse's astute observations can lead to the accurate assessment of and prompt intervention in problems related to environment injuries. Patient education is a key responsibility and involves informing patients and caregivers about hazards in the environment and how to protect themselves.

Associated Clinical Problems

- Contamination Exposure: exposure to environment contaminants at a level that can cause adverse health effects
- Risk of Poisoning: increased risk of injury from swallowing, inhaling, or having contact with a toxic substance
- Risk of Radiation Exposure: increased risk of exposure to potentially hazardous levels of ionizing radiation
- Risk of Radiation Injury: increased risk for adverse health effects caused by exposure to ionizing radiation

Common Risk Factors

- Age
- Bioterrorism and warfare
- Exposure to pesticides, radiation, pollution, chemicals (e.g., lead-based paint)
- Improperly stored chemicals and medications
- Indoor smoke
- Lack of or inappropriate use of personal protective equipment (PPE)
- Living conditions, contaminated water, and poor sanitation
- Natural disasters, such as earthquakes, hurricanes, tornadoes, and flooding
- Self-report of exposure

Radiation Exposure/Radiation Injury

- Living at a high altitude
- Multiple radiographs
- Radiologic medical tests and procedures
- Radon in the home or workplace

Manifestations

- Changes in cognition
- Clusters of family or community members with similar illness
- Specific symptoms associated with the causative agent
  - Flulike symptoms
  - Gastrointestinal: nausea, anorexia, vomiting
  - Muscle weakness
  - Self-reports of fatigue and tiredness
- Laboratory testing: abnormal complete blood count (CBC), chemistry, toxicology, urine studies

Pediatric

- Congenital defects
- Impaired growth and development
- School problems

Radiation Exposure/Radiation Injury

- Acute radiation syndrome
- Cancer
- Hair loss
- Radiation burns
- Skin redness

Key Conceptual Relationships

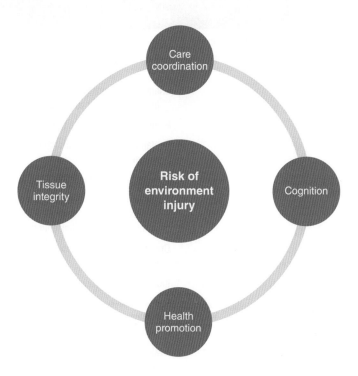

ASSESSMENT OF ENVIRONMENT SAFETY	RATIONALE
Identify patients in need of emergency management for an environment injury or toxicity so that they can be stabilized.	Identifying an injury allows for the initiation of emergency management procedures.
Assess personal and environment factors that place the patient at risk for an environment injury.	Identifying factors that place the patient at risk for an environment injury allows for early intervention.
Obtain an environment history: • Current and past longest-held jobs • Where they spend their days and what they do there • Recent exposure to chemicals or radiation • Relationship noted between symptoms and their activities • Living environment	Through the environment history, a nurse may uncover exposures to hazardous substances that the patient did not suspect as a cause of illness.
Obtain a thorough exposure history: • Agent • Amount of exposure • Source of contact • When exposure occurred • Length of time of exposure • Route of exposure	Identifying the causative agent is important in understanding how a person became exposed and the subsequent potential health effects.
Obtain a thorough history of manifestations of a potential environment injury, including: • Onset, sudden or gradual • Symptoms experienced • Duration of symptoms • Severity of reaction • Frequency of occurrence • Reproducibility of symptoms with repeated exposure	A thorough history aids in evaluating the patient's injury and helps direct the assessment and treatment.

Continued

ASSESSMENT OF ENVIRONMENT SAFETY	RATIONALE
Perform a physical assessment and obtain diagnostic tests based on the patient's history, monitoring for indicators of an environment injury on an ongoing basis:	
• Vital signs	Changes in vital signs, particularly heart and respiratory rates, reflect impaired cardiac and respiratory function.
• Neuromuscular manifestations	Many contaminants are associated with neuromuscular manifestations.
• **TISSUE INTEGRITY:** Skin	Contaminants that are absorbed through the skin often produce immediate manifestations.
• Blood and urine toxicology screens	Toxicology and urine studies can show the presence of contaminants.
• Lead levels, as needed	Those who should be tested include children at risk at 1 and 2 years old or 3 and 6 years old, those with signs of lead toxicity, and recent immigrants from other countries.
Determine whether others share the risk of the same environment injury and notify appropriate authorities of concerns.	Groups of persons exposed to the same contaminant share similar health risks.
HEALTH PROMOTION: Screen for smoking and smoke in the patient's environment.	Indoor smoke is a significant contributor to respiratory injuries.
Assess for a history of radiation exposure.	Radiation exposure must be considered to weigh cumulative risk versus benefit accurately.
Evaluate the effectiveness of measures used to promote environment safety through ongoing assessment.	Evaluating the effectiveness of measures to promote environment safety allows for changes in plans.
Women's Health Determine pregnancy status before medically related radiation exposure.	The effects of radiation are more profound in early pregnancy and less significant as pregnancy progresses.

Expected Outcomes

The patient will:

- be free from an environment-related injury.
- implement strategies to reduce the risk for environment injury.
- identify how an environment injury occurred.

INTERVENTIONS TO PROMOTE ENVIRONMENT SAFETY	RATIONALE
Perform decontamination procedures if needed.	Decontamination physically removes toxic substances.
Institute resuscitation protocols according to the type of exposure if the patient has an acute environment-related injury.	The goal of emergency management is to prevent life-threatening complications that occur from contamination.
Administer prescribed medication that acts as an antidote.	Antidotes can counteract or neutralize the effects of contaminants.
Implement collaborative interventions aimed at treating the manifestations of an environment injury.	Care is needed to address the manifestations and prevent further complications.
Implement needed isolation precautions.	Isolation may be needed to protect the patient and others from contaminants.
Strategize with the patient to reduce or eliminate exposure to potential contaminants.	Aim to reduce the exposure to potential contaminants.
Provide a safe environment for the patient with neurologic or neuromuscular manifestations by initiating fall and seizure precautions.	Changes in cognition and the potential for seizures may accompany an environment injury.

INTERVENTIONS TO PROMOTE ENVIRONMENT SAFETY	RATIONALE
Develop a monitoring plan with the patient if long-term evaluation and treatment are needed.	Follow-up care may be needed to identify complications and initiate treatment.
CARE COORDINATION: Assist the patient in obtaining and using needed PPE and making environment adaptations.	PPE use and environment modifications reduce the risk of injury.
COGNITION: Implement measures to address impaired cognition.	Changes in cognition and the potential for seizures may accompany an environment injury.
HEALTH PROMOTION: Discuss with the patient and persons living in the home ways to decrease the risk of exposure to secondhand smoke.	Smoking is a key indoor air pollutant that contributes to respiratory injuries.
Pediatric Advise parents to limit children's play in certain situations: • Do not allow play in basements with radon. • Limit outdoor time when air pollution levels are high.	These limits reduce the child's exposure to air pollution, decreasing the risk of injury.

COLLABORATION	RATIONALE
Poison control center	Poison control centers provide advice on managing exposure, collect information to assess poison exposure, and exchange patient information, treatment recommendations, and clinical information with the health care provider (HCP).
Social services	The health department or a professional contractor may need to be involved with removing lead-based paint or other contaminants from the environment.

PATIENT AND CAREGIVER TEACHING

- Common environment safety risks
- Factors that place the patient at risk for environment injury
- What to do if an exposure occurs
- Where to find more information
- Manifestations of an environment injury
- Diagnostic and laboratory tests used to detect an environment injury
- Management of an environment injury
- Measures to decrease environment safety risks
- Modifications in the environment to promote safety
- When to notify the HCP

DOCUMENTATION

Assessment

- Assessments performed
- Diagnostic and laboratory test results
- Manifestations of an environment injury
- Safety screening test results

Interventions

- Discussions with other interprofessional team members
- Environment modifications made
- Medications given
- Notification of HCP about patient status
- Notification of the proper authorities
- Therapeutic interventions and the patient's response
- Teaching provided
- Referrals initiated
- Safety measures implemented

Evaluation

- Patient's status: occurrence of environment injury
- Manifestations of an environment injury
- Response to teaching provided
- Response to therapeutic interventions

Risk for Injury 68

Definition

State in which a person is at an increased risk for harm

Fall and injury prevention pose a considerable challenge across the care continuum. The interaction of multiple factors causes most injuries. Reducing the risk of harm from falls and other injuries requires the attention of all health care team members. Assessing fall risk and implementing prevention strategies are key in preventing many incidents. Some aspects of fall prevention plans are routine. Others are tailored to the patient's specific risk profile. Providing patient education about measures to reduce the risk for injury can have a significant impact.

Injury prevention in the community involves teaching patients to take safety precautions to prevent injuries while at home or work, driving, or taking part in sports. The risk of injury can be reduced if we teach people about environment hazards, the proper use of safety equipment, and the importance of following safety and traffic rules. In the occupation setting, teach employees and employers how to avoid hazardous working situations and encourage the use of safety equipment.

Associated Clinical Problems

- Risk for Falls: increased risk for falling
- Risk of Occupational Injury: increased risk for experiencing an injury at work
- Risk for Trauma: increased risk for accidental injury
- Wandering: aimless movement

Common Risk Factors

- Age
- Balance problems
- Cancer
- Diabetes
- Environment hazards
- Fatigue
- History of falls and accidents
- Impaired cognition
- Impaired mobility
- Improper use of assistive devices
- Incontinence
- Lack of or improper use of personal protection equipment (PPE)
- Lack of supervision
- Medications: anticoagulants, antihypertensives, hypoglycemics, psychotropics, sedative-hypnotics
- Not following safety precautions
- Peripheral neuropathy
- Postural hypotension
- Sedation
- Stroke
- Substance use
- Vision problems

Risk of Occupational Injury

- Exposure to chemicals, fumes, and vibration
- High noise levels
- Operating heavy machinery
- Overexertion
- Physically demanding work
- Type of work, such as low-wage or temporary

Manifestations

- Falls
- Injuries, including fractures and visible wounds

Risk of Occupational Injury

- Hearing loss

Wandering

- Elopement
- Frequent activity
- Hyperactivity
- Pacing
- Scanning and searching

Key Conceptual Relationships

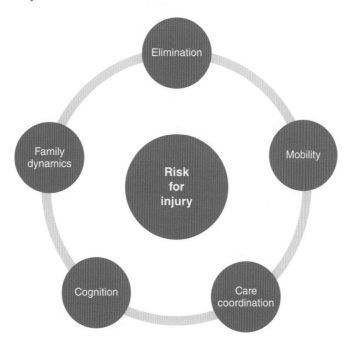

ASSESSMENT OF RISK FOR INJURY	RATIONALE
Assess factors that place the patient at risk for injury.	Identifying specific factors that place the patient at risk for injury allows for the development of a customized safety plan.
Evaluate the patient's underlying health status.	Health status has a significant influence on the risk for injury.
Use a valid, reliable tool, appropriate for the patient's age and cognition, to perform a fall risk assessment, such as the Morse Fall Scale (Table 68.1).	The consistent use of fall risk rating scales identifies the level of risk and helps determine the prevention plan.
Perform a physical assessment and obtain diagnostic tests based on the history, including:	Physical assessment and diagnostic tests are used to evaluate risk factors for injury so treatment can be initiated.
• **COGNITION:** Cognitive and mental status	Cognitive impairments directly increase the risk for injury.
• **MOBILITY:** Mobility and musculoskeletal function	Physical mobility problems have a significant impact on the risk of injury.
• **SENSORY PERCEPTION:** Sensory deficits	The presence of sensory deficits directly increases risk for injury.
• Perform the Timed Get Up and Go test (https://www.cdc.gov/steadi/pdf/TUG_test-print.pdf).	The Timed Get Up and Go test measures mobility, with a higher score reflecting an increased risk of falling.
Refer the patient for a formal physical therapy evaluation, as appropriate.	Physical therapists assess, plan, and implement interventions that improve a person's muscle strength and balance.
Perform a comprehensive assessment if a patient falls and monitor them as needed, including: • Vital signs • Neurologic status and a determination of loss of consciousness • Wounds, visible injuries	An assessment after a fall identifies injuries, allowing for appropriate treatment.
Screen for general safety risks in the environment and safety precautions in use.	Identifying specific factors that place the patient at risk for injury allows for the development of a safety plan.
Evaluate the effectiveness of measures used to decrease the risk of injury through ongoing assessment.	Ongoing monitoring allows for evaluation of the effectiveness of the prevention plan.

Table 68.1 Morse Fall Risk Assessment

Risk Factor	Scale	Score
History of falls	Yes	25
	No	0
Secondary diagnosis	Yes	15
	No	0
Ambulatory aid	Furniture	30
	Crutches/cane/walker	15
	None/bed rest/wheelchair/nurse	0
IV/heparin lock	Yes	20
	No	0
Gait/transferring	Impaired	20
	Weak	10
	Normal/bed rest/immobile	0
Mental status	Forgets limitations	15
	Oriented to own ability	0

To obtain the Morse Fall Score, add the scores from each category: 0, no risk for falls; <25, low risk for falls; 25–45, moderate risk for falls; >45, high risk for falls.
From Morse JM, Morse RM, Tylko SJ. Development of a scale to identify the fall-prone patient. *Canadian Journal on Aging*. 1989;8(4): 366–377. Canadian Association on Gerontology.

Expected Outcomes

The patient will:

- be free from injury.
- identify factors that increase the risk of injury.
- identify how an injury occurred.
- describe and implement strategies to reduce the risk of injury.

INTERVENTIONS TO REDUCE RISK FOR INJURY	RATIONALE
Provide care for injuries that are incurred after a fall or trauma.	An injured patient needs to be stabilized before further evaluation can proceed.
Implement collaborative interventions aimed at treating factors contributing to the risk for injury.	Treatment of contributing factors may reduce the risk of injury.
Discuss potential medication adjustments with the health care provider (HCP).	Several medication categories are associated with an increased risk of falling.
Assist with implementing the plan of care developed by physical therapy.	The physical therapist's plan of care is designed to promote optimal mobility and physical function, reducing the risk of injury.
Encourage the patient to take part in an exercise plan that includes leg strengthening and balance training.	Exercise helps maintain and improve balance and muscle strength, decreasing the risk of falls.
Encourage the patient to discuss their concerns about falling and injuries.	Discussing the patient's concerns can help the nurse confirm the patient's understanding of their risk factors and the need for interventions.
Implement universal fall precautions, including: • Appropriate footwear • Maintain clear paths • Have adequate lighting • Keep the call light and personal possessions within reach • Keep floors clean and dry • Use low-rise beds with locked brakes	Implementing universal fall precautions is the best way to reduce the risk of injury; they apply to all patients.
Encourage the use of needed adaptive devices for mobility and activities of daily living (ADLs).	The use of adaptive devices reduces the risk of injury and promotes independence.

INTERVENTIONS TO REDUCE RISK FOR INJURY	RATIONALE
Assist with implementing the plan of care developed by occupational therapy.	The occupational therapist's plan of care is designed to promote the performance of ADLs and reduce the risk of injury.
SLEEP: Ensure that the patient whose sleep is impaired is not driving, operating heavy machinery, or participating in dangerous activities.	Impaired sleep may alter the usual cognitive ability, which increases the risk of injury.
CARE COORDINATION: Assist the patient in obtaining needed PPE and making environment adaptations.	Using PPE and making environment modifications can reduce the risk of injury.
COGNITION: Implement measures to address impaired cognition.	Impaired cognitive function directly increases the patient's risk for injury.
MOBILITY: Implement measures to address impaired mobility.	Improving the patient's level of mobility directly decreases the risk of injury.
ELIMINATION: Institute measures to address incontinence.	Incontinence is a risk factor for falls.
Encourage the patient to follow precautions at home, at work, and in the community, reviewing measures about: • Bathroom safety • Bicycles • Electricity and electrical devices • Fire safety • Kitchen safety • Motor vehicles • Outdoors and recreation	Specific safety instructions can reduce the risk of injury from trauma.
Encourage caregivers to maintain an appropriate level of supervision.	Anticipatory safety guidance reduces the risk of injury to a person who requires supervision.
Implement an eye care protocol as needed: • Manually close or tape the eyes closed. • Administer eye ointment as ordered.	An eye care protocol protects the eyes of vulnerable patients, thus preventing corneal injuries.
Pediatric **FAMILY DYNAMICS:** Institute measures to support positive parenting and the provision of appropriate supervision.	Positive parenting strategies with anticipatory safety guidance can reduce the risk of injury to a child from a lack of supervision.
Provide the parent/caregiver anticipatory guidance regarding injury prevention strategies tailored to the patient/child's development stage and curiosity level.	Anticipatory guidance helps prevent common injuries.

INTERVENTIONS TO REDUCE THE RISK FOR OCCUPATIONAL INJURY	RATIONALE
Encourage the patient to participate in an employer-sponsored injury prevention program.	Injury prevention programs address occupation hazards and provide education and training aimed at reducing injuries.
Have the patient use designated PPE properly.	PPE use is a critical factor in reducing occupational injury.

INTERVENTIONS TO REDUCE WANDERING	RATIONALE
Implement measures to decrease the risk of elopement with wandering: • Place mirrors on exit doors. • Apply a personal alarm device. • Install locks and alarms on exits.	A wide range of interventions can be used to manage wandering behavior and prevent elopement.
Provide a safe area for the patient to move and encourage them to take part in activities requiring movement.	Structured movement may fulfill the patient's need to wander while remaining safe.

COLLABORATION	RATIONALE
MOBILITY: Physical therapy	Physical therapists assess, plan, and implement interventions that can reduce the risk of injury.
Home safety evaluation	A home safety evaluator assesses a patient's home environment and provides recommendations for enhanced safety.
Occupational therapy	Occupational therapists can recommend assistive devices and help with developing skills that decrease the patient's risk for injury.
CARE COORDINATION: Social work or case management	A social worker or case manager can help the patient and caregiver secure PPE and make modifications to reduce the risk of injury.

PATIENT AND CAREGIVER TEACHING

- Factors that contribute to the patient's specific risks for injury
- Management of a condition contributing to risk for injury
- General safety measures at work, at home, and in the community
- Measures to take to avoid falls
- Lifestyle changes to decrease the risk of injury
- Anticipatory guidance about problematic situations
- Community and self-help resources available
- Where to find additional information
- When to notify the HCP

DOCUMENTATION

Assessment

- Assessments performed
- Circumstances surrounding an injury
- Manifestations of an injury
- Screening test results

Interventions

- Discussions with other interprofessional team members
- Environment modifications made
- Notification of HCP about patient status
- Therapeutic interventions and the patient's response
- Teaching provided
- Referrals initiated
- Safety measures implemented, including fall precautions

Evaluation

- Patient's status: improved, stable, declined
- Manifestations of an injury
- Response to teaching provided
- Response to therapeutic interventions

Exemplars With Common Clinical Problems 69

Clinical Problems Applicable to All Exemplars

Deficient Knowledge

Clinical Problems Applicable Dependent on the Patient Situation

Continuity of Care Problem
Cultural Belief Conflict
Decision Conflict
Inadequate Community Resources
Literacy Problem
Risk for Disease
Socioeconomic Difficulty

Achalasia

Difficulty Coping
Impaired Gastrointestinal Function
Impaired Respiratory Function
Nutritionally Compromised
Pain

Acromegaly

Activity Intolerance
Altered Glucose
Impaired Cardiac Problem
Impaired Endocrine Function
Impaired Respiratory Function
Impaired Sexual Function
Negative Self-Image
Risk for Injury

Acute Coronary Syndrome

Activity Intolerance
Altered Blood Pressure
Anxiety
Impaired Cardiac Function
Impaired Respiratory Function
Impaired Tissue Perfusion
Pain
Risk for Clotting

Acute Kidney Injury

Activity Intolerance
Altered Blood Pressure
Difficulty Coping
Electrolyte Imbalance
Fluid Imbalance
Health Care–Associated Complication
Impaired Cognition
Impaired Urinary Elimination
Risk for Infection

Acute Respiratory Distress Syndrome (ARDS)/ Acute Respiratory Failure (ARF)

Acid-Base Imbalance
Activity Intolerance
Altered Blood Pressure
Fluid Imbalance
Impaired Communication
Impaired Respiratory Function
Infection
Nutritionally Compromised
Risk for Infection

Addison Disease

Activity Intolerance
Altered Blood Pressure
Electrolyte Imbalance
Fluid Imbalance
Impaired Cardiac Function
Impaired Cognition
Impaired Endocrine Function
Impaired Tissue Perfusion
Negative Self-Image

Adjustment Disorder

Depressed Mood
Difficulty Coping
Grief
Impaired Family Function

Impaired Role Performance
Impaired Socialization

Acute Alcohol Intoxication

Impaired Cognition
Impaired Psychological Status
Impaired Respiratory Function
Neurologic Problem
Risk for Injury
Substance Use

AIDS

Activity Intolerance
Caregiver Role Strain
Continuity of Care Problem
Difficulty Coping
Dying Process
Fatigue
Grief
Impaired Bowel Elimination
Impaired Cognition
Impaired Growth and Development
Impaired Immunity
Impaired Respiratory Function
Impaired Sexual Function
Impaired Sleep
Impaired Socialization
Infection
Nutritionally Compromised
Pain
Risk for Infection
Spiritual Problem

Alcohol Use Disorder

Altered Blood Pressure
Anxiety
Body Weight Problem
Depressed Mood
Difficulty Coping
Fatigue
Impaired Family Function
Impaired Fertility
Impaired Gastrointestinal Function
Impaired Immunity
Impaired Role Performance
Impaired Socialization
Parenting Problem
Nutritionally Compromised
Risk for Impaired Skin Integrity
Risk for Infection
Sensory Deficit
Substance Use

Alcohol Withdrawal

Altered Glucose Level
Anxiety
Difficulty Coping
Impaired Cognition
Impaired Psychological Status
Impaired Sleep
Neurologic Problem
Nutritionally Compromised
Personal Care Problem
Risk for Injury
Violent Behavior

Alzheimer Disease

Caregiver Role Strain
Depressed Mood
Difficulty Coping
Dying Process
Emotional Problem
Impaired Bowel Elimination
Impaired Cognition
Impaired Communication
Impaired Family Function
Impaired Psychological Status
Impaired Sexual Function
Impaired Sleep
Impaired Urinary Elimination
Neurologic Problem
Nutritionally Compromised
Personal Care Problem
Risk for Injury
Sensory Deficit

Amputation

Decision Conflict
Difficulty Coping
Grief
Impaired Role Performance
Impaired Socialization
Impaired Tissue Integrity
Impaired Tissue Perfusion
Musculoskeletal Problem
Negative Self-Image
Pain
Risk for Infection
Risk for Injury

Amyotrophic Lateral Sclerosis (ALS)

Caregiver Role Strain
Difficulty Coping
Dying Process
Grief
Impaired Communication
Impaired Respiratory Function
Impaired Socialization
Musculoskeletal Problem
Negative Self-Image
Neurologic Problem
Personal Care Problem

Risk for Impaired Integrity
Risk for Infection
Risk for Injury
Spiritual Problem

Anal Cancer

Continuity of Care Problem
Difficulty Coping
Impaired Bowel Elimination
Impaired Sexual Function
Impaired Tissue Integrity
Negative Self-Image
Pain
Risk for Infection

Anaphylaxis/Anaphylactic Shock

Allergy
Anxiety
Health Care–Associated Complication
Impaired Cardiac Function
Impaired Respiratory Function
Impaired Tissue Perfusion
Inflammation
Risk for Injury

Anemia

Activity Intolerance
Fatigue
Impaired Fertility
Impaired Growth and Development
Impaired Respiratory Function
Impaired Tissue Perfusion
Nutritionally Compromised
Risk for Disease
Risk for Impaired Skin Integrity
Risk for Perinatal Problems

Anemia, Aplastic

Activity Intolerance
Difficulty Coping
Fatigue
Impaired Tissue Perfusion
Nutritionally Compromised
Risk for Infection

Anemia, Cobalamin (Vitamin B_{12}) Deficiency

Activity Intolerance
Fatigue
Impaired Tissue Integrity
Impaired Tissue Perfusion
Neurologic Problem
Nutritionally Compromised
Risk for Injury

Anemia, Folic Acid Deficiency

Activity Intolerance
Fatigue
Impaired Tissue Perfusion
Nutritionally Compromised
Risk for Perinatal Problems

Anemia, Iron-Deficiency

Activity Intolerance
Fatigue
Impaired Respiratory Function
Impaired Tissue Perfusion
Nutritionally Compromised

Aneurysm, Aortic

Altered Blood Pressure
Fluid Imbalance
Impaired Urinary Elimination
Impaired Tissue Perfusion
Pain

Angina, Chronic Stable

Activity Intolerance
Altered Blood Pressure
Anxiety
Health Maintenance Alteration
Impaired Cardiac Function
Impaired Sexual Function
Pain

Anorexia Nervosa

Activity Intolerance
Altered Temperature
Anxiety
Body Weight Problem
Difficulty Coping
Impaired Bowel Elimination
Impaired Fertility
Impaired Growth and Development
Negative Self-Image
Nutritionally Compromised

Antepartum Hemorrhage

Anxiety
Fluid Imbalance
Grief
Impaired Cardiac Function
Impaired Tissue Perfusion
Pain
Risk for Infection
Risk for Perinatal Problems

Aortic Dissection

Altered Blood Pressure
Fluid Imbalance
Impaired Urinary Elimination
Impaired Tissue Perfusion
Pain
Risk for Infection
Risk for Injury

Appendicitis/Appendectomy
Altered Temperature
Fluid Imbalance
Impaired Gastrointestinal Function
Impaired Skin Integrity
Inflammation
Pain
Risk for Infection

Arthroplasty, Knee/Hip
Impaired Role Performance
Impaired Tissue Integrity
Impaired Tissue Perfusion
Musculoskeletal Problem
Pain
Risk for Clotting
Risk for Infection
Risk for Injury

Asthma
Acid-Base Imbalance
Activity Intolerance
Allergy
Anxiety
Difficulty Coping
Health Maintenance Alteration
Impaired Respiratory Function
Impaired Sleep
Inflammation
Risk for Infection

Attention Deficit Hyperactivity Disorder (ADHD)
Caregiver Role Strain
Impaired Family Function
Impaired Growth and Development
Impaired Role Performance
Impaired Socialization
Negative Self-Image
Parenting Problem
Risk for Injury

Autism Spectrum Disorder
Caregiver Role Strain
Emotional Problem
Functional Ability
Impaired Communication
Impaired Family Function
Impaired Growth and Development
Impaired Role Performance
Impaired Socialization
Negative Self-Image
Parenting Problem
Risk for Injury

Bariatric Surgery
Activity Intolerance
Body Weight Problem
Electrolyte Imbalance
Fluid Imbalance
Impaired Cardiac Function
Impaired Gastrointestinal Function
Impaired Respiratory Function
Nutritionally Compromised
Pain
Risk for Impaired Skin Integrity
Risk for Infection

Benign Prostatic Hyperplasia (BPH)
Difficulty Coping
Impaired Sleep
Impaired Sexual Function
Impaired Urinary Elimination
Negative Self-Image
Risk for Infection

Bipolar Disorder
Anxiety
Depressed Mood
Difficulty Coping
Emotional Problem
Health Maintenance Alteration
Impaired Communication
Impaired Family Function
Impaired Psychological Status
Impaired Role Performance
Impaired Sleep
Impaired Socialization
Nutritionally Compromised
Personal Care Problem
Risk for Injury
Violent Behavior

Bladder Cancer
Continuity of Care Problem
Difficulty Coping
Impaired Tissue Integrity
Impaired Urinary Elimination
Negative Self-Image
Pain
Risk for Infection

Bone Cancer
Activity Intolerance
Continuity of Care Problem
Depressed Mood
Difficulty Coping
Impaired Role Performance
Impaired Tissue Integrity
Musculoskeletal Problem
Pain

Borderline Personality
Anxiety
Depressed Mood

Difficulty Coping
Emotional Problem
Impaired Communication
Impaired Psychological Status
Impaired Role Performance
Impaired Socialization

Bowel Resection

Activity Intolerance
Difficulty Coping
Electrolyte Imbalance
Fluid Imbalance
Impaired Bowel Elimination
Impaired Gastrointestinal Function
Impaired Respiratory Function
Impaired Tissue Integrity
Negative Self-Image
Nutritionally Compromised
Pain
Risk for Infection
Risk for Injury

Brain Tumor

Altered Temperature
Difficulty Coping
Grief
Impaired Cognition
Impaired Communication
Impaired Gastrointestinal Function
Impaired Socialization
Increased Intracranial Pressure
Neurologic Problem
Pain
Personal Care Problem
Risk for Impaired Skin Integrity
Risk for Injury

Bradycardia

Activity Intolerance
Altered Blood Pressure
Fatigue
Impaired Cardiac Function
Impaired Respiratory Function
Impaired Role Performance
Impaired Tissue Perfusion

Breast Cancer

Continuity of Care Problem
Difficulty Coping
Health Care–Associated Complication
Impaired Sexual Function
Impaired Tissue Integrity
Musculoskeletal Problem
Negative Self-Image
Pain
Risk for Infection

Bronchiolitis

Altered Temperature
Fluid Imbalance
Impaired Respiratory Function
Infection
Inflammation
Nutritionally Compromised

Bronchopulmonary Dysplasia

Activity Intolerance
Fluid Imbalance
Impaired Cardiac Function
Impaired Growth and Development
Impaired Respiratory Function
Infant Feeding Problem
Nutritionally Compromised
Risk for Infection

Bulimia

Activity Intolerance
Anxiety
Body Weight Problem
Difficulty Coping
Electrolyte Imbalance
Fluid Imbalance
Impaired Bowel Elimination
Impaired Family Function
Impaired Fertility
Negative Self-Image
Nutritionally Compromised

Burns

Acid-Base Imbalance
Altered Blood Pressure
Altered Temperature
Difficulty Coping
Electrolyte Imbalance
Fluid Imbalance
Impaired Bowel Elimination
Impaired Cardiac Function
Impaired Immunity
Impaired Respiratory Function
Impaired Sleep
Impaired Socialization
Impaired Tissue Integrity
Impaired Urinary Elimination
Impaired Tissue Perfusion
Negative Self-Image
Nutritionally Compromised
Pain
Sensory Deficit
Risk for Infection

Cardiac Catheterization

Anxiety
Health Care–Associated Complication

Impaired Cardiac Function
Impaired Tissue Perfusion
Pain
Risk for Clotting
Risk for Infection

Cardiogenic Shock

Acid-Base Imbalance
Altered Blood Pressure
Anxiety
Fluid Imbalance
Impaired Cardiac Function
Impaired Respiratory Function
Impaired Urinary Function
Impaired Tissue Perfusion
Nutritionally Compromised
Risk for Clotting
Risk for Injury

Cardiomyopathy

Activity Intolerance
Altered Blood Pressure
Fluid Imbalance
Health Maintenance Alteration
Impaired Cardiac Function
Impaired Respiratory Function
Impaired Tissue Perfusion

Carotid Endarterectomy

Impaired Respiratory Function
Impaired Tissue Integrity
Impaired Tissue Perfusion
Risk for Infection
Risk for Injury

Cataract Surgery

Pain
Risk for Infection
Risk for Injury
Sensory Deficit

Celiac Disease

Body Weight Problem
Fluid Imbalance
Impaired Gastrointestinal Function
Impaired Growth and Development
Health Maintenance Alteration
Nutritionally Compromised

Cellulitis

Activity Intolerance
Altered Temperature
Impaired Tissue Integrity
Impaired Tissue Perfusion
Infection
Inflammation
Pain
Risk for Impaired Skin Integrity

Cerebral Palsy

Activity Intolerance
Caregiver Role Strain
Difficulty Coping
Impaired Family Function
Impaired Growth and Development
Impaired Respiratory Function
Impaired Role Function
Musculoskeletal Problem
Negative Self-Image
Neurologic Problem
Nutritionally Compromised
Personal Care Problem
Risk for Injury
Sensory Deficit

Cervical Cancer

Continuity of Care Problem
Difficulty Coping
Impaired Fertility
Impaired Sexual Function
Impaired Tissue Integrity
Negative Self-Image
Pain

Cesarean Delivery

Activity Intolerance
Altered Temperature
Depressed Mood
Fluid Imbalance
Grief
Health Care–Associated Complication
Impaired Gastrointestinal Function
Impaired Respiratory Function
Impaired Skin Integrity
Impaired Sleep
Impaired Urinary Elimination
Impaired Tissue Perfusion
Pain
Risk for Infection
Risk for Injury
Risk for Perinatal Problems

Chemotherapy

Activity Intolerance
Difficulty Coping
Electrolyte Imbalance
Fatigue
Fluid Imbalance
Health Care–Associated Complication
Impaired Bowel Elimination
Impaired Endocrine Function
Impaired Fertility
Impaired Gastrointestinal Function
Impaired Immunity
Impaired Socialization
Impaired Tissue Integrity
Impaired Tissue Perfusion

Negative Self-Image
Nutritionally Compromised
Pain
Risk for Infection
Sensory Deficit

Chest Trauma

Acid-Base Imbalance
Altered Blood Pressure
Fluid Imbalance
Impaired Cardiac Function
Impaired Respiratory Function
Impaired Tissue Integrity
Musculoskeletal Problem
Pain
Risk for Clotting
Risk for Infection

Chest Tubes and Pleural Drainage

Health Care–Associated Complication
Impaired Cardiac Function
Impaired Respiratory Function
Impaired Sleep
Impaired Tissue Integrity
Musculoskeletal Problem
Pain
Risk for Clotting
Risk for Infection

Chlamydia Infection

Impaired Fertility
Impaired Sexual Function
Infection
Negative Self-Image
Risk for Infection
Risk for Perinatal Problems

Cholelithiasis/Cholecystitis

Altered Temperature
Impaired Gastrointestinal Function
Impaired Tissue Integrity
Inflammation
Nutritionally Compromised
Pain

Chronic Obstructive Pulmonary Disease (COPD)

Acid-Base Imbalance
Activity Intolerance
Continuity of Care Problem
Difficulty Coping
Electrolyte Imbalance
Fatigue
Fluid Imbalance
Health Maintenance Alteration
Impaired Immunity
Impaired Respiratory Function
Impaired Role Performance
Impaired Sexual Function
Impaired Sleep
Inflammation
Nutritionally Compromised
Risk for Infection

Chronic Pain

Difficulty Coping
Depressed Mood
Fatigue
Impaired Role Performance
Impaired Sleep
Pain
Substance Use

Cirrhosis

Activity Intolerance
Alcohol Use Disorder
Altered Blood Pressure
Continuity of Care Problem
Difficulty Coping
Electrolyte Imbalance
Fatigue
Fluid Imbalance
Impaired Bowel Elimination
Impaired Gastrointestinal Function
Impaired Respiratory Function
Impaired Role Performance
Impaired Tissue Integrity
Impaired Tissue Perfusion
Inflammation
Nutritionally Compromised
Risk for Infection

Cleft Lip/Cleft Palate

Impaired Communication
Impaired Family Function
Impaired Respiratory Function
Impaired Tissue Integrity
Infant Feeding Problem
Nutritionally Compromised
Pain
Risk for Infection

Colorectal Cancer

Continuity of Care Problem
Difficulty Coping
Impaired Bowel Elimination
Impaired Gastrointestinal Function
Impaired Sexual Function
Impaired Tissue Integrity
Nutritionally Compromised
Pain

Coma

Impaired Bowel Elimination
Impaired Urinary Elimination
Impaired Tissue Perfusion

Increased Intracranial Pressure
Musculoskeletal Problem
Neurologic Problem
Personal Care Problem
Risk for Clotting
Risk for Impaired Skin Integrity
Risk for Infection

Congenital Heart Disease

Activity Intolerance
Altered Blood Pressure
Electrolyte Imbalance
Fatigue
Fluid Imbalance
Impaired Cardiac Function
Impaired Family Function
Impaired Growth and Development
Impaired Respiratory Function
Impaired Role Performance
Impaired Sleep
Impaired Tissue Perfusion
Infant Feeding Problem
Nutritionally Compromised
Risk for Infection
Risk for Injury

Conjunctivitis

Allergy
Impaired Role Performance
Infection
Pain
Risk for Injury
Sensory Deficit

Constipation

Fluid Imbalance
Impaired Bowel Elimination
Impaired Gastrointestinal Function
Musculoskeletal Problem

Cor Pulmonale

Activity Intolerance
Altered Blood Pressure
Difficulty Coping
Fluid Imbalance
Impaired Cardiac Function
Impaired Respiratory Function
Impaired Tissue Perfusion

Coronary Artery Bypass Graft/Valve Surgery

Activity Intolerance
Altered Blood Pressure
Fluid Imbalance
Health Care–Associated Complication
Impaired Cardiac Function
Impaired Respiratory Function
Impaired Sleep
Impaired Tissue Integrity
Impaired Tissue Perfusion
Musculoskeletal Problem
Pain
Personal Care Problem
Risk for Clotting
Risk for Infection

Coronary Artery Disease (CAD)

Activity Intolerance
Anxiety
Health Maintenance Alteration
Impaired Cardiac Function
Impaired Tissue Perfusion
Nutritionally Compromised
Pain

COVID-19 Infection

Acid-Base Imbalance
Activity Intolerance
Altered Temperature
Difficulty Coping
Fluid Imbalance
Health Maintenance Alteration
Impaired Cardiac Function
Impaired Respiratory Function
Impaired Sleep
Infection
Nutritionally Compromised
Pain
Risk for Clotting
Risk for Injury

Crohn Disease

Difficulty Coping
Fluid Imbalance
Impaired Bowel Elimination
Impaired Gastrointestinal Function
Nutritionally Compromised
Pain

Cushing Syndrome

Activity Intolerance
Altered Glucose Level
Body Weight Problem
Electrolyte Imbalance
Fluid Imbalance
Impaired Endocrine Function
Impaired Immunity
Negative Self-Image
Risk for Impaired Skin Integrity
Risk for Infection
Sensory Deficit

Cystic Fibrosis

Activity Intolerance
Altered Glucose Level

Body Weight Problem
Caregiver Role Strain
Difficulty Coping
Grief
Fluid Imbalance
Health Maintenance Alteration
Impaired Family Function
Impaired Fertility
Impaired Growth and Development
Impaired Respiratory Function
Impaired Role Performance
Impaired Sleep
Nutritionally Compromised
Risk for Infection

Cystitis

Altered Temperature
Fluid Imbalance
Impaired Urinary Elimination
Infection
Inflammation
Pain

Dehydration

Activity Intolerance
Altered Blood Pressure
Altered Glucose Level
Altered Temperature
Electrolyte Imbalance
Fluid Imbalance
Impaired Cardiac Function
Impaired Cognition
Impaired Elimination
Impaired Infant Feeding
Impaired Urinary Elimination
Risk for Impaired Skin Integrity

Delirium

Health Care–Associated Complication
Impaired Cognition
Impaired Communication
Impaired Psychological Status
Impaired Sleep
Neurologic Problem
Personal Care Problem
Risk for Injury
Substance Use

Dementia

Caregiver Role Strain
Emotional Problem
Impaired Bowel Elimination
Impaired Cognition
Impaired Psychological Status
Impaired Sleep
Impaired Urinary Elimination
Neurologic Problem
Nutritionally Compromised
Personal Care Problem
Risk for Injury
Sensory Deficit

Depression

Anxiety
Body Weight Problem
Depressed Mood
Difficulty Coping
Emotional Problem
Fatigue
Grief
Health Maintenance Alteration
Impaired Cognition
Impaired Endocrine Function
Impaired Family Function
Impaired Growth and Development
Impaired Psychological Status
Impaired Role Performance
Impaired Sleep
Impaired Socialization
Negative Self-Image
Neurologic Problem
Pain
Parenting Problem
Personal Care Problem
Risk for Perinatal Problems
Spiritual Problem

Diabetic Ketoacidosis

Acid-Base Imbalance
Altered Glucose Level
Altered Blood Pressure
Electrolyte Imbalance
Fatigue
Fluid Imbalance
Impaired Cognition
Impaired Endocrine Function
Risk for Impaired Tissue Integrity
Risk for Infection

Diabetes Insipidus (DI)

Altered Blood Pressure
Electrolyte Imbalance
Fatigue
Fluid Imbalance
Impaired Endocrine Function
Neurologic Problem

Diabetes

Acid-Base Imbalance
Altered Glucose Level
Altered Blood Pressure
Continuity of Care Problem
Difficulty Coping
Electrolyte Imbalance

Fatigue
Fluid Imbalance
Impaired Gastrointestinal Function
Impaired Endocrine Function
Impaired Sexual Function
Impaired Urinary Elimination
Impaired Tissue Perfusion
Neurologic Problem
Nutritionally Compromised
Risk for Impaired Skin Integrity
Risk for Infection
Risk for Injury
Risk for Perinatal Problems
Sensory Deficit

Diarrhea

Acid-Base Imbalance
Altered Blood Pressure
Electrolyte Imbalance
Fluid Imbalance
Impaired Bowel Elimination
Impaired Gastrointestinal Function
Infection
Nutritionally Compromised
Pain
Risk for Impaired Skin Integrity

Disseminated Intravascular Coagulation (DIC)

Altered Blood Pressure
Fluid Imbalance
Impaired Respiratory Function
Impaired Tissue Perfusion
Risk for Impaired Skin Integrity

Diverticulosis/Diverticulitis

Fluid Imbalance
Impaired Bowel Elimination
Impaired Gastrointestinal Function
Infection
Inflammation
Nutritionally Compromised
Pain

Domestic Violence

Anxiety
Depressed Mood
Difficulty Coping
Impaired Family Function
Impaired Growth and Development
Impaired Sleep
Negative Self-Image
Parenting Problem
Spiritual Problem
Substance Use
Victim of Violence
Violent Behavior

Dysrhythmias

Activity Intolerance
Altered Blood Pressure
Anxiety
Impaired Cardiac Function
Impaired Tissue Perfusion
Risk for Clotting

Ear Surgery

Impaired Tissue Integrity
Pain
Sensory Deficit
Risk for Injury

Ectopic Pregnancy

Altered Blood Pressure
Fluid Imbalance
Grief
Impaired Sexual Function
Impaired Tissue Integrity
Infertility
Pain
Risk for Infection
Risk for Perinatal Problems

Elder Abuse and Neglect

Depressed Mood
Difficulty Coping
Emotional Problem
Impaired Family Function
Impaired Growth and Development
Impaired Psychological Function
Impaired Socialization
Negative Self-Image
Spiritual Problem
Substance Use
Victim of Violence

Endocarditis, Infective

Activity Intolerance
Altered Temperature
Impaired Cardiac Function
Impaired Respiratory Function
Impaired Tissue Perfusion
Infection
Pain
Risk for Clotting

Endometrial Cancer

Continuity of Care Problem
Difficulty Coping
Impaired Fertility
Impaired Sexual Function
Impaired Tissue Integrity
Negative Self-Image
Pain

Endometriosis
Difficulty Coping
Impaired Fertility
Impaired Sexual Function
Negative Self-Image
Pain

End-Stage Renal Disease
Acid-Base Imbalance
Activity Intolerance
Altered Blood Pressure
Altered Glucose Level
Difficulty Coping
Dying Process
Electrolyte Imbalance
Fatigue
Fluid Imbalance
Impaired Cognition
Impaired Immunity
Impaired Role Performance
Impaired Tissue Integrity
Impaired Urinary Elimination
Musculoskeletal Problem
Nutritionally Compromised
Risk for Injury

Enteral Nutrition
Altered Glucose Level
Body Weight Problem
Diarrhea
Electrolyte Imbalance
Fluid Imbalance
Health Care–Associated Complication
Impaired Bowel Elimination
Impaired Respiratory Function
Impaired Tissue Integrity
Nutritionally Compromised
Risk for Infection

Epididymitis
Anxiety
Impaired Fertility
Impaired Sexual Function
Infection
Inflammation
Pain

Erectile Dysfunction
Altered Blood Pressure
Difficulty Coping
Impaired Family Function
Impaired Fertility
Impaired Role Performance
Impaired Sexual Function
Impaired Urinary Elimination
Negative Self-Image

Esophageal Cancer
Continuity of Care Problem
Difficulty Coping
Impaired Communication
Impaired Gastrointestinal Function
Impaired Respiratory Function
Impaired Tissue Integrity
Nutritionally Compromised
Pain
Risk for Infection

Facial Trauma
Impaired Communication
Impaired Respiratory Function
Impaired Tissue Integrity
Negative Self-Image
Nutritionally Compromised
Pain
Risk for Infection

Fat Embolism
Anxiety
Impaired Cardiac Function
Impaired Cognition
Impaired Respiratory Function
Impaired Tissue Integrity
Impaired Tissue Perfusion Pain

Fever/Hyperthermia
Acid-Base Imbalance
Altered Blood Pressure
Altered Temperature
Fluid Imbalance
Impaired Cardiac Function
Impaired Cognition
Impaired Sleep
Infection
Inflammation
Neurologic Problem
Pain
Risk for Injury

Fibromyalgia
Depressed Mood
Difficulty Coping
Fatigue
Impaired Role Performance
Impaired Sleep
Inflammation
Musculoskeletal Problem
Negative Self-Image
Pain

Flail Chest/Rib Fracture
Anxiety
Impaired Cardiac Function

Impaired Respiratory Function
Pain

Foodborne Illness

Altered Temperature
Electrolyte Imbalance
Fluid Imbalance
Impaired Bowel Elimination
Impaired Gastrointestinal Function
Infection
Pain

Fracture

Impaired Role Performance
Impaired Tissue Integrity
Impaired Tissue Perfusion
Musculoskeletal Problem
Neurologic Problem
Pain
Risk for Clotting
Risk for Infection
Risk for Injury

Fracture, Hip

Impaired Tissue Integrity
Impaired Tissue Perfusion
Musculoskeletal Problem
Neurologic Problem
Pain
Personal Care Problem
Risk for Clotting
Risk for Infection
Risk for Injury

Fracture, Humerus

Impaired Role Performance
Impaired Tissue Integrity
Impaired Tissue Perfusion
Musculoskeletal Problem
Neurologic Problem
Pain
Personal Care Problem
Risk for Infection
Risk for Injury

Fracture, Pelvis

Impaired Tissue Perfusion
Musculoskeletal Problem
Neurologic Problem
Pain
Personal Care Problem
Risk for Clotting
Risk for Impaired Skin Integrity
Risk for Infection
Risk for Injury

Gastroenteritis

Electrolyte Imbalance
Fluid Imbalance
Impaired Bowel Elimination
Impaired Gastrointestinal Function
Infection
Inflammation
Pain
Risk for Impaired Skin Integrity

Gastrectomy

Activity Intolerance
Body Weight Problem
Difficulty Coping
Electrolyte Imbalance
Fluid Imbalance
Impaired Gastrointestinal Function
Impaired Respiratory Function
Impaired Tissue Integrity
Negative Self-Image
Nutritionally Compromised
Pain
Risk for Infection
Risk for Injury

Gastroesophageal Reflux Disease (GERD)

Fluid Imbalance
Impaired Gastrointestinal Function
Impaired Respiratory Function
Impaired Sleep
Infant Feeding Problem
Nutritionally Compromised
Pain

Gastrointestinal Bleeding, Upper

Altered Blood Pressure
Fluid Imbalance
Impaired Cardiac Function
Impaired Gastrointestinal Function
Impaired Tissue Perfusion
Nutritionally Compromised

Glaucoma

Impaired Role Performance
Sensory Deficit
Risk for Injury

Glomerulonephritis

Altered Temperature
Altered Blood Pressure
Electrolyte Imbalance
Fluid Imbalance
Impaired Urinary Elimination
Infection
Inflammation
Pain

Gonorrhea
Impaired Fertility
Impaired Sexual Function
Impaired Tissue Integrity
Infection
Negative Self-Image
Pain

Gout
Difficulty Coping
Impaired Role Performance
Impaired Sleep
Musculoskeletal Problem
Pain

Guillain-Barre Syndrome
Caregiver Role Strain
Difficulty Coping
Impaired Communication
Impaired Respiratory Function
Impaired Socialization
Musculoskeletal Problem
Neurologic Problem
Pain
Personal Care Problem
Risk for Impaired Skin Integrity
Risk for Injury

Head and Neck Cancer
Continuity of Care Problem
Difficulty Coping
Grief
Impaired Communication
Impaired Respiratory Function
Impaired Socialization
Impaired Tissue Integrity
Negative Self-Image
Nutritionally Compromised
Pain
Risk for Infection

Head Injury
Altered Temperature
Caregiver Role Strain
Difficulty Coping
Emotional Problem
Impaired Cognition
Impaired Growth and Development
Impaired Family Function
Impaired Psychological Status
Impaired Respiratory Function
Impaired Role Performance
Increased Intracranial Pressure
Neurologic Problem
Personal Care Problem
Risk for Injury
Violent Behavior

Headache
Difficulty Coping
Impaired Role Performance
Impaired Sleep
Increased Intracranial Pressure
Neurologic Problem
Pain

Heart Failure
Activity Intolerance
Altered Blood Pressure
Difficulty Coping
Electrolyte Imbalance
Fatigue
Fluid Imbalance
Health Maintenance Alteration
Impaired Cardiac Function
Impaired Respiratory Function
Impaired Role Performance
Impaired Sleep
Impaired Tissue Perfusion
Impaired Urinary Elimination
Nutritionally Compromised

Hemodialysis
Difficulty Coping
Electrolyte Imbalance
Fatigue
Fluid Imbalance
Health Care–Associated Complication
Health Maintenance Alteration
Impaired Gastrointestinal Function
Impaired Role Performance
Impaired Tissue Integrity
Pain
Risk for Clotting
Risk for Infection
Risk for Injury

Hemophilia and von Willebrand Disease
Difficulty Coping
Impaired Tissue Perfusion
Musculoskeletal Problem
Pain

Hemorrhoids
Impaired Bowel Elimination
Impaired Tissue Integrity
Pain
Risk for Infection

Hemothorax
Altered Blood Pressure
Fluid Imbalance
Impaired Cardiac Function
Impaired Respiratory Function
Pain

Hepatitis, Viral
Activity Intolerance
Altered Temperature
Electrolyte Imbalance
Fatigue
Fluid Imbalance
Impaired Bowel Elimination
Impaired Gastrointestinal Function
Impaired Respiratory Function
Impaired Tissue Integrity
Infection
Nutritionally Compromised
Risk for Infection
Risk for Perinatal Problems

Herpes, Genital
Difficulty Coping
Impaired Sexual Function
Impaired Tissue Integrity
Infection
Inflammation
Negative Self-Image
Pain
Risk for Perinatal Problems

Herpes Zoster
Impaired Sleeping
Impaired Tissue Integrity
Inflammation
Negative Self-Image
Pain

Hiatal Hernia
Health Maintenance Alteration
Impaired Gastrointestinal Function
Nutritionally Compromised
Pain

Hirschsprung Disease
Body Weight Problem
Fluid Imbalance
Impaired Bowel Elimination
Impaired Gastrointestinal Function
Impaired Tissue Integrity
Infant Feeding Problem
Nutritionally Compromised
Pain
Risk for Infection

Hodgkin Lymphoma
Difficulty Coping
Fatigue
Health Care–Associated Complication
Impaired Immunity
Nutritionally Compromised
Risk for Infection

Human Immunodeficiency Virus (HIV) Infection
Continuity of Care Problem
Difficulty Coping
Impaired Immunity
Impaired Respiratory Function
Impaired Sexual Function
Impaired Socialization
Infection
Negative Self-Image
Nutritionally Compromised
Risk for Infection
Risk for Perinatal Problems

Huntington Disease (HD)
Caregiver Role Strain
Difficulty Coping
Dying Process
Fatigue
Grief
Impaired Cognition
Impaired Communication
Impaired Respiratory Function
Impaired Role Performance
Impaired Socialization
Musculoskeletal Problem
Neurologic Problem
Personal Care Problem
Risk for Impaired Skin Integrity
Risk for Injury

Hydrocephalus
Fluid Imbalance
Impaired Cognition
Impaired Growth and Development
Increased Intracranial Pressure
Infant Feeding Problem
Musculoskeletal Problem
Neurologic Problem
Nutritionally Compromised
Pain
Risk for Impaired Skin Integrity
Risk for Infection
Risk for Injury

Hyperbilirubinemia
Acid-Base Imbalance
Altered Temperature
Fluid Imbalance
Health Care–Associated Complication
Impaired Gastrointestinal Function
Infant Feeding Problem
Neurologic Problem
Nutritionally Compromised
Parenting Problem
Risk for Impaired Skin Integrity
Risk for Injury

Hypercalcemia

Acid-Base imbalance
Electrolyte Imbalance
Impaired Cardiac Function
Impaired Gastrointestinal Function
Impaired Urinary Elimination
Musculoskeletal Problem
Neurologic Problem
Risk for Injury

Hyperglycemic Hyperosmolar Nonketotic Syndrome (HHNS)

Altered Glucose Level
Altered Blood Pressure
Altered Temperature
Electrolyte Imbalance
Fluid Imbalance
Impaired Cardiac Function
Impaired Cognition
Impaired Endocrine Function
Impaired Respiratory Function
Impaired Tissue Perfusion
Neurologic Problem
Risk for Injury

Hyperkalemia

Acid-Base Imbalance
Altered Glucose Level
Electrolyte Imbalance
Impaired Cardiac Function
Musculoskeletal Problem
Neurologic Problem
Risk for Injury

Hyperlipidemia

Altered Blood Pressure
Body Weight Problem
Difficulty Coping
Health Maintenance Alteration
Impaired Cardiac Function
Impaired Sexual Function
Impaired Tissue Perfusion
Nutritionally Compromised
Risk for Clotting
Risk for Disease

Hyperparathyroidism

Acid-Base imbalance
Electrolyte Imbalance
Impaired Cardiac Function
Impaired Endocrine Function
Impaired Gastrointestinal Function
Impaired Urinary Elimination
Musculoskeletal Problem
Neurologic Problem
Risk for Injury

Hypertension

Altered Blood Pressure
Body Weight Problem
Difficulty Coping
Fluid Imbalance
Health Maintenance Alteration
Impaired Cardiac Function
Impaired Sexual Function
Impaired Tissue Perfusion
Nutritionally Compromised
Risk for Disease

Hyperthyroidism

Activity Intolerance
Altered Blood Pressure
Altered Temperature
Anxiety
Body Weight Problem
Impaired Bowel Elimination
Impaired Cardiac Function
Impaired Endocrine Function
Impaired Respiratory Function
Nutritionally Compromised
Risk for Impaired Skin Integrity
Risk for Infection
Risk for Injury

Hypoglycemia

Altered Glucose Level
Health Maintenance Alteration
Impaired Cognition
Neurologic Problem
Risk for Injury

Hypotension

Acid-Base Imbalance
Activity Intolerance
Altered Blood Pressure
Fluid Imbalance
Health Case–Associated Complication
Impaired Cardiac Function
Impaired Cognition
Impaired Tissue Perfusion
Impaired Urinary Elimination
Risk for Injury

Hypothermia

Altered Temperature
Impaired Cardiac Function
Impaired Respiratory Function
Impaired Tissue Integrity
Impaired Tissue Perfusion
Risk for Impaired Skin Integrity

Hypothyroidism

Activity Intolerance
Altered Temperature

Body Weight Problem
Fatigue
Impaired Bowel Elimination
Impaired Cardiac Function
Impaired Endocrine Function
Impaired Role Performance

Hypovolemic Shock

Acid-Base Imbalance
Altered Blood Pressure
Altered Temperature
Electrolyte Imbalance
Fluid Imbalance
Impaired Cardiac Function
Impaired Gastrointestinal Function
Impaired Urinary Elimination
Impaired Tissue Perfusion
Impaired Urinary Elimination
Nutritionally Compromised
Risk for Clotting
Risk for Injury

Hysterectomy

Grief
Impaired Sexual Function
Impaired Tissue Integrity
Impaired Urinary Elimination
Negative Self-Image
Pain
Risk for Infection

Immobility

Activity Intolerance
Impaired Bowel Elimination
Impaired Urinary Elimination
Impaired Respiratory Function
Impaired Sleep
Impaired Socialization
Impaired Tissue Perfusion
Musculoskeletal Problem
Personal Care Problem
Risk for Clotting
Risk for Impaired Skin Integrity
Risk for Infection

Impetigo

Altered Temperature
Impaired Skin Integrity
Infection
Negative Self-Image
Personal Care Problem

Increased Intracranial Pressure (ICP)

Impaired Cognition
Impaired Respiratory Function
Impaired Tissue Perfusion
Increased Intracranial Pressure
Musculoskeletal Problem
Neurologic Problem
Personal Care Problem
Risk for Injury

Inflammatory Bowel Disease (IBD)

Difficulty Coping
Fatigue
Fluid Imbalance
Impaired Bowel Elimination
Impaired Gastrointestinal Function
Impaired Socialization
Infection
Inflammation
Nutritionally Compromised
Pain

Influenza

Altered Temperature
Fatigue
Fluid Imbalance
Impaired Gastrointestinal Function
Impaired Respiratory Function
Infection
Pain
Risk for Injury

Intervertebral Disc Disease

Activity Intolerance
Depressed Mood
Difficulty Coping
Impaired Role Performance
Musculoskeletal Problem
Neurologic Problem
Pain
Risk for Injury

Intestinal Obstruction

Fluid Imbalance
Impaired Bowel Elimination
Impaired Gastrointestinal Function
Nutritionally Compromised
Pain
Risk for Infection

Irritable Bowel Syndrome (IBS)

Difficulty Coping
Fatigue
Impaired Bowel Elimination
Impaired Gastrointestinal Function
Impaired Socialization
Impaired Sleep
Nutritionally Compromised
Pain

Kawasaki Disease

Altered Temperature
Fluid Imbalance
Impaired Cardiac Function

Impaired Tissue Integrity
Impaired Tissue Perfusion
Inflammation
Nutritionally Compromised
Pain

Kidney Cancer

Acid-Base Imbalance
Altered Blood Pressure
Continuity of Care Problem
Difficulty Coping
Fatigue
Impaired Immunity
Impaired Respiratory Function
Impaired Tissue Integrity
Impaired Urinary Elimination
Pain
Risk for Injury

Kidney Disease, Chronic

Acid-Base Imbalance
Activity Intolerance
Altered Blood Pressure
Continuity of Care Problem
Depressed Mood
Difficulty Coping
Electrolyte Imbalance
Fatigue
Fluid Imbalance
Impaired Cognition
Impaired Health Maintenance
Impaired Immunity
Impaired Role Performance
Impaired Tissue Integrity
Impaired Urinary Elimination
Musculoskeletal Problem
Negative Self-Image
Risk for Injury

Labor and Delivery

Anxiety
Difficulty Coping
Fatigue
Fluid Imbalance
Health Care–Associated Complication
Impaired Gastrointestinal Function
Impaired Urinary Elimination
Pain
Risk for Impaired Skin Integrity
Risk for Infection
Risk for Injury
Risk for Perinatal Problems

Laminectomy

Activity Intolerance
Impaired Tissue Integrity
Impaired Urinary Elimination
Impaired Tissue Perfusion
Musculoskeletal Problem
Neurologic Problem
Pain
Risk for Clotting
Risk for Infection
Risk for Injury

Laryngectomy

Difficulty Coping
Grief
Impaired Communication
Impaired Respiratory Function
Impaired Socialization
Impaired Tissue Integrity
Negative Self-Image
Pain
Risk for Infection

Laryngotracheobronchitis/Croup

Altered Temperature
Fluid Imbalance
Impaired Respiratory Function
Infant Feeding Problem
Infection
Inflammation
Nutritionally Compromised
Pain

Latex Allergy

Allergy
Health Care–Associated Complication
Impaired Respiratory Function
Impaired Tissue Integrity
Inflammation
Risk for Impaired Skin Integrity

Leukemia

Activity Intolerance
Altered Temperature
Anxiety
Difficulty Coping
Fatigue
Health Care–Associated Complication
Nutritionally Compromised
Pain
Risk for Impaired Skin Integrity
Risk for Infection

Liver Cancer

Acid-Base Imbalance
Activity Intolerance
Altered Blood Pressure
Altered Glucose Level
Continuity of Care Problem
Difficulty Coping
Electrolyte Imbalance
Fatigue
Fluid Imbalance

Grief
Impaired Bowel Elimination
Impaired Gastrointestinal Function
Impaired Respiratory Function
Impaired Tissue Integrity
Impaired Tissue Perfusion
Nutritionally Compromised
Risk for Infection

Low Back Pain, Acute

Difficulty Coping
Impaired Role Performance
Inflammation
Musculoskeletal Problem
Neurologic Problem
Pain
Risk for Injury

Low Back Pain, Chronic

Activity Intolerance
Depressed Mood
Difficulty Coping
Impaired Role Performance
Inflammation
Musculoskeletal Problem
Neurologic Problem
Pain
Risk for Injury

Lung Cancer

Activity Intolerance
Continuity of Care Problem
Depressed Mood
Difficulty Coping
Grief
Impaired Respiratory Function
Impaired Tissue Integrity
Nutritionally Compromised
Pain
Risk for Infection
Substance Use

Lyme Disease

Altered Temperature
Fatigue
Impaired Cardiac Function
Impaired Psychological Status
Infection
Musculoskeletal Problem
Neurologic Problem
Pain

Macular Degeneration

Depressed Mood
Difficulty Coping
Impaired Role Performance
Impaired Socialization
Sensory Deficit
Risk for Injury

Malabsorption

Body Weight Problem
Electrolyte Imbalance
Fluid Imbalance
Impaired Elimination
Impaired Gastrointestinal Function
Impaired Growth and Development
Nutritionally Compromised
Risk for Impaired Skin Integrity

Mastitis

Altered Temperature
Impaired Tissue Integrity
Infant Feeding Problem
Infection
Inflammation
Pain
Parenting Problem

Melanoma

Difficulty Coping
Impaired Tissue Integrity
Negative Self-Image
Risk for Infection

Mechanical Ventilation

Acid-Base Imbalance
Anxiety
Fluid Imbalance
Health Care–Associated Complication
Impaired Communication
Impaired Respiratory Function
Musculoskeletal Problem
Nutritionally Compromised
Risk for Infection

Ménière Disease

Neurologic Problem
Risk for Injury
Sensory Deficit

Meningitis

Altered Temperature
Fluid Imbalance
Impaired Cognition
Impaired Communication
Impaired Gastrointestinal Function
Impaired Growth and Development
Impaired Psychological Status
Impaired Respiratory Function
Increased Intracranial Pressure
Infection
Musculoskeletal Problem
Neurologic Problem

Pain
Risk for Impaired Skin Integrity
Risk for Injury

Menopause

Altered Temperature
Body Weight Problem
Decision Conflict
Difficulty Coping
Impaired Family Function
Impaired Role Performance
Impaired Sexual Function
Impaired Sleep
Impaired Urinary Elimination
Negative Self-Image

Metabolic Syndrome

Activity Intolerance
Altered Glucose Level
Altered Blood Pressure
Body Weight Problem
Difficulty Coping
Risk for Disease

Mononucleosis

Activity Intolerance
Altered Temperature
Fatigue
Impaired Respiratory Function
Infection
Pain
Risk for Injury

Multiple Gestation

Anxiety
Continuity of Care Problem
Fatigue
Fluid Imbalance
Impaired Bowel Elimination
Impaired Gastrointestinal Function
Impaired Role Performance
Impaired Sleep
Impaired Urinary Elimination
Infant Feeding Problem
Musculoskeletal Problem
Nutritionally Compromised
Risk for Perinatal Problems

Multiple Sclerosis (MS)

Caregiver Role Strain
Continuity of Care Problem
Difficulty Coping
Emotional Problem
Fatigue
Impaired Communication
Impaired Gastrointestinal Function
Impaired Immunity
Impaired Psychological Status
Impaired Role Performance
Impaired Socialization
Impaired Urinary Elimination
Inflammation
Musculoskeletal Problem
Negative Self-Image
Neurologic Problem
Nutritionally Compromised
Personal Care Problem
Risk for Impaired Skin Integrity
Risk for Infection
Sensory Deficit

Muscular Dystrophy

Caregiver Role Strain
Continuity of Care Problem
Difficulty Coping
Impaired Growth and Development
Impaired Respiratory Function
Impaired Role Performance
Impaired Socialization
Musculoskeletal Problem
Negative Self-Image
Neurologic Problem
Nutritionally Compromised
Personal Care Problem
Risk for Impaired Skin Integrity
Risk for Infection
Risk for Injury

Myasthenia Gravis

Difficulty Coping
Fatigue
Impaired Communication
Impaired Respiratory Function
Impaired Socialization
Inflammation
Musculoskeletal Problem
Negative Self-Image
Neurologic Problem
Nutritionally Compromised
Pain
Risk for Impaired Skin Integrity
Risk for Injury

Myocardial Infarction (MI)

Activity Intolerance
Altered Blood Pressure
Anxiety
Difficulty Coping
Fluid Imbalance
Health Maintenance Alteration
Impaired Cardiac Function
Impaired Respiratory Function
Impaired Sexual Function
Impaired Tissue Perfusion

Pain
Risk for Clotting

Myocarditis

Anxiety
Impaired Cardiac Function
Impaired Respiratory Function
Infection
Inflammation
Pain

Nausea and Vomiting

Acid-Base Imbalance
Altered Blood Pressure
Body Weight Problem
Electrolyte Imbalance
Fatigue
Fluid Imbalance
Impaired Gastrointestinal Function
Impaired Sleep
Infant Feeding Problem
Nutritionally Compromised

Necrotizing Enterocolitis

Altered Temperature
Body Weight Problem
Electrolyte Imbalance
Fluid Imbalance
Impaired Bowel Elimination
Impaired Gastrointestinal Function
Impaired Growth and Development
Infant Feeding Problem
Infection
Nutritionally Compromised
Pain
Parenting Problem
Risk for Infection

Neonatal Abstinence Syndrome

Altered Glucose Level
Altered Temperature
Fluid Imbalance
Impaired Bowel Elimination
Impaired Family Function
Impaired Gastrointestinal Function
Impaired Growth and Development
Impaired Parenting
Impaired Respiratory Function
Impaired Sleep
Infant Feeding Problem
Neurologic Problem
Pain
Parenting Problem
Risk for Infection
Risk for Injury
Substance Use

Nephrectomy

Fluid Imbalance
Health Care–Associated Complication
Impaired Respiratory Function
Impaired Tissue Integrity
Impaired Urinary Elimination
Impaired Tissue Perfusion
Pain
Risk for Infection
Risk for Injury

Nephrotic Syndrome

Acid-Base Imbalance
Altered Blood Pressure
Depressed Mood
Difficulty Coping
Electrolyte Imbalance
Fatigue
Fluid Imbalance
Impaired Cognition
Impaired Immunity
Impaired Urinary Elimination
Impaired Tissue Perfusion
Negative Self-Image
Nutritionally Compromised
Risk for Infection

Neural Tube Defect

Allergy
Caregiver Role Strain
Difficulty Coping
Impaired Bowel Elimination
Impaired Growth and Development
Impaired Role Performance
Impaired Urinary Elimination
Musculoskeletal Problem
Negative Self-Image
Neurologic Problem
Personal Care Problem
Risk for Impaired Skin Integrity
Risk for Infection

Newborn Care

Altered Glucose Level
Altered Temperature
Impaired Endocrine Function
Impaired Gastrointestinal Function
Impaired Growth and Development
Impaired Respiratory Function
Infant Feeding Problem
Infection
Parenting Problem
Risk for Infection
Risk for Injury
Risk for Perinatal Problems
Substance Use

Non-Hodgkin Lymphoma
Difficulty Coping
Fatigue
Health Care–Associated Complication
Nutritionally Compromised
Risk for Infection

Obesity
Activity Intolerance
Altered Glucose Level
Body Weight Problem
Health Care–Associated Complication
Health Maintenance Alteration
Impaired Fertility
Impaired Gastrointestinal Function
Impaired Respiratory Function
Impaired Socialization
Musculoskeletal Problem
Negative Self-Image
Risk for Disease
Risk for Impaired Skin Integrity
Risk for Infection
Risk for Perinatal Problems
Socioeconomic Difficulty

Obsessive-Compulsive Disorder
Anxiety
Difficulty Coping
Emotional Problem
Impaired Socialization
Risk for Injury

Obstructive Sleep Apnea
Altered Blood Pressure
Fatigue
Impaired Respiratory Function
Impaired Cardiac Function
Impaired Sleep

Oppositional Defiant Disorder
Anxiety
Difficulty Coping
Emotional Problem
Impaired Family Function
Impaired Socialization
Violent Behavior

Oral Cancer
Body Weight Problem
Continuity of Care Problem
Difficulty Coping
Impaired Tissue Integrity
Negative Self-Image
Nutritionally Compromised
Pain
Sensory Deficit

Organ Transplantation
Continuity of Care Problem
Decision Conflict
Difficulty Coping
Health Care–Associated Complication
Impaired Immunity
Pain
Risk for Infection

Osteoarthritis
Difficulty Coping
Impaired Home Maintenance
Impaired Role Performance
Impaired Sleep
Impaired Socialization
Inflammation
Musculoskeletal Problem
Pain
Personal Care Problem

Osteomyelitis
Altered Temperature
Fluid Imbalance
Impaired Tissue Integrity
Infection
Inflammation
Musculoskeletal Problem
Pain
Risk for Impaired Skin Integrity

Osteoporosis
Impaired Role Performance
Impaired Sleep
Musculoskeletal Problem
Pain

Ostomy
Fluid Imbalance
Health Maintenance Alteration
Impaired Bowel Elimination
Impaired Gastrointestinal Function
Impaired Tissue Integrity
Impaired Urinary Elimination
Negative Self-Image

Otitis Media
Allergy
Infection
Pain
Risk for Injury
Sensory Deficit

Ovarian Cancer
Continuity of Care Problem
Difficulty Coping
Grief

Health Care–Associated Complication
Impaired Fertility
Impaired Sexual Function
Impaired Tissue Integrity
Negative Self-Image
Pain

Pacemaker/Cardioverter-Defibrillator

Activity Intolerance
Anxiety
Health Care–Associated Complication
Impaired Cardiac Function
Impaired Skin Integrity
Impaired Tissue Perfusion
Pain
Risk for Infection
Risk for Injury

Pancreatic Cancer

Altered Glucose Level
Continuity of Care Problem
Difficulty Coping
Grief
Impaired Gastrointestinal Function
Impaired Respiratory Function
Impaired Tissue Perfusion
Nutritionally Compromised
Pain

Pancreatitis, Acute

Altered Glucose Level
Altered Blood Pressure
Electrolyte Imbalance
Fluid Imbalance
Impaired Gastrointestinal Function
Impaired Respiratory Function
Impaired Tissue Perfusion
Infection
Inflammation
Nutritionally Compromised
Pain

Pancreatitis, Chronic

Altered Glucose Level
Difficulty Coping
Electrolyte Imbalance
Fluid Imbalance
Impaired Gastrointestinal Function
Inflammation
Nutritionally Compromised
Pain

Paralytic Ileus

Electrolyte Imbalance
Fluid Imbalance
Impaired Bowel Elimination
Impaired Gastrointestinal Function
Nutritionally Compromised
Pain

Paranoia

Anxiety
Impaired Cognition
Depressed Mood
Difficulty Coping
Emotional Problem
Health Maintenance Alteration
Impaired Family Function
Impaired Psychological Status
Impaired Role Performance
Impaired Sleep
Impaired Socialization
Violent Behavior

Parenteral Nutrition

Altered Glucose Level
Body Weight Problem
Continuity of Care Problem
Electrolyte Imbalance
Fluid Imbalance
Health Care–Associated Complication
Impaired Gastrointestinal Function
Nutritionally Compromised
Risk for Infection

Parkinson Disease (PD)

Caregiver Role Strain
Difficulty Coping
Impaired Communication
Impaired Musculoskeletal Function
Impaired Role Performance
Impaired Socialization
Musculoskeletal Problem
Negative Self-Image
Neurologic Problem
Nutritionally Compromised
Risk for Injury
Sensory Deficit

Patent Ductus Arteriosus

Acid-Base Imbalance
Altered Blood Pressure
Fluid Imbalance
Impaired Cardiac Function
Impaired Growth and Development
Impaired Respiratory Function
Impaired Tissue Perfusion
Risk for Clotting

Pelvic Inflammatory Disease (PID)

Impaired Fertility
Impaired Sexual Function
Infection
Inflammation
Pain

Peptic Ulcer Disease
Difficulty Coping
Impaired Gastrointestinal Function
Infection
Nutritionally Compromised
Pain

Pericarditis
Activity Intolerance
Anxiety
Impaired Cardiac Function
Impaired Respiratory Function
Nutritionally Compromised
Pain

Perinatal Loss
Difficulty Coping
Grief
Impaired Family Function
Spiritual Problem

Peripheral Artery Disease (PAD)
Activity Intolerance
Impaired Tissue Integrity
Impaired Tissue Perfusion
Pain
Risk for Clotting
Risk for Impaired Skin Integrity
Risk for Injury
Sensory Deficit

Peripheral Artery Revascularization
Activity Intolerance
Impaired Tissue Integrity
Impaired Tissue Perfusion
Pain
Risk for Clotting
Risk for Injury
Sensory Deficit

Peripheral Neuropathy
Activity Intolerance
Altered Glucose Level
Neurologic Problem
Pain
Risk for Impaired Skin Integrity
Risk for Injury
Sensory Deficit

Peritoneal Dialysis
Altered Glucose
Difficulty Coping
Electrolyte Imbalance
Fatigue
Fluid Imbalance
Health Care–Associated Complication
Health Maintenance Alteration
Impaired Gastrointestinal Function
Impaired Role Performance
Impaired Sleep
Impaired Tissue Integrity
Pain
Risk for Infection
Risk for Injury

Peritonitis
Altered Temperature
Altered Blood Pressure
Fluid Imbalance
Impaired Gastrointestinal Function
Impaired Respiratory Function
Infection
Inflammation
Nutritionally Compromised
Pain

Pertussis
Altered Temperature
Fluid Imbalance
Impaired Respiratory Function
Infant Feeding Problem
Infection
Inflammation
Nutritionally Compromised
Pain

Placental Abruption
Anxiety
Fluid Imbalance
Impaired Respiratory Function
Impaired Tissue Perfusion
Pain
Risk for Perinatal Problems

Placenta Previa
Anxiety
Difficulty Coping
Fluid Imbalance
Impaired Respiratory Function
Impaired Role Performance
Impaired Tissue Perfusion
Risk for Perinatal Problems
Risk for Injury

Pneumonia
Acid-Base Imbalance
Activity Intolerance
Altered Temperature
Fatigue
Fluid Imbalance
Health Care–Associated Complication
Impaired Immunity
Impaired Respiratory Function
Impaired Sleep

Infection
Nutritionally Compromised
Pain

Pneumothorax

Activity Intolerance
Fatigue
Health Care–Associated Complication
Impaired Cardiac Function
Impaired Respiratory Function
Pain

Poisoning

Acid-Base Imbalance
Electrolyte Imbalance
Fluid Imbalance
Impaired Cognition
Impaired Respiratory Function
Neurologic Problem
Risk for Environment Injury
Risk for Injury

Polycystic Kidney Disease

Acid-Base Imbalance
Activity Intolerance
Altered Blood Pressure
Continuity of Care Problem
Depressed Mood
Difficulty Coping
Electrolyte Imbalance
Fatigue
Fluid Imbalance
Impaired Health Maintenance
Impaired Immunity
Impaired Role Performance
Impaired Urinary Elimination
Negative Self-Image
Risk for Injury

Polycythemia

Fatigue
Impaired Tissue Perfusion
Pain
Risk for Infection
Risk for Injury

Postoperative Care

Activity Intolerance
Altered Glucose Level
Altered Temperature
Electrolyte Imbalance
Fatigue
Fluid Imbalance
Health Care—Associated Complication
Impaired Communication
Impaired Gastrointestinal Function
Impaired Respiratory Function
Impaired Role Performance
Impaired Sleep
Impaired Tissue Integrity
Impaired Tissue Perfusion
Impaired Urinary Elimination
Nutritionally Compromised
Pain
Personal Care Problem
Risk for Clotting
Risk for Infection
Risk for Injury

Postpartum Care

Depressed Mood
Fatigue
Fluid Imbalance
Impaired Bowel Elimination
Impaired Family Function
Impaired Sexual Function
Impaired Sleep
Impaired Tissue Integrity
Impaired Urinary Elimination
Infant Feeding Problem
Negative Self-Image
Nutritionally Compromised
Pain
Parenting Problem
Risk for Infection
Risk for Injury
Risk for Perinatal Problems

Posttraumatic Stress Disorder (PTSD)

Depressed Mood
Difficulty Coping
Impaired Role Performance
Impaired Sleep
Impaired Socialization
Negative Self-Image
Spiritual Problem
Substance Use
Victim of Violence

Preeclampsia

Activity Intolerance
Anxiety
Altered Blood Pressure
Difficulty Coping
Fluid Imbalance
Impaired Family Function
Impaired Tissue Perfusion
Neurologic Problem
Risk for Infection
Risk for Injury
Risk for Perinatal Problems

Pregnancy (Normal)

Continuity of Care Problem
Fatigue
Fluid Imbalance

Impaired Bowel Elimination
Impaired Endocrine Function
Impaired Gastrointestinal Function
Impaired Immunity
Impaired Role Performance
Impaired Sleep
Impaired Urinary Elimination
Nutritionally Compromised
Risk for Infection
Risk for Perinatal Problems

Pregnancy Loss

Anxiety
Decision Conflict
Depressed Mood
Difficulty Coping
Grief
Impaired Family Function
Impaired Role Performance
Impaired Sexual Function
Pain
Risk for Infection
Spiritual Problem

Premature Rupture of Membranes

Anxiety
Difficulty Coping
Infection
Risk for Infection
Risk for Perinatal Problems

Preterm Labor

Anxiety
Decision Conflict
Difficulty Coping
Impaired Endocrine Function
Impaired Family Function
Impaired Sexual Function
Risk for Infection
Risk for Perinatal Problems

Preterm Newborn

Acid-Base Imbalance
Altered Glucose Level
Altered Temperature
Electrolyte Imbalance
Fluid Imbalance
Impaired Cardiac Function
Impaired Family Function
Impaired Gastrointestinal Function
Impaired Growth and Development
Impaired Respiratory Function
Impaired Sleep
Impaired Tissue Integrity
Impaired Tissue Perfusion
Impaired Urinary Elimination
Increased Intracranial Pressure
Infant Feeding Problem
Infection
Neurologic Problem
Nutritionally Compromised
Parenting Problem
Risk for Impaired Skin Integrity
Risk for Infection
Risk for Injury
Sensory Deficit

Pressure Injury

Continuity of Care Problem
Impaired Tissue Integrity
Impaired Tissue Perfusion
Inflammation
Musculoskeletal Problem
Negative Self-Image
Nutritionally Compromised
Pain
Personal Care Problem
Risk for Infection
Sensory Deficit

Prostate Cancer

Continuity of Care Problem
Depressed Mood
Difficulty Coping
Impaired Family Function
Impaired Fertility
Impaired Role Performance
Impaired Sexual Function
Impaired Urinary Elimination
Negative Self-Image
Pain
Risk for Infection

Psoriasis

Difficulty Coping
Impaired Home Maintenance
Impaired Role Performance
Impaired Socialization
Impaired Tissue Integrity
Inflammation
Musculoskeletal Problem
Negative Self-Image
Pain

Pulmonary Edema

Acid-Base Imbalance
Activity Intolerance
Allergy
Electrolyte Imbalance
Fatigue
Fluid Imbalance
Impaired Cardiac Function
Impaired Cognition
Impaired Respiratory Function
Impaired Sleep
Nutritionally Compromised

Pulmonary Embolism
Acid-Base Imbalance
Activity Intolerance
Anxiety
Impaired Cardiac Function
Impaired Cognition
Impaired Respiratory Function
Impaired Sleep
Impaired Tissue Perfusion
Pain
Risk for Clotting
Risk for Infection

Pulmonary Hypertension
Activity Intolerance
Anxiety
Continuity of Care Problem
Fatigue
Fluid Imbalance
Impaired Cardiac Function
Impaired Respiratory Function
Impaired Role Performance
Pain

Pyelonephritis
Altered Temperature
Altered Blood Pressure
Electrolyte Imbalance
Fluid Imbalance
Impaired Urinary Elimination
Infection
Inflammation
Pain

Pyloric Stenosis
Body Weight Problem
Electrolyte Imbalance
Fluid Imbalance
Impaired Growth and Development
Impaired Sleep
Infant Feeding Problem
Nutritionally Compromised
Pain
Risk for Infection

Radiation Therapy
Fatigue
Health Care–Associated Complication
Impaired Bowel Elimination
Impaired Gastrointestinal Function
Impaired Growth and Development
Impaired Fertility
Impaired Immunity
Impaired Tissue Integrity
Inflammation
Pain
Risk of Clotting
Risk of Environment Injury
Risk for Infection

Respiratory Failure, Acute
Acid-Base Imbalance
Activity Intolerance
Anxiety
Fluid Imbalance
Health Care—Associated Complication
Impaired Cardiac Function
Impaired Communication
Impaired Respiratory Function
Musculoskeletal Problem
Nutritionally Compromised
Risk for Infection

Retinal Detachment
Anxiety
Impaired Role Performance
Risk for Injury
Sensory Deficit

Rheumatic Fever, Rheumatic Heart Disease
Activity Intolerance
Altered Blood Pressure
Altered Temperature
Continuity of Care Problem
Impaired Cardiac Function
Impaired Growth and Development
Impaired Respiratory Function
Impaired Tissue Perfusion
Infection
Pain
Risk for Clotting
Risk for Injury

Rheumatoid Arthritis (RA)
Difficulty Coping
Impaired Home Maintenance
Impaired Immunity
Impaired Role Performance
Impaired Socialization
Inflammation
Musculoskeletal Problem
Negative Self-Image
Pain
Personal Care Problem

Schizophrenia
Depressed Mood
Difficulty Coping
Emotional Problem
Health Maintenance Alteration
Impaired Cognition
Impaired Communication

Impaired Family Function
Impaired Psychological Status
Impaired Role Performance
Impaired Socialization
Personal Care Problem

Scleroderma

Impaired Communication
Impaired Immunity
Impaired Tissue Integrity
Negative Self-Image
Nutritionally Compromised
Pain

Scoliosis

Impaired Respiratory Function
Musculoskeletal Problem
Negative Self-Image
Neurologic Problem
Pain
Risk for Injury

Seizure Disorder

Altered Glucose Level
Difficulty Coping
Electrolyte Imbalance
Impaired Respiratory Function
Impaired Role Performance
Impaired Socialization
Increased Intracranial Pressure
Neurologic Problem
Risk for Injury
Substance Use

Sepsis/Septic Shock

Acid-Base Imbalance
Altered Blood Pressure
Altered Temperature
Electrolyte Imbalance
Fluid Imbalance
Impaired Cardiac Function
Impaired Cognition
Impaired Urinary Function
Impaired Tissue Perfusion
Infection
Nutritionally Compromised
Risk for Clotting
Risk for Impaired Skin Integrity
Risk for Injury

Sexual Assault

Difficulty Coping
Impaired Sexual Function
Negative Self-Image
Risk for Infection
Spiritual Problem
Victim of Violence

Sexually Transmitted Infections (STI)

Altered Temperature
Difficulty Coping
Impaired Fertility
Impaired Sexual Function
Infection
Pain
Risk for Disease
Risk for Perinatal Problems

Short Bowel Syndrome

Body Weight Problem
Electrolyte Imbalance
Fluid Imbalance
Impaired Elimination
Impaired Gastrointestinal Function
Impaired Growth and Development
Nutritionally Compromised
Risk for Impaired Skin Integrity

Sickle Cell Disease

Activity Intolerance
Altered Temperature
Continuity of Care Problem
Difficulty Coping
Fluid Imbalance
Impaired Growth and Development
Impaired Respiratory Function
Impaired Tissue Perfusion
Musculoskeletal Problem
Pain
Negative Self-Image
Risk for Clotting
Risk for Infection

Spinal Cord Injury (SCI)

Altered Blood Pressure
Caregiver Role Strain
Depressed Mood
Difficulty Coping
Grief
Impaired Bowel Elimination
Impaired Musculoskeletal Function
Impaired Respiratory Function
Impaired Role Performance
Impaired Sexual Function
Impaired Urinary Elimination
Musculoskeletal Problem
Neurologic Problem
Personal Care Problem
Risk for Clotting
Risk for Impaired Skin Integrity
Risk for Injury
Sensory Deficit
Spiritual Problem

Spinal Cord Tumors

Depressed Mood
Difficulty Coping
Impaired Bowel Elimination
Impaired Musculoskeletal Function
Impaired Respiratory Function
Impaired Role Performance
Impaired Sexual Function
Impaired Urinary Elimination
Musculoskeletal Problem
Neurologic Problem
Pain
Risk for Injury
Sensory Deficit

Stomach Cancer

Continuity of Care Problem
Difficulty Coping
Fluid Imbalance
Impaired Gastrointestinal Function
Impaired Tissue Integrity
Nutritionally Compromised
Pain

Stroke

Acid-Base Imbalance
Altered Blood Pressure
Altered Glucose Level
Altered Temperature
Caregiver Role Strain
Continuity of Care Problem
Difficulty Coping
Emotional Problem
Impaired Cognition
Impaired Communication
Impaired Gastrointestinal Function
Impaired Psychological Status
Impaired Respiratory Function
Impaired Role Performance
Impaired Sexual Function
Impaired Socialization
Impaired Tissue Perfusion
Increased Intracranial Pressure
Musculoskeletal Problem
Negative Self-Image
Neurologic Problem
Nutritionally Compromised
Personal Care Problem
Risk for Impaired Skin Integrity
Risk for Injury
Sensory Deficit

Substance Withdrawal

Acid-Base Imbalance
Continuity of Care Problem
Difficulty Coping
Impaired Cognition
Impaired Psychological Status
Impaired Sleep
Neurologic Problem
Personal Care Problem
Risk for Injury
Substance Use
Violent Behavior

Suicide, Risk for/Attempted

Anxiety
Depressed Mood
Difficulty Coping
Emotional Problem
Health Maintenance Alteration
Impaired Family Function
Impaired Psychological Status
Impaired Role Performance
Impaired Sleep
Negative Self-Image
Spiritual Problem
Victim of Violence
Violent Behavior

Syncope

Altered Blood Pressure
Altered Glucose Level
Fluid Imbalance
Impaired Cardiac Function
Impaired Tissue Perfusion
Neurologic Problem
Risk for Injury
Sensory Deficit

Syndrome of Inappropriate Antidiuretic Hormone (SIADH)

Altered Blood Pressure
Electrolyte Imbalance
Fluid Imbalance
Impaired Cardiac Function
Impaired Cognition
Impaired Endocrine Function
Neurologic Problem
Risk for Injury

Syphilis

Difficulty Coping
Impaired Fertility
Impaired Sexual Function
Infection
Pain
Risk for Disease
Risk for Perinatal Problems

Systemic Inflammatory Response Syndrome (SIRS)/Multiple Organ Dysfunction Syndrome (MODS)

Acid-Base Imbalance
Altered Blood Pressure
Electrolyte Imbalance

Fluid Imbalance
Impaired Cardiac Function
Impaired Cognition
Impaired Respiratory Function
Impaired Tissue Perfusion
Impaired Urinary Elimination
Neurologic Problem
Nutritionally Compromised
Personal Care Problem
Risk for Clotting
Risk for Injury

Systemic Lupus Erythematosus (SLE)

Activity Intolerance
Caregiver Role Strain
Difficulty Coping
Fatigue
Impaired Cognition
Impaired Communication
Impaired Immunity
Impaired Role Performance
Impaired Tissue Integrity
Impaired Urinary Elimination
Inflammation
Musculoskeletal Problem
Negative Self-Image
Neurologic Problem
Nutritionally Compromised
Pain
Personal Care Problem
Risk for Clotting
Risk for Infection

Testicular Cancer

Continuity of Care Problem
Depressed Mood
Difficulty Coping
Impaired Fertility
Impaired Role Performance
Impaired Sexual Function
Impaired Tissue Integrity
Negative Self-Image
Pain
Risk for Infection

Thalassemia

Activity Intolerance
Continuity of Care Problem
Impaired Tissue Perfusion
Pain
Risk for Infection

Thoracic Surgery

Activity Intolerance
Altered Blood Pressure
Fatigue
Health Care–Associated Complication
Impaired Cardiac Function
Impaired Respiratory Function
Impaired Sleep
Impaired Tissue Integrity
Impaired Tissue Perfusion
Musculoskeletal Problem
Pain
Personal Care Problem
Risk for Clotting
Risk for Infection
Risk for Injury

Thromboangiitis Obliterans

Impaired Tissue Perfusion
Inflammation
Pain
Risk for Impaired Skin Integrity
Risk for Injury

Thrombocytopenia

Impaired Tissue Perfusion
Pain
Risk for Injury

Thyroid Cancer

Altered Temperature
Continuity of Care Problem
Difficulty Coping
Fatigue
Impaired Endocrine Function
Impaired Respiratory Function
Impaired Tissue Integrity
Risk for Infection

Thyroidectomy

Altered Temperature
Continuity of Care Problem
Difficulty Coping
Electrolyte Imbalance
Fatigue
Impaired Communication
Impaired Endocrine Function
Impaired Respiratory Function
Impaired Sleep
Impaired Tissue Integrity
Nutritionally Compromised
Pain
Risk for Infection

Tonsillectomy/Adenoidectomy

Altered Temperature
Fluid Imbalance
Impaired Respiratory Function
Impaired Sleep
Impaired Tissue Integrity
Infant Feeding Problem
Pain
Risk for Infection

Tracheoesophageal Fistula/Esophageal Atresia

Fluid Imbalance
Impaired Communication
Impaired Gastrointestinal Function
Impaired Respiratory Function
Impaired Tissue Integrity
Infant Feeding Problem
Nutritionally Compromised
Risk for Infection
Risk for Injury

Tracheostomy

Continuity of Care Problem
Difficulty Coping
Health Care–Associated Complication
Health Maintenance Alteration
Impaired Communication
Impaired Respiratory Function
Impaired Socialization
Impaired Tissue Integrity
Negative Self-Image
Nutritionally Compromised
Risk for Infection
Risk for Injury

Traumatic Brain Injury (Acute)

Caregiver Role Strain
Difficulty Coping
Emotional Problem
Impaired Cognition
Impaired Family Function
Impaired Growth and Development
Impaired Psychological Status
Impaired Respiratory Function
Impaired Role Performance
Increased Intracranial Pressure
Neurologic Problem
Personal Care Problem
Risk for Injury
Violent Behavior

Transient Ischemic Attack

Altered Blood Pressure
Altered Glucose Level
Impaired Cognition
Impaired Tissue Perfusion
Increased Intracranial Pressure
Neurologic Problem
Risk for Injury
Sensory Deficit

Trigeminal Neuralgia

Difficulty Coping
Neurologic Problem
Nutritionally Compromised
Pain

Tuberculosis

Activity Intolerance
Altered Temperature
Continuity of Care Problem
Fatigue
Health Maintenance Alteration
Impaired Respiratory Function
Impaired Role Performance
Impaired Sleep
Infection
Inflammation
Nutritionally Compromised

Ulcerative Colitis

Difficulty Coping
Fatigue
Fluid Imbalance
Impaired Bowel Elimination
Impaired Gastrointestinal Function
Impaired Socialization
Inflammation
Nutritionally Compromised
Pain

Upper Respiratory Infection (Croup, Pharyngitis, Tonsillitis)

Altered Temperature
Fluid Imbalance
Impaired Respiratory Function
Impaired Sleep
Infant Feeding Problem
Infection
Inflammation
Nutritionally Compromised
Risk for Infection

Urethritis

Altered Temperature
Impaired Sexual Function
Impaired Urinary Elimination
Infection
Inflammation
Pain

Urinary Catheterization

Health Care–Associated Complication
Health Maintenance Alteration
Impaired Urinary Elimination
Neurologic Problem
Pain
Risk for Infection

Urinary Incontinence

Impaired Role Performance
Impaired Urinary Elimination
Negative Self-Image

Personal Care Problem
Risk for Impaired Skin Integrity
Risk for Infection

Urinary Retention

Impaired Urinary Elimination
Neurologic Problem
Risk for Infection

Urinary Tract Calculi

Fluid Imbalance
Impaired Urinary Elimination
Pain
Risk for Infection

Urinary Tract Infections (UTIs)

Altered Blood Pressure
Altered Temperature
Electrolyte Imbalance
Fluid Imbalance
Impaired Urinary Elimination
Infection
Pain

Urologic Surgery

Difficulty Coping
Fluid Imbalance
Health Care–Associated Complication
Impaired Respiratory Function
Impaired Sexual Function
Impaired Tissue Integrity
Impaired Urinary Elimination
Negative Self-Image
Pain
Risk for Infection
Risk for Injury

Vaginal, Cervical, Vulvar Infections

Altered Temperature
Difficulty Coping
Impaired Fertility
Impaired Sexual Function
Impaired Urinary Elimination
Infection
Negative Self-Image
Pain
Risk for Disease
Risk for Perinatal Problems

Valvular Heart Disease

Activity Intolerance
Anxiety
Continuity of Care Problem
Fatigue
Fluid Imbalance
Impaired Cardiac Function
Impaired Respiratory Function
Impaired Tissue Perfusion
Risk for Clotting
Risk for Infection

Varicose Veins

Activity Intolerance
Impaired Tissue Perfusion
Negative Self-Image
Pain
Risk for Clotting
Risk for Impaired Skin Integrity

Venous Thromboembolism (VTE)/Deep Vein Thrombosis (DVT)

Activity Intolerance
Altered Blood Pressure
Health Care–Associated Complication
Impaired Cardiac Function
Impaired Respiratory Function
Impaired Tissue Integrity
Impaired Tissue Perfusion
Inflammation
Musculoskeletal Problem
Pain
Risk for Clotting
Risk for Impaired Skin Integrity
Risk for Injury

Warts, Genital

Difficulty Coping
Impaired Fertility
Impaired Sexual Function
Impaired Tissue Integrity
Impaired Urinary Elimination
Infection
Negative Self-Image
Pain
Risk for Disease
Risk for Perinatal Problems

Wound/Ulcer, Chronic

Continuity of Care Problem
Impaired Tissue Integrity
Impaired Tissue Perfusion
Infection
Inflammation
Nutritionally Compromised
Musculoskeletal Problem
Pain
Risk for Infection
Risk for Injury
Sensory Deficit

Bibliography

General

Ball JW, Dains JE Flynn JA, Solomon BS, Stewart R. *Seidel's Guide to Physical Examination*, ed 10. St. Louis: Elsevier; 2022.

Butcher H, Bulechek G, Dochterman J, Wagner, M: *Nursing Interventions Classification*, ed 7. St. Louis: Elsevier Health Sciences; 2018.

Ferri F. *Ferri's Clinical Advisor 2023*. St. Louis: Elsevier; 2023.

Giddens J. *Concepts for Nursing Practice*, ed 4. St. Louis: Elsevier; 2023.

Halter MJ. *Varcarolis' Foundations of Psychiatric-Mental Health Nursing: A Clinical Approach*, ed 9. St. Louis: Elsevier Health Sciences; 2022.

Harding M, Kwong J, Hagler D, Reinisch C, eds. *Lewis's Medical-Surgical Nursing: Assessment and Management of Clinical Problems*, ed 12. St. Louis: Elsevier Health Sciences; 2022.

Hartjes T. *AACN's Core Curriculum for Progressive and Critical Care Nursing*. St. Louis: Elsevier; 2022.

Makic MB, Martinez-Kratz M. *Nursing Diagnosis Handbook: An Evidence-Based Guide to Planning Care*, ed 13. St. Louis: Mosby-Elsevier; 2023.

Mosby's Dictionary of Medicine, Nursing, & Health Professions, ed 11. St. Louis: Elsevier Health Sciences; 2021.

Pagana KD, Pagana TJ, Pagana TN. *Mosby's Manual of Diagnostic and Laboratory Tests*, ed 16. St. Louis: Elsevier Health Sciences; 2023.

Perry SE, Hockenberry MJ, Cashion MC, Alden KR, Olshansky EF. *Maternal Child Nursing Care*, ed 7. St. Louis: Elsevier Health Sciences; 2023.

Potter PA, Perry AG, Stockert PA, Hall A. *Fundamentals of Nursing*, ed 11. St. Louis: Elsevier Health Sciences; 2023.

Raymond JL, Morrow K. *Krause and Mahan's Food and the Nutrition Care Process*, ed 23. St. Louis: Elsevier, 2023.

Touhy T, Jett K. *Ebersole and Hess' Gerontologic Nursing and Healthy Aging*, ed 6. St. Louis: Elsevier Health Sciences; 2022.

Urden LD, Stacy KM, Lough ME. *Critical Care Nursing*, ed 9. St. Louis: Elsevier; 2022.

Yoost B, Crawford LR. *Fundamentals of Nursing*, ed 3. St. Louis: Elsevier Health Sciences; 2023.

Concept Specific

Acid-Base Balance

- Bruno JJ, Canada T, Canada N, Tucker A. *ASPEN Fluids, Electrolytes, and Acid-Base Disorders Handbook*, ed 2. Silver Spring: Aspen; 2020.
- Bergman M, Miyakawa L, Lee YI. Acid–base disorders. *Mount Sinai Expert Guides: Critical Care*. 2021;Jan 19:537.
- Tinawi M. Respiratory acid-base disorders: respiratory acidosis and respiratory alkalosis. *Arch Clin Biomed Res*. 2021;5:158.
- Tinawi M. Pathophysiology, evaluation, and management of metabolic alkalosis. *Cureus*. 2021;13.

Anxiety

- Álvarez-García C, Yaban ZŞ. The effects of preoperative guided imagery interventions on preoperative anxiety and postoperative pain: a meta-analysis. *Complementary Therapies [AE1]in Clinical Practice*. 2020;38:101077.
- Beck AT, Epstein N, Brown G, Steer RA. An inventory for measuring clinical anxiety: psychometric properties. *Journal of Consulting and Clinical Psychology*. 1988;56:893.
- Sampaio F, Gonçalves P, Parola V, Sequeira C, Lluch Canut T. Nursing process addressing the focus "anxiety": a scoping review. *Clinical Nursing Research*. 2021;30: 001.
- Weathers F. Posttraumatic stress disorder checklist. In Reyes G, Elhai JD, Ford J (eds): *Encyclopedia of Psychological Trauma*. Hoboken, NJ: Wiley, 2008.

Care Coordination

- Anderson A, Hewner S. Care coordination: a concept analysis examining the value nursing brings to this critical clinical role. *The American Journal of Nursing*. 2021;121:30.
- Joo JY, Liu MF. The experience of chronic illness transitional care: a qualitative systematic review. *Clinical Nursing Research*. 2022;31: 163.
- New York State Department of Health. *Suggested model for transitional care planning*. Retrieved from https://www.health.ny.gov/professionals/patients/discharge_planning /discharge_transition.htm.
- Peart A, Barton C, Lewis V, Russell G. A state-of-the-art review of the experience of care coordination interventions for people living with multimorbidity. *Journal of Clinical Nursing*. 2020; 29:1445.

Clotting

- Alblaihed L, Dubbs SB, Koyfman A. Long B. High risk and low prevalence diseases: Hemophilia emergencies. *The American Journal of Emergency Medicine*. 2022;56:21.
- Etxeandia-Ikobaltzeta I, Zhang Y, Brundisini F, Florez ID, Wiercioch W, Nieuwlaat R, et al. Patient values and preferences regarding VTE disease: a systematic review to inform American Society of Hematology guidelines. *Blood Advances*. 2022;4:953.
- Hu J, Geng Y, Ma J, Dong X, Fang S, Tian J. The best evidence for the prevention and management of lower extremity deep venous thrombosis after gynecological malignant tumor surgery: a systematic review and network meta-analysis. *Frontiers in Surgery*. 2022;9:841275.
- Nemetski S, Ip A, Josephs J, Hellmann M. Clotting events among hospitalized patients infected with COVID-19 in a large multisite cohort in the United States. *PLoS One*. 2022;17:e0262352.

Cognition

- Borson S, Scanlan J, Brush M, et al. The Mini-Cog: a cognitive "vital signs" measure for dementia screening in multi-lingual elderly. *International Journal of Geriatric Psychiatry*. 2000;15:1021.
- Eagles D, Cheung WJ, Avlijas T, Yadav K, Ohle R, Taljaard M, et al. Barriers and facilitators to nursing delirium screening in older emergency patients: a qualitative study using the theoretical domains framework. *Age and Ageing*, 2022;51:1.
- ldwikat RK, Manias E, Tomlinson E, Amin M, Nicholson P. Delirium screening tools in the post-anaesthetic care unit: a systematic review and meta-analysis. *Aging Clinical and Experimental Research*. 2022; 34:1225.

- Inouye S, van Dyck C, Alessi C, et al. Clarifying confusion: the Confusion Assessment Method. *Annals of Internal Medicine* 1990; 113:941.
- Wolff L, Benge J. Everyday language difficulties in Parkinson's disease: caregiver description and relationship with cognition, activities of daily living, and motor disability. *American Journal of Speech-Language Pathology*. 2019;28:165.

Communication

- Fogelson D, Brown BB, Gustin T, Goode V. Hearing impaired older adults in the acute care setting: an innovation solution to improve care. *Geriatric Nursing*. 2022;44:272.
- Happ MB. Giving voice: nurse-patient communication in the intensive care unit. *American Journal of Critical Care*. 2021;30:256.
- Lam W, Wong FY, Chan AE. Factors affecting the levels of satisfaction with nurse-patient communication among oncology patients. *Cancer Nursing*. 2020;43:E186.

Culture

- Dorrance Hall E, Ma M, Azimova D, Campbell N, Ellithorpe M, Plasencia J, et al. The mediating role of family and cultural food beliefs on the relationship between family communication patterns and diet and health issues across racial/ethnic groups. *Health Communication*. 2021, 36:593.
- Mayes J, Castle EM, Greenwood J, et al. Cultural influences on physical activity and exercise beliefs in patients with chronic kidney disease: 'The Culture-CKD Study'—a qualitative study. *BMJ Open*. 2022;12:e046950. doi:10.1136/ bmjopen-2020-046950
- Narayan MC, Mallinson RK. Transcultural nurse views on culture-sensitive/patient-centered assessment and care planning: a descriptive study. *Journal of Transcultural Nursing*. 2022;33:150.

Development

- Macdonald SH, Travers J, Shé ÉN, Bailey J, Romero-Ortuno R, Keyes M, et al. Primary care interventions to address physical frailty among community-dwelling adults aged 60 years or older: a meta-analysis. *PLoS One*. 2020;15:e0228821.
- Smith KA, Samuels AE. A scoping review of parental roles in rehabilitation interventions for children with developmental delay, disability, or long-term health condition. *Research in Developmental Disabilities*. 2021;111:103887.
- Studzińska K, Studnicki R, Adamczewski T, Hansdorfer-Korzon R. Criteria for diagnosis and evaluation of frailty syndrome. *Journal of Health Study and Medicine*. 2021;3:5.
- Tam W, Poon SN, Mahendran R, Kua EH, Wu XV. The effectiveness of reminiscence-based intervention on improving psychological well-being in cognitively intact older adults: a systematic review and meta-analysis. *International Journal of Nursing Studies*. 2021;114:103847.
- Tang MN, Adolphe S, Rogers SR, Frank DA. Failure to thrive or growth faltering: medical, developmental/behavioral, nutritional, and social dimensions. *Pediatrics in Review*. 2021;42:590.
- Zuair AA, Sopory P. Effects of media health literacy school-based interventions on adolescents' body image concerns, eating concerns, and thin-internalization attitudes: a systematic review and meta-analysis. *Health Communication*. 2022;37:20.

Elimination

- Desprez C, Turmel N, Chesnel C, Mistry P, Tamiatto M, Haddad R, et al. Comparison of clinical and paraclinical characteristics of patients with urge, mixed, and passive fecal incontinence: a systematic literature review. *International Journal of Colorectal Disease*. 2020;36:633.
- Dunlap JJ, Dunlap BS. Constipation. *Gastroenterology Nursing*. 2021;44:361.
- Lane, Hagan K, Erekson E, Minassian VA, Grodstein F, Bynum J. Patient-provider discussions about urinary incontinence among older women. *The Journals of Gerontology. Series A, Biological Sciences and Medical Sciences*. 2021;76:463.
- Sussman SR, Brucker BM. Guideline of guidelines: urinary incontinence in women. *BJU International*. 2020;125:638.

Family Dynamics

- Gregory M, Kannis-Dymand L, Sharman R. A review of attachment-based parenting interventions: recent advances and future considerations. *Australian Journal of Psychology*. 2020;72:109.
- Shorey S, Ng ED. The efficacy of mindful parenting interventions: a systematic review and meta-analysis. *International Journal of Nursing Studies*. 2021;121:103996.
- Walker DK. Parenting and social determinants of health. *Archives of Psychiatric Nursing*. 2021;35:134.

Fatigue

- Alleva JM, Tylka TL. Body functionality: a review of the literature. *Body Image*. 2021;36:149.
- Hersche R, Roser K, Weise A, Michel G, Barbero M. Fatigue self-management education in persons with disease-related fatigue: a comprehensive review of the effectiveness on fatigue and quality of life. *Patient Education and Counseling*. 2021;105:1362.
- Lerdal A. Fatigue Severity Scale. *Encyclopedia of Quality of Life and Well-Being Research*. 2021;Nov 1.
- Loades ME, Chalder T. Chronic fatigue in the context of pediatric physical and mental illness. *Mental Health and Illness of Children and Adolescents*. 2020:1.

Fluids and Electrolytes

- Alexander M, Gorski L, Vizcarra C, Perucca R, Czaplewski L. *Infusion Nursing*, ed 3. St. Louis: Elsevier Health Sciences; 2020.
- Bruno JJ, Canada T, Canada N, Tucker A. *ASPEN Fluids, Electrolytes, and Acid-Base Disorders Handbook*, ed 2. Silver Spring: Aspen; 2020.
- Bruno C, Collier A, Holyday M, Lambert K. Interventions to improve hydration in older adults: a systematic review and meta-analysis. *Nutrients*. 2021;13:3640.
- Reintam Blaser A, van Zanten AR, de Man AM. Electrolytes in the ICU. *Annual Update in Intensive Care and Emergency Medicine*. 2022;183.

Functional Ability

- Buma LE, Vluggen S, Zwakhalen S, Kempen GI, Metzelthin SF. Effects on clients' daily functioning and common features of reablement interventions: a systematic literature review. *European Journal of Ageing*. 2022;3: 1.
- Edemekong PF, Bomgaars DL, Sukumaran S, Levy SB. Activities of daily living. Retrieved from https://www.ncbi.nlm.nih.gov/books/NBK470404/.
- Hartford Institute for Geriatric Nursing. Assessment Tools for Best Practices of Care for Older Adults. Retrieved from https://hign.org/consultgeri/try-this/general-assessment.
- Motamed-Jahromi M, Kaveh MH. Effective interventions on improving elderly's independence in activity of daily living: a systematic review and logic model. *Frontiers in Public Health*. 2021;8:824.

- Patrizio E, Calvani R, Marzetti E, Cesari M. Physical functional assessment in older adults. *The Journal of Frailty & Aging*. 2021; 10:141.
- Williams T, Lakhani A, Spelten E. Interventions to reduce loneliness and social isolation in rural settings: a mixed- methods review. *Journal of Rural Studies*. 2022;90:76.

Gas Exchange

- Feng Z, Wang J, Xie Y, Li J. Effects of exercise-based pulmonary rehabilitation on adults with asthma: a systematic review and meta-analysis. *Respiratory Research*. 2021;22:33.
- Gol RM, Rafraf M. Association between abdominal obesity and pulmonary function in apparently healthy adults: a systematic review. *Obesity Research & Clinical Practice*. 2021;15:415.
- Rosenberg K. High-flow nasal oxygen vs. noninvasive ventilation or conventional oxygen therapy in acute respiratory failure. *AJN*. 2021;121: 55.
- Vieira LF, Fernandes VR, Papathanassoglou E, Azzolin K de O. Accuracy of defining characteristics for nursing diagnoses related to patients with respiratory deterioration. *International Journal of Nursing Knowledge*. 2020;31:262.

Glucose Regulation

- American Diabetes Association. Standards of medical care in diabetes 2022. *Diabetes Care*. 2022;45:Suppl 1.
- Teo HN, Tam W, Koh S. Effectiveness of continuous glucose monitoring in maintaining glycaemic control among people with type 1 diabetes mellitus: a systematic review of randomised controlled trials and meta-analysis. *Diabetologia*. 2022;65(4):604-619. https://doi.org/10.1007/s00125-021-05648-4.

Health Equity

- PRAPARE. Retrieved from: http://www.nachc.org/wp-content/uploads/2019/04/NACHC_PRAPARE_Full-Toolkit.pdf
- Kuehnert P, Fawcett J, DePriest K, Chinn P, Cousin L, Ervin N, et al. Defining the social determinants of health for nursing action to achieve health equity: a consensus paper from the American Academy of Nursing. *Nursing Outlook*. 2022;70:10.
- U.S. Department of Health and Human Services, Office of Disease Prevention and Health Promotion. *Healthy People 2030*. Retrieved from https://health.gov/healthypeople/priority-areas/health-equity-healthy-people-2030
    - Wakefield MK, Williams DR, Le Menestrel S, Flaubert JL. *The fute of nursing 2020-2030: Charting a path to achieve health equity*. 2021; The National Academies Press.

Health Promotion

- Moon RY, Carlin RF, Hand I; AAP Task Force on Sudden Infant Death; AAP Committee on Fetus and Newborn. Evidence base for 2022 updated recommendations for a safe infant sleeping environment to reduce the risk of sleep-related infant deaths. *Pediatrics*. 2022;150(1):e2022057991.
- U.S. Department of Health and Human Services, Office of Disease Prevention and Health Promotion. *Healthy People 2030*. Retrieved from https://health.gov/healthypeople/priority-areas/health-equity-healthy-people-2030.

Hormonal Regulation

- Cruz-Flores S. Neurological complications of endocrine emergencies. *Current Neurology and Neuroscience Reports*. 2021;21:1.
- Doherty AM, Dinneen SF. Depression across endocrine disorders. *Mental Health, Diabetes and Endocrinology*. 2021;Oct 28:7.
- Nasrullah A, Azharuddin S, Young M, Kejas A, Dumont T. Endocrine emergencies in the medical intensive care unit. *Critical Care Nursing Quarterly*. 2022;45:266.
- Salvador J, Gutierrez G, Llavero M, Gargallo J, Escalada J, López J. Endocrine disorders and psychiatric manifestations. *Endocrinology and Systemic Diseases*. 2021:311.

Immunity

- American Academy of Allergy Asthma & Immunology: Food allergy. Retrieved from https://www.aaaai.org/Conditions-Treatments/Allergies/Food-Allergy.
- American Academy of Allergy Asthma & Immunology: Anaphylaxis. Retrieved from https://www.aaaai.org/conditions-treatments/allergies/anaphylaxis.
- Barrea L, Muscogiuri G, Frias-Toral E, Laudisio D, Pugliese G, Castellucci B, et al. Nutrition and immune system: from the Mediterranean diet to dietary supplementary through the microbiota. *Critical Reviews in Food Science and Nutrition*. 2021;61:3066.
- Baveja UK, Mehta Y. *Prevention of Healthcare Associated Infections: Infection Prevention and Control*. New Delhi: Jaypee Brothers; 2021.
- Centers for Disease Control and Prevention. Preventing allergic reactions to natural rubber latex in the workplace. Retrieved from http://www.cdc.gov/niosh/docs/97-135/pdfs/97-135.pdf.
- Muraro A, Worm M, Alviani C, Cardona V, Dunn Galvin A, Garvey LH, et al. EAACI guidelines: anaphylaxis. *Allergy: European Journal of Allergy and Clinical Immunology*. 2022;77:357.
- Rossi CM, Lenti MV, Di Sabatino A. Adult anaphylaxis: a state-of-the-art review. *European Journal of Internal Medicine*. 2022:100;5.

Infection

- Berkley JA: Bacterial infections and nutrition: a primer. *Nutrition and Infectious Diseases* 2021;9:113.
- Centers for Disease Control and Prevention: Healthcare-associated infections. Retrieved from www.cdc.gov/HAI.
- Centers for Disease Control and Prevention: Transmission-based precautions. Retrieved from https://www.cdc.gov/infectioncontrol/basics/transmission-based-precautions.html.
- Wilson J. *Infection Control in Clinical Practice*, ed 3. St. Louis: Elsevier Health Sciences; 2019.

Inflammation

- Bautmans I, Salimans L, Njemini R, Beyer I, Lieten S, Liberman K. The effects of exercise interventions on the inflammatory profile of older adults: a systematic review of the recent literature. *Experimental Gerontology*. 2021;146:111236.
- Givens DL, McMorris M. Rehabilitation of musculoskeletal injuries. *Clinical Foundations of Musculoskeletal Medicine*. 2021;255.
- Hannoodee S, Nasuruddin DN. Acute inflammatory response. Retrieved from https://www.ncbi.nlm.nih.gov/books/NBK556083/.
- Upadhyay A, Amanullah A, Joshi V, Dhiman R, Prajapati VK, Poluri KM, Mishra A. Ibuprofen-based advanced therapeutics: breaking the inflammatory link in cancer, neurodegeneration, and diseases. *Drug Metabolism Reviews*. 2021;53:100.

Interpersonal Violence

- AHRQ. Intimate partner violence screening. Retrieved from: https://www.ahrq.gov/ncepcr/tools/healthier-pregnancy/fact-sheets/partner-violence.html.
- Cleek EA, Totka JP, Sheets LK, Mersky JP, Haglund KA. Helping nurses identify and report sentinel injuries of child abuse in infants. *Pediatric Nursing*. 2022;48:123.

- Joint Commission. De-escalation in health care. Retrieved from: https://www.jointcommission.org/resources/news-and-multimedia/newsletters/newsletters/quick-safety/quick-safety-47-deescalation-in-health-care/#.YpvIlqjMJPY
- Mancini MA. Integrated behavioral health approaches to interpersonal violence. *Integrated Behavioral Health Practice*. 2021:155.
- Saxton A, Resnick P. Patient violence. *Malpractice and Liability in Psychiatry*. 2022:97.
- Shirdel H, Ghasempour S, Esmaeili Shandiz E, Shamabadi R, Dolatabadi Z, Attaei Nakhaei AR, et al. Prevalence and risk factors for parental violence against children: a review study. *International Journal of Pediatrics*. 2021;9:13127.
- Stapleton S, Bradford J, Horigan A, Barnason S, Foley A, Johnson M, et al. Clinical practice guideline: Intimate partner violence. *Journal of Emergency Nursing*. 2019;45:191.
- Whiting D, Lichtenstein P, Fazel S. Violence and mental disorders: a structured review of associations by individual diagnoses, risk factors, and risk assessment. *The Lancet Psychiatry*. 2021; 8:150.

Intracranial Regulation

- Kolmos M, Christoffersen L, Kruuse C. Recurrent ischemic stroke – a systematic review and meta-analysis. *Journal of Stroke and Cerebrovascular Disease*. 2021;30:105935.
- Norager NH, Olsen MH, Pedersen SH, Riedel CS, Czosnyka M, Juhler M. Reference values for intracranial pressure and lumbar cerebrospinal fluid pressure: a systematic review. *Fluids and Barriers of the CNS*. 2021:18:19.
- Sacco TL, Davis JG. Management of intracranial pressure part II: Nonpharmacologic interventions. *Dimensions of Critical Care Nursing*, 2019;38:61.

Mobility

- Boynton T, Kumpar D,VanGilder C. The Bedside Mobility Assessment Tool 2.0. *American Nurse*. 2020;15.
- Coppola C, Lizardi V, Ribsam V. Mobility. *Orthopaedic Nursing*. 2021:40 4.
- Delgado B, Novo A, Lopes I, Rebelo C, Almeida C, Pestan S, et al. The effects of early rehabilitation on functional exercise tolerance in decompensated heart failure patients: results of a multicenter randomized controlled trial (ERIC-HF study). *Clinical Rehabilitation*. 2022;36:813.
- Jones RA, Merkle S, Ruvalcaba L, Ashton P, Bailey C, Lopez M. Nurse-led mobility program: driving a culture of early mobilization in medical-surgical nursing. *Journal of Nursing Care Quality*. 2020;35:2026.
- Katsi V, Georgiopoulos G, Mitropoulou P, Kontoangelos K, Kollia Z, Tzavara C, et al. Exercise tolerance and quality of life in patients with known or suspected coronary artery disease. *Quality of Life Research*. 2021;30:2541.
- Olson L , Zonsius M , Rodriguez-Morales G, Emery-Tiburcio E. Promoting safe mobility. *AJN, American Journal of Nursing*. 2022;122:46.

Mood and Affect

- American Foundation for Suicide Prevention. Retrieved from https://afsp.org/.
- Fineberg NA, Hollander E, Pallanti S, Walitza S, Grünblatt E, Dell'Osso BM, et al. Clinical advances in obsessive-compulsive disorder: a position statement by the International College of Obsessive-Compulsive Spectrum Disorders. *International Clinical Psychopharmacology*. 2020;35:173.
- Hoare E, Collins S, Marx W, Callaly E, Moxham-Smith R, Cuijpers P, et al. Universal depression prevention: an umbrella review of meta-analyses. *Journal of Psychiatric Research*. 2021; 144:483.
- Lee EE, Bangen KJ, Avanzino JA, Hou B, Ramsey M, Eglit G, et al. Outcomes of randomized clinical trials of interventions to enhance social, emotional, and spiritual components of wisdom: a systematic review and meta-analysis. *JAMA Psychiatry*. 2020; 77:925.
- National Alliance on Mental Illness. Retrieved from https://www.nami.org/#.
- National Institute of Mental Health. Retrieved from https://www.nimh.nih.gov/index.shtml.

Nutrition

- American Academy of Pediatrics. Breastfeeding. Retrieved from https://www.aap.org/breastfeeding.
- Cristina NM, Lucia DA. Nutrition and healthy aging: Prevention and treatment of gastrointestinal diseases. *Nutrients*. 2021; 13:4337.
- Malone A, Mogensen KM. Key approaches to diagnosing malnutrition in adults. *Nutrition in Clinical Practice*. 2022;37:23.
- NIDDK. Weight management. Retrieved from https://www.niddk.nih.gov/health-information/weight-management.
- Schuetz P, Seres D, Lobo DN, Gomes F, Kaegi-Braun N, Stanga Z. Management of disease-related malnutrition for patients being treated in hospital. *The Lancet*. 2021;398:1927.
- USDA. Dietary guidelines for Americans 2020-2025. Retrieved from: https://www.dietaryguidelines.gov/resources/2020-2025-dietary-guidelines-online-materials.

Pain

- Amaechi O, Huffman MM, Featherstone K. Pharmacologic therapy for acute pain. *American Family Physician*. 2021;104:63.
- Centers for Disease Control and Prevention. Opioid prescribing guideline resources. Retrieved from https://www.cdc.gov/opioids/providers/prescribing/index.html.
- Czarnecki M, Turner HN. *Core Curriculum for Pain Management Nursing*. St. Louis: Elsevier; 2018.
- Gülnar E, Özveren H, Tüzer H, Yılmazer T. An investigation of pain beliefs, pain coping, and spiritual well-being in surgical patients. *Journal of Religion and Health*. 2021;Jul 16:1.
- International Association for the Study of Pain. Retrieved from https://www.iasp-pain.org/.
- Joint Commission. Pain management standards for accredited organizations. Retrieved from https://www.jointcommission.org/resources/patient-safety-topics/pain-management-standards-for-accredited-organizations/.

Palliative Care

- American Association of Colleges of Nursing. CARES: Competencies and recommendations for educating undergraduate nursing students: Preparing nurses to care for the seriously ill and their families. Retrieved from https://www.aacnnursing.org/Portals/42/ELNEC/PDF/New-Palliative-Care-Competencies.pdf.
- Balante J, Broek D, White K. Mixed-methods systematic review: Cultural attitudes, beliefs and practices of internationally educated nurses towards end-of-life care in the context of cancer. *Journal of Advanced Nursing*, 2021;77(9):3618-3629. https://doi.org/10.1111/jan.14814.
- World Health Organization. *Palliative care*. Retrieved from https://www.who.int/news-room/fact-sheets/detail/palliative-care.

Patient Education

- Agency for Healthcare Research and Quality. *Health Literacy Measurement Tools (Revised)*. Retrieved from: https://www.ahrq.gov/health-literacy/quality-resources/tools/literacy/index.html.
- Choi S, Choi J. Effects of the teach-back method among cancer patients: a systematic review of the literature. *Supportive Care in Cancer*. 2021;29:7259.
- Durand M, Yen RW, O'Malley J, Elwyn G, Mancini J. Graph literacy matters: examining the association between graph literacy, health literacy, and numeracy in a Medicaid eligible population. *PLoS One*. 2020;15:e0241844.
- Nash R, Patterson K, Flittner A, Elmer S, Osborne R. School-based health literacy programs for children (2-16 years): an international review. *The Journal of School Health*. 2021;91:632.
- Shersher V, Haines TP, Sturgiss L, Weller C, Williams C. Definitions and use of the teach-back method in healthcare consultations with patients: a systematic review and thematic synthesis. *Patient Education and Counseling*. 2021;104:118.

Perfusion

- American Heart Association. *High blood pressure*. Retrieved from https://www.heart.org/en/health-topics/high-blood-pressure.
- D'Elia L, La Fata E, Giaquinto A, Strazzullo P, Galletti F. Effect of dietary salt restriction on central blood pressure: a systematic review and meta-analysis of the intervention studies. *The Journal of Clinical Hypertension*. 2022;22:814.
- Fabbri M, Murad MH, Wennberg AM, Turcano P, Erwin PJ, Alahdab F, et al. Health literacy and outcomes among patients with heart failure: a systematic review and meta-analysis. *JACC. Heart Failure*. 2020;8451.
- Heidenreich PA, Bozkurt B, Aguilar D, Allen LA, Byun JJ, Colvin MM, et al. 2022 AHA/ACC/HFSA Guideline for the Management of Heart Failure: a Report of the American College of Cardiology/American Heart Association Joint Committee on Clinical Practice Guidelines. *Journal of the American College of Cardiology*. 2022;79:e263.
- Zhao Q, Chen C, Zhang J, Ye Y, Fan X. Effects of self-management interventions on heart failure: systematic review and meta-analysis of randomized controlled trials. *International Journal of Nursing Studies*. 2021;116:103909.

Population Health

- Distelhorst KS, Graor CH, Hansen DM. Upstream factors in population health: a concept analysis to advance nursing theory. *Advances in Nursing Science*. 2021;44:210.
- Pan American Health Organization. *Healthy cities action toolkit*. Retrieved from https://paho.ctb.ku.edu/#toolkit.
- U.S. Department of Health & Human Services. *Population health*. Retrieved from https://www.cdc.gov/populationhealth/.

Psychosis

- Alyahya NM, Munro I, Moss C. The experience of psychosis and recovery from consumers' perspectives: an integrative literature review. *Journal of Psychiatric and Mental Health Nursing*. 2022; 29:99.
- Courvoisie H, Labellarte MJ, Riddle MA. Psychosis in children: diagnosis and treatment. *Dialogues in Clinical Neuroscience*. 2022;3:79.
- National Institute of Mental Health. Schizophrenia. Retrieved from https://www.nimh.nih.gov/health/topics/schizophrenia/index.shtml.

Reproduction

- American College of Obstetricians and Gynecologists. Medications for pain relief during labor and delivery. Retrieved from https://www.acog.org/Patients/FAQs/Medications-for-Pain-Relief-During-Labor-and-Delivery?IsMobileSet=false.
- Armah D, van der Wath AE, Yazbek M, Naab F. Development of holistic health care interventions for women with infertility: a nominal group technique. *Holistic Nursing Practice*. 2022;36:85.
- Ciebiera M, Esfandyari S, Siblini H, Prince L, Elkafas H, Wojtyła C, et al. Nutrition in gynecological diseases: Current perspectives. *Nutrients*. 2021;13:1178.
- Mayo Clinic. Female infertility. Retrieved from https://www.mayoclinic.org/diseases-conditions/female-infertility/symptoms-causes/syc-20354308.

Safety

- Agency for Healthcare Research and Quality. Preventing falls in hospitals. Retrieved from: https://www.ahrq.gov/patient-safety/settings/hospital/fall-prevention/toolkit/index.html.
- American Academy of Pediatrics. Lead exposure. Retrieved from https://www.aap.org/en/patient-care/lead-exposure/.
- Baveja UK, Mehta Y. *Prevention of Healthcare Associated Infections: Infection Prevention and Control*. New Delhi: Jaypee Brothers; 2021.
- Fuller R, Landrigan PJ, Balakrishnan K, Bathan G, Bose-O'Reilly S, Brauer M, et al. Pollution and health: a progress update. *The Lancet Planetary Health*. 2022;6;e535.
- Li Y, Zhang X, Yang L, Yang Y, Qiao G, Lu C, Liu K. Association between polypharmacy and mortality in the older adults: a systematic review and meta-analysis. *Archives of Gerontology and Geriatrics*. 2022:100;104630.
- World Health Organization. Radiation health effects. Retrieved from https://www.who.int/news-room/fact-sheets/detail/ionizing-radiation-health-effects-and-protective-measures.

Self Management

- Cox C, Fritz Z. Presenting complaint: use of language that disempowers patients. *BMJ*. 2022;377:e066720 doi:10.1136/bmj-2021-066720.
- Krist AH, Davidson KW, Mangione CM, Barry MJ, Cabana M, Caughey AB, et al. Behavioral counseling interventions to promote a healthy diet and physical activity for cardiovascular disease prevention in adults with cardiovascular risk factors: US Preventive Services Task Force Recommendation Statement. *JAMA*. 2020;324:2069.
- Sanford K, Rivers AS. Treatment adherence perception questionnaire: assessing patient perceptions regarding their adherence to medical treatment plans. *Psychological Assessment*. 2020:32.
- van der Gaag M, Heijmans M, Spoiala C, Rademakers J. The importance of health literacy for self-management: a scoping review of reviews. *Chronic Illness*. 2022;18:234.

Sensory Perception

- Campos JL, Launer S. From healthy hearing to healthy living: a holistic approach. *Ear and Hearing*. 2020;41:99S.
- Hearing Loss Association of America. Retrieved from http://hearingloss.org.
- Hopkins C, Alanin M, Philpott C, Harries P, Whitcroft K, Qureishi A, et al. Management of new onset loss of sense of smell during the COVID-19 pandemic-BRS Consensus Guidelines. *Clinical Otolaryngology*. 202146:16.
- Link T. Common causes of hearing loss in adults. *American Nurse Journal*. 2021:16:26.

Sexuality

- Cattani L, De Maeyer L, Verbakel JY, Bosteels J, Deprest J. Predictors for sexual dysfunction in the first year postpartum: a systematic review and meta-analysis. *BJOG: an International Journal of Obstetrics and Gynaecology*. 2022;129:1017.
- Cleveland Clinic. *Sexual dysfunction*. Retrieved from https://my.clevelandclinic.org/health/diseases/9121-sexual-dysfunction.
- National Cancer Institute. *Self-image and sexuality*. Retrieved from https://www.cancer.gov/about-cancer/coping/self-image.
- National Center on the Sexual Behavior of Youth. Retrieved from: http://ncsby.org/.
- Smith AB, Barton DL, Davis M, Jackson EA, Smith J, Wittmann D. A preliminary study of short-term sexual function and satisfaction among men post-myocardial infarction. *Journal of Holistic Nursing*. 2021; https://doi.org/10.1177/08980101211038085.
- Williams M, Addis G. Addressing patient sexuality issues in cancer and palliative care. *British Journal of Nursing*. 2021;30:S24.

Sleep

- Akashiba T, Inoue Y, Uchimura N, Ohi M, Kasai T, Kawana F, et al. Sleep apnea syndrome clinical practice guidelines 2020. *Sleep and Biological Rhythms*. 2022;20:5.
- Bender E. New guidelines for behavioral treatment of chronic insomnia in adult patients. *Neurology Today*. 2021;21:6.
- Law EF, Kim A, Ickmans K, Palermo TM. Sleep health assessment and treatment in children and adolescents with chronic pain: state of the art and future directions. *Journal of Clinical Medicine*. 2022;11:1491.
- National Sleep Foundation. Sleep solutions and sleep disorders. Retrieved from: https://www.sleepfoundation.org/.
- Rosenberg R, Citrome L, Drake CL. Advances in the treatment of chronic insomnia: a narrative review of new nonpharmacologic and pharmacologic therapies. *Neuropsychiatric Disease and Treatment*. 2021;17:2549.
- Szpalher AS, Cardoso RB, da Silva NC, da Silva Ramos LM, de Souza PA, Weiss C. Assessment and diagnosis of insomnia for clinical and research practice: a scoping review protocol. *Research, Society and Development*. 2021;10:e2810413736.
- Willard AF, Ferris AH. Solving the problem of insomnia in clinical practice. *Medical Clinics*. 2021;105:107.

Spirituality

- Anandarajah G, Hight E. Spirituality and medical practice. *American Family Physician*. 2001;63:81.
- Bożek A, Nowak PF, Blukacz M. (2020). The relationship between spirituality, health-related behavior, and psychological well-being. *Frontiers in Psychology*. 2020;11:1997.
- Hughes BP, DeGregory C, Elk R, Graham D, Hall EJ, Ressallat J. *Spiritual Care and Nursing: A Nurse's Contribution and Practice*. New York: Health Care Chaplaincy Network; 2017.
- Litalien M, Atari, DO, Obasi I. The influence of religiosity and spirituality on health in Canada: a systematic literature review. *Journal of Religion and Health*. 2021;61:373.
- The George Washington Institute for Spirituality and Health. *FICA spiritual history tool*. Retrieved from: http://smhs.gwu.edu/gwish/clinical/fica/spiritual-history-tool

Stress and Coping

- Alzheimer's Association: Staying strong: Stress relief for a caregiver. Retrieved from http://www.alz.org/national/documents/aa_brochure_stressrelief.pdf.
- Carver CS. You want to measure coping but your protocol's too long: consider the Brief COPE. *International Journal of Behavioral Medicine*. 1997;4:92.
- Goddard JR, Etcher L. Trauma informed care in nursing: a concept analysis. *Nursing Outlook*. 2022;70(3):429-439. https://doi.org/10.1016/j.outlook.2021.12.010
- Helpguide.org International. *Caregiver stress and burnout*. Retrieved from https://www.helpguide.org/articles/stress/caregiver-stress-and-burnout.htm.
- Holmes TH, Rahe RH. The social readjustment rating scale. *Journal of Psychosomatic Research*. 1967:11;213.
- Mason TM, Szalacha LA, Tofthagen CS, Buck HG. quality of life of older adults with complicated grief: a mixed methods exploration. *Journal of Gerontological Nursing*. 2022;48:19.
- Tracewski M, Scarlett K. Grief in children. *Advances in Family Practice Nursing*. 2022;4:203.
- National Alliance for Caregiving National Alliance for Caregiving. *Executive summary: Caregiving in the U.S*. Retrieved from http://www.caregiving.org/pdf/research/CaregivingUSAllAgesExecSum.pdf.

Substance Use

- Krist AH, Davidson KW, Mangione CM, Barry MJ, Cabana M, Caughey AB, et al. Interventions for tobacco smoking cessation in adults, including pregnant persons: USPSTF recommendation statement. *JAMA*. 2021;325:265.
- Kurup U, Merchant N. Neonatal abstinence syndrome: management and current concepts. *Paediatrics and Child Health*. 2021;31:24.
- Modified Finnegan Neonatal Abstinence Score. Retrieved from: https://www.mdcalc.com/modified-finnegan-neonatal-abstinence-score-nas.
- National Institute on Drug Abuse: Retrieved from: https://www.drugabuse.gov/.
- SAMSA-HRSA Center for Integrated Health Solutions: SBIRT. Retrieved from https://www.samhsa.gov/sbirt.
- University of Maryland School of Medicine. Clinical Institute Withdrawal Assessment of Alcohol Scale, Revised (CIWA-Ar). Retrieved from http://umem.org/files/uploads/1104212257_CIWA-Ar.pdf.

Thermoregulation

- Périard JD, Eijsvogels TMH, Daanen H. Exercise under heat stress: thermoregulation, hydration, performance implications, and mitigation strategies. *Physiological Reviews*. 2021;101:1873.
- Simegn GD, Bayable SD, Fetene MB. Prevention and management of perioperative hypothermia in adult elective surgical patients: a systematic review. *Annals of Medicine and Surgery*. 2021;72:103059.

Tissue Integrity

- Agency for Healthcare Research and Quality. Preventing pressure ulcers in hospitals. Retrieved from https://www.ahrq.gov/patient-safety/settings/hospital/resource/pressureulcer/tool/pu7b.html.
- Burke G, Faithfull S, Probst H. Radiation induced skin reactions during and following radiotherapy: a systematic review of interventions. *Radiography*. 2022;28:232.
- Mileski M, McClay R, Natividad J. Facilitating factors in the proper identification of acute skin failure: a systematic review. *Critical Care Nurse*. 2021;41:36.
- Pusey-Reid E, Quinn L, Samost M, Reidy P. Skin assessment in patients with dark skin tone. *AJN*. 123;3:36.

Index

Page numbers followed by *b*, *f*, and *t* indicate boxes, figures, and tables respectively

D

E

G

R

S